Radioactive Isotopes in Clinical Medicine and Research XXIII

Edited by
H. Bergmann
H. Köhn
H. Sinzinger

Springer Basel AG

Editors:

Professor Dr. Helmar Bergmann
Institut für Biomedizinische Technik
und Physik
Allgemeines Krankenhaus Wien
Währinger Gürtel 18-20
A-1090 Wien

Professor Dr. Horst Köhn
Institut für Nuklearmedizin
Wilhelminenspital
Montleartstrasse 37
A-1171 Wien

Professor Dr. Helmut Sinzinger
Universitäts-Klinik für Nuklearmedizin
Allgemeines Krankenhaus Wien
Währinger Gürtel 18-20
A-1090 Wien

A CIP catalogue record for this book is available from the Library of Congress, Washington D.C., USA

Deutsche Bibliothek Cataloging-in-Publication Data
Radioactive isotopes in clinical medicine and research XXIII:
proceedings of the 23rd International Badgastein Symposium / ed. by
H. Bergmann ... - Basel ; Boston ; Berlin : Birkhäuser, 1999
ISBN 978-3-0348-9772-3 ISBN 978-3-0348-8782-3 (eBook)
DOI 10.1007/978-3-0348-8782-3

The publisher and editor can give no guarantee for the information on drug dosage and administration contained in this publication. The respective user must check its accuracy by consulting other sources of reference in each individual case.

Originally published by Birkhäuser Verlag in 1999
Softcover reprint of the hardcover 1st edition 1999

Camera-ready copy prepared by the editors and authors
Printed on acid-free paper produced from chlorine-free pulp. TCF ∞

ISBN 978-3-0348-9772-3

9 8 7 6 5 4 3 2 1

Table of contents

Preface

These proceedings of the Badgastein Symposium, being the 23rd in an uninterrupted series, offer a complete review over the scientific events.
Professor Peter Ell was presenting an outstanding introductory (Badgastein) lecture, outlining developments and chances for Nuclear Medicine in the next century.
Highlights this time were certainly different topics dealing with PET, due to the opening of respective units here in Austria, and the application of various cationic tracers.
According to the traditional style of the symposium there was a wide range of topics covered in both basic sciences and clinical application of Nuclear Medicine.

The Austrian Nuclear Medicine Society acted again as a co-organizer, together with the Departments of Nuclear Medicine and Biomedical Engineering and Physics of the Medical Faculty of the University of Vienna. Special thanks again to all our referees, who edited all the manuscripts picking up inconsistencies, errors, omissions etc. in order to improve further substantially the scientific standard of the proceedings and to our staff arranging a smooth organization in the usual atmosphere of the meeting
Finally, we appreciate the perfect cooperation of Birkhäuser-publisher for the third time presenting the proceedings in a high quality standard.

We are looking forward to meeting you again on the next occasion in January 2000.

Helmar Bergmann | Horst Köhn | Helmut Sinzinger

List of Chairmen

W.Becker	(Göttingen)
H.Bergmann	(Vienna)
H.J.Biersack	(Bonn)
A.Bischof-Delaloye	(Lausanne)
T.Brücke	(Vienna)
T.Budinger	(Berkely, U.S.A)
U.Büll	(Aachen)
M.Clausen	(Kiel)
T.D.Cradduck	(London, Ontario)
P.J.Ell	(London)
L.Fridrich	(Steyr)
G.Fueger	(Graz)
G.Galvan	(Salzburg)
K.Hahn	(Munich)
E.Henze	(Kiel)
W.H.Knapp	(Leipzig)
H.Köhn	(Vienna)
A.Kroiss	(Vienna)
J.T.Kuikka	(Kuopio)
G.Limouris	(Athens)
P.Lind	(Klagenfurt)
J.Makaiova	(Bratislava)
J.Martin-Comin	(Barcelona)
V.R.McCready	(Sutton)
G.Muehllehner	(Philadelphia, U.S.A)
E.Ogris	(Vienna)
R.Palumbo	(Perugia)
L.Pávics	(Szégéd)
G.Riccabona	(Innsbruck)
C.Reiners	(Würzburg)
S.N.Reske	(Ulm)
M.Schwaiger	(Munich)
H.Sinzinger	(Vienna)
S.-E.Strand	(Lund)
A.E.Todd-Pokropek	(London)

List of Participants

Aas Magne, Dr. Norwegian Radium Hospital, N-0310 Montebello, Oslo, Norway

Ahonen Aapo Kaarlo Aapeli, Dr., Division of Nuclear Medicine, Oulu University Hospital, FIN-90220 Oulu, Finland

Aigner Reingard, Dr., Klinische Abteilung für Nuklearmedizin, LKH-ZRI Graz, A-8010 Graz, Austria

Alexander Christof, Dr., Nuklearmedizin, Univ.Klinikum Homburg/Saar, D-66421 Homburg/Saar, Germany

Als Claudine, Dr., Institute of Pathology, University of Berne, CH-3010 Berne, Switzerland,

Anayat Reza, Dr., Medical Radiation Science, University of Newcastle, Callaghan NSW 2308, Australia

Andreeff Michael, Dipl.-Physik., Klinik für Nuklearmedizin, Universität Dresden, D-01307 Dresden, Fetscherstr. 74, Germany

Aprile Carlo, Dr., Nuclear Medicine Service, Fondazione S.Maugeri, I-27100 Pavia, Via Ferrata 8, Italy

Arnold, A., ELSCINT Central & Eastern Europe Ges.m.b.H., A-1150 Vienna, Nobileg.23-25, Austria

Artner Christoph, Mag., IASON Labormedizin KEG, A-8010 Graz, Rechbauerstr. 3, Austria

Atefie Khosrow, Dr., Nuklearmedizinisches Institut, A-1220 Vienna, Arnikaweg 99, Austria

Auinger Christian, Dr., Institut für Nuklearmedizin, KA Rudolfsstiftung, A-1030 Vienna, Juchg. 25, Austria

Avcin Jurij, Dr., Klinicni Center Ljubljana, SLO-1000 Ljubljana, Klinicni Center Ljubljana, Slovenia

Bachmayr Siegfried, Dr., Nuklearmed.Institut, KH Elisabethinen Linz, A-4010 Linz, Fadingerstr.1, Austria

Bako Andreas, PICKER Deutschland, D-32339 Erlangen, Marienwerder Str.2, Germany

Balogh Ildiko, Dr., MEDISO, Alsotörökvesz 14, Hungary

Barthel Henryk, Dr., Dept. of Nuclear Medicine, University of Leipzig, D-04103 Leipzig, Liebigstr.20A, Germany

Bartosch Rainer, Dept. of Nuclear Medicine, University of Vienna, A-1090 Vienna, Waehringer Guertel 18-20, Austria

Basmanov Vassily, Dr., Radiopharmaceutical Laboratory, Institute of Physics and Power Engineering, Obninsk, 249020, Bondarenko sq. 1, Russia

Bauer Ulrike, Dr., Zentrum für Psychiatrie, D-35385 Giessen, Am Steg 32, Germany

Bauer Richard, Prof., Klinik für Nuklearmedizin, Justus-Liebig-Universität, D-35385 Giessen, Friedrichstr.25, Germany

Bauer Harald, Dr., Klinik für Nuklearmedizin, Hanusch-Krankenhaus, A-1140 Vienna, Heinrich-Collinstr.30, Austria

Becker Wolfgang, Prof., Dept. of Nuclear Medicine, University of Göttingen, D-37075 Göttingen, Robert-Koch-Str. 40, Germany

Behr Thomas, Dr., Abtl. für Nuklearmedizin, Universität Göttingen, D-37075 Göttingen, Robert-Koch-Str. 40, Germany

Ber Gérard, CIS MEDIPRO SA, CH-1214 Vernier/Genève, Case postale 530, Switzerland

Bergmann Helmar, Prof., Dept. of Biomedical Engineering & Physics, Vienna University Hospital AKH, A-1090 Vienna, Waehringer Guertel 18-20, Austria

Bergström Kim, Dr., Dept. of Clinical Physiology, Kuopio University Hospital, FIN-70211 Kuopio, P.O.Box 1777, Finland

Bertling Jan, NUCLEAR DIAGNOSTICS AB, S-126 30 Hägersten, Elektravägen 5, Sweden
Biersack H.J., Prof., Klinik und Poliklinik für Nuklearmedizin, Universität Bonn, D-53127 Bonn, Siegmund-Freud-Str. 25, Germany
Bischof-Delaloye Angelika, Prof., Service de Medecine Nucleaire, Centre Hospitalier Universitaire Vaudois, CH-1011 Lausanne, Rue de Bugnon 46, Switzerland
Blajs Karoline, Dept. of Nuclear Medicine and Special Endocrinology, LKH-Klagenfurt, A-9020 Klagenfurt, St.Veiter-Str.47, Austria
Blajs Brigitte, A-8020 Graz, Finkeng. 3/24, Austria
Bohuslavizki, Karl H., Dr., Clinic of Nuclear Medicine, Christian-Albrechts-University, D-24105 Kiel, Arnold-Heller-Str. 9, Germany
Boni Giuseppe, Dr., Div. of Nuclear Medicine, Dept. of Oncology, S.Chiara Hospital, University of Pisa, I-56100 Pisa, Via Roma 67, Italy
Börner Anne Rose, Dr., Institute of Medicine, Research Center Jülich, D-52425 Jülich, Germany
Bredow Jan, Klinik und Poliklinik für Nuklearmedizin, Univ.-Klinikum Carl Gustav Carus, TU-Dresden, D-01307 Dresden, Fetscherstr. 74, Germany
Bremer Per Oscar, ISOPHARMA AS, N-2007 Kjeller, P.O.Box 65, Norway
Brill Stefanie, SWK, D-66119 Saarbrücken, Haus-Dietter-Weg 4, Germany
Brücke Thomas, Prof., Dept. of Neurology, Wilhelminenspital, A-1160 Vienna, Montleartstr. 37, Austria
Bubeck Bernd, Prof., Institut f. Nuklearmedizin, Kantonspital, CH-9007 St.Gallen, Switzerland
Bucher Christian, SCHOELLER PHARMA Ges.m.b.H., A-1231 Vienna, Industrieg. 7, Austria
Buchinger Wolfgang, Dr., BMB-Eggenberg, A-8020 Graz, Bergstr. 27, Austria
Budinger Thomas, Prof., Lawrence Berkeley National Laboratory, 1 Cyclotron Road, Berkeley, California 94720, U.S.A
Büll U., Prof., Klinik F. Nuklearmedizin, RWTH, D-52057 Aachen, Pauwelstr. 1, Germany
Burroni Luca, Dr., Dept. of Nuclear Medicine, Policlinic „Le Scotte“, University of Siena, I-53100 Siena, Viale Bracci, Italy
Buscombe John Richard, Dr., Nuclear Medicine Dept., Royal Free Hospital, GB-London NW3 2OW, Pond Street, Great Britain

Cardinali Laura, Dr., Dept. of Nuclear Medicine, Policlinico Monteluce, I-06100 Perugia, Via Brunamonti, Italy
Carnell Dawn, Dr., Royal Marsden Hospital, Sutton , Surrey SM2 5PT, United Kingdom
Carrai Franco, COMECER, I-48018 Castelbolognese (RA), V.Emilia Ponente 390, Italy
Chinol Marco, Dr., European Institute of Oncology, I-20141 Milano, Via Ripamonti 435, Italy
Clausen Malte, Prof., Abteilung Nuklearmedizin, UKE, D-20246 Hamburg, Martinistr. 52, Germany
Cradduck Trevor D., Prof., Victoria Hospital, CAN-London, Ontario N6A 4G5, 375 South Street, Canada

Dahlström Jan, Dr., Hospital of Helsingborg, S-25187 Helsingborg, Fysiologiska Avdelningen, Lasarettet, Sweden
Dannenberg Claudia, Klinik für Nuklearmedizin, Universität Leipzig, D-04103 Leipzig, Liebigstr. 20a, Germany
De Haas M.J., Dr., Dept. of Nuclear Medicine, Hospital Eemland, NL-3518 ES Amersfoort, Utrechtseweg 160, The Netherlands
De Vos Filip, Dr., Dept. of Radiopharmacy, University of Ghent, S-25187 Ghent, Harelbekestraat 79, Belgium
Deckart Harald, Prof., D-13187 Berlin, Mendelstr. 19, Germany
Deckart Eva, Dr., D-13187 Berlin, Mendelstr. 19, Germany

Deininger Heinz K., Prof., Institut für Strahlendiagnostik & Nuklearmedizin, Städt.Klinikum Darmstadt, D-64283 Darmstadt, Grafenstr. 9, Germany

Delree Marc, Dr., N.V. Radiologie & Medische Beeldvorming, B-1500 Halle, 48 Ninoofse Steenweg, Belgium

Denk Eva, BIOCIS Handels.Ges.m.b.H., A-1210 Vienna, Divischgasse 4, Austria

Dielemann J., Dept. of Nuclear Medicine, Hospital Eemland, NL-3518 ES Amersfoort, Utrechtseweg 160, The Netherlands

Diemling Markus, Dipl.Phys., Dept.of Biomedical Engineering & Physics, University of Vienna, A-1090 Vienna, Waehringer Guertel 18-20, Austria

Donaldson John, Dr., X-Ray Department, Maidstone Hospital, GB-Kent ME16 9OO, Great Britain

Donnemiller Eveline, Dr., Dept. of Nuclear Medicine, Innsbruck University Hospital, A-6020 Innsbruck, Anichstr. 35, Austria

Doppler Katja, A, ELSCINT Central & Eastern Europe Ges.m.b.H, A-1150 Vienna, Nobileg. 23-25, Austria

Dorn Gerald, Ing., B.R.A.H.M.S. Diagnostica GmbH, A-1070 Vienna, Zollergasse 2/18, Austria

Eckholt Markus, Dipl.-Phys., Dept. of Biomedical Engineering & Physics, Vienna University Hospital AKH, A-1090 Vienna, Waehringer Guertel 18-20, Austria

Ell Peter J., Prof., Institute of Nuclear Medicine, Middlesex Hospital, GB-London W1N 8AA, Mortimer St., Great Britain

Ellam Susan, NUCLEAR DIAGNOSTICS Ltd., GB-Kent DA11 8HH, Unit E1, Springhead Enterprise Park, Northfleet, Gravesend, Great Britain

Erler Hermann, Dr., Univ.Klinik für Nuklearmedizin, A-6020 Innsbruck, Anichstr. 35, Austria

Eschner Wolfgang, Dr., Clinic for Nuclear Medicine, University of Cologne, D-50924 Cologne, Germany

Falk Christian, ELIMPEX-Medizintechnik Ges.m.b.H., A-2340 Mödling, Spechtg. 32, Austria

Fettich Jurij, Doz.Dr., Klinicni Center Ljubljana, SLO-1000 Ljubljana, Klinicni Center Ljubljana, Slovenia

Fischer Sybille, Dept. of Nuclear Medicine, LMU Munich, D-80336 Munich, Ziemssenstr. 1, Germany

Fitz Friedrich, Dr., Nuklearmedizin, KH Melk, A-3390 Melk, Austria

Florkowski Maciej, ELSCINT Central & Eastern Europe Ges.m.B.H., A-1150 Vienna, Nobilegasse 23-25, Austria

Frassine Harald, Department of Nuclear Medicine, University of Vienna, A-1090 Vienna, Waehringer Guertel 18-20, Austria

Fridrich Leo, Prof., Dept. of Nuclear Medicine, LKH-Steyr, A-4400 Steyr, Sierningerstr. 141, austria

Friesacher Karoline, Abtl. für Nuklearmedizin, LKH-Klagenfurt, A-9020 Klagenfurt, St.Veiter-Str. 7, Austria

Fritzsche Heinz, Prof., Nuklearmedizin, LKH-Feldkirch, A-6800 Feldkirch, Carinag. 45, Austria

Fröhlich Jürgen, Dr., B.R.A.H.M.S. Diagnostica GmbH, D-12099 Berlin, Komturstr. 19-20, Germany

Fueger Gerhard F., Prof., A-8010 Graz, Jakob-Redtenbacher-G. 10, Austria

Fürlinger Martina, Institut für Nuklearmedizin, KH Lainz, A-1130 Vienna, Wolkersbergenstr. 1, Austria

Füzy Márton, Dr., Institut of Isotopes Co. Ltd., H-1121 Budapest, Konkoly Thege 29-33, Hungary

Gaede A., ELSCINT Central & Eastern Europe Ges.m.b.H., A-1150 Vienna, Nobilegasse 23-25, Austria

Gallowitsch Hans-Jürgen, Dr., Abtl. für Nuklearmedizin, LKH-Klagenfurt, A-9020 Klagenfurt, St.Veiter-Str. 47, Austria

Galvan Günther, Prof., Institut für Nuklearmedizin und Endokrinologie, LKA -Salzburg, A-5020 Salzburg, Müllner Hauptstr. 48, Austria

Garvie Neil, Isotope Dept., Royal London Hospital, London E1 1BB, Great Britain

Gattinger Arno, Dr., Institut für Nuklearmedizin, LKH-Salzburg, A-5020 Salzburg, Müllner Hauptstr. 48, Austria

Giovanella Luca, Dr., Nuclear Medicine Dept., Ospedale Universitario, I-21100 Varese, Viale Borri, Italy

Goransson Meta, Dept. of Nuclear Medicine, Huddinge University Hospital, S-14186 Huddinge, Sweden

Gottschild Dietmar, Prof., Abtl. für Nuklearmedizin, Friedrich-Schiller-Universität, D-07740 Jena, Bachstr. 18, Germany

Gradwohl Martha, Geb. Gyn. Univ.-Klinik, LKH-Graz, A-8036 Graz, Auenbruggerplatz, Austria

Gräf Mathias, AMERSHAM, D-83250 Marquartstein, Oberfeldstr. 1, Germany

Granegger Susanne, Dept. of Nuclear Medicine, University of Vienna, A-1090 Vienna, Waehringer Guertel 18-20, Austria

Gregoire Jean, Dr., Montreal Heart Institute, Montreal, Quebec H1T 1C8, 5000 East, Belanger, Canada

Groth Steffen, Prof.DDr., Division of Human Health, IAEA, A-1220 Wagramerstr. 5, P.O.Box 100, Austria

Gruber Beate, Dept. of Nuclear Medicine, LKH Klagenfurt, A-9020 Klagenfurt, St.Veiter-Str. 47, Austria

Günalp Bengül, Gülhane Medical School, TR-06530 Ankara, 36.C 432.S Ezgi Evleri B/5 Blok, Turkey

Haas Christian, Dipl.-Ing., Dept. of Medical Physics, LKH Feldkirch, A-6800 Feldkirch, Carinag. 47, Austria

Hahn Klaus, Prof., Dept. of Nuclear Medicine, LMU Munich, D-80336 Munich, Ziemssenstr. 1, Germany

Hämisch York, ADAC Laboratories Europe B.V., NL-3600 BK Maarssen, Zonnebaan 34, P.O.Box 1419, The Netherlands

Handgriff Dafne, Dr., Inst. für Nuklearmedizin, Kaiserin Elisabeth-Spital, A-1150 Wien, Huglgasse 1-3, Austria

Hantelle Marie-Claude, CIS bio international, F-91192 Gif-sur-Yvette Cédéx, BP No.32, France

Häusler Dagmar, Institut für Nuklearmedizin & Endokrinologie, LKA Salzburg, A-5020 Salzburg, Müllner Hauptstr. 48, Austria

Havlik Ernst, Univ.Doz.Dr., Dept. of Biomedical Engineering & Physics, Vienna University Hospital AKH, A-1090 Vienna, Waehringer Guertel 18-20, Austria

Haydl Johannes, Dr., A.ö. Krankenhaus Schwarzach, A-5620 Schwarzach, Austria

Heckenberg Dick, DIGIMED-ADAC, A-1030 Vienna, Landstraßer Hauptstr. 146/6A/B2, Austria

Heckenberg Andrea, Mag., Dept. for Biomedical Engineering & Physics, Vienna University Hospital AKH, A-1090 Vienna, Waehringer Guertel 18-20, Austria

Heiden Ursula, MALLINCKRODT Deutschland, D-53115 Bonn, Kaufmannstr. 81a, Germany

Heinisch Martin, Dr., Institut für Nuklearmedizin, KH Melk, A-3390 Melk, Krankenhausstr. 11, Austria

Henze Eberhard, Prof., Dept. of Nuclear Medicine, University of Kiel, D-24105 Kiel, Arnold-Heller-Str. 9, Germany

Hiltunen Jukka, MAP-Medical Technologies Oy, FIN-41160 Tikkakoski, Elementtitie 27, Finland

Höbarth Josef, ELSCINT Central & Eastern Europe Ges.m.b.H., A-1150 Vienna, Nobileg. 23-25, Vienna

Hoeflin Friedrich, Dr., Nukelarmedizin, Kantonspital, CH-7000 Chur, Switzerland

Hojker Sergej, Doz.Dr., Klinicni Center Ljubljana, SLO-1000 Ljubljana, Zaloska 2, Slovenia

Huber Erich, Dr., A-1120 Vienna, Nauheimerg. 6, Austria

Hurtl Ingrid, Dr., Institut für Nuklearmedizin, KH Lainz, A-1130 Vienna, Wolkersbergenstr. 1, Austria

Jank Julia, Dipl.Ing., Dept. of Nuclear Medicine, University of Vienna, A-1090 Vienna, Waehringer Guertel 18-20, Austria

John-Scheder Alexander, ELSCINT Central & Eastern Europe Ges.m.b.H., A-1150 Nobileg. 23-25, Austria

Junik Roman, Dr., Dept. of Endocrinology, PL-60 355 Poznan, Ul. Przybyszewskiego 49, Poland

Kairemo Kalervi, Dr., Dept. of Clinical Chemistry, Helsinki University Central Hospital, Haartmaninkattu 4, FIN-00029 Hyks Helsinki, Finland

Karanikas Georgios, Dr., Dept. of Nuclear Medicine, University of Vienna, A-1090 Vienna, Waehringer Guertel 18-20, Austria

Karvonen Anna-Liisa, Dr., University Hospital of Tampere, FIN-33100 Tampere, Otavalankatu 8 B 9, Finland

Karvonen Juha, Dr., National Board of Medicolegal Affairs, FIN-00531 Helsinki, P.O.Box 265 Finland

Kauders Harald, Ing., SIEMENS Medizintechnik AG, A-1030 Vienna, Erdberger Lände, Austria

Kenda Rajko, Dr., Pediatric Hospital, University Medical Center Ljubljana, SLO-1000 Ljubljana, Stare pravde 4, Slovenia

Kendler Dorota, Dr., Univ.Klinik für Nuklearmedizin, A-6020 Innsbruck, Anichstr. 35, Austria

Kirsch C.M., Prof., Abteilung für Nuklearmedizin, Univ.Kliniken d.Saarlandes, D-66421 Homburg/Saar, Germany

Kirsten Beatrix, Dr., B.R.A.H.M.S. Diagnostica GmbH, A-1070 Vienna, Zollerg. 2/18, Austria

Kivimäki Kalervo, Dr., Keski-Pohjanmaa Central Hospital, Mariankatu 16-20, FIN-67200 Kokkola, Finland

Kletter Kurt, Prof.DDr., Department of Nuclear Medicine, University of Vienna, A-1090 Vienna, Waehringer Guertel 18-20, Austria

Klug-Schalud Waltraud, KH Barmherzige Brüder, A-1020 Vienna, Gr.Mohreng. 9-11, Austria

Kluge Regine, Dr., Klinik für Nuklearmedizin, D-04103 Leipzig, Liebigstr. 20a, Germany

Klutmann Susanne, Dr. Clinic of Nuclear Medicine, Christian-Albrechts-University, D-24105 Kiel, Arnold-Heller-Str. 9, Germany

Knapp W.H., Prof., Nuklearmed. Klinik und Poliklinik, Universität Leipzig, D-04103 Leipzig, Liebigstr. 20A, Germany

Knierim Andreas, Dr., Praxis für Nuklearmedizin, D-74523 Schwäbisch Hall, Spitalmühlenstr. 3, Germany

Knoll Peter, Mag., Instit. für Nuklearmedizin, Wilhelminenspital, A-1160 Vienna, Montleartstr. 37, Austria

Köhn Horst, Prof., Dept. of Nuclear Medicine, Wilhelminenspital, A-1160 Vienna, Montleartstr. 37, Austria

König Beatrix, Dr., Nuklearmedizin, Hanusch-Krankenhaus, A-1140 Vienna, Heinrich-Collin-Str.30, Austria

Könne Werner, Dr., D-30635 Hannover, Wieselpfad 1, Germany
Konrad Gertrude, Dept. of Nuclear Medicine, LKH Klagenfurt, A-9020 Klagenfurt, St.Veiter-Str. 47, Austria
Korenjak Claudia, Dept. of Nuclear Medicine, LKH Klagenfurt, A-9020 Klagenfurt, St.Veiter-Str. 47, Austria
Környei József, Dr., Institute of Isotopes Co. Ltd, H-1121 Budapest, Konkoly Thege 29-33, Hungary
Kresnik Ewald, Dr., Abtl. für Nuklearmedizin & Spezielle Endokrinologie, LKH Klagenfurt, A-9020 Klagenfurt, St.Veiter-Str. 47, Austria
Kritz Harald, Dr., Kurhaus Engelsbad/Baden, A-2522 Oberwaltersdorf, Badenerstr. 20, Austria
Kroiss Alois, Univ.Doz.Dr., Institute of Nuclear Medicine, KA Rudolfstiftung, A-1030 Vienna, Juchg. 25, Austria
Krotla Gabriele, Dr., Nuklearmedizin, Kaiserin Elisabeth Spital, A-1150 Vienna, Huglg. 1-3, Austria
Kuba Andràs, Dr., Dept. of Nuclear Medicine, Albert Szent-Györgyi Medical University, H-6720 Szeged, Koranyi Fasor 8, Hungary
Kuckeland Michael, Dr., IMMUNOMEDICS Europe, D-79206 Breisach, Gewerbestr. 8, Germany
Kuikka Jyrki T., Dr., Kuopio University Hospital, FIN-70210 Kuopio, P.O.Box 1777, Finland
Kusic Zvonko, Prof., University Hospital „Sestre Milosrdnice“, CRO-10000 Zagreb, Vinogradska 29, Croatia
Kvaternik Herbert, Dr., Forschungszentrum Seibersdorf, A-2444 Seibersdorf, Austria

Lauterbach Hubert, Dr. Abtl. Nuklearmedizin, Klinik für Radiologie, Klinikum d.FSU Jena, D-07740 Jena, Bachstr. 18, Germany
Leb Georg, Dr., Med.Univ.Klinik, A-8036 Graz, Auenbruggerplatz, Austria
Ledermann Bert, Mag., DPC-Bühlmann, A-1110 Vienna, Austria
Leisner Bernhard, Prof., Allg.Krankenhaus St.Georg, D-20149 Hamburg, Oberfelderstr. 42, Germany
Lengyel Zsolt, Dr., PET Centre, Univ.Medical School of Debrecen, H-4026 Debrecen, Hungary
Leppänen Esa, Dr., Helsinki City Hospital, Laboratory, FIN-002730 Espoo, Laaksonpohjantie 3A, Finland
Lewander Rolf, Dr., Radiology Dept. St.Göran Hospital, S-11281 Stockholm, P.O.Box 12500, Sweden
Liepe Knut, Dr., Nuclear Medicine, Dept., University Hospital Dresden, D-01307 Dresden, Fetscherstr. 13, Germany
Limouris Georgios, Prof., Athens University Medical Faculty, Areteion Hospital, GR-11528 Athens, 76 Vas Sophias Ave, Greece
Lincke Hans-Joachim, Dipl.-Ing., Hans-Wällischmiller GmbH, Betriebsstätte Dresden, D-01474 Schönfeld, Rossendorfer Ring 42, Germany
Lind Peter, Prof, Dept. of Nuclear Medicine & Special Endocrinology, LKH Klagenfurt, A-9020 Klagenfurt, St.Veiter-Str. 47, Austria
Ljungberg Michael, Prof, Dept. of Physiology, Helsingborgs Lasarett, Physiologiska Avd, S-25185 Helsingborg, Sweden
Lorenz Walter, Prof., German Cancer Research Center (DKFZ), D-69009 Heidelberg, Germany
Lörinczy Endre, Dr., Institute of Isotopes Co. Ltd, H-1121 Budapest, Konkoly Thege 29-33, Hungary

Lübeck Martin, Dr., Dept. of Nuclear Medicine, Univ.Hospital UKE, D-20246 Hamburg, Martinistr. 52, Germany

Makaiova Izabela, Doz.Dr., National Oncological Institute, Clinic of Nuclear Medicine, Medical Faculty, SK-81250 Bratislava, Heydukova 10, Slovak Republic
Makowiecka Izabela, Dr., Medical Centre, Dept. of Radiology, FIN-67200 Kokkola, Kokkolan Terv.Kesk.Rtg., Mariankatu 28, Finland
Mann Heinz-Peter, POLAROID GmbH, D-63069 Offenbach, Sprendlinger Landstr. 109, Germany
Manzl Monika, Dr., Institut für Nuklearmedizin, A-5020 Salzburg, Müllner Hauptstr. 48, Austria
Márián Teréz, Dr., PET Centre, Univ. Medical School of Debrecen, H-4026 Debrecen, Hungary
Maringer Adelheid, Dept. of Nuclear Medicine, University of Vienna, A-1090 Vienna, Waehringer Guertel 18-20, Austria
Markt Bernhard, Dr., KH Elisabethinen Linz, A-4010 Linz, Fadingerstr. 1, Austria
Martin-Comín José, Prof, Servicio Medicina Nuclear, Hospital de Bellvitge CSVB, E-08907 Barcelona, Feixa Llarga s/n, Spain
Maschek Wilhelmine, Dr.,Abtl. für Nuklearmedizin, AKH-Linz, A-4020 Linz, Krankenhausstr. 9, Austria
Mather Stephen J., Dr., Dept. of Nuclear Medicine, St.Bartholomews' Hospital, GB-London EC1A 7BE, Great Britain
Mayer Sebastian, Dr., Department of Nuclear Medicine, University of Vienna, A-1090 Vienna, Waehringer Guertel 18-20, Austria
McCready Ralph, Prof., Royal Marsden Hospital, GB-Sutton, Surrey SM2 5PT, Great Britain
Meghdadi Susan, Dr., Dept. of Nuclear Medicine, University of Vienna, A-1090 Vienna, Waehringer Guertel 18-20, Austria
Mesicek Heinz, ELSCINT Central & Eastern Europe Ges.m.b.H., A-1150 Vienna, Nobileg. 23-25, Austria
Mester Janos, Dr., Abtl. f. Nuklearmedizin, UKE, D-20246 Hamburg, Martinistr. 52, Germany
Meyer Geerd-J., Prof., Medizinische Hochschule Hannover, D-30623 Hannover, Germany
Mihailovic Jasna, Dr., Dept. of Nuclear Medicine, Institute of Oncology, YU-21204 Sremska Kamenica, Institutski put 4, Yugoslavia
Mikosch Peter, Dr., Dept. of Nuclear Medicine & Special Endocrinology, LKH Klagenfurt, A-9020 Klagenfurt, St.Veiter-Str. 47, Austria
Milcinski Metka, Doz.Dr., Klinicni Center Ljubljana, SLO-1000 Ljubljana, Zaloska 2, Slovenia
Minchev Dimitar, Doz.Dr., Dept. of Neurology, Medical University of Varna, BG-9002 Varna, Marin Drinov Str. 55A, Bulgaria
Minear Greg, B.Sc., Dept. of Biomedical Engineering & Physics, Vienna University Hospital AKH, A-1090 Vienna, Waehringer Guertel 18-20, Austria
Mirzaei Siroos, Dr., Institute of Nuclear Medicine, Wilhelminenspital, A-1160 Vienna, Montleartstr. 37,. Austria
Moka Detlef, Dr., Klinik für Nuklearmedizin, Univ.Klinik Köln, D-50924 Cologne, Josef Stelzmann Str. 9, Germany
Moldrich Waltraud, Dr., Wilhelminenspital, A-1160 Vienna, Montleartstr. 37, Austria
Morneburg Heinz, Dipl.Ing., Fachakademie für Medizintechnik, Ansbach, D-91080 Munich, Höhenweg 12, Germany
Muehllehner Gerd, Dr., UGM Medical Systems, Philadelphia, 3401 Market Street, Suite #222, U.S.a.
Muth Jochen, Dr., Nuklearmedizin, Universität Ulm, D-89081 Ulm, Robert-Koch-Str. 8, Germany

Najemnik Claudia, Dr., Nuklearmedizin, KH-Lainz, A-2522 Oberwaltersdorf, Badenerstr. 20, Austria

Nedelchev Krassen, Dr., Dept. of Neurology, Medical University of Varna, BG-9002, Marin Drinov Str. 55 A, Bulgaria
Nicoletti Rudolf, Prof., Univ.Klinik f. Radiologie - Nuklearmedizin, LKH Graz, A-8036 Auenbruggerplatz 9, Austria
Nooitgedacht E.A., Dr., Dept. of Nuclear Medicine, Hospital Eemland, NL-3518 ES Amersfoort, Utrechtseweg 160, The Netherlands
Nordgren Jan, Dr., Radiological Science HMQ, FIN-02200 Espoo, Rennaniitty 405, Finland
Nosslin Bertil, Prof., S-223 66 Lund, Knut Wicksells väg 19, Sweden
Novak Johann, Nuklearmedizin, LKH Salzburg, Müllner Hauptstr. 48, Austria

Oberladstätter Michael Dr., Univ.Clinic for Nuclear Medicine,, A-6020 Innsbruck, Anichstr. 35, Austria
Oehr Peter, Dr., PET-Zentrum Bonn, D-5311 Bonn, Münsterstr. 20, Germany
Ogris Emil, Prof., Abtl. f.Nuklearmed. Diagnostik und Therapie, Donauspital - SMZ-Ost, A-1220 Langobardenstr. 122, Austria
Öhman Kai, Dr., Radiological Science HMQ, FIN-02200 Espoo, Rennaniitty 405, Finland

Palumbo Renato, Prof., Cattedra di Medicina Nucleare, Università di Perugia, I-06100 Perugia, Cattedra di Medicina Nucleare, Italy
Palumbo Barbara, Dr., Cattedra di Medicina Nucleare, Università di Perugia, I-06100 Perugia, Cattedra di Medicina Nucleare, Italy
Papòs Miklòs, Dr., Dept. of Nuclear Medicine, Albert-Szent-Györgyi Medical University, H-6720 Szeged, Koranyi Fasor 8, Hungary
Pávics Làszlò, Prof., Dept. of Nuclear Medicine, Albert-Szent-Györgyi Medical University, H-6720 Szeged, Koranyi Fasor 8, Hungary
Penttilä Pirkko, MAP - Medical Technologies Oy, FIN-4116 Tikkakoski, Elementtitie 27, Finland
Petritsch Sylvia, Ing., BSM-Diagnostica GesmbH, A-1090 Vienna, Alserstr. 25, Austria
Pinkert Jörg, Dr., Klinik für Nuklearmedizin, Universitätsklinikum d.TU-dresden, D-01279 Dresden, Hermannstädter Str. 17, Germany
Pirich Christian, Dr., Dept. of Nuclear Medicine, University of Vienna, A-1090 Vienna, Waehringer Guertel 18-20, Austria
Plachcinska Anna, Dr., Akademia Medyczna W Lodzi, PL-90419 Lodz, Al Kosciuszki 4, Poland
Podreka Ivo, Prof., Neurologische Abteilung, KH Rudolfstiftung, A-1030 Vienna, Juchg. 25, Austria
Pohner Anita, Dr., Nuklearmed.Abtl., Zentralkrankenhaus Gauting, D-82131 Gauting/Munich, Robert-Koch-Allee 2, Germany
Pollak Manfred, Dipl.-Ing., PHARMACIA & UPJOHN GesmbH, A-1101 Vienna, Oberlaaerstr. 251, Austria
Pollheimer Gerald, Dr., MEDPRO GmbH, A-1180 Vienna, Gersthoferstr. 9, Austria
Prohaska Rudolf, Dr., A-3390 Melk, Austria
Puklavec Ludvik, Dr., Splosna Bolnisnica Maribor, SLO-2000 Maribor, Ljubljanska 5, Slovenia
Püls Eike, Klinikum rechts der Isar München, D-81675 Munich, Ismaningerstr. 69, Germany

Ramschak-Schwarzer Sigrid, Dr. Klin. Abtl. f.Endokrinologie/Nuklearmed., Univ.Klinik Graz, A-8010 Graz, Auenbruggerplatz 15, Austria
Rehefeldt Dieter, Nuklearmedizin, Kantonspital Luzern, CH-6000 Luzern, Switzerland
Rehmann Coen, Dr., Rijnstate Hospital, NL-6800 TA Arnhem, P.O.Box 9555, The Netherlands
Reiners C., Prof., Klinik und Poliklinik f.Nuklearmedizin, D-97080 Würzburg, Josef-Schneider-Str. 2, Germany

Reske S.N.,Prof., Abteilung für Nuklearmedizin, Univ.Klinikum Ulm, D-89070 Ulm, Robert-Koch-Str. 8, Germany
Reyes Renate, Dr., DGN/BDN, D-10589 Berlin, Goslauer Platz 6, Germany
Riccabona Georg, Prof., Univ.Klinik für Nuklearmedizin Innsbruck, A-6020 Innsbruck, Anichstr. 35, Austria
Rickers Carsten, Dr., Dept. of Paediatric Cardiology, Pav. 56, D-20246 Hamburg, Martinistr. 56, Germany
Riedl Peter, Dr., MEDPRO GmbH, A-1180 Vienna, Gersthoferstr. 9, Austria
Riehs Gerhard, Dr., Department of Nuclear Medicine, University of Vienna, A-1090 Vienna, Waehringer Guertel 18-20, Austria
Riihimäki Esko, Dr., Radiological Science HMQ, FIN-02200 Espoo, Rennaniitty 405, Finland
Riva Pietro, Dr., M.Bufalini Hospital, I-47023 Cesena, Via Ghirotti 286, Italy
Rothland Michael, AMERSHAM, D-59425 Unna, Mühlhausener Dorfstr. 26, Germany

Šámal Martin, Dr., Dept. of Nuclear Medicine, 1st Fac of Med., Charles University Prague, CZ.120 00 Praha 2, Salmovska 3, Czech.Rep.
Sarby Bert, Dr., Avd för sjukhusfysik, Huddinge Hospital, S-141 86 Huddinge Sweden
Sasse Karin, Dept. of Paediatric Cardiology, D-20246 Hamburg, Martinistr. 56, Pavillon 56, Germany
Sattler Bernhard, Dipl.Ing., Klinik f. Nuklearmedizin, Universität Leipzig, D-04103 Leipzig, Germany
Sauer Jürgen, Dr., Nuklearmedizin.Radiol.Klinik, LKH Bremen, D-28205 Bremen, St.Jürgen-Str., Germany
Scherer Oskar, BSM- Diagnostica GmbH, A-1080 Vienna, Alserstr. 25, Austria
Schmaljohann Jörn, Dr., Dept. of Nuclear Medicine, University of Vienna, A-1090 Vienna, Waehringer Guertel 18-20, Austria
Schmid Peter, Prof., Rehabilitationszentrum Austria, A-4701 Bad Schallerbach, Austria
Schmidlin Peter, Dr., DKFZ, D-69120 Heidelberg, Im Neuenheimer Feld 280, Germany
Schmidt Hermann, B.R.A.H.M.S. Diagnostica GmbH, A-1070 Vienna, Zollerg. 2/18, Austria
Schöppy Herbert, Dipl.Ing., PICKER INTERNATIONAL GmbH, D-32339 Espelkamp, Marienwerder Str. 2, Germany
Schröttle Wilhelm, Dr., Medizinische Klinik II, Klinikum Ingolstadt, D-85049 Ingolstadt, Krumenauerstr. 25, Germany
Schwaiger M., Prof., Dept. of Nuclear Medicine, Nuklearmed. Klinik rechts der Isar, D-81675 Munich, Ismaningerstr. 22, Germany
Sinzinger Helmut, Prof., Dept. of Nuclear Medicine, University of Vienna, A-1090 Vienna, Waehringer Guertel 18-20, Austria
Skretting Arne, Prof., Dept. of Medical Physics & Technology, The Norwegian Radium Hospital, N-8310 Oslo, Norway
Slomka Piotr, Dr., Nuclear Medicine Dept., London Health Sciences Centre, Victoria Campus Ontario N6A 4G5, 375 South Street, Canada
Smith Timothy A.D., Dr., Dept. of Nuclear Medicine, Royal Marsden NHS Trust, GB-Sutton, Surrey SM2 5PT, Great Britain
Sobal Grazyna, Dr., Department of Nuclear Medicine, University of Vienna, A-1090 Vienna, Waehringer Guertel 18-20, Austria
Soldner Jürgen, SIEMENS Medizintechnik AG, D-91052 Erlangen, Henkestr. 127, Germany
Somer Kalevi, Dr., Radiological Science HMQ, Fin-02200 Espoo, Rennaniitty 405, Finland
Sonderkamp Horst-M, Dr., Abtl. für Nuklearmedizin und Strahlentherapie, Kreiskrankenhaus Heide, D-25746 Heide, Esmarchstr. 50, Germany
Sonderkamp Annegret S., Dr., D-25746 Heide, Esmarchstr. 50, Germany

Stabell Uwe, Dr., Praxis für Nuklearmedizin, D-14199 Berlin, Dillenburgerstr. 1, Germany
Stach Lisa, Med.Univ.Klinik, LKH Graz, A-8036 Graz, Auenbruggerplatz 15, Austria
Standke Rudolf, Dr., ICT GmbH, A-1180 Vienna, Trazerbergg. 76, Austria
Stockhammer M., Dr., AÖ Krankenhaus Wels, A-4600 Wels, Grieskirchnerstr. 42, Austria
Strand Sven-Erik, Prof. Radiation Physics Dept., Lund University Hospital, S-22185 Lund, Sweden
Stuller Yvonne, Dept. of Nuclear Medicine and Special Endocrinology, LKH Klagenfurt, A-9020 Klagenfurt, St.Veiter-Str. 47, Austria
Svensson Leif, Dr., Avd för sjukhusfysik, Huddinge Hospital, S-141 86 Huddinge, Sweden,
Szakáll Szabolcs jr., Dr., PET Centre, University Medical School Debrecen, H-4026 Debrecen, Bem tér 18/C, Hungary
Szemety Gabriela, Dr., SCHOELLER-PHARMA Ges.m.b.H, A-1231 Vienna, Industrieg. 7, Austria
Szilvasi Julia, Dr., Dept. of Radiology, Semmelweis University, H-1126 Budapest, Barthastr. 31/c, Hungary
Szilvási István, Dr., Dept. of Nuclear Medicine, Haynal University, H-1389 Budapest, P.O.Box 112, Hungary

Talbot Jean-Noel, Prof., Hopital Tenon, F-75970 Paris CX 20, 4 Rue de Chine, France,
Teule G.J.J., Dr., AMERSHAM, NL-3079 AK Rotterdam, Spuikreek 321, The Netherlands
Theissen Peter, Dr., Universität zu Köln, D-50924 Cologne, Joseph-Stelzmann-Str. 9, Germany
Thierfelder Hans, Dr., GKH Berlin, D-10707 Berlin, Sächsische Str. 49, Germany
Thomas Robert James, Dr., Adderbrookes Hospital Cambridge, GB-Cambridge, Hills Rd., Great Britain
Thomson William H., Dr., Physics and Nuclear Medicine Dept., City Hospital NHS Trust, GB-Birmingham B18 7QH, Great Britain,
Thurner-Reichmann Doris, Dr., Rehabilitationszentrum Austria, A-4701 Bad Schallerbach, Austria
Todd-Pokropek Andrew E., Prof., Medical Physics Dept., GB-London WC1E 6BT, Gower St., Great Britain
Trimmel Jolanta, Abtl. f.Nuklearmedizin, Diagnostik & Therapie, Donauspital - SMZ-Ost, A-1220 Vienna, Langobardenstr. 122, Austria
Trón Lajos, Prof. PET Centre, University Medical School of Debrecen, H-4026 Debrecen, Bem tér 18/C, Hungary

Unterluggauer Paula, KH Barmh.Brüder, A-1020 Vienna, Gr.Mohreng. 9-11, Austria

Van Klaveren Ronald, NYCOMED AMERSHAM International, NL-3079 AK Rotterdam, Spuikreek 321, The Netherlands
Vanninen Esko, Dr., Dept. of Clinical Physiology & Nuclear Medicine, Kuopio University Hospital, FIN-70211 Kuopio, P.O.Box 1777, Finland
Varoglu Erhan, Dr., Dept. of Nuclear Medicine, Atatürk University Medical School, TR-25240 Erzurum, Turkey
Verbruggen Rudi, IBA, B-1348 Louvain-la Neuve, Chemin du cyclotron, 3, Belgium
Visser Frans, Dr. Dept. of Cardiology, Free University Hospital, NL-1081 HV Amsterdam, De Boekelaan 1117, The Netherlands
Volterrani Duccio, Dr., Dept. of Nuclear Medicine, Policlinico „Le Scotte", University of Siena, I-53100 Siena, Viale Bracci, Italy

Wagner Gabriele, Dept. of Nuclear Medicine, Vienna University Hospital AKH, A-1090 Vienna, Waehringer Guertel 18-20, Austria

Wallis Jerold, Prof., Mallinckrodt Institute of Radiology, Wahington Univ. School of Medicine, Div of Nuclear Medicine, St.Louis, Missouri 63110, 510 South Kingshighway Blvd., U.S.A

Weber Andrea, Geb.Gyn.Univ.Klinik, LKH-Graz, A-8036 Graz, Auenbruggerplatz 14, Austria

Weblacher Michaela, Dr., BIOMEDICA Ges.m.b.H., A-8043 Graz, Joseph-Marx-Str. 5, Austria

Wegener Bernd, Dr., B.R.A.H.M.S Diagnostica GmbH, D-12099 Berlin, Komturstr. 19-20, Germany

Weller Rolf, Dr., Abtl. f. Nuklearmedizin, Universität Ulm, D-89070 Ulm, Robert-Koch-Str. 8, Germany

Wenger Martin, Dr., Dept. of Nuclear Medicine, University of Innsbruck, A-6020 Innsbruck, Anichstr. 35, Austria

Wengler Cornelia, IMMUNOMEDICS Europe, D-07639 Bad Klosterlausnitz, Waldstr. 14, Germany

Westhoff Dieter, Dr., D-31303 Bürgdorf, Von der Höfen 26, Germany

Wielepp Peter, Dr., Nuclear Medicine, Inselspital, University of Berne, Ch-3010 Berne, Switzerland

Wizsy Dolores, Nuklearmedizin, LKH Graz, A-8045 Graz, Andr.Reichsstr. 58/d, Austria

Xie Yanfen, Dr., Division of Human Health, IAEA, A-1220 Wagramerstr. 5, Austria

Yvan David, CIS-Diagnostik (Deutschland), F-91192 Gif-sur-Yvette Cédéx, BP No. 32, France

Zakarias Herbert, BIOMEDICA Ges.m.b.H., A-8043 Graz, Joseph-Marx-Str. 5, Austria

Zaknun John, Dr., Univ.Klinik für Nuklearmedizin, A-6020 Innsbruck, Anichstr. 35, Austria,

Ziegler S., Dr., Nuklearmedizin. Klinik rechts der Isar, Technische Universität München, D-81674 Munich, Ismaningerstr. 22, Germany

Zimmermann Gudrun, KH Barmh.Brüder, A-8020 Graz, Bergstr. 27, Austria

Zink Hannelore, KH Barmh.Brüder Graz Eggenberg, A-8054 Graz, Bergstr. 27, Austria

Zolle Ilse, Prof., Department of Nuclear Medicine, University of Vienna, A-1090 Vienna, Waehringer Guertel 18-20, Austria

23rd International Symposium

„Radioactive Isotopes in Clinical Medicine and Research"

International Scientific Committee

H.Bergmann (Vienna)
H.J.Biersack (Bonn)
A.Bischof-Delaloye (Lausanne)
P.J.Ell (London)
H.Köhn (Vienna)
A.Kroiss (Vienna)
P.Lind (Klagenfurt)
J.Martin-Comín (Barcelona)
R.Palumbo (Perugia)
G.Riccabona (Innsbruck)
M.Schwaiger (Munich)
H.Sinzinger (Vienna)
A.E.Todd-Pokropek (London)

Organizing Committee

Honorary President :

R.Höfer

Chairmen Organizing Committee :

H.Bergmann
H.Köhn
H.Sinzinger

Staff Members of Congress Office :

R.Bartosch
Susanne Granegger
E.Havlik
Andrea Heckenberg
Julia Jank
Bärbel John
G.Karanikas
Adelheid Maringer
G.Minear
W.Piller
Ch.Pirich
J.Schmaljohann
Gabriela Vida

List of exhibitors

ADAC Laboratories Europe B.V.
Zonnebaan 34
P.O.Box 1419
NL-3600 BK Maarssen

BERTHOLD-Analytische Instrumente
Vertriebs-Ges.m.b.H
Ameisgasse 49-51
A-1140 Vienna

BIOCIS Handelsges.m.b.H.
Divischgasse 4
A-1210 Vienna

B.R.A.H.M.S. Diagnostica GmbH
Zollergasse 2/18
A-1070 Vienna

DPC Bühlmann GmbH
Hauffgasse 3-5/2/H
A-1110 Vienna

ELIMPEX - Medizintechnik Ges.m.b.H
Spechtgasse 32
A-2340 Mödling

ELSCINT Central & Eastern Europe
Handelsges.m.b.H
Nobilegasse 23-25
A-1150 Vienna

IASON Labormedizin GesmbH & CO.KG
Rechbauerstraße 3
A-8010 Graz

ICT Chemikalien, Handelsges.m.b.H.
Trazerberggasse 76
A-1130 Vienna

KLIMONITORS OEG
Am Hundsturm 2-4/6
A-1050 Vienna

MEDISO Ltd
Alsótörökvész út 14
H-1022 Budapest

MED PRO - Vertrieb f.Med.-Diagnost.
Produkte Ges.m.b.H.
Gersthoferstr. 9
A-1180 Vienna

NOVARTIS Pharma GmbH
Brunnerstr. 59
A-1235 Vienna

NUCLEAR DIAGNOSTICS AB
Elektravägen 5
S-12630 Hägersten

PHARMACIA &UPJOHN GesmbH
Oberlaaer Straße 251
A-1101 Vienna

PICKER INTERNATIONAL GmbH
Marienwerder Straße 2
D-32339 EspelkaMp

POLAROID GmbH
Sprendlinger Landstraße 109
D-63069 Offenbach/M.

SCHOELLER Pharma Ges.m.b.H.
Industriegasse 7
A-1231 Vienna

SIENENS AG - Bereich Med.Technik
Henkestraße 127
D-91052 Erlangen

TOSHIBA Medical Systems GmbH
IZ NÖ-Süd
Ricoweg 40
A-2351 Wr.Neudorf

THE BADGASTEIN LECTURE

Radioactive Isotopes in
Clinical Medicine and Research XXIII
ed. by H. Bergmann, H. Köhn and H. Sinzinger

THE CHALLENGE OF THE 21st CENTURY

The 23rd International Symposium of Radioactive Isotopes in Clinic and Research

Professor PJ Ell
Institute of Nuclear Medicine, Middlesex Hospital, UCL, London, UK

INTRODUCTION

This is the 12th Bad Gastein lecture, a prestigious international series which began in 1982 when Nigel Trott was invited to deliver his lecture entitled „The safe and effective use of radiopharmaceuticals". These lectures became embedded and a main feature of the International Symposium of Radioactive Isotopes in Clinic and Research, a series of international meetings at 2 year intervals which began in 1954 (see Table 2 for the Bad Gastein lectures). As we approach the 21st century (only 717 and 5 and ½ hours were left on the day of the delivery of this lecture on 13 January 1998) it is appropriate to attempt an overview, if not an informal SWOT analysis of the possible implications for the practice of Nuclear Medicine as technology and health care and delivery systems envolve. In this context of gazing into the crystal ball of the future, it may be sobering to be reminded of two citations. „The future ain't what it used to be" by Josie Berra in 1925 and „I never think of the future. It comes soon enough" by Albert Einstein in 1930. The conflict is already apparent. We know that what is will not be and we also know how hard it will be to anticipate change.

Table 1
BADGASTEIN LECTURES

1976	Veall, Norman Prospects today for Radioisotope Techniques in Clinical Research
1978	Lassen, Niels A Mapping of the Function of the Cortex in Normal and Diseased Brain: Regional Blood Flow Studies by the Intraarterial 133-Xenon Method
1980	Kellershohn, C Compartmental Analysis
1982	Trott, Nigel G The Safe and Effective Use of Radiopharmaceuticals
1984	Feinendegen, LE The Dual Parameter Analysis for In Vivo Measuring Metabolic Reactions
1986	Beckers, C The Impact of Thyroid in Nuclear Medicine
1988	Biersack, HJ The Answer of Nuclear Medicine to Health Problems of the Nineties
1990	Rosler, H Self-limiting Hyperthyroidism
1992	Britton, KE Nuclear Endocrinology
1994	Höfer, R Nuclear Medicine - Tool of Specialty
1996	Rigo, P, Paulus, P, Jerusalem, G, Benoit, T, Larock, MP, Foidart, J Clinical PET in Oncology
1998	Ell, PJ The Challenge of the 21st Century

In this era where science has become a predominant force in the practice of medicine and science degrees are cherished diamonds in the career of a bright, young doctor aspiring to make an impact in health care, it is sobering to quote from recent literature.

„The commonly used criteria for diagnosis can differ by factor of 10 in the number of subjects classified as having dementia". „Serious implications for research and treatment as well as for the right of many elderly to drive, make a will and handle financial affairs."

(From NEJM 337:1667-74,1997)

Ring, PA (in Diagnostic Imaging 1997) states „The penetration and acceptance of the technique or modality do not seem to depend much on scientific results or costs, but rather on local culture, politics and lobbying". This conflict between technological potential, science and daily practice is further contrasted when one finds that eminent scientists such as Lauterbur can operate an MRI scanner over the Web (animal scale, 4T, 31cm bore with signal and image processing at a distance) and that educational establishments (University of Newcastle, NSW, Australia) can offer Nuclear Medicine postgraduate degree courses on the WWW. One feels flooded with information, with an ever greater difficulty of distinguishing the trees from the bushes (in modern scientific language distinguishing the signal from noise). Society leaders are therefore looking for new mechnisms to categorise knowledge and seek a solution to the gathering of evidence. The American College of Physicians and the British Medical Journal have teamed up with the production of a new publication „Evidence-based Medicine“ which seeks to guide health care delivery through the publication of data which is based on sound premise from which guidelines for practice can be derived. That this difficult to achieve can be seen in one of the abstracts or articles quoted in the November/December 97 issue of this journal. It refers to a publication by Turkstra T et al (in Annals of Internal Medicine, 126, 775-81, 199/) where in a teaching hospital apparently 357 patients suspected of having pulmonary embolism had a non-diagnostic lung scan carried out in 155 of these. The questions which, of course, arise immediately from this citation are: Is this data representative of general practice? If yes, why are lung scans still performed? If not, where is the bias in patient selection? Or are there other factors: inappropriate referrals, reporting, etc? Often, data whose purpose is to gather evidence, leaves too many questions unanswered.

GENERAL CONSIDERATION ON THE MARKET AND PRACTICE

In the October issue of Diagnostic Imaging in 1997, Rink states an estimate for instrumentation in the US, Japan and Europe with 150.000 ultrasound scanners performing approximately 115 million investigations per annum, 20.000 CT scanners performing 63 million investigations, 9.000 MRI scanners performing approximately 18 million investigations and 750.000 Nuclear Medicine cameras performing 35 million investigations. As the author states, these figures are an estimate and may require major readjustments. Nevertheless, we know a little bit more accurately that the clinical practice of Nuclear Medicine involves 2 major topics (Cardiology 40% and Oncology 40%) with all other acitivities representing one fifth of today's Nuclear Medicine practice. We also kow that like with other imaging procedures there are huge variations in the number of procedures per million population as practiced in the US and different European countries. A reasonable guess estimate allows us to document these differences and naturally to raise the question as tho whether those nations at the bottom of the list are simply not offering adequate patient care to their patient population or whether those at the top of the list are in default by over-utilisation. As often in medicine as in life, the appropriate answer would be found somewhere in between the extremes of the figures quoted. The trends of the submission of scientific work to European Conferences was analysed by I.Carrio at last year's Annual Conference of the European Association of Nuclear Medicine in

Glasgow, and his Highlights Lecture published in the December 1997 issue of the European Journal of Nuclear Medicine clearly shows that there is a reasonable plateauing of the submissions in the fields of Cardiology when surveyed from 1990 up to 1997 whilst there is an almost doubling of submissions over this same period of time in respect to work which reflect applications in Oncology and in Therapy. Slow trends upwards for data in respect to tracers and instrumentations was also seen.

Worrying is the apparent concentration of the industry dedicated to Nuclear Medicine activity. Whilst in 1985 possible 10 relevant radiopharamceutical companies could have been found, it is arguable that there are now less half of this number. At the same time there is huge activity in the field as witness by the numerous efforts to develop new tracers. 16 potentially new radiopharmaceuticals were discussed at the World Federation Meeting in Sydney in 1994, it would be feasible to list another 16 tracer for imaging of infection (see Table 2) and all this activity contrasts with the relative paucity of tracers introduced and registered in the market for approved clinical indications. Too many small scale initiatives are being developed in a radiopharmaceutical market which pales in comparison with the gigantic pharmaceutical market dominated by the major drug companies. Similar trends of fusions and merges are to be seen in the equipment industry, the number of major manufacturers has also been reduced significantly over the last 5 years. The electronic world through the INTERNET (a global web of interconnecting computer networks developed 25 years ago) now poses the potential and the threat of a distant expert on call for the reporting of medical data.

Table 2

INFECTION IMAGING

^{111}In - WBC's	^{67}Ga - Citrate
^{99m}Tc - WBC's	^{18}FDG
^{99m}Tc - Colloids	
^{99m}Tc - MoAB's	

	Fragments
	Anti-E Selectin
Peptides	
	IL-1, IL-2, IL-8
	f-Meltlen Phe
	Tuftsin
Antibodies	(Ciprofloxacin)
Others	

PRESENT PRACTICE

The following 5 tables provide an overwiew for the present clinical practice of clinical Nuclear Medicine as it affects diagnosis, staging, treatment and monitoring of the evolution of disease in a number of important pathologies.

Table 3

NUCLEAR MEDICINE	
Diagnosis	: Has the patient an ischaemic heart ?
Staging	: Is more than one territory involved ?
Monitoring	: Has CABG caused a drop in RV function ?
Treatment	: Is a stent appropriate? And where?
Prognosis	: What is the risk of a future event ?

Table 4

NUCLEAR MEDICINE	
Diagnosis	: Is there a functioning neuroendocrine mass ?
Staging	: Are there functioning metastases ?
Monitoring	: Has conventional treatment failed ?
Treatment	: Initiate specific ^{131}I-MIBG

Table 5

NUCLEAR MEDICINE	
Diagnosis	: Is there a Ca Breast ? (Conventional diagnostic triad uncertain)
Staging	: Is the axilla free of disease ?
Therapy	: - Has the radiotherapy field been adequately dimensioned ? - Is pain palliation appropriate ?
Monitoring	: What is the response to therapy ?

Table 6

NUCLEAR MEDICINE	
Diagnosis	: Is there a functioning or non-functioning thyroid nodule ?
Staging	: Has the disease progressed beyound the neck ?
Therapy	: What is the appropriate Iodine treatment ?
Monitoring	: Is the patient free from disease ?

Table 7

NUCLEAR MEDICINE

Diagnosis	: Is the kidney scarred ? Does it respond to diuresis ? Is it obstructed or just dilated ? Is there a non-functioning organ ? Is there ATN ?
Monitoring	: What is the GFR ? Has it changed ?
Treatment	: Is the transplant perfused ? Has the transplant deteriorated ? Is tracer in the bladder ? Is there a leak ?

KEY ISSUE AND KEY CHOICES

The tables above, whilst not a comprehensive description of present clinical practice in the field, give a very good indication as to the range of breadth and indeed depth of clinical activity when the radioactive tracer methodology is applied to medicine. As in other fields, the pace of change determines the need for choices to be made and new strategic directions to be identified. Rega rdless of the prevailing choices or avenues to be pursued, it is clear nevertheless, that the major tools for successful implementation are to be found in TEAMWORK. This is applicable locally, regionally or indeed nationally and internationally. Scientific progress and medical progress recognises no boundaries and ultimately also impacts on resource. It is inconceivable that ultimately Nuclear Medicine will succeed at a local or national level whilst failing at a regional or international level. It has been a significant failure of the recent past that leaders in the field have not addressed this issue with significant determination, purpose and vigour. Some leaders have even advocated regional or national policies as the key for success. This strategy is doomed to failure. It is therefore not surprising how little attention has been paid by the specialised community on the training required to implement, monitor and apply international criteria for multicentre trials. There is a vast learning deficit here which needs to be filled and rapidly! We could list the key choices for Nuclear Medicine as follows: service versus research, pathology versus physiology, diagnostic versus therapeutics, inward looking (national) efforts and outward looking (international) efforts. At the same time key issues for Nuclear Medicine have remained over the years in terms of the internal organisation of the activity. The issues that we confront today are those of a centralised department and its continuity, those of the development of a spoke and hub organisation, those which relate from a fragmented medical speciality-driven facility (as if Nuclear Cardiology can ever survive on its own) and those of volume.

Table 8

KEY SOLUTIONS	
* Patient Lobby	Patient/Doctor Associations (Cardiac, Breast, Alzheimer's Stroke, Osteoporosis, etc.)
* Volume Strategy	
* Instant Availability	
* Instant Reporting	
* Team Practices	Cardiology Oncology Rheumatology Endocrinology etc.

Table 9

KEY CHOICES FOR NUCLEAR MEDICINE		
* Service	-	Research
* Pathology	-	Physiology
* Diagnostic	-	Therapeutics
* Inward Looking (National)	-	Telemedicine (International)

Policy makers will not reduce their efforts to determine cost benefit and we in the field must find the appropriate answers. No one else will find those for us. It is also abundantly clear that such efforts cannot be found with inward looking efforts only.

MAJOR OPPORTUNITIES AND KEY SOLUTIONS

Nuclear Medicine is now presented with major new opportunities for growth. The main growth areas include Neurology and Psychiatry where over 30% of Nuclear Medicine research and development are focused, the surgical management of a variety of cancer diseases, infection rheumatology and the general field of oncology and radionuclide therapy. Let us not forget that one in three patients eventually will present with cancer. In keeping with growth, major new opportunities are available for Nuclear Medicine in drug discovery, in organ specific tools (detectors and tracers), in the need for new medical therapy and in the potential of tele-medicine as a whole. In the pursuit of appropriate solutions or strategies which will deal with the perceived challenge which Nuclear Medicine is facing from competing technologies, the following approach as described in Tables X to XIII is presented as the most likely model for success of the speciality in the future. The model clearly appreciates the need for an increase in overall volume of procedures, without which industrial support is difficult to sustain. The model clearly identifies that medicine is evolving from the classification of groups of patients into the individual detailed assessment of the response of an individual patient to a particular specific treatment. The model recognises the huge deficit in knowledge which patients and doctors alike face in the crucial distinction between responders and non-responders to treatment, and the urgent need to identify early markers which will permit the monitoring of disease. The model recognises the importance of patient lobbies and associations and the crucial determining factors of instant availability, instant reporting and team practices. Diagrams are presented which explain pathways for successful interaction between Nuclear Medicine and referring physicians.

Table 10

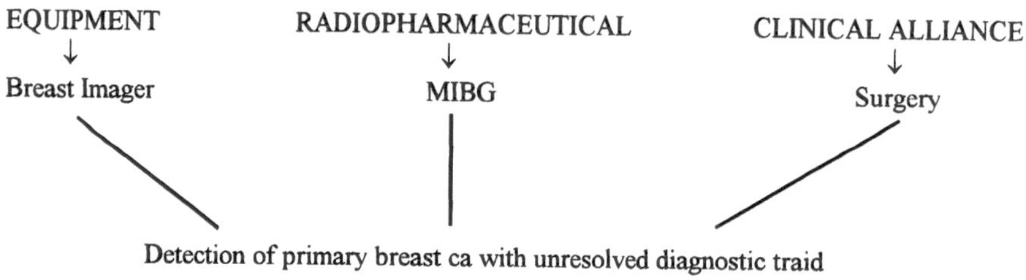

Table 11

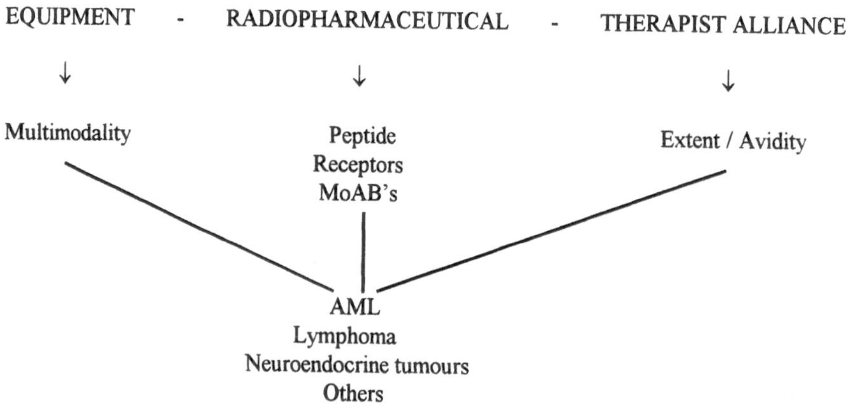

Table 12

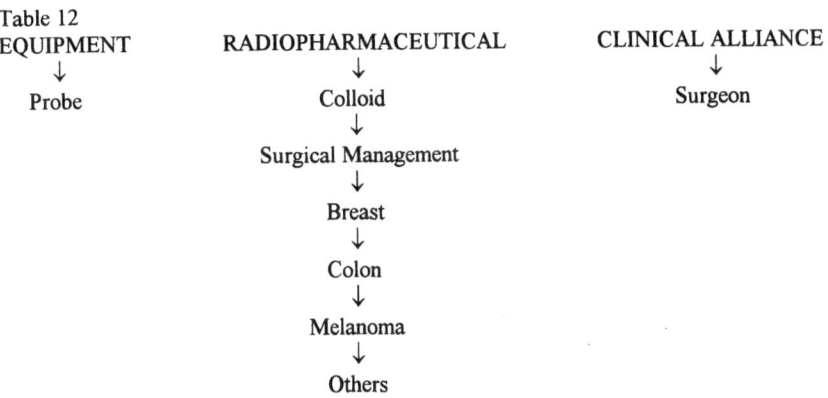

EQUIPMENT	RADIOPHARMACEUTICAL	CLINICAL ALLIANCE
↓	↓	↓
Probe	Colloid	Surgeon
	↓	
	Surgical Management	
	↓	
	Breast	
	↓	
	Colon	
	↓	
	Melanoma	
	↓	
	Others	

Table 13

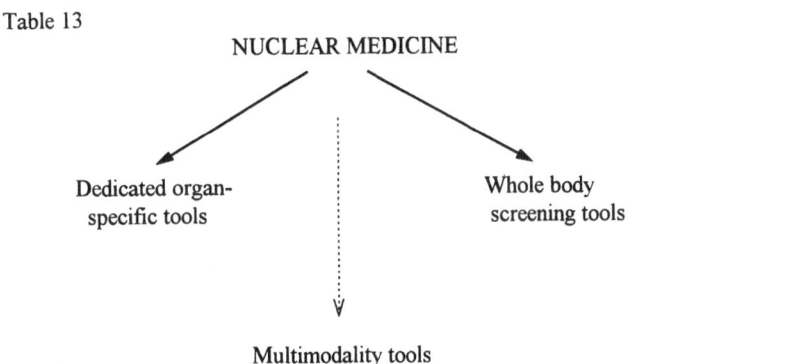

NUCLEAR MEDICINE

↙ ↘

Dedicated organ-specific tools

Whole body screening tools

↓

Multimodality tools

PRESENT TRENDS AND DEVELOPMENTS

At the time of the last World Federation in Nuclear Medicine and Biology conference in Sydney in 1994, I set a challenge for the Nuclear Medicine Industry in identifying the requirements for a single instrument for planar and tomographic imaging, for fast and slow data acquisition, for the imaging of energies between 80 and 511 KeV, with spatial resolution of 5mm FWHM and superior sensitivity, for single and coincidence counting for 1998! Were these prophetic words? If we watch the detector developments over the last 20 years (approximate dates) we see the arrival of single photon emission tomography in 1981, that of multi-detector SPET in 1989, that of multi-detector Sodium Iodide based PET in 1990, the dual detector and variable angle SPET systems in 1994 and the gamma camera PET imaging with Sodium Iodide in 1996. Finally over the last two years we have actually seen the arrival of new detector technology! Melcher and Schweitzer published in 1992 in Nuclear Instruments

and Methods in Physics Research (Section A - A314, 1, 212-214), their paper entitled, „ A promising new scintillator: cerium-doped lutetium oxyorthosilicate." The new LSO detector has exciting characteristics for radiation detection including high light output, fast decay time, high atomic number. This new material is being actively investigated with both Siemens and CTI leading this technological development. The lead is substantial and the introduction of new instrumentation for the clinical user is expected soon. Instrumentation with dual capability for SPET and PET imaging is therefore appearing on the practical horizon. Hybrid systems are also being designed and researchers at the Crump Institute for Biological Imaging at UCLA have developed a high resolution PET scanner that can fit inside the bore of an MRI system. This micro PET system utilises small and more sensitive scintillation crystals also made from LSO. In parallel, other developments with radiation detector technology make use of Cd, Zn, Te detectors which inherently can be made small, portable with high count rate capabilities and are designed for dedicated organ imaging. As an example the Digirad system has won FDA approval for the company's solid state, digital gamma camera. Images can be produced throughout the entire energy spectrum from low energy SPET to high energy PET imaging.
Again during the Conference in Sydney in 1994 I challenged the Industry for a new tracer for Oncology for general application, a superior tracer for infection imaging and a new tracer for coronary artery disease and the localisation of atherosclerosis. The unmet challenge is the imaging of the lesion of the arterial wall! The new Nuclear Medicine pipeline which appears on the market or is near to approaching market recognition includes a new tracer for infection imaging, a marker for tissue hypoxia, an Iodine-123 or indeed a Tc-99m labelled dopamine transporter agent, a new agent for radiation synovectomy and a number of new agents for the treatment of oncological patients.

The special impact of Nuclear Medicine in drug discovery and drug action studies is highlighted by a review article entitled," More choices for treating voices" by Flaum and Andreasen, published in *The Lancet*, S322, End of year review 1997. Our group confirmed the limbic selectivity of Clozapine in *The Lancet* (3502, 490-491, 19997) and the work on the newer neurotransmission agent such as Iodine-123 labelled epidepride are opening new avenues for research and clinical investigation. This particular probe for imaging striatal and extrastriatal and dopamine D2 receptor sites exhibits peak striatal activity at 3 hours, peak extrastriatal activity at approximately one hour in the temporal cortex and clearly demonstrates improved affinity for D2 over IBZM. Our own group is active in this field investigating the role of epidepride in the evaluation of D2 light receptor blockade, evaluating Iodine-123 labelled iomazenil in alcohol-dependency and participating in a multi-centre trial evaluating the role of Iodine-123 labelled FP CIT as a dopamine transporter ligang (work in progress and/or in press).

NUCLEAR MEDICINE IN ONCOLOGY

It represents conventional wisdom to describe the role of Nuclear Medicine in Oncology as one which impacts on diagnosis, staging, re-staging, treatment monitoring, treatment and prediction of treatment outcome, organ function measurements and drug efficacy studies. The known areas of application of Nuclear Medicine treatment in Oncology include thyroid cancer, the palliation of bone pain, the treatment of neural crest tumours, the antibody therapy of some lymphomas, the antibody guided treatment of high grade gliomas and a splattering of other rarer indications and treatments. Whilst a detailed analysis of all of these indications and roles falls outside the scope of this presentation, we will highlight some important new avenues for work which will change definitely the present impact of Nuclear Medicine in the general area of Oncology.

BREAST IMAGING (AN UNRESOLVED CONTROVERSY)

There are a huge range of techniques employed for the diagnosis of primary breast carcinoma. Whilst Nuclear Medicine has focused its interest over the last 5 years in this area and we will be able to play a role in al limited number of patients where the conventional diagnostic triad (clinical examination, mammography and fine needle biopsy) will still leave a definite though smaller number of patients undiagnosed, a most exciting and perhaps more relevant role will be the surgical management of patients presenting for the first time with operable carcinoma of the breast. We know that the definition of axillary lymph node status of these patients is the most important prognostic factor and we know that the determination of the status of the axillary lymph nodes is crucial in patient management. Post-operative adjuvant chemotherapy is different in ALN positive patients and ALN negative patients, we know that conventional axillary sampling is inaccurate, if not abandoned, in view of a high false negative rate, we know that the resection of level 1 nodes is not widely accepted and that the resection of level 1 and 2 nodes is usually part of the procedure. We also know that ALN positive patients are likely to develop metastases, that they die earlier and the post-operative adjuvant chemotherapy significantly reduces the risk of dissemination.

Nuclear Medicine is now addressing the concept of sentinel lymph node detection aiming at detecting the first regional lymph node which drains lymph from the primary tumour. It will be (by definition) the first node to receive malignant cells from lymph node borne spread. The seminal paper by Veronese at al. in *The Lancet* 1997, 349-1864-1867 entitled „Sentinel node biopsy to avoid axillary dissection in breast carcinoma with clinically negative lymph nodes" clearly defines the exciting potential of Nuclear Medicine in this field. In a sample of 163 patients, Nuclear Medicine was able to accurately predict the status of axillary lymph nodes in 97.5% of all cases. In 38% of patients with metastatic axillary nodes, SLN status and the negative status of axillary nodes as examined histologically. This field will undergo an explosive discussion throughout Europe and we will await the outcome of several trials which are now extending this already important database with increasing enthusiasm. It is also clear that sentinel lymph node scintigraphy will be applied to a variety of other tumours (head and neck, colorectal, penis, melanoma).

We will finish this presentation with a more detailed discussion on the upcoming role of radionuclide therapy with alpha emitters.

Table 14

USEFUL ALPHA PARTICLE EMITTERS

	T1/2	KeV	MeV(α)
Bi-213	46'	440 (imaging)	5.8
Ac-225	10 days		5.8
At-211	7 hours		

Both obtained from decay of Th-229. Obtained from natural decay of U-233 or neutron irradiation of Ra-226.

Table 15

THERAPY WITH ALPHA-EMITTERS (II)

- 30x greater energy than that of a Beta Particle (6 MeV versus 200 KeV).
- +2 charge versus -1 charge of Beta Particle.
- 7.000x heavier mass (4 units versus 1/1.600 for Beta).
- 1000x more energy dissipated per unit track length versus Beta.
- Non-elastic collisions cause 3x greater cell killing / Unit of engery dissipated versus Beta.

The merit of this approach includes a high LET over a few cell diameters versus hundreds of cell diameters for beta particles, the highest dose dependent cell mortality achievable with alpha emitters in view of the much greater energy deposited per cell in comparison with what is achievable with beta particles. Therapy applications for alpha emitters could include the treatment of micrometastases in patients with relapsing AML, NH lymphoma, and multiple myeloma, the intracavitary teatment of patients with ovarian carcinoma and the adjuvant treatment of prostate, colon and breast carcinoma. Naturally there is potential for combined alpha and beta particle therapy where appropriate. This area deserves careful monitoring since real progress in being made in the USA and throughout Europe.

Finally, the concept of labelled peptides to be used both in diagnosis and in treatment is gaining increasing importance. Recent progress made with somatostatin and analogues labelled with Yttrium-90 point to the new promising area opened for medical treatment of cancer.

CONCLUSION

The future is a bright one. Change will come and the field will respond. We have pointed the way forward. In pointing let us be reminded of the aphorism:

„Quand le savant montre la lune, l'idiot regarde le doigt"

NEUROLOGY, PSYCHIATRY

Radioactive Isotopes in
Clinical Medicine and Research XXIII
ed. by H. Bergmann, H. Köhn and H. Sinzinger

FIRST EVALUATION IN HUMANS OF [^{123}I]PE2I: A SELECTIVE RADIOLIGAND FOR VISUALIZATION OF THE STRIATAL DOPAMINE TRANSPORTER DENSITY

K.A. Bergström[1], J.T. Kuikka[1], P. Emond[2], J. Hiltunen[3], C. Halldin[4], D. Guilloteau[2], L. Mauclaire[5], M. Yu[1], J. Karhu[1], E. Tupala[6], J. Tiihonen[6]

[1]Department of Clinical Physiology, Kuopio University Hospital, Kuopio, Finland; [2]Laboratoire de Biophysique Médicale et Pharmaceutique, Université François Rabelais, Tours, France; [3]MAP Medical Technologies Inc., Tikkakoski, Finland; [4]Department of Clinical Neuroscience, Psychiatry Section, Karolinska Institute, Stockholm, Sweden; [5]CIS-Bio industrie, Gif-sur-Yvette, France; [6]Department of Forensic Psychiatry, University of Kuopio, Niuvanniemi Hospital, Kuopio, Finland.

SUMMARY: (E)-N-(3-iodoprop-2-enyl)-2β-Carbomethoxy-3β-(4-methylphenyl)nortropane (PE2I) is recently synthesised selective compound for the dopamine transporter. In the present study ^{123}I-labelled PE2I were prepared for SPET studies with healthy volunteers. There was a rapid uptake of radioactivity in brain (3% of ID at 1 hour) and a high accumulation of radioactivity in the striatum. In the thalamus and in cortical regions no visible uptake of radioactivity was observed. Striatum-to-cerebellum ratio was 5 at 70 min. Percentage of unchanged [^{123}I]PE2I in plasma was less than 20% at 1 h post injection. In conclusion, [^{123}I]PE2I is a potential radioligand for the dopamine transporter imaging with SPET.

INTRODUCTION

Radiolabelled β-CIT and analogues have been used for the imaging of the dopamine transporter (DAT) with single-photon emission tomography (SPET) or positron emission tomography (PET) (1-4). (E)-N-(3-iodoprop-2-enyl)-2β-Carbomethoxy-3β-(4-methylphenyl)-nortropane (PE2I) is recently synthesised selective compound for DAT, which *in vitro* has similar affinity to DAT ($K_i = 17$ nM) as β-CIT whereas affinity to serotonin and noradrenalin transporters is 500 and >1000 nM, respectively (5). In the present study ^{123}I-labelled PE2I were prepared for SPET studies with 2 healthy volunteers.

MATERIALS AND METHODS

Radiolabelling. The iodination of PE2I was performed from the tributyltin precursor by MAP Medical Technologies Inc. (Tikkakoski, Finland) by the chloramine-T method. Carrier free Na^{123}I was obtained from CIS (CIS bio international, Gif-sur-Yvette, France). The specific radioactivity of [^{123}I]β-CIT was estimated to be same as that of Na^{123}I, i.e. 8.7 TBq/μmol (237 Ci/μmol) and the radiochemical purity was > 98 %.

Subjects. Two healthy male volunteers (31 and 37 years) were studied. Subjects gave their informed consent for the study. The study was approved by the Ethical Committee of Kuopio University Hospital.

SPET Brain Imaging. A 215 MBq dose of [^{123}I]PE2I was used. The dose was injected into the right antecubital vein. SPET imaging was performed on the Siemens MultiSPECT 3 gamma camera with fan-beam collimators. Dynamic SPET was started immediately after the injection. In total, 9-11 scans per study subjects were performed within 7 hours. The energy window (15 %) was centred around the photopeak of ^{123}I (159 keV). During 360° rotation (120° per camera head), 40 views/head were acquired in a 128 x 128 matrix mode (pixel size of 2.8 mm). The raw data were reconstructed with the filtered back-projection technique (Butterworth: order 8 and a cut-off frequency 0.75 cm-1). The transaxial slices were corrected for the Chang's attenuation method with the uniform attenuation coefficient of 0.10 cm^{-1}. The imaging resolution was 7-8 mm. Transaxial, sagittal and coronal slices were visually surveyed and two slices were consecutively summarised (slice thickness of 5.6 mm). Irregular regions of interest were drawn onto the cerebellum, the midbrain, the thalamus, cortical regions, and the striatum. Average regional counts (counts/voxel) were used in calculations, and time-activity curves were printed out (Fig. 1).

Blood analysis. Blood analysis was performed with a gradient HPLC method which is similar to the one used earlier (7). Blood samples (5 ml) were drawn in heparin coated tubes.

One sample just prior to the administration of [^{123}I]PE2I and 7-8 samples after injection of the tracer (2, 5, 10, 30, 60, 120, 160, and 220 min). After centrifugation, plasma (0.5 ml) was removed and mixed with acetonitrile (0.7 ml) containing PE2I as a reference compound. The mixture was centrifuged at 1000 g for ten minutes and the supernatant (>1 ml) was removed and used for the gradient HPLC separation. After protein precipitation the radioactivity recovered in the supernatant was more than 85%. The gradient HPLC (Waters) consisted of a UV detector operated at 254 nm followed by a Packard radioisotope detector with computer data acquisition. The analysis was performed on a Waters μBondapak C18 300 x 7.8 mm (10 μm) column eluted with a mixture of acetonitrile in phosphoric acid (0.01 M) from 25% acetonitrile to 60%. The flow was 6 ml/min and a 1 ml sample loop was used. The radioactivity of whole blood and plasma was counted in equal volume aliquots (1 ml) in a well NaI detector.

RESULTS AND DISCUSSION

There was a rapid uptake of radioactivity in brain (3% of injected dose at 1 hour) and a high accumulation of radioactivity in the striatum. In the midbrain, the thalamus and in cortical regions no visible uptake of radioactivity was observed. The highest uptake of [^{123}I]PE2I in the striatum was at 60-80 min after injection of tracer (Fig. 1). Striatum-to-cerebellum ratio was 5 at 70 min representing transient equilibrium. The results are in line with recent studies *in vivo* in primates which indicate the specificity of PE2I for the dopamine transporter (8). The previous *in vitro* autoradiographic studies using [^{125}I]PE2I on post-mortem human brain have shown that DAT is mainly present in the striatum and in less amount into the subtantia nigra, but not in other regions such as the thalamus and cortical regions (9). The results of the present study confirm that [^{123}I]PE2I accumulates only into the striatum (Fig. 1), no other brain regions are visible 1 h after injection of tracer as found with other β-CIT analogues. PE2I seems to be a selective compound for the DAT that can be used with both PET (8) and SPET.

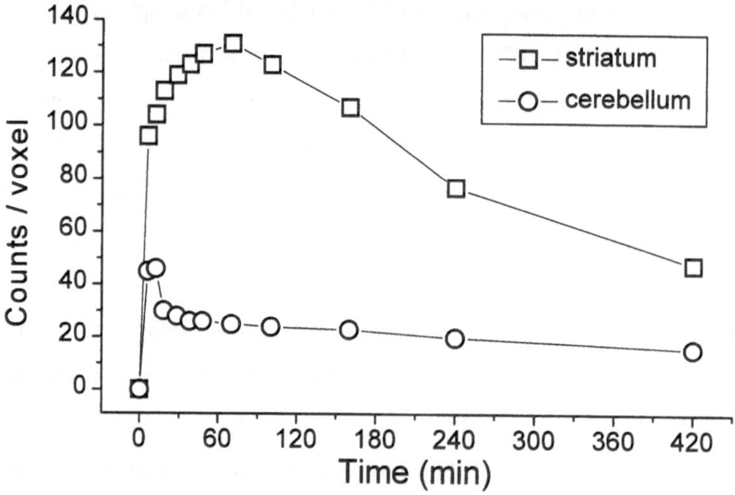

Fig. 1. Regional time-activity curves of a [^{123}I]PE2I study.

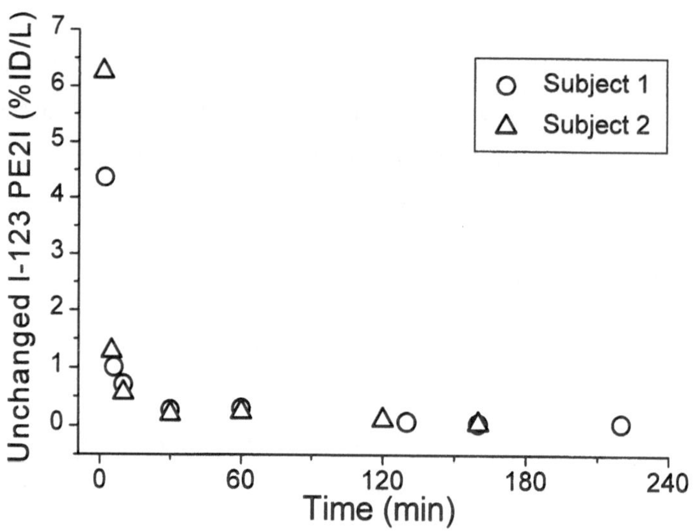

Fig. 2. Unchanged [^{123}I]PE2I in plasma along with time.

Percentage of unchanged [^{123}I]PE2I in plasma was < 20% at 1 h post injection. The whole blood to plasma ratio was about 0.75 indicating most blood radioactivity was in plasma fraction. [^{123}I]PE2I transforms rapidly to one main polar metabolite (Fig. 2). The polar metabolites are unlikely to enter brain tissue at least prior to the suggested scan time of 60-100 min.

Imaging properties of [^{123}I]PE2I favour its use in clinical practice compared to that of [^{123}I]β-CIT. One SPET scan performed between 70-100 min after injection instead of 24 hours with [^{123}I]β-CIT. In conclusion, [^{123}I]PE2I appears to be a specific SPET ligand with very low non-specific binding for imaging DAT density.

REFERENCES

1. Innis RB, Seibyl JP, Wallace E, et al. Single photon emission computed tomographic imaging demonstrates loss of striatal dopamine transporters in Parkinson's disease. Proc Natl Acad Sci 1993; 90:11965-11969.
2. Farde F, Halldin C, Müller L, et al. PET study of [^{11}C]β-CIT binding to monoamine transporters in the monkey and human brain. Synapse 1994; 16:93-103.
3. Kuikka JT, Åkerman K, Bergström KA, et al. Iodine-123 labelled N-(2-fluoroethyl)-2β-carbomethoxy-3β-(4-iodophenyl)nortropane for dopamine transporter imaging in the living brain. Eur J Nucl Med 1995; 22:682-686.
4. Halldin C, Farde L, Lundkvist C, et al. [^{11}C]β-CIT-FE, a radioligand for quantitation of the dopamine transporter in the living brain using positron emission tomography. Synapse 1996; 22:386-390.
5. Emond P, Garreau L, Chalon S, et al. Synthesis and ligand binding of nortropane derivatives: N-substituted-2β-carbomethoxy-3β-(4-iodophenyl)nortropane and N-(3-iodoprop-2E-enyl)-2β-carbomethoxy-3β-(3',4'-disubstituted-phenyl)nortropane. New high affinity and selective compounds for the dopamine transporter. J Med Chem 1997; 40:1366-1372.
6. Guilloteau D, Emond P, Baulieu J-L, et al. Exploration of the dopamine transporter: In vitro and in vivo characterization of a high affinity and high specificity iodinated tropane derivative (E)-N-(3-iodoprop-2-enyl)-2β-carbomethoxy-3β-(4'-methylphenyl)nortropane or PE2I. Nucl Med Biol (in press).
7. Bergström KA, Halldin C, Lundkvist C, et al. Characterization of C-11 or I-123 labelled β-CIT-FP and β-CIT-FE metabolism measured in monkey and human plasma. Identification of two labelled metabolites with HPLC. Hum Psychopharmacol 1996; 11:483-490.
8. Halldin C, Lundkvist C, Guilloteau D, et al. The first selective dopamine transporter radioligand suitable for quantitation with both PET and SPET. Eur J Nucl Med 1997; 24:1057.
9. Hall H, Halldin C, Guilloteau D, et al. Dopamine transporters in the post-mortem human brain. Autoradiographic localisation using [^{125}I]PE2I. Eur J Nucl Med 1997; 24:880.

Radioactive Isotopes in
Clinical Medicine and Research XXIII
ed. by H. Bergmann, H. Köhn and H. Sinzinger

COMPARISON OF IODINE-123 LABELLED NOR-β-CIT AND β-CIT AS POTENTIAL RADIOLIGANDS FOR SEROTONIN TRANSPORTER IMAGING

Jyrki T. Kuikka, Kim A. Bergström, Kari Åkerman and Jari Tiihonen

Departments of Clinical Physiology and Forensic Psychiatry, University of Kuopio, Kuopio, Finland

SUMMARY: Iodine-123 labelled nor-β-CIT has a high in vitro affinity for the serotonin transporter. In the present study initial SPET studies with [^{123}I]nor-β-CIT were performed in 5 healthy subjects and the results were compared with those of [^{123}I]β-CIT. The dynamic SPET studies demonstrated a high and rapid uptake of tracer in the brain (6 %/ID at 30 min). Highest uptake was observed in the striatum, the thalamus and in the mid-brain. The specific binding of [^{123}I]nor-β-CIT in the mid-brain was 20 % higher than that of [^{123}I]β-CIT. The high radioactivity in the mid-brain is assumed to represent the accumulation of [^{123}I]nor-β-CIT in the serotonin transporter.

INTRODUCTION

Serotonin (5-HT) and dopamine (DA) transporters have been intensively studied in recent years. The successful development of new cocaine analogs and availability of dedicated imaging devices both for single photon emission tomography (SPET) and positron emission tomography (PET) have made possible to study DAT density in the living human brain (1-3). One potentially important tracer is iodine-123 labelled 2β-carbomethoxy-3β-(4-iodophenyl) tropane, ([^{123}I]β-CIT), which can be used for dopamine and serotonin transporter imaging in the living human brain (4,5). However, its affinity and accumulation to the serotonin rich-regions is relatively low.

We introduce here 2β-carbomethoxy-3β-(4-iodophenyl)nortropane ([^{123}I]nor-β-CIT) (6) for SPET imaging of the serotonin transporter. In addition, we compare the findings of [^{123}I]nor-β-CIT with those of [^{123}I]β-CIT.

MATERIAL AND METHODS

Four healthy males and one female were studied with [^{123}I]nor-β-CIT SPET. Their mean age was 30 years (range: 25-35 years). Before the tracer injection 400 mg potassium perchlorate was given per os in order to reduce thyroid uptake of ^{123}I. Informed consent was obtained from the subjects and the nature of the studies was fully explained. The Ethical Committee of Kuopio University Hospital has approved the research project.

The radiolabelling of [^{123}I]nor-β-CIT was performed by MAP Medical Technologies, Inc. (Tikkakoski, Finland) with the iododestannylation method as described earlier [7]. After purification with semi-preparative HPLC and formulation to an injectable solution, the final product was sterilized by filtration through 0.2 μm filter. The radiochemical purity of [^{123}I] nor-β-CIT was determined before injection with similar HPLC conditions as the product purification was performed.

A dose of 187-220 MBq of [^{123}I]nor-β-CIT was diluted in a volume of 10 ml physiological saline. The dose was slowly injected into the right antecubital vein in a dark and quiet imaging room. Dynamic SPET brain imaging was performed on the dedicated Siemens MultiSPECT 3 gamma camera with fan beam collimators. The energy window was centered around the photopeak of ^{123}I (148 - 170 keV). Full 360° rotations (120°/camera head) were used. The imaging resolution was 7 - 8 mm.

Four other study subjects were previously studied with dynamic [^{123}I]β-CIT SPET using the same camera and computer settings. Camera quality control values did not reveal significant differences between these studies.

Transaxial oriented in the orbito-meatal line, sagittal and coronal slices, 3 mm thick, were reconstructed after Butterworth filtering (cut-off frequency 0.4 cm^{-1} and order of 5) and Chang's uniform attenuation correction (μ = 0.10 cm^{-1}). Two consecutive transaxial slices were summarized and regions of interest (ROIs) were drawn onto the cerebellum, the temporal lobes, the mid-brain, the anterior gingulate gyrus, the thalamus, the basal ganglia and onto the white matter. The cerebellum served as a non-specific + free binding region. The mean counts/voxel of each region were used for analysis. Time activity curves of the mid-brain, the basal ganglia, and the cerebellum of [^{123}I]nor-β-CIT are illustrated in Fig. 1.

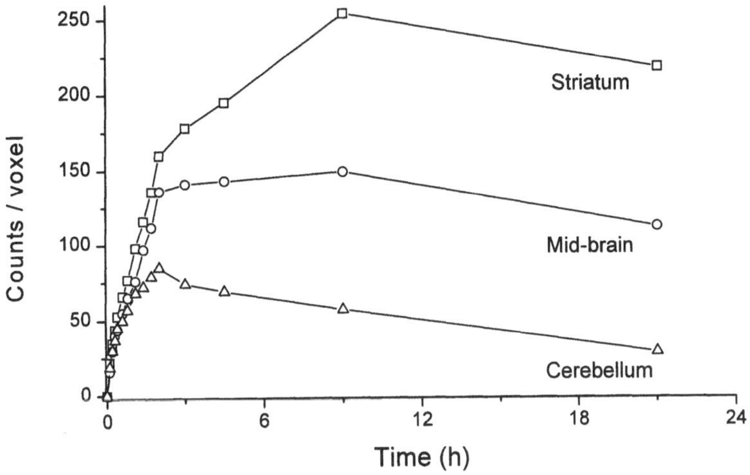

Figure 1. Time activity curves after injection of 185 MBq of [^{123}I]nor-β-CIT in a healthy male.

The modified formula presented by Costa and co-workers (8) was used to determine the specific 5-HT and DAT binding of [^{123}I]nor-β-CIT in the given region i, i.e. total binding (= specific + non-specific + free) minus cerebellum (= non-specific + free) related to total:

$$\text{specific binding of } ROI_i = (ROI_i - CER)/ROI_i = 1 - CER/ROI_i \,, \qquad (1)$$

The specific binding was calculated at the time of peak tracer uptake of each region i. The time of the peak uptake varied between the regions of interest as well as between the two tracers. It might be also dependent on the age of the study subjects/patients and on the severity of the disease.

RESULTS

The highest accumulation of [^{123}I]nor-β-CIT was observed in the striatum, the mid-brain and in the thalamus. The peak brain uptake was 6 % of the dose injected. Lung activity was higher than that of [^{123}I]β-CIT probably reflecting accumulation of the tracer into the serotonin-rich lung capillaries. The specific binding of [^{123}I]nor-β-CIT was 0.88 ± 0.04 in the basal ganglia (DAT) and 0.52 ± 0.03 in the mid-brain (5-HT). Corresponding figures for [^{123}I]β-CIT were 0.92 ± 0.03 and 0.43 ± 0.03, respectively. In the male subject pretreated with 30 mg of citalopram, the specific binding in the mid-brain (0.32) was 37 % less than that of the untreated subjects. Figure 2 shows transaxial slices scanned 4 hours after injection of 185 MBq of [^{123}I]nor-β-CIT without and with 30 mg citalopram.

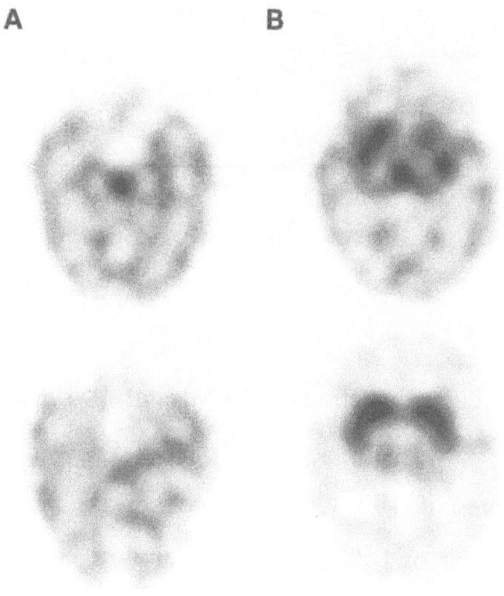

Figure 2. Transaxial slices oriented in orbito-meatal line at the level of the mid-brain (**A**) and at the level of the striatum (**B**) in healthy subjects without (upper row) and with pretreatment of 30 mg citalopram (lower row). Note a reduced tracer uptake in the mid-brain and in the thalamus of the pretreated subject whereas his striatal uptake is increased. The scans were performed 4 hours after injection.

The radiation exposure to the study subjects was 0.035 mSv/MBq (effective dose equivalent).

DISCUSSION

The present study illustrates for the first time the use of [^{123}I]nor-β-CIT for imaging monoamine transporter re-uptake sites in the living human brain. The initial results showed that the 5-HT specific binding of this tracer in the mid-brain was 20 % higher than that of [^{123}I]β-CIT [7]. Preliminary studies suggested that [^{123}I]nor-β-CIT is a promising agent for selective serotonin transporter imaging in the living human brain. The dynamic SPET studies demonstrated a high and rapid uptake of radioactivity in the brain. Highest accumulation was observed in the striatum, the mid-brain, and in the thalamus. The high radioactivity in the mid-brain is assumed to represent the accumulation of [^{123}I]nor-β-CIT in the serotonin transporter rich regions which indicates that [^{123}I]nor-β-CIT might be a potential tracer for visualization of serotonin transporter sites in the human brain with SPET. However, the high and long-lasting lung uptake (serotonin specific uptake) introduces more or less cumbersome tracer input to the brain and thus makes semi-quantification and visual interpretation difficult in clinical practice. The elimination of this effect needs blood sampling and serial SPET scans.

CONCLUSION

In conclusion, we initially suggest that [^{123}I]nor-β-CIT is a useful radioligand for imaging of re-uptake sites of monoamine transporters in the living human brain. Imaging quality (contrast) is higher in the mid-brain but poorer in the striatum than that of [^{123}I]β-CIT.

REFERENCES

1. Innis RB, Baldwin RM, Sybirska E, et al. Single photon emission computed tomography imaging of monoamine reuptake sites in primate brain with [^{123}I]β-CIT. *Eur J Pharmacol* 1991; 200: 369-370.
2. Neumeyer JL, Wang S, Milius RA, et al. [^{123}I]-2β-carbomethoxy-3β-(4-iodophenyl)tropane: High-affinity SPECT radiotracer of monoamine reuptake sites in brain. *J Med Chem* 1991; 34: 3144-3146.
3. Kuikka JT, Bergström KA, Vanninen E, et al. Initial experience with SPET examinations using [^{123}I]-2β-carbomethoxy-3β(4-iodophenyl) tropane in human brain. *Eur J Nucl Med* 1993; 20: 783-786.
4. Brücke T, Kornhuber J, Angelberger P, et al. SPECT imaging of dopamine and serotonin transporters with [^{123}I]β-CIT. Binding kinetics in the human brain. *J Neural Transm [Gen Sect]* 1993; 94: 137-146.
5. Farde L, Halldin C, Müller L, et al. PET study of [^{11}C]β-CIT binding to monoamine transporters in the monkey and human brain. *Synapse* 1994; 16: 93-103.
6. Bergström KA, halldin C, Hall H, et al. In vitro and in vivo characterisation of nor-β-CIT: a potential radioligand for visualisation of the serotonin transporter in the brain. *Eur J Nucl Med* 1997; 24: 596-601.
7. Kuikka JT, Bergström KA, Ahonen A et al. Comparison of iodine labelled 2β-carbomethoxy-3 β-(4-iodophenyl)tropane (β-CIT) and 2β-carbomethoxy-3β-(4-iodophenyl-N-(3-fluoropropyl)-nortropane (β-CIT-FP) for the dopamine transporter imaging in the living human brain. *Eur J Nucl Med* 1995; 22: 356-360.
8. Costa DC, Verhoeff NPLG, Cullum ID, et al. In vivo characterisation of 3-iodo-6-methoxybenzamide [^{123}I]IBZM in humans. *Eur J Nucl Med* 1990; 16: 813-816.

Radioactive Isotopes in
Clinical Medicine and Research XXIII
ed. by H. Bergmann, H. Köhn and H. Sinzinger

BRAIN SEROTONIN AND DOPAMINE TRANSPORTERS IN DEPRESSIVE CHILDREN

Ahonen A[1], Dahlström M[2], Moilanen I[2], Torniainen P[1], Heikkilä J[1].
[1]Division of Nuclear Medicine, Oulu University Hospital, 90220 Oulu, Finland
[2]Department of Paediatrics, Oulu University Hospital, 90220 Oulu, Finland

Summary

Until now 22 children with neuropsychiatric disorders have been imaged for brain dopamine and serotonin transporters using [^{123}I] β–CIT. Imaging was carried out using dual head gamma camera equipped with fan beam collimators. The thalamic serotonin transporter density index 4 hours after injection was significantly lower ($p<0.001$) in depressive children with multifactorial courses (14 pts) compared to a group of non–depressive children (8 pts). Surprisingly no difference could be found in the middle brain, region known to have plenty of serotonin transporters. Based on Cipramil displacement and human autoradiographic studies, we are convinced that our abnormal findings in the thalamic area really reflect serotonin transporters.

Introduction

Brain monoamines, especially the lack of serotonin, has been an object of extensive interest in biological psychiatry during the last decades. Both human and animal research connect reduced brain serotonin activity to an aggressive model of behaviour. In addition to this novel selective serotonin re–uptake inhibitors (SSRI) have shown their efficiency in treatment of depressive patients thus implicating the lack of serotonin not only in aggressive behaviour but also in depressive episodes. The mechanism of SSRI drug action leads the interest from post synaptic serotonin receptors to the presynaptic regulation of the monoamine transmission, transporter molecules on the presynaptic cell surface.

New biochemical imaging techniques provide local measurements of monoamines in brain. In the past years, only the PET techniques were available for this purpose, but now along the developing resolution power of gamma–cameras, the presynaptic monoamine transporters can be imaged using a single photon emission tomography (SPET)[1]. For visualisation of monoamine transporters a radio labelled cocaine derivate, 2–β–carbomethoxy–3–β(4–tromethlystannylphenyl)tropane, 123–I–β–CIT is available. This compound binds dopamine and serotonin transporters in brain.[2] This method is suitable for visualisation of abnormal changes in dopamine and serotonin transporters in adult patients suffering from Parkinson's disease, Tourette's syndrome, alcoholism and social phobia.

There is reason to assume that the depression in children and adolescents would be connected to the function of brain dopamine and serotonin transporters, as it occurs in adults. Prospective studies have shown that children with conduct disorders and hyperactivity–attention deficit disorder often develop antisocial personality disorder by adulthood align with impulsive aggression and drug– or alcohol dependency. Whether this is due to the genetically transmitted traits, such as dopamine–D2–receptor genes, remains an object of controversies.

The purpose of the study was to find out whether there are differences in the function of brain dopamine and serotonin transporters in children and adolescents suffering from major depressive disease, hyperactivity–attention deficit disorder, conduct disorder, obsessive–compulsive disorder, pervasive developmental disorder, childhood psychosis and many mixture of these along with the learning disabilities. In addition the dopamine–D2–receptor genes and possible changes in quantitative EEGs are being measured.

Patients and methods

The study is a collaboration between The Child Psychiatric Clinic and Division of Nuclear Medicine in the Oulu University Hospital. The permission to start the study was obtained from the ethic committee of the Oulu University on the 28th February, 1996. Until now 22 children of ages 7–17 are studied, 17 boys and 5 girls. There were 7 depressive children with conduct disorders and 7 pure depression, whereas non–depressive group (8 pts) consisted of children with pervasive developmental disorder, hypomanic, intoxication, conduct disorder and obsessive–compulsive disorder. The study is offered to the children and adolescents under the permission from their parents. Children who were drug abusers or who were on medication affecting on central nervous system were excluded. No normal children were included into study due to the small radiation load induced by receptor SPET imaging.

A thorough paediatric medical examination was performed for all the children and adolescents in the study. For the hospitalised patients the diagnoses were determined on common clinical ways. In addition to this a standard diagnostic interview C–SSAGA according to DSM IV criteria was performed to all probands and Clonongers tridimensional Personality Questionnaire for those above age of 15 years. The probands, their parents and teachers fill in Achenbach's questionnaires Youth Self Report Children's Behaviours Checklist and Teachers Report Forms. The probands also filled in Kovacs questionnaire, the Children's Depression Inventory in order to focus on one's depression. Just before the imaging process, the urine samples were taken to exclude drug abusing subjects from probands.
Because there were no normal controls available for the SPET imaging in this study we compared probands with different symptoms with each others – internalising or externalising, low or high impulse control, Multidimensionality of symptoms will be considered as one part of this study.

SPECT scanning
SPECT was performed using a dual head gamma camera (ADAC Vertex) equipped with high resolution fan beam collimators. The scans were made 1, 4 and 24 hours after the injection of [^{123}I]β–CIT [2β–carbomethoxy–3β–(4–iodophenyltropane)], obtained from MAP Medical Technologies Inc (Tikkakoski, Finland) and having a specific radioactivity of >180 GBq/μmol and a radiochemical purity >98%. No–carrier–added [^{123}I] was purchased from PSI, Switzerland, and from Medgemix, Belgium. The ligand was synthesised as described previously in detail.[2]

After blockade of thyroid uptake with 400 mg potassium perchlorate taken orally 30 min before tracer application, the subjects received a slowly injected intravenous dose of 120–185 MBq [^{123}I]β–CIT diluted in 10 ml of physiological saline.

The head was positioned in a head holder using a crossed laser beam system for repositioning. Raw data were obtained from photopeak counts within a 20% symmetric energy window centred around 159 KeV. 4.6 mm cross–sections parallel to the cantomeatal plane were reconstructed by filtered backprojection in a 128x128 matrix using a Butterworth filter (power factor 5, cutoff 0.22 Nq). Attenuation correction was then performed using Chang zero–order correction based on an ellipse fitted to the brain using an empirically determined linear attenuation factor (=0.09 cm^{-1}).

The physicist who performed the regions–of–interest analyses was blind to the demographic data on the subjects. Transaxial slices oriented along the orbitomeatal line were reconstructed and the two slices corresponding to the highest striatal uptake were summed digitally, yielding a final slice of 9.3 mm (pixel size 4.64 mm, voxel volume 99.9 mm^3). The regions of interest were drawn over the right and left striatum (STR) using a colour scale with about 60% isocontour cutoff boundaries for delineation. The size of the average striatal area of interest was about 20 pixels ≈ 431 mm^2, corresponding to a volume of 4.0 cm^3. Frontal white matter (FWM) regions of interest were drawn on the slice about 60 mm superior to the orbitomeatal line. FWM values were used for reference (non–displaceable activity) because post–mortem studies have shown a very low density of DA transporters in this region. Occipital white matter (OWM) values were also determined, and were not significantly different from the FMW values, but they were rejected because of greater variability and possible artefacts. The cerebellar region was not taken as a reference for non–displaceable activity, because this region is situated close to the bed surface and could cause an artefact in the raw SPET data. For estimation of serotonin transporter density following regions of interest were drawn: medial prefrontal cortex (MFC), thalamic area (Th), middle–brain (MB).

Striatal DA transporter binding was calculated as the ratio of the total binding in STR minus the non–displaceable binding in FWM to the non–displaceable binding in FWM, i.e. (STR–FWM)/FWM. As it has been shown that a state of equilibrium exists in the striatal and occipital areas 24 hours after the injection, the ratio at this time point can be used as an estimate of the Binding Potential.[3] We call this estimate the Binding Potential Index (BPI) and consider it to reflect the equilibrium partition coefficient described by Salmon et al.[4] Following serotonin transporter indexes were calculated: MFC/FWM, Th/FWM and MB/FWM.

Results

The thalamic serotonin transporter density index 4 hours after injection was significantly lower ($p<0.001$) in depressive children with multifactorial courses (14 pts) compared to a group of non–depressive children (8 pts). Surprisingly no difference could be found in the middle brain, region known to have plenty of serotonin transporters. Results of various serotonin transporter indexes are shown in details in table 1. There was no statistically significant difference in striatal dopamine transporter level between depressive and non–depressive groups. The thalamic serotonin transporter density index was lower in children showing aggressive behaviour compared to those without any aggressive features. However, no statistical difference was reached. Highest serotonin transporter indexes were found in two children with pervasive development disorder and in one hypomanic child.

Table 1. Serotonin transporter indexes in depressive (14 pts) and non–depressive (8pts) children (I–123 β–CIT)

		Depressive	Non–depressive
Th/FWM	x	1.64	1.61
1 h	SD	0.10	0.20
	P	0.64	
Th/FWM	x	1.97	2.22
4 h	SD	0.11	0.12
	P	<0.001	
MFC/FWM	x	1.09	1.13
1 h	SD	0.07	0.10
	P	0.289	
MFC/FWM	x	1.09	1.19
4 h	SD	0.14	0.12
	P	0.109	
MB/FWM	x	1.26	1.24
1 h	SD	0.09	0.15
	P	0.703	
MB/FWM	x	1.45	1.36
4 h	SD	0.20	0.24
	P	0.334	

Th= thalamus, FWM= frontal white matter, MB= middle brain, MFC= medial prefrontal cortex

Discussion

Earlier studies in Finland have shown diminished liquor serotonin metabolites in impulsive violent, depressive and suicidal adult patients. The SPET findings in Kuopio have shown not only high striatal dopamine in violent alcoholics but also low serotonin transporter levels in the very same individuals, although this takes place in prefrontal cortex.

Depressive episodes of children and adolescents often consist of lowered mood and irritability and co-occur in conjunction with conduct problems. Along with the conduct problems the adolescent himself may loose his sensitivity to describe his vulnerable feelings. He may also be reluctant to report about his problems. That is why it is important to use several information sources: the child and adolescent himself, the parents and the fosterparents, teachers and not least, the professional clinical assessment. In our study the low serotonin transporter levels were detected in thalamus, where the ascending somatosensoric pathways cross to continue their way up to the frontal cortex. The thalamus also serves an alike function for the pathways from hippocampus and amygdala, the developmentally earliest emotional parts of brain, on their way to cortical associative areas on frontal cortex.

For ethical reasons we don't have normal controls in this study. It is not easy to find a patient or an institutionalised adolescent without depressive symptoms. Still those having other than depressive disorders make a reliable comparison group.

In general, it is of great importance that human behaviour and feelings are shown to be connected with brain receptors and transmitters. Our SPET method provides direct measuring of brain dopamine and serotonin transporter proteins with a low and temporary radiation load. It would be essential also in neuropsychiatric disorders to learn the biological background of each symptomology, especially when any medication would be administered or any medication would be preferred to an other. On this base it might be possible to develop medications that would, starting at childhood, make an essential factor in preventing psychiatric diseases such as schizophrenia, MDD, violence or alcoholism.

Brain serotonin transporter density index in thalamus was significantly lower in depressive than in non-depressive children and adolescents.

Our results are very preliminary. More patients must be imaged before any definitive conclusions can be drawn. Our early results support the idea that serotonergic malfunction in at least one factor behind the depression in children. Serotonin transporter index is very arbitrary unit. Pseudoequilibrium time is not exactly documented. Therefore the binding potential index for serotonin is not so reliable as in the case of dopamine transporter measurements. However, based on Cipramil displacement and human autoradiographic studies we are convinced that our abnormal findings in the thalamic area really reflect serotonin transporters.

References:

1. Ahonen A, Dahlström M, Moilanen I, Torniainen P, Heikkilä J. Brain serotonin transporters in depressive children. Eur J Nucl Med 1997;24:945.

2. Hiltunen J, Åkerman KK, Kuikka JT et al. Iodine–123 labeled nor–ß–CIT as a potential tracer for serotonin transporter imaging in the human brain with single–photon emission tomography. Eur J Nucl Med 1998;25:19–23.

3. Laruelle M, Wallace E, Seibyl JP, Baldwin RM, Zea–Ponce Y, Zoghbi SS, Neymeyer JL, Charney DS, Hoffer PB, Innis RB. Graphical, kinetic, and equilibrium analyses of in vivo [^{123}I]ß–CIT binding to dopamine transporters in healthy human subjects. J Cereb Blood Flow Metab 1994;14:982–994.

4. Salmon E, Brooks DJ, Leenders KL et al. A two compartment description and kinetic procedure for measuring regional cerebral [^{11}C]nomifensine uptake using positron emission tomography. J Cereb Blood Flow Metab 1990;10: 307–316.

5. Tiihonen J et al. Altered striatal dopamine re–uptake site densities in habitually violent and non–violent alcoholics. et al. Nature Med 1(7):654–4,1995

Radioactive Isotopes in
Clinical Medicine and Research XXIII
ed. by H. Bergmann, H. Köhn and H. Sinzinger

PROGNOSTIC POTENTIAL OF Tc-99m-ECD-SPET WITHIN 6 HOURS AFTER ONSET OF STROKE SYMPTOMS

H. Barthel, J. Berrouschot*, S. Hesse, C. Dannenberg, D. Schneider*,
W.H. Knapp, W. Burchert

Departments of Nuclear Medicine and *Neurology, University of Leipzig, Germany

SUMMARY: The aim of this present study was to evaluate the prognostic impact of early SPET after stroke. 108 patients underwent SPET (400 - 600 MBq Tc-99m-ECD, brain dedicated camera) within 6h after onset of stroke symptoms. In follow-up period CT revealed no hypodensities (n = 20), subtotal medial cerebri artery territory (MCA) hypodensities (n = 78) or total MCA territory hypodensities (n = 10). Sensitivity and specificity of visual SPET analysis equaled 96.1% and 90.0%. Semiquantitative SPET analysis revealed significant group differences regarding size and depth of early activity deficits. Using cut-off values for these parameters, clinical outcome after 5d was correctly predicted in 89/108 patients.

INTRODUCTION

Since some years new aggressive therapies for acute cerebral infarction, for instance thrombolysis, have been tested [1]. Adequate treatment of cerebral infarction should be started within 6 hours after onset of symptoms. Therefore, within this time window diagnosis as well as prediction of clinical outcome is required [2]. However, early morphological imaging like CT or conventional MRI often fails to identify ischemia [3,4]. This even appears in case of total infarction of medial cerebri artery (MCA) territory, which is associated with lethality of about 80%, even under maximal conservative intensive care [5].

In a previous study we demonstrated, that high-resolution Tc-99m-ECD-SPET within 6 hours after stroke onset is able to differentiate between reversible and irreversible cerebral ischemia [6]. The aim of this present study was to evaluate the diagnostic potential of early SPET for differentiation between subtotal and total ("malignant") MCA infarctions and for prediction of clinical outcome.

MATERIALS AND METHODS

Subjects and protocol: 108 patients (44 f, 64 m; age: 27 - 88 years, m.v. 65 ± 13 y) were enrolled in the study. All patients had acute ischemia in the MCA territory, no stroke history, Scandinavian stroke scale (SSS) < 40 points and CT and SPET within 6 hours after onset of stroke symptoms. SSS scoring, CT and SPET directly followed each other. Neurological scoring and CT were repeated after 5 days. Patients were classified according to the results of follow-up CT after 5d:

group 1 (n = 20): no hypodensities,

group 2 (n = 78): hypodensities in subtotal MCA territory and

group 3 (n = 10): hypodensities in total MCA territory.

SPET: Imaging was carried out 30 minutes after injection of 400-600 MBq Tc-99m-ECD using the brain dedicated Ceraspect camera (DSI). Photons were registered over 30min in 120 projections (360°) and using a 128 x 128 x 64 matrix. Data were reconstructed by standard filtered back projection using a butterworth filter (cut-off 0.95, order 10). For attenuation correction Chang's first order method (μ = 0.15/cm) was used. The transverse slices were reorientated to the AC-PC- line corresponding to the stereotactical system of Talairach and Tournoux.

The SPET data were analysed visually and semiquantitatively. For visual analysis the images were interpreted by 3 independent experts regarding the occurrence of local activity deficits. Quantitative analysis was performed using 89 regular regions of interests (ROIs) in 5 transverse and 3 coronal slices. The count density of the ROIs of symptomatic hemisphere was related to that of corresponding contralateral ROIs. An asymmetry over 10% was defined as abnormal. Additional, ROI indices were calculated as recommended by Hanson et al., considering both size and depth of activity deficits [7].

Statistical analysis: Group differences in semiquantitative SPET parameters were tested for significance using Student's t test for independent samples, after verification of normal distribution. Results of visual SPET analysis were evaluated using chi-quadrate-testing. Receiver operating characteristic (ROC) curves for semiquantitative SPET parameters were calculated and fitted using the programs CLABROC (maximum likelihood operation) and ROCFIT. Differences between the indices of the area under ROC curves were tested for significance using a univariate z-score area test operation.

RESULTS

1. Visual SPET analysis: There were significant differences between the 3 patient groups regarding visual SPET analysis ($p < 0.001$, Table 1). Combination of the data of all patients with hypodensity at follow-up CT (groups 2 and 3) resulted in sensitivity of 96.1 %, specificity of 90.0 % and accuracy of 95.4 % for detection of cerebral infarction.

Table 1. Visual analysis of SPET data by 3 independent experts in patients of group 1 (no hypodensity in CT after 5d), group 2 (subtotal MCA territory hypodensity) and group 3 (total MCA territory hypodensity).

Activity deficit	no	yes
group 1 (n = 20)	18	2
group 2 (n = 78)	3	75
group 3 (n = 10)	0	10

2. Semiquantitative SPET analysis: Concerning number of abnormal ROIs as well as maximal ROI activity asymmetry and ROI index the values of patients of group 2 and 3 significantly exceeded those of patients of group 1. Smallest group differences were found analysing the number of abnormal ROIs, however, largest group differences were detected analysing the ROI indices (Figure 1).

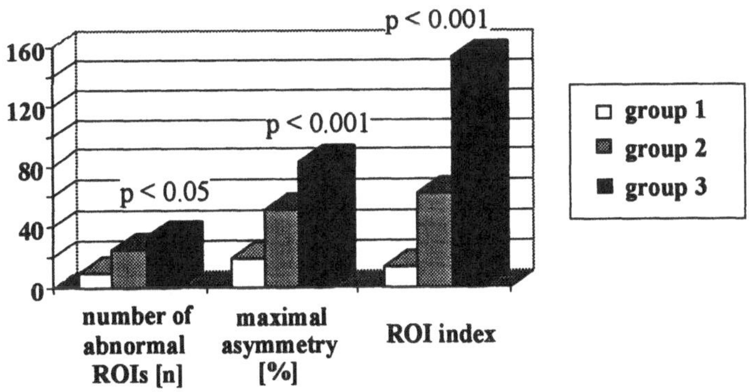

Figure 1. Results of semiquantitative SPET analysis.

3. ROC analysis: In order to predict clinical outcome cut-off values were defined for each ROI parameter by means of ROC curves. Whereas for separation between group 1 and 2 no significant differences were found between the areas under the ROC curves of the 3 ROI parameters, for separation between group 2 and 3 significantly ($p < 0.05$) larger areas under the ROC curves were detected for maximal ROI activity asymmetry (area index under ROC curve = 0.92) and ROI index (0.91) in comparison to that for number of abnormal ROIs (0.82). The marks on the ROC curves with the best relation between sensitivity and specificity were used for calculation of cut-off values. Resulting cut-off values of ROI index equaled 23 for separation between group 1 and 2 and 120 for separation between group 2 and 3, respectively (Figure 2).

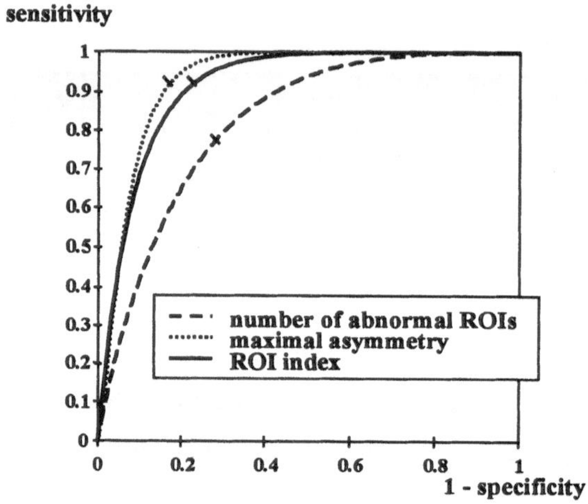

Figure 2. ROC analysis of semiquantitative SPET parameters for separation between patients of group 2 and 3.

According to the above cut-off values of ROI index the patients were separated into 3 outcome groups: Group A = ROI index < 23 (n = 29), group B = ROI index 23 - 120 (n = 63), group C = ROI index > 120 (n = 16). In outcome group A 21 patients completely and 8 patients incompletely recovered (moderate symptoms, SSS > 16 pt.) after 5 days. In contrary, in outcome group B only 8 patients completely recovered after 5d, however, 50 patients had moderate and 4 patients severe symptoms (SSS < 16 pt.) at follow-up evaluation and 1 patient died within this period. In case of outcome group C, 5 patient had severe symptoms after 5 days and 9 patients died within the follow-up period. Altogether, outcome was successfully predicted using the ROI index and the quoted cut-off values in 85 of the 108 patients (78.7%).

DISCUSSION AND CONCLUSION

This present study was carried out to define the potential of early SPET for differentiation between subtotal and total ("malignant") MCA infarctions and for prediction of clinical outcome. Using high resolution Tc-99m-ECD-SPET within 6 hours after onset of stroke symptoms we were able to differentiate between evolving cerebral infarction and reversible ischemia with sensitivity of 96.1% and specificity of 90.0%, respectively. Analysing the SPET data semiquantitatively, high significant differences were found between subtotal and total MCA infarctions regarding both size and depth of early perfusion deficits.

Different studies were carried out performing SPET for early diagnosis after stroke [8,9,10]. However, until now no data are available using the newer cerebral perfusion marker Tc-99m-ECD. On the other side, the patient group of this study represents the largest number of stroke patients which ever has been investigated using SPET within the therapeutical time-window of 6 hours. Although comparison with the quoted studies is limited, our results of very high accuracy of early SPET for diagnosis of evolving cerebral infarction are in accordance with those of Baird et al. and Brass et al., who found sensitivity of 79 % and specificity of 95% (86 and 98%, respectively) for diagnosis of cerebral infarction [9,10].

Since Weir et al. concluded from their Tc-99m-HMPAO study within 40 hours after stroke onset, that accuracy of prediction of clinical outcome decreases the longer SPET is delayed [11], ultra early imaging - like performed in our study - might deliver reliable prognostication. Really, in this study clinical outcome after stroke was successfully predicted in 79% of the patients by early SPET and semiquantitative analysis. Best prognostication was achieved combining data on size and depth of early perfusion deficit. Giubilei et al. firstly investigated prognostic value of SPET within 6 hours after onset of stroke symptoms using Tc-99m-HMPAO in 32 patients. They analysed depth of perfusion deficits and thus were able to predict outcome after 1 month successfully in 22 of the 32 patients (69%) [12]. Our higher value of correct outcome prediction could be attributed to better image quality of Tc-99m-ECD compared to that of Tc-99m-HMPAO, which was applied by Giubilei, or to the high spatial resolution of our brain dedicated camera (6-7mm).

From the results of our study is concluded, that brain perfusion SPET within 6 hours after onset of stroke symptoms is able to differentiate not only between reversible and irreversible cerebral ischemia, but also between evolving subtotal and total MCA infarction. Quantification in Tc-99m-ECD-SPET can improve prediction of prognosis after ischemia. The data demonstrate, that clinical outcome after cerebral infarction is codetermined by size and depth of early perfusion deficits.

REFERENCES

1. Hacke W, Kaste M, Fiesche C et al. Intravenous thrombolysis with recombinant tissue plasminogen activator for acute hemispheric stroke: the European Cooperative Acute Stroke Study (ECASS). JAMA 1995; 274: 1017-25.
2. Brass LM. Brain SPECT in clinical neurology: Stroke. In: Assessment of brain SPECT. Report of the therapeutics and technology assessment subcommittee of the American Academy of Neurology.
   American Academy of Neurology 49th Annual Meeting, Boston; 1997, 333: 39-51.
3. von Kummer R, Nolte PN, Schnittger H et al. Detectability of cerebral hemisphere ischaemic infarcts by CT within 6 h of stroke. Neurology 1996; 38: 31-33.
4. Alberts MJ, Faulstich ME, Gray L. Stroke with negative brain magnetic resonance imaging. Stroke 1992; 23: 663-7.
5. Hacke W, Schwab S, Horn M et al. "Malignant" middle cerebri artery infarction. Arch Neurol 1996; 53: 309-15.
6. Berrouschot J, Barthel H, Hesse S et al. Differentiation between TIA and ischemic stroke within the first six hours after onset of symptoms by using Tc-99m-ECD-SPECT. J Cerebr Blood F Met 1998 (in press).
7. Hanson SK, Grotta JC, Rhoades H et al. Value of Single-Photon Emission-Computed Tomography in acute stroke therapeutic trials. Stroke 1993; 24: 1322-9.
8. Shimosegawa E, Hatazawa J, Inugami A et al. Cerebral infarction within six hours after onset: Prediction of completed infarction with Technetium-99m-HMPAO SPECT. J Nucl Med 1994; 35: 1097-1103
9. Brass LM, Walowich RC, Joseph JL et al. The role of Single Photon Emission Computed Tomography brain imaging with Tc-99m-Bicisate in the localisation and definition of mechanism of ischemic stroke. J Cereb Blood Flow Metab 1994; 14(1): 91-98.
10. Baird AE, Austin MC, McKay WJ et al. Sensitivity and specificity of Tc-99m-HMPAO SPECT cerebral perfusion measurements during the first 48 hours for the localization of cerebral infarction. Stroke 1997; 28: 976-980.
11. Weir CJ, Bolster AA, Tytler S et al. Prognostic value of single-photon emission tomography in acute ischaemic stroke. Eur J Nucl Med 1997; 24: 21-26.
12. Giubilei F, Lenzi GL, Di Piero V et al. Predictive value of brain perfusion Single-Photon Emission Computed Tomography in acute ischemic stroke. Stroke 1990; 21: 895-900.

Radioactive Isotopes in
Clinical Medicine and Research XXIII
ed. by H. Bergmann, H. Köhn and H. Sinzinger

BRAIN PERFUSION IN PATIENTS WITH SEVERE SLEEP APNEA SYNDROME (SAS) BEFORE AND AFTER n-CPAP-THERAPY

Dannenberg C., Bosse-Henck A. *, Weiser A., Barthel H., Schedel U., Sattler B., Dietrich J., Knapp W.H., Burchert W.

Departments of Nuclear Medicine and *Internal Medicine, University of Leipzig, Germany

Summary: The aim of the study was to evaluate the therapeutic potential of nocturnal transnasal continuous positive airway pressure breathing (n-CPAP-therapy) with respect to regional cerebral blood flow. 30 patients with severe sleep apnea syndrome (SAS) underwent daytime Tc-99m-ECD SPET before and after 6 month n-CPAP-therapy and brain CT (n = 25) to evaluate atrophy. SPET data were analysed visually by 3 experts: Perfusion deficits were mainly located in frontal and temporal lobes. Frontal ($p < 0.01$) and temporal ($p < 0.05$) activity significantly increased after therapy. In 10 patients with brain atrophy activity did not change significantly, what probably reflects morphological changes induced by hypoxemia and/or sleep fragmentation.

INTRODUCTION

Incidence of SAS is comparable to that of diabetes mellitus: 2 % of women and 4 % of men in the age of 30 to 60 years suffer from SAS [1]. Excessive daytime sleepiness and disturbances in ability of concentration, short time memory and learning functions are common symtoms of the disease. Since neuronal activity is closely related to brain perfusion, measurement of local cerebral blood flow may help to describe the severity of the disease.

Neuropsychological data suggest, that cognitive dysfunction is only partially reversible after efficient n-CPAP-therapy [2,3]. The aim of the study was to evaluate the therapeutic potential of n-CPAP-therapy with respect to regional cerebral blood flow.

MATERIALS AND METHODS

Subjects. 30 patients (age 52 ± 11 a; 27 male, 3 female) with severe SAS (respiratory distress index: 52.05 ± 23.7, $O_2\downarrow$-time < 90 %: 169 ± 56 min) were enrolled in the study.

Protocol. Polysomnography and daytime brain SPET before and after 6 month of n-CPAP-therapy. Additional brain CT (SOMATOM PLUS/PLUS S; SIEMENS) to evaluate atrophy in 25 patients.

SPET. Resting patients in supine position with eyes opened were injected at 8 a.m. in a quiet dimly lit room via a prefixed butterfly cannula with 600 MBq Tc-99m-ECD and were kept in the same conditions for 5 minutes post injection. Data acquisition was started 30 minutes later using a high resolution brain dedicated system(CERASPECT, DSI). Counts were collected in a 128 x 128 x 64 matrix. Data were reconstructed by a standard filtered back projection using a 2-D Butterworth filter (cut-off 0.95, order 10). Attenuation correction was performed with Chang`s first order method. Reorientation was carried out corresponding to the stereotactic atlas of the human brain by Talairach and Tournoux [4]. Emission tomograms were analysed by visual scoring of 3 independent experts with a scale from 0 to 3 [5]: 0 = normal local activity, 1 = non significant activity deficit, 2 = significant activity deficit (abnormal), 3 = large activity defect.

Statistical analysis. Inter-observer reliability for visual scores was assessed by determining the degree of concordance by using Kendal's W-test. Differences in mean values of visual scores of the three experts before and after therapy were proved for significance performing the two-tailed

Wilcoxon rank test.

RESULTS

Before n-CPAP-therapy 27 % of patients showed definitely pathological activity deficits which were mainly located in frontal and temporal lobes (figure 1).

Inter-rater degree of concordance of visual scores was $W = 0.82$ ($p < 0.0001$).

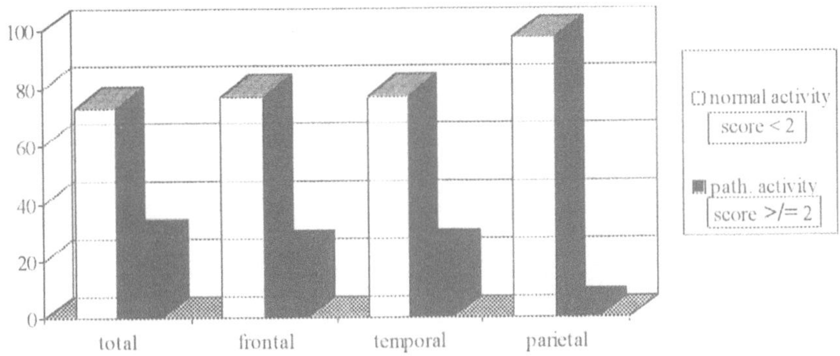

Figure 1. Percentage of patients with normal/definitely abnormal visual scores of cortical activity distribution

Polysomnographic data before and after 6 month n-CPAP-therapy demonstrate the efficient nocturnal breathing (figure 2).

After therapy frontal ($p = 0.009$) and temporal ($p = 0.026$) activity scores were significantly decreased. CT revealed brain atrophy in 10 patients. Atrophy was predominantly located in the majority bifrontal cortices. In this subgroup of patients changes in mean values of visual scores after therapy were non significant. In the second subgroup of 15 patients with normal brain CT cortical activity significantly increased ($p_{frontal} = 0.0023$; $p_{temporal} = 0.0031$) (figure 3).

There was no significant difference between the mean age of the patients with atrophy compared to that patients without atrophy.

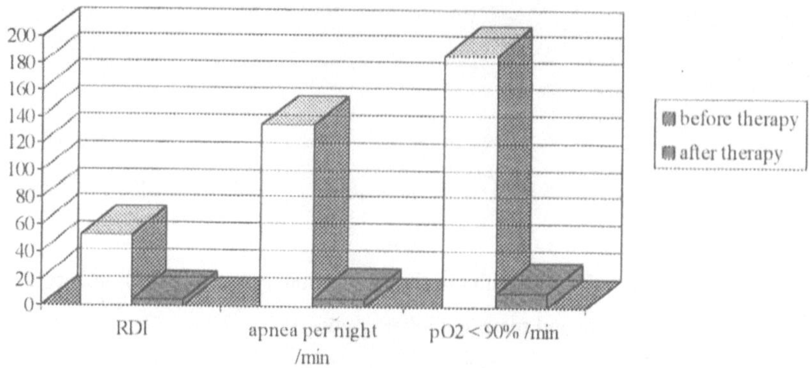

Figure 2. Mean value of respiratory distress index (RDI), duration of apnea per night and time with oxygen saturation below 90 % per night in SAS patients before and after n-CPAP-therapy

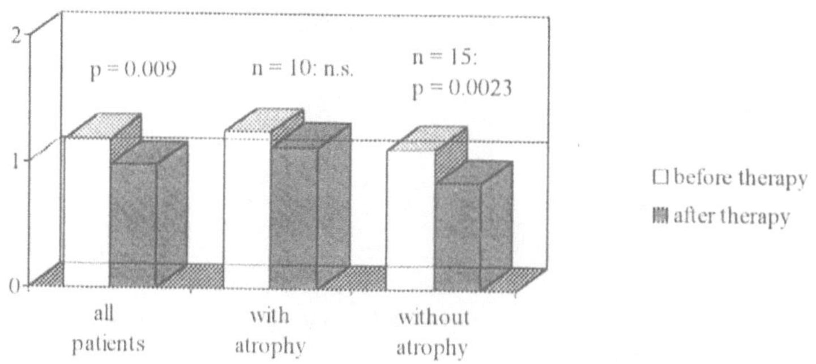

Figure 3. Mean value of visual scores of frontal activity uptake in SAS patients before and after 6 month efficient n-CPAP-therapy

DISCUSSION AND CONCLUSION

Daytime cortical perfusion deficits in our patients were predominantly localised in frontal and temporal lobes. Our results are in accordance with these of Feistel et al. [6], who found nocturnal perfusion abnormalities in frontal lobes in some SAS patients, which normalised after n-CPAP-therapy. In another study frontal daytime hypoperfusion was measured using Xenon-CT in a small SAS patient group [7].

Cognitive dysfunction in SAS related to hypoxemia is not reversible after efficient n-CPAP-n-CPAP-therapy [8]. This may be caused by hypoxic brain damage. 1/3 of our patients had abnormal brain CT-scans, probably induced by hypoxemia and/or sleep fragmentation. In that patients perfusion abnormalities did not change significantly after n-CPAP-therapy. Cognitive dysfunction related to vigilance, however, is partially reversible after therapy [8]. Cerebral perfusion deficits in our patients - especially in patients without atrophy according to brain CT - were partially reversible after n-CPAP-therapy. This may be due to functional neuronal deactivation caused by vigilance disturbances.

REFERENCES

1. Young T, Palta M, Dempsey J, Skatrud J, Weber S, Badr S. The occurence of sleep disordered breathing among middle aged adults. New Engl J Med 1993; 328: 1230-1235.
2. Feuerstein C, Naegle B, Pepin JL, Levy P. Frontal lobe-related cognitive functions in patients with severe sleep apnea syndrome before and after treatment. Acta Neurol Belg 1997; 97: 96-107.
3. Montplaisir J, Bedard MA, Richer F, Rouleau I. Neurobehavioral manifestations in obstructive sleep apnea syndrome before and after treatment with continuous positive airway pressure. Sleep 1992; 15: S17-19.
4. Talairach J, Tournoux P. Co-planar stereotaxic atlas of the human brain. Stuttgard, New York: Thieme, 1988.
5. Knapp WH, Dannenberg C, Marschall B, Zedlick D, Löschmann K, Bettin S, Barthel H, Seese A: Changes in local cerebral blood flow by neuroactivation and vasoactivation in patients with impaired cognitive function. Eur J Nucl Med 1996; 23: 878-888.
6. Feistel H, Merkl M, Siegfried W, Möller C, Dertinger S, Ficker JH, Platsch G, Hahn EG, Wolf F. Brain perfusion during sleep apnea - a study with Tc-99m-HMPAO in sleep laboratory. Eur J Nucl Med 1994; 21: 183.
7. Meyer JS, Yshikawa Y, Hata T, Karacan I. Cerebral blood flow in normal and abnormal sleep and dreaming. Brain and Cognition 1987; 6: 266-294.
8. Valencia-Flores M, Bliwise DL, Guilleminault C, Cilveti R, Clerk A. Cognitive function in patients with sleep apnea after acute nocturnal nasal continuous positive airway pressure (CPAP) treatment: sleepiness and hypoxemia effects. J Clin Exp Neuropsychol 1996; 18: 197-210.

THERAPY

Radioactive Isotopes in
Clinical Medicine and Research XXIII
ed. by H. Bergmann, H. Köhn and H. Sinzinger

RADIOIMMUNOTHERAPY OF COLORECTAL CANCER IN SMALL VOLUME DISEASE: PRECLINICAL EVALUATION IN COMPARISON TO EQUITOXIC CHEMOTHERAPY AND PRELIMINARY RESULTS OF AN ONGOING PHASE-I/II CLINICAL TRIAL

T.M. Behr[1], S. Memtsoudis[1], V. Vougioukas[1], T. Liersch[2], S. Gratz[1], F. Schmidt[3], T. Lorf[3], S. Post[2], B. Wörmann[4], W. Hiddemann[4], B. Ringe[3] and W. Becker[1]

[1]Department of Nuclear Medicine, [2]General and [3]Transplantation Surgery, and [4]Hematology-Oncology of the Georg-August-University of Göttingen, Robert-Koch-Str. 40, D - 37075 Göttingen, Germany.

SUMMARY: The aim of the present study was to compare, in preclinical models, the therapeutic efficacy of radioimmunotherapy in colorectal cancer to equitoxic chemotherapy, as well as to evaluate, in a pilot clinical trial, their efficacy in small volume disease. The data suggest that radioimmunotherapy may be a viable therapeutic option in colorectal cancer patients with limited disease. Myelotoxicity is the only dose-limiting organ toxicity. Although most patients were treated below the maximum tolerated dose, encouraging anti-tumor effects have been observed.

INTRODUCTION

With 15% of all malignancies, colorectal cancer is one of the most frequent cancer types in both sexes [1]. To date, surgery is the only potentially curative therapeutic modality [1]. However, in unresectable cases, the five-year survival is close to zero despite several new chemotherapeutic developments [1]. In this context, radioimmunotherapy appears as an attractive therapeutic concept, aiming to deliver tumoricidal radiation doses to the tumors [2]. We have shown earlier, that the tumor uptake, thus, the radiation dose to the tumor increases exponentially with decreasing tumor size [2]. The aim of the present study was, therefore, to compare the therapeutic efficacy of radiolabeled monoclonal antibodies to equitoxic "standard" chemotherapy with 5-fluorouracil / folinic acid in a human colon cancer xenograft model in nude mice, and to evaluate, in a pilot clinical trial in colorectal cancer patients, the efficacy of radioimmunotherapy in small volume disease.

MATERIALS, PATIENTS AND METHODS

Antibodies and radiolabeling

The murine monoclonal antibody CO17-1 was obtained from GlaxoWellcome (Hamburg, Germany). It belongs to the IgG_{2a} isotype and was shown to be internalized after antigen binding [3]. Its affinity was determined as 5×10^7 l/mol. The anti-CEA antibody, clone F023C5, was obtained from Sorin Biomedica (Saluggia, Italy). It is not internalized to a significant extent. Its affinity constant is, with approximately 0.5×10^7 l/mol, in the same range as for CO17-1A [4]. Radioiodination was performed using the iodogen method as described previously [5].

Animal models, experimental radioimmuno- and chemotherapy

The human colon carcinoma cell line, GW-39, was serially propagated in nude mice as described in detail earlier [6]. For the pulmonary metastatic model, intravenous injection of the GW-39 human colon cancer cell was performed in nude mice, as has been described previously in detail [7].

Tumor sizes of subcutaneous tumors were determined by caliper measurement immediately before therapy and at weekly intervals thereafter [6]. Tumors were either left untreated (controls) or injected with a single dose of radiolabeled antibody, with the activities indicated. Eight to twenty animals were studied in each treatment group. For chemotherapy, the mice received an intravenous injection of 1.8 mg leucovorin, followed by 0.6 mg 5-fluorouracil one hour later, for five consecutive days each in 200 μl saline. The maximum tolerated dose (MTD) was defined as the highest possible activity under the respective conditions that did not result in any animal deaths [6].

Initial clinical phase-I/II radioimmunotherapy in patients with small volume disease

So far, ten colorectal cancer patients with minimal residual metastatic disease (all lesions $\leq$ 3 cm) have been entered in the ongoing mCi/m^2-based dose escalation study with the ^{131}I-labeled anti-CEA MAb, F023C5 (IgG_1 subtype). The patients were given single injections, starting at 50 mCi/m^2, and escalating in 10 mCi/m^2 increments. The maximum tolerated dose is defined as the dose level where $\leq$ 1/6 patients develop a myelotoxicity > grade 3. Therapeutic responses were graded according to oncological standard criteria.

RESULTS

Therapeutic efficacy of radioimmunotherapy as compared to treatment with unconjugated immunoglobulins or chemotherapy with 5-fluorouracil / leucovorin in the subcutaneous tumor model

Splenic IgG_{2a}-receptor mediated clearance is a phenomenon which has been described earlier in nude mice [5,8], and which has been shown to be overcome by higher protein doses. We have determined 200 μg as the optimal protein dose of CO17-1A [5]. In contrast, no such prominent protein influence was seen over a wide range of protein doses with the anti-CEA Mab, F023C5, which belongs to the IgG_1 subtype.

In order to establish the MTD of ^{131}I-labeled CO17-1A and F023C5, varying amounts of activity were injected, starting at 250 μCi each, and proceeding in 10- to 20-percent increments. The MTD of ^{131}I-labeled CO17-1A was reached at 300 μCi, the MTD of ^{131}I- F023C5 at 600 μCi. In accordance to radiation doses to the blood of approximately 15 Gy each, comparably severe myelosuppression occurred in both groups (data not shown), and a further 10-% increase in the administered activity resulted in 10 - 30% deaths within 3 to 4 weeks p.i. each. No signs of second-organ toxicity were observed. In untreated controls, the subcutaneous human colon cancer xenografts grew rapidly with a mean tumor volume doubling time of less than one week (Figure 1a). Whereas, at the 200-μg protein level, no significant anti-tumor effects were observed with unlabeled 17-1A ($p=0.72$), ^{131}I-labeled CO17-1A, at its MTD (300 μCi), led to a significant ($p=0.04$) growth retardation for approximately 7 - 8 weeks (Figure 1b). Similar anti-tumor effects were observed with ^{131}I-labeled F023C5. Differences between both radiolabeled antibodies were not statistically significant.

Since chemotherapy with 5-fluorouracil / leucovorin is regarded as the "gold standard" therapeutic regimen in metastatic colorectal cancer [1], we undertook a comparison of the therapeutic effects of chemo- and radioimmunotherapy in the subctaneous GW-39 model at equitoxic doses. Mice were given 1.8 mg leucovorin intravenously, followed one hour later by 0.6 mg 5-fluorouracil, which has been shown as the maximum tolerated dose earlier [9]. This regimen induces only very mild myelotoxicity (data not shown), but causes dose-limiting mucositis [9]. Figure 1a as compared to 1b shows the therapeutic efficacy of this chemotherapeutic regimen as compared to untreated controls or animals treated with both radiolabeled antibodies. Although there seemed to be a trend versus tumor growth retardation with 5-

FU/leucovorin, the difference was not statistically significant as compared to the controls (p=0.31).

Therapeutic efficacy of radioimmunotherapy versus 5-fluorouracil / leucovorin chemotherapy in a (micro-)metastatic animal model

Pulmonary metastases of a human colon cancer were induced by intravenous injection of the GW-39 human colon cancer cell in nude mice. Multiple microscopic tumor colonies develop in the lungs of such animals, reaching a size of approximately 1 - 3 mm at 4 weeks after tumor cell inoculation. Treatment was initiated on day 7 after tumor cell inoculation. Animals either received chemotherapy with 5-fluorouracil / folinic acid, or were given equitoxic radioimmunotherapy, each at its respective maximum tolerated dose. Untreated animals died from rapidly progressing pulmonary metastases within 5 to 8 weeks after tumor inoculation (Figure 2). Histologically, the lung parenchyma was almost completely replaced by tumor. Whereas 5-FU/leucovorin chemotherapy led to a mean prolongation of survival of only 3-4 weeks, the tumor-specific radiolabeled antibodies performed significantly ($p<0.001$) better, with 35-55% long term survival (Fig. 2). Animals surviving 25 weeks were sacrificed and their lungs were examined histologically. No signs of vital tumor residues were found in these mice.

Initial clinical phase-I/II radioimmunotherapy in patients with small volume disease

A total of ten patients with small volume metastatic disease of metastatic colorectal cancer has been enroled so far in a phase-I/II dose escalation study with the ^{131}I-labeled anti-CEA MAb, F023C5. All known tumor lesions were targeted. As we have shown earlier for other anti-CEA antibodies [2], tumor doses increased exponentially with decreasing tumor size (highest observed dose: 185 cGy/mCi in a 0.5-cm lung lesion). At mean red marrow doses of 0.45 cGy/mCi, myelotoxicity seems to become dose-limiting, although the MTD has not yet been reached at 80 mCi/m^2. In these ten assessable patients with small volume disease, one had a complete, two patients partial remissions (corresponding to an objective response rate of 30%) (Figure 3), and four patients experienced stabilization of previously rapidly progressing disease, lasting for up to 12+ months.

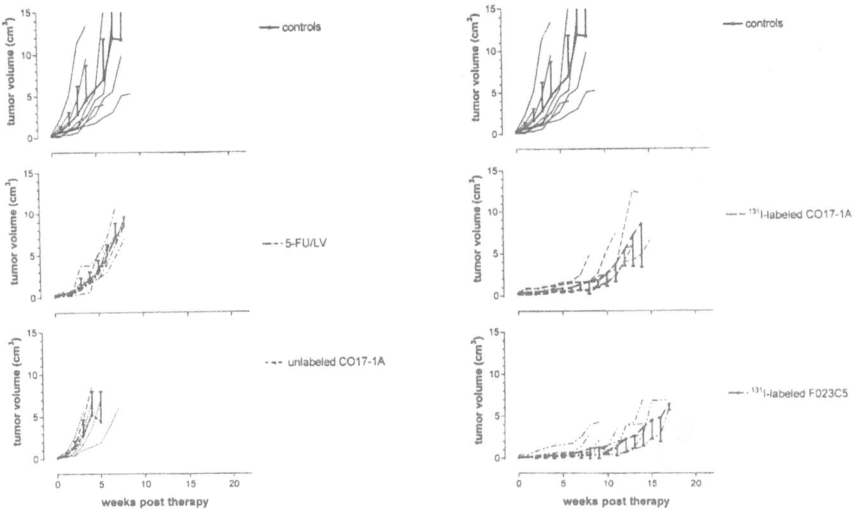

Figure 1
Therapeutic efficacy of (a) chemotherapy with 5-FU/leucovorin at its maximum tolerated dose (0.6mg/1.8mg×5d), as compared to 200 μg of unlabeled CO17-1A or to untreated controls. (b) ^{131}I-labeled CO17-1A or F023C5 at their respective maximum tolerated doses (300 vs. 600 μCi) as compared to untreated controls.

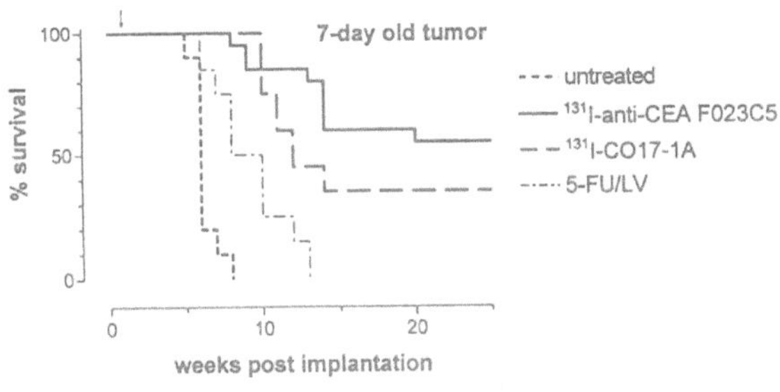

Figure 2
Therapeutic efficacy of ^{131}I-labeled CO17-1A or F023C5 IgG, as compared to chemotherapy with 5-FU/leucovorin on the survival of animals bearing multiple pulmonary metastases.

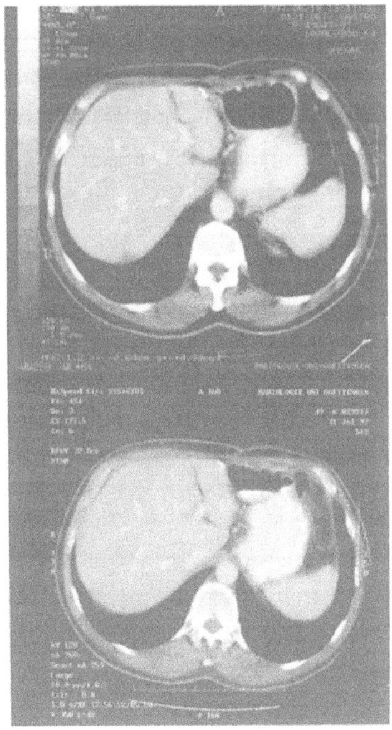

Figure 3
Therapeutic effect of 149 mCi of ^{131}I-labeled F023C5 in a patient with colorectal cancer metastatic to the liver before (upper panel) and six weeks after radioimmunotherapy.

DISCUSSION

We and others have shown earlier that tumor uptake and radiation doses to the tumor in radioimmunotherapy are inveresely correlated to the tumor size [2]. This led to the hypothesis that radioimmunotherapy may be viable therapeutic option in small volume metastatic disease, even though it may not be a very effective treatment modality in "bulky" disease. Indeed, the preclinical data, as presented in this communication, suggest that radioimmunotherapy may be therapeutically superior, in this setting, to standard 5-FU/leucovorin chemotherapy.

Anti-tumor effects with both, ^{131}I-labeled CO17-1A and F023C5, appear surprisingly good given the comparably low affinity, thus low tumor uptake. An inverse relationship between tumor size and uptake is a well known phenomenon [2,10]. We have shown earlier that this dependency of uptake upon size is the more pronounced, the lower the affinity of the antibody [10]. On the other hand, low affinity may favor a more homogenous antibody and dose distribution in the tumor which may have some advantage with respect to the comparably short path length of the ^{131}I radiation. Further studies will show whether combination strategies of radioimmuno- and chemotherapy will help to further improve the therapeutic results.

In accordance to these preclinical data, toxicity in the pilot clinical radioimmunotherapy studies, was restricted to a transient myelosuppression. Despite the fact that the MTD has not been reached yet at 80 mCi/m^2, encouraging anti-tumor effects have been observed.

Summarizing, our data suggest that radioimmunotherapy may be a viable therapeutic option in colorectal cancer patients with limited disease. Myelotoxicity is the only dose-limiting toxicity. Although the patients were treated below the respective maximum tolerated dose, anti-tumor effects are encouraging. Further studies are ongoing in order to show whether combination approaches of radioimmunotherapy with potentially radiosensitizing chemotherapeutic agents may further enhance the therapeutic efficacy [11,12].

ACKNOWLEDGEMENTS

The authors express their gratitude to Dr. D.M. Goldenberg (Garden State Cancer Center, Belleville, NJ) for providing us with the GW-39 cell line. Part of this work was supported by grant Be 1689/4-1 from the Deutsche Forschungsgemeinschaft (DFG).

REFERENCES

1. DeVita VT, Hellman S, Rosenberg SA (eds.): Cancer - Principles and Practice of Oncology (5th edition). Philadelphia: Lippincott-Raven, 1997.
2. Behr TM, Goldenberg DM, Becker WS: Radioimmunotherapy of solid tumors: a review "Of Mice and Men". Hybridoma *16:* 101-107, 1997.
3. Woo DV, Li D, Mattis JA, Steplewski Z: Selective chromosomal damage and cytotoxicity of ^{125}I-labeled monoclonal antibody 17-1a in human cancer cells. Cancer Res *49:* 2952-2958, 1989.
4. Behr T, Becker W, Bair HJ, Klein M, Stühler CM, Cidlinsky KP, Scheele JR, Wolf FG: Comparison of complete versus fragmented ^{99m}Tc-labeled anti-CEA monoclonal antibodies for immunoscintigraphy in colorectal cancer. J Nucl Med *36:* 430-441, 1995.
5. Behr TM, Sgouros G, Vougioukas V, Memtsoudis S, Gratz S, Nebendahl K, Schmidberger H, Becker W: Therapeutic efficacy and dose-limiting toxicity of Auger-electron versus beta emitters in radioimmunotherapy with internalizing antibodies: evaluation of ^{125}I- versus ^{131}I-labeled CO17-1A in a colorectal cancer model. Int J Cancer: *in press*, 1998.
6. Behr TM, Sgouros G, Sharkey RM, Dunn RM, Blumenthal RD, Kolbert K, Juweid ME, Siegel JA, Goldenberg DM: ^{90}Y-Dosimetry in the nude mouse: evaluation of three dosimetry models in relation to the observed biological effects in the radioimmunotherapy of human colon cancer xenografts. Proc 6th Int Radiopharm Dosim Symp Gatlinburg (TN) 1996, *in press:* 1997.
7. Blumenthal RD, Sharkey RM, Haywood L, Natale AM, Wong GY, Siegel JA, Kennel SJ, Goldenberg DM: Targeted therapy of athymic mice bearing GW-39 human colonic cancer micrometastases with ^{131}I-labeled monoclonal antibodies. Cancer Res *52:* 6036-6044, 1992.
8. Sharkey RM, Natale A, Goldenberg DM, Mattes MJ: Rapid blood clearance of immunoglobulin G2a in nude mice. Cancer Res *51:* 3102-3107, 1991.
9. Blumenthal RD, Sharkey RM, Natale AM, Kashi R, Wong G, Goldenberg DM: Comparison of equitoxic radioimmunotherapy and chemotherapy in the treatment of human colonic cancer xenografts. Cancer Res *54:* 142-151, 1994.
10. Behr TM, Sharkey RM, Juweid ME, Dunn RM, Siegel JA, Goldenberg, DM: Variables influencing tumor dosimetry in radioimmunotherapy of CEA-expressing ,cancers with anti-CEA and anti-mucin monoclonal antibodies. J Nucl Med *38:* 409-418, 1997.
11. Behr TM, Wulst E, Radetzky S, Blumenthal RD, Dunn RM, Gratz S, Rave-Fränk M, Schmidberger H, Raue F, Becker W: Improved treatment of medullary thyroid cancer in a nude mouse model by combined radioimmunochemotherapy: doxorubicin potentiates the therapeutic efficacy of radiolabeled antibodies in a radioresistant tumor type. Cancer Res *57:* 5309-5319, 1997.
12. Tschmelitsch J, Barendswaard E, Williams Jr C, Yao TJ, Cohen AM, Old LJ, Welt S: Enhanced antitumor activity of combination radioimmunotherapy (^{131}I-labeled monoclonal antibody A33) with chemotherapy (fluorouracil). Cancer Res *57:* 2181-2186, 1997.

Radioactive Isotopes in
Clinical Medicine and Research XXIII
ed. by H. Bergmann, H. Köhn and H. Sinzinger

Radioimmunotherapy of glioblastoma by using I-131 and Y-90 labeled anti-tenascin Monoclonal Antibodies.

Pietro Riva ^, Giancarlo Franceschi ^, Massimo Frattarelli°, Nada Riva^, Guiducci °, Anna Maria Cremonini°, Giuliano Giuliani°, Michela Casi^, Rossella Gentile^. ^Nuclear Medicine Dept. and Istituto Oncologico Romagnolo; °Neurosurgery Dept.; "M.Bufalini" Hospital 47023 Cesena (Italy).

Summary

BC-2 and BC-4 Mabs labelled with I-131, were given directly in the tumoral bed. 81 glioblastoma evaluable cases were treated. Adverse effects were very few. The treatment lengthened the patients' median survival (22 months in total). 11 PR, 1 CR and 24 NED (No Evidence of Disease) were recorded. The response rate was 44.4 %. Then a new isotope, Y-90, has been employed. Following a phase I trial, a phase II study was initiated in 22 cases with malignant glioma (anaplastic astrocytoma n.6 and glioblastoma n.16). In 16 evaluable patients (12 glioblastoma and 4 anaplastic astrocytoma) the objective response consisted in 1 PD, 4 SD, 7 PR, 2 CR and 2 NED. The global response rate (PR + CR + NED) was 68.75% (66.6% in glioblastoma and 75% in anaplastic astrocytoma group).

Introduction

High grade malignant gliomas are tumours which cannot be controlled with the current therapeutical regimens. This is due by their aggressive infiltrating attitude toward the adjacent normal brain, and more in particular , by the microscopic diffusion of a large population of neoplastic cells which spread in an area all around the main lesion: the so called BAT (Brain Adjacent Tissue). The are not detectable by means of radiological (CT scan, MRI, SPECT) tools and cannot be entirely eradicated by surgery nor by external radiotherapy . Thus in a quite short time (12 months, as median time) they give rise to a lethal recurrence[1]. The local application of a therapeutical agent capable to reach and destroy part or all these malignant elements, may improve the control of the disease. The use of monoclonal antibodies (Mabs) armed with suitable nuclides could represent a useful therapeutic approach able to lessen or to completely arrest the tumour growth[2]. More in particular, if the radioactive Mabs are locally injected, directly in the site of tumoral bed after operation, they diffuse through the remaining malignant tissue and react with their specific antigenic receptors. By this way a large amount of radioactivity can be concentrated selectively into the neoplastic area, completely sparing the normal elements[3]. The loco-regional administration of radiolabelled Mabs presents several handy advantages as to be applied in clinical practice. The immunoglobulins are given in a solution form, thus they easily scatter across the zone of disease overcoming possible anatomic obstacles; the modality of injection is quite simple, and it is not time consuming. Moreover the application of intralesional Radioimmunotherapy (IL-RIT) can be repeated many times (up to 9, in our experience) without any significant damage to healthy surrounding brain[4].

Material and methods

Monoclonal antibodies

Two murine Mabs BC2 and BC4 were utilised . They are directed against tenascin (TN) which is a glycoprotein abundantly and homogeneously expressed by the cells and mainly by the stroma of malignant glioma tissue [5]. Owing to the presence of large quantity of antigenic sites the tumour targeting is remarkably intense. The whole IgGs were employed. The dose of proteins injected was, on mean 3.19 mg. (range 0.73-8.87).

Isotopes

In the fist group of cases the antibodies were conjugated to I-131 by means of the Iodogen method, achieving a good labelling efficiency (>95%), while preserving the immunoreactivity of immunoglobulins (> 80%). The mean dose of I-131 given per RIT cycle was 1809.3 MBq, corresponding to 48.9 mCi. More recently a new trial, by using Y-90 has begun. In this cases the Mabs were firstly linked to the chelator Benzyl-DTPA and, then conjugated to Y-90, obtaining high levels (>97%) of labelling efficiency. The mean dose of Y-90 was 666 MBq (18 mCi).

Radioimmunotherapy protocol

In all cases IL-RIT was given after an operation as radical as possible. In cases bearing a recurrent lesion a second surgical approach was applied. When possible the surgeon produced a postoperative cavity and always implanted an indwelling Rickam or Ommaya catheter with its internal tip in the core of the surgical crater, as to yield a regular diffusion of radioactive solution. Moreover all patients were previously submitted to external radiotherapy at the maximum tolerated doses (55-60 Gy). Finally the anti-tenascin antibodies were infused, within 30 days after the completion of radiotherapy courses, or, in cases of recurrent tumour, 20-30 days after the second operation. The patients' preparation consisted in antiepileptic drugs and in steroids (dexamethasone 4-8 mg per day) starting from day - 3 and continuing up to day +10. The cases who received I-131 labelled antibodies received, in addition, thyroid blocking agents (tiroxine and potassium iodide). The administration of the radiopharmaceutical, was bolus performed through the subcutaneous reservoir of the indwelling catheter. After the infusion of the radioactive compound the patients were isolated in a shielded room. Their stay in hospital lasted on mean 10 days (range 7-15 days) for I-131 group and 4 days (range 3-5) for patients who received Y-90 labelled antibodies. The IL-RIT applications were generally given more times. The first 3 cycles were carried out at a 30-40 days interval, then further infusions, if required, were given after longer periods (2-3 months).

Our cases had a accurate follow up, which consisted in monthly clinical examination, and a radiological (CT scan or MRI) brain images every three months. The objective response to RIT was defined according to the WHO[6] criteria. More in particular the cases who had IL-RIT when their disease was remarkably or totally reduced by precedent regimens and did not present, for a long period of time, clinical or radiological sign of disease, were considered positive responders to the treatment and were classified as NED (Not Evidence of Disease)[7].

Dosimetry evaluations

The dose to the target neoplastic tumour and to the healthy organs was calculated before the administration of the therapeutical dose, following the intralesional injection of a tracer dose (1 mg of protein and 37 Mbq of I-131) according to both MIRD and Monte Carlo formalisms[8]. By contrast in the cases who received Y-90 antibodies, the biodistribution and the dosimetry were calculated following the infusion of the therapeutic dose, by utilising the bremsstrahlung emissions of radioyttrium. In patients who received intralesional RIT following a complete surgical tumour removal, in whom the presence of disease was not radiologically assessable the tumour area was theoretically assumed as a restricted zone with an extension of 1.5 mm. situated around the bed of the primary glioblastoma and incorporating hidden tumour cell clusters (BAT). In this case both the dose to the entire cavity and the BAT were separately computed.

Patients

a) I-131 labelled Mabs: 122 cases have received IL-RIT since 1990. 15 patients were accrued in a phase I trial. Then 107 (12 with anaplastic astrocytoma and 95 with glioblastoma) were enrolled in a phase II study. Only the outcomes observed in 81 glioblastoma evaluable cases, which received IL-RIT at least 6 months before, are reported here. 41 out of 81 were affected by newly diagnosed malignant gliomas and received all customary regimens before the antibody infusion, while the remaining 40 were bearing recurrent lesions and were operated again before the application of IL-RIT. At the time IL-RIT was given, 32 out of 81 had a macroscopic disease and 49 resulted bearers of minimal or microscopic lesion.

b) Y-90 labelled Mabs: in a phase I trial 15 patients received escalating dose (185, 370, 555, 740, 925 MBq) of BC2-DTPA-^{90}Y which was locally given in the site of the disease, according the same modalities utilised in the I-131 group. 3 patients were studied at each incremental level to assess the maximum tolerated dose. At the same time the biodistribution, the pharmacokinetics and the dosimetry were evaluated. Subsequently a phase II has started including, so far 22 cases (anaplastic astrocytoma n.6 and glioblastoma n.16) already submitted to conventional treatments: 8 were newly diagnosed tumours and 14 recurrent malignancies. 9 patients has been treated with small (diameter < 1.5 cm) or minimal lesion, conversely 13 presented a macroscopic (diameter >2.5 cm) neoplastic remnant. The Y-90 dose was, on mean 747.03 Mbq. Multiple cycles were done.
All patients gave their informed, signed consent to receive the radiolabelled Mabs intralesionally. The RIT protocol had previously been approved by the Ethical Committee of M.Bufalini Hospital.

Results

Biodistribution and dosimetry

Both in I-131 and Y-90 groups, the local administration of Mabs led to a high uptake in the site of their deposition. The percentage of the injected dose concentrated per gram of tumour after 24 hours, was on mean 3.1% in I-131 class, and 3.5 in Y-90 subset. The effective half life of Mabs in the tumour was on mean 57.1 hours in I-131 group and 43 hours in Y-90 subset. The tumour radiation dose was 1006.4 cGy/mCi of radioiodine and 1805.6 cGy/mCi of radioyttrium administered. More in particular the dose delivered to the walls of postoperative cavity, which embodied several occult neoplastic cells clusters resulted about 4 times higher in patients who were given the Y-90 conjugates. This was due to the strong beta energy of this isotope which allows a deeper penetration into neoplastic milieu, as well as into the brain adjacent tissue (BAT). For this reason the possibility to reach most or all neoplastic cells scattered outside the main tumour mass was enhanced. The cumulative dose, in patients who underwent multiple RIT applications, progressively increased after each subsequent administration, and reached very high values in cases who had had more than 5 courses (> 2000 Gy).

Adverse effects

No significant haematologic, renal, hepatic early or late side effects were observed, both after single and multiple RIT applications. 4 patients of Y-90 group presented a transient brain oedema. More than 85% of cases developed HAMA after the first infusion of monoclonal antibodies. Nevertheless the presence of HAMA did not preclude further and repeated local MAbs infusions nor did change the immunoglobulins pharmacokinectics.

Clinical outcomes

a) I-131 group (81 glioblastoma):

The treatment yielded a significant extension of the patients' median survival (22 months in total, 25 months in cases with minimal lesion, 16 months in patients with macroscopic remnant).
At the same time the disease free time up to relapse was favourably prolonged : 12 months versus 5 months which was observed in a group of cases with similar characteristics, who did not receive radioimmunotherapy. Favourable objective responses were recorded: 11 PR, 1 CR and 24 NED (No Evidence of Disease) which were achieved in patients submitted to therapy with minimal tumour burden. The response rate was 44.4 %. The limited extension of the neoplasm at the time of therapy was the most important factor in order to obtain beneficial outcomes. No significant dissimilarity was observed between the group of newly diagnosed tumours and the patients who had RIT in a recurrent phase of glioblastoma, following a second operation.

b) Y-90 group:

In 16 evaluable patients (12 glioblastoma and 4 anaplastic astrocytoma) the objective response consisted in 1 PD, 4 SD, 7 PR, 2 CR and 2 NED. The global response rate (PR + CR + NED) was 68.75% (66.6% in glioblastoma and 75% in anaplastic astrocytoma group). In 4 cases (2 glioblastoma and 2 anaplastic astrocytoma) a complete tumour shrinking was radiologically (MRI) demonstrated. Not enough time has been elapsed , from the beginning of the trial, to allow the calculation of the median survival.

Discussion and conclusions.

After 7 years clinical experience the effectiveness of this approach in order to cure or to block the progression of this otherwise untreatable neoplastic disease, has been assessed in many cases, whose number can be judged statistically significant[9]. The direct infusion of the radioactive antibodies represents one of the steps of a multimodality strategy, whose cornerstones are the radical surgery and external radiotherapy which can destroy the major quantity of neoplastic cell but which need a further therapeutic agent to complete the tumour killing. The treatment is safe and does not alter the normal cerebral tissue, even if in some patients treated with Y-90 compound, a brain oedema was recorded. The normal major organs are completely spared. The possibility to accumulate, for a quite long time an high amount of radioactivity in the tumour zone, accounts for the promising clinical outcomes so far observed. The radiation dose delivered to glioma tissue and, the consequent clinical results of this approach, are more consistent the less is the tumour burden at the time of RIT application. For this reason the IL-RIT should be given as adjuvant setting following previous cyto-reducing procedures. On the other hand even when the lesion is minimal or microscopic thanks to previous regimens, the disease remains very risky and its prognosis is always ominous. In all cases the IL-RIT represent a rescue approach aiming to stop or delay the progression of the tumour. Moreover the possibility to carry out multiple IL-RIT cycles, without any untoward reaction , ameliorates the effects of this therapy and allows to lengthen for an extended period of time the control of the disease. The preliminary results observed in the Y-90 group, can be considered encouraging, but a longer time has to pass and more patients have to be recruited, in order to draw more significant conclusions. The radiation dose conveyed by this nuclide to the tumour area is notably higher in comparison to I-131 and, what is very important, the strong beta particles produced by this nuclide can run for a longer path inside the BAT, thus the probability to reach and damage the microscopic focuses of glioma cells migrated in this area is improved. Our aim is to complete the Y-90 phase II study, then, to carry out a phase III randomised trial in which a group of cases treated only with surgery and radiotherapy will be compared with a second subset who, in addition, will receive IL-RIT, should be done.

Acknowledgement: Work supported by Istituto Oncologico Romagnolo, by AIRC (Italian Association on Cancer Research), and by Cassa di Risparmio di Cesena.

References

1. Ransonhoff J., Kelly P., Laws E. The role of intracranial surgery for the treatment of malignant gliomas. Semin in Oncology 1986; 13:27-37.
2. Goldenberg D.M., Griffith G.L. Radioimmunotherapy of cancer: arming the missiles. J.Nucl.Med 1992;33: 1110-12.
3. Riva P., Arista A., Mariani M., Seccamani E., Sturiale C., Tison V., et al. Radioimmunotherapy of brain glioblastoma by direct intratumor injection of ^{131}I labelled BC-2 monoclonal antibody: Clinical experience in 11 patients. In :R.Hofer,H.Bergmenn,H.Sinzinger (eds.) Radio-active Isotopes in Clinical Medicine and Research, Stuttgart, New York: Scattauer; 1992:40-44.
4. Riva P., Franceschi G., Arista A., Frattarelli M., Riva N., Cremonini A.M.,, Giuliani G., Casi M. Local application of radiolabeled mabs for the treatment of high grade malignant gliomas: a six year clinical experience. Cancer suppl., 80,12, 2733-2742,1997.

5.Siri A.., Carnemolla B., Saginati M., Leprini A., Casari G., BaralleF.et al. Human Tenascin: primary structure, pre-mRNA splicing patterns and localization of the epitopes recognized by two monoclonal antibodies. Nuclear Acids Research.1991;19:525-31.

6.World Health Organization handbook for reporting results of cancer treatments. Offsets Publication n.40,1979.Geneva,Switzerland:WHO,1979.

7. Riva P.,Arista A:,Tison V.,Sturiale C.,Franceschi G.,Spinelli A.et al. Intralesional Radioimmunotherapy of Malignant Glioma: an effective treatment in recurrent tumors. Cancer suppl. 1994;73:1076-82.

8. Loevinger, R.,Berman, M..A schema for absorbed dose calculation for biologically distributed radionuclides. MIRD pamphlet n.1. New York:J Nucl Med.

9. Riva P., Arista A., Sturiale C., Tison V., Frattarelli M., Lazzari S. et al. Radioimmunotherapy of CNS malignant gliomas by direct intralesional injection of specific ^{131}I radiolabeled monoclonal antibodies. In: Cancer therapy with radiolabeled antibodies. D. M. Goldenberg (ed .) pp.203-216. Boca Raton, Ann Arbor, London, Tokyo. CRC Press,1994.

Radioactive Isotopes in
Clinical Medicine and Research XXIII
ed. by H. Bergmann, H. Köhn and H. Sinzinger

I-131-LIPIODOL THERAPY IN LIVER NEOPLASMS

Risse JH, Grünwald F, Strunk H, Bultmann T and Biersack HJ.

Nuclear Medicine Dep. and Radiology Dep., University of Bonn,
Sigmund-Freud-Str. 25, D - 53105 Bonn

SUMMARY: 11 patients with liver neoplasms (9 HCC, 1 CCC, 1 multiple breast cancer metastases (BCM)) were treated by transarterial I-131-Lipiodol. CT and SPECT showed pronounced I-131-Lipiodol accumulation in the tumor tissue in all cases. In 2 HCC a significant reduction of tumor size was achieved. Of the patients with big tumor mass, 5 (4 HCC, 1 CCC) had stable disease, and 2 HCC were progressive. 1 patient died. The BCM proved significant reduction in number and size. 18-FDG-PET and CT controls showed in part different results with pretherapeutic PET proving high interindividual variability in tumor activity. Side effects were tolerabel.

INTRODUCTION

Hepatocellular carcinoma (HCC) is a common malignant tumor worldwide, leading to one million deaths each year (1). Only surgical therapy may lead to long-term survival, but the resectability rate in HCC may be as low as 1 % (2). Non-surgical regional therapy like transarterial chemoembolisation (TACE) has shown some effect (3). Percutaneous ethanol injection (PEI) as an alternative to transarterial therapy is usually limited to one or few lesions (4). Intraarterial I-131-Lipiodol has been shown to be effective in HCC (5). In contrast to TACE, I-131-Lipiodol therapy is also suitable in portal vein thrombosis because it does not cause relevant embolisation (6). Since many HCC patients initially present with portal vein thrombosis and multinodular disease, the treatment with I-131-Lipiodol may primarily be the only regional therapy option.

Although the I-131-Lipiodol treatment in liver malignancies is well introduced in France and Asia, no experience has been reported in Middle Europe. Our objective was to introduce this therapy in Germany and to assess safety and effectiveness with special care to side effects.

MATERIALS AND METHODS

11 patients with liver malignancies were treated by selective intraarterial (i.a.) administration of I-131-labeled Lipiodol (Lipiocis[R]) during hepatic angiography. 10 patients had primary liver cancer, i.e. 9 hepatocellular cancer with or without portal vein thrombosis (HCC; 6 male, 3 female, age 50 - 82 years) and 1 cholangiocellular cancer (CCC; male, 61). 1 patient suffered from multiple liver metastases due to chemotherapy resistent breast cancer (BCM; female, 41).

The mean administered I-131 dose was 45.4 ± 5.6 mCi (1680 ± 207 MBq) with a range from 30 - 52 mCi (1110 - 1924 MBq). Repeated administrations were done every 2 months. In total, 17 applications have been done with 3 therapies in 1 HCC patient and 2 therapies in 4 patients each (3 HCC, 1 CCC), respectively. For radiation protection reasons the patients had an 8 days hospital stay for each therapy cycle, during which sodium perchlorate for prophylactical thyroid blockage was prescribed.

Monitoring for the I-131-Lipiodol distribution in the liver and whole body was achieved by computed tomography (CT) 7 days after administration because of the high X-ray density of Lipiodol and by planar scintigraphy of the thorax and abdomen and SPECT of the liver on days 4 and 7. For evaluation of therapy success all patients underwent a pretherapeutic 3-phase helical liver CT as well as a 18-FDG-PET (positron emission tomography with Fluor-18-deoxy-glucose; except the BCM patient and one of the HCC group) of the whole body. Imaging follow-up consisted of 3-phase helical liver CT after 6 weeks and, if the disease was not progressive, 18-FDG-PET before the next therapy application. All CT scans were done on a „fourth generation" scanner (Philips Tomoscan[R]) as helical CT with 7 mm slice thickness, 10 mm table feed (pitch factor 1.4), reconstruction interval 7 mm, 120 kV and 250 mA. The PET scanner was a CTI ECAT Exact[R] ; all patients had 18-FDG-activities between 6 and 8 mCi (222-296 MBq). Imaging included transmission corrigated tomograms of the whole body in all 3 standard planes as well as coronal emission tomograms. In the meantime the patients had a close monitoring program with history evaluation, physical examination, blood samples for all pertinent laboratory values, planar scintigraphy of thorax and abdomen and SPECT of the liver on an outpatient basis every two weeks after therapy.

RESULTS

Pretherapeutic CT scans revealed HCC diameters of more than 8 cm and in part additional multinodular disease in 6 patients. One HCC was multinodular with nodule diameters up to 5 cm. Only 2 HCC patients had smaller unifocal tumors with diameters of 3.2 and 5 cm, respectively. In the CCC patient, the tumor tissue left virtually no normal liver parenchyma except some few remainders in the left liver lobe. The BCM patient suffered from multiple liver metastases with diameters between 0.5 and 3 cm. Pretherapeutic PET scans revealed a high interindividual variability in tumor tracer accumulation, ranging from 3 lesions equivalent to normal liver tissue (3 HCC) to different grades of hot lesions (5 HCC, 1 CCC).

CT follow-up one week after administration of I-131-lipiodol showed pronounced accumulation in the tumor tissue in 9 patients. The lipiodol distribution pattern varied between solid high-density lipiodol aggregations and diffuse discrete uptake with all combinations between. In 2 patients the lipiodol was hardly visible in the liver CT due to ist diffuse discrete uptake; in those cases, scintigraphy and SPECT proved the predominant liver uptake of I-131. Planar scintigraphy of the thorax and abdomen revealed a high liver I-131 uptake in all patients. In the cases with primary liver cancer there was always some slight activity in the lungs on day 4 which disappeared quickly in the first 1 - 2 weeks after therapy. Liver SPECT showed pronounced I-131 uptake in the tumor tissue as known by pretherapeutic CT and PET. The scintigraphic findings became even more striking during the further 2-weekly follow-up program since the non-tumoral liver cleared completely of activity while the tumor tissue proved prolonged activity retention.

Therapy success after the first treatment as controlled by CT was dependent on initial tumor mass. In 2 HCC (one multinodular with nodules up to 5 cm; one unifocal of 3.2 cm) a significant reduction of tumor size was achieved (responder). One of these has been stable for 7 months after having received two further treatments. 5 patients (4 HCC, 1 CCC) had stable disease. 2 HCC were progressive. One HCC patient is not evaluable for therapy success because he died 13 days after application; in this case a pretherapeutic bad condition due to advanced tumor stage and age (82 years) was complicated by renal failure. The BCM patient liver metastases again proved significant reduction in number and size.

Control PET scans could be achieved in 5/10 primary liver cancer patients. After the first treatment PET revealed no change in 2 patients and a glucose utilisation increase in 2 indicative of progressive disease. One HCC (responder) without pretherapeutic PET control showed no change of the cool lesion in all further PET controls despite obvious tumor changes in the CT controls. The second responder also had no PET change. In contrast, PET showed progression of the CCC earlier than CT. In 2 patients control findings of PET and CT were concordant with progressive disease in both.

Side effects occured as the so-called post embolisation syndrome in 7 patients (6 mild, 1 moderate) with high temperature up to 40° C, transient leucocytosis and abdominal tension feeling. All patients had a transient rise in liver enzymes for few days. 2 patients with huge tumors showed a transient elevation of pancreatic enzymes. In 7 cases there was a thyroid I-131 uptake in the meantime beginning 2 - 4 weeks after treatment.

DISCUSSION

In previous studies safety and effectiveness of i.a. I-131-Lipiodol therapy for HCC have been investigated (5, 6). Most of the experience worldwide has been gained in France and Asia and to a lesser extent in Great Britain, but the whole patient number does not reach 200 worldwide yet (6 - 8). In Germany there is also some experience in i.a. radionuclide therapy for liver cancer with Yttrium-90 which has been widely abandoned (9). Nevertheless, the i.a. I-131-Lipiodol therapy has not yet been introduced in Germany or Middle Europe. Several reasons may be responsible for this lack of use of a liver cancer therapy option: First, HCC is an uncommon malignancy in these countries; second, there is need for long hospital stays for radiation protection reasons due to rigid laws in Germany; third, in many instances the application procedure requires a radiologist and a nuclear medicine physician because the application procedure requires both radiological skills and the permission of open radionuclide handling with the two specialties strictly separated in Germany; and last but not least the injection procedure itself carries some risk for the medical staff because of high radiation load particularly to the fingers.

Our experience with the first 11 patients with liver neoplasms treated by i.a. I-131-Lipiodol confirm the intratumoral uptake and retention kinetics as well as the good results known from the literature concerning tumor response in HCC up to some size. Nevertheless, our investigation yields new results. We found that a tumor size above 8 cm correlated with virtually no therapy response. In the literature, such big tumors probably have not been treated. Other authors report much better responses, but the tumor size is much smaller than in our population (e.g., 3-6 cm in (10)). This finding is consistent with the results of YOO et al. who found a tumor reduction rate depending on primary tumor size (11); there again no tumor diameter exceeded 8 cm.

In many reports side effects are not discussed or tolerance is described as excellent (6). In contrast to this we found considerable side effects. We believe that the post embolisation syndrome - which is well known from the TACE literature -, the altered liver enzymes and the raise of pancreatic enzymes all are at least in part due to some transient liver swelling because of the internal liver radiation; both pancreas enzyme cases had no clinical or CT evidence of pancreatitis but huge liver tumors compressing the pancreas body. Thyroid I-131 uptake has been negotiated by some authors and the manufacturer (12); our findings may in part be due to the two-weekly control monitoring program for our patients. As a consequence, all patients are continously treated with a combination of thyroxin and iodine now (in addition to sodium perchlorate during the hospital stay). The side effects described here have not yet been reported but are tolerable and in most instances even asymptomatic.

CONCLUSION

Our first 11 patients with liver neoplasms treated by transarterial I-131-Lipiodol in Germany show tumor mass dependent therapy response. Side effects are tolerabel. The procedure is safe, effective, and the results are encouraging for cancer tissue up to a moderate mass.

REFERENCES

1. London W. Primary hepatocellular carcinoma - etiology, pathogenesis and prevention. Hum Pathol 1981; 12: 1085-1097.

2. Maraj R, Kew MC, Hyslop RJ. Resectability rate of hepatocellular carcinoma in rural southern Africans. Br J Surg 1988; 75: 335-338.

3. Groupe d`étude et de traitement du carcinome hepatocellulaire. A comparison of Lipiodol chemoembolisation and conservative treatment for unresectable hepatocellular carcinoma. N Engl J Med 1995; 332: 1256-1261.

4. Livraghi T, Bolondi L, Lazzaroni S et al. Percutaneous ethanol injection in the treatment of hepatocellular carcinoma in cirrhosis: a study on 207 patients. Cancer 1992; 69: 925-929.

5. Bretagne JF, Raoul JL, Bourguet P et al. Hepatic artery injection of I-131-labeled Lipiodol. Part 2: Preliminary results of therapeutic use in patients with hepatocellular carcinoma and liver metastases. Radiology 1988; 168: 547-550.

6. Raoul JL, Guyader D, Bretagne JF et al. Randomized controlled trial for hepatocellular carcinoma with portal vein thrombosis: intra-arterial iodine-131-iodized oil versus medical support. J Nucl Med 1994; 35: 1782-1787.

7. Leung WT, Lau WY, Ho S et al. Selective internal radiation therapy with intra-arterial Iodine-131-Lipiodol in inoperable hepatocellular carcinoma. J Nucl Med 1994; 35: 1313-1318.

8. Novell R, Hilson A and Hobbs K. Ablation of recurrent primary liver cancer using ^{131}I-lipiodol. Postgrad Med J 1991; 67: 393-395.

9. Schild HH, Kutzner J. Intraarterielle Applikation von Radionukliden. In: Interventionelle Radiologie. Günther RW, Thelen M, editors. Stuttgart New York: Thieme, 1996: 336-339.

10. Kobayashi H, Hidaka H, Kajiya Y et al. Treatment of hepatocellular carcinoma by transarterial injection of anticancer agents in iodized oil suspension or of radioactive iodized oil solution. Acta Radiol [Diagn] 1986; 27: 139-147.

11. Yoo HS, Lee JT, Kim KW et al. Nodular hepatocellular carcinoma. Treatment with subsegmental intraarterial injection of iodine-131-labeled oil. Cancer 1991; 68: 1878-1884.

12. Raoul JL, Bourguet P, Bretagne JF et al. Hepatic artery injection of I-131-labeled Lipiodol. Part 1: Biodistribution study results in patients with hepatocellular carcinoma and liver metastases. Radiology 1988; 168: 541-545.

Radioactive Isotopes in
Clinical Medicine and Research XXIII
ed. by H. Bergmann, H. Köhn and H. Sinzinger

INDIVIDUALIZED DOSE ESTIMATION FOR Sr-89 WITH THE USE OF DIAGNOSTIC Tc-99m MDP BONE SCINTIGRAPHY

Ageliki Manetou*, Georgios S Limouris**
* NIMTS Hospital, Med Phys Unit, Athens, Greece
** Areteion Univ Hospital, Rad Dept, Athens, Greece

SUMMARY: A simplified model for the kinetics of both Sr-89 and Tc-99m-MDP was assumed. Normal adult data on time retention of the two radiopharmaceuticals in the whole skeleton were combined together and a linear relationship was derived between the time required for the same percentage uptake of the two radiopharmaceuticals after single injection. The same relationship was assumed to hold for metastatic sites. Tc-99m -MDP sequential quantitative images of the metastases were used to derive an individualized Sr-89 time retention curve.

INTRODUCTION

The control of pain in patients with multiple skeletal metastases is the major clinical problem especially in patients with carcinoma of the breast and the prostate. Sr-89 radiotherapy is becoming an important treatment for the palliation of pain of those patients [1]. Sr-89 is a pure beta-emitter; the mean energy of the particles emitted is 0.583 MeV and the range of the beta-particles in the soft tissue is less than 8 mm. The short range of the particles emitted makes it impossible for an external radiation detector to be used in order to estimate the tumor uptake of Sr-89 and therefore the tumor absorbed dose.

Sr-85 is a beta-emitter which is often administrated at the same time with Sr-89. It allows imaging of the kinetics of Sr-89 and provides useful data for the calculation of the tumor absorbed dose.

The main drawback of the use of Sr-85 for the estimation of the dose delivered to the tumor by Sr-89, is that the therapeutic results of the applied therapy are not predictable. This lack of predictability reflects the inability to select those patients whose lesions will receive adequate radiation doses from Sr-89 therapy.

In this study a technique for a first order approximation of the tumor absorbed dose from Sr-89, prior to the administration of the radiopharmaceutical, is presented. This technique involves the quantitative scintigraphic follow-up of Tc-99m-MDP tumor uptake for a period of 8 hours after the injection. It is based a) on the observation that patients who underwent bone scanning with Sr-85 and Tc-99m-MDP showed a close qualitative correlation [2-4] and b) on the fact that a quantitative comparative study of the percentage skeleton uptake of Sr-89 and Tc-99m-MDP in normal adults revealed a linear relationship between the times required for the same percentage of skeleton uptake from the two radiopharmaceuticals.

Estimations of the tumor absorbed dose based on this technique for three patients with extensive metastatic prostate cancer are also reported.

MATERIALS AND METHODS

A simplified four-compartment model was used to describe the kinetic pathways of both Sr-89 and Tc-99m-MDP [5-6]. Both tracers entering blood are transferred to soft tissue and bone space and are excreted through the urinary track. Bone surface and bone space are treated as a single compartment, attributed the term "skeleton" elsewhere in this study. In this model no distinction is made between compact and cancellous bone, eventhough the amount of bone formation per unit area of bone surface is approximately the same for both types of bone and the removal rate for strontium from cancellous bone must be 4 times the removal rate from compact bone [5]. The latter does not introduce any mistake in the model when the data used concern the skeleton as a whole.

In order to express quantitatively the similar biodistribution of the two radiopharmaceuticals, normal adult data of the skeleton uptake after single injection were used. Data for Sr-89 were obtained from ICRP No 20, Table 29 [7] and data for Tc-99m-MDP were given by Mele et.al.,1983 [6]. They were both corrected for time decay and expressed as percentage of the injected activity.

A linear relationship (R^2=0.99) which is described by Equation 1, was found between the time required for certain percentage uptake of Sr-89 by the whole skeleton following single injection and the time required for the same percentage uptake of the administrated activity of Tc-99m-MDP, after single injection.

$t_{Sr-89} = 1.2t_{Tc-99m-MDP} - 0.009$ for $t_{Tc-99m-MDP} < 8h$ (1)

where t_{Sr-89} the time after the injection of Sr-89 (d)

and $t_{Tc-99m-MDP}$ the time after the injection of Tc-99m-MDP (h)

Equation 1 implies that by measuring the percentage uptake of Tc-99m-MDP of a normal bone region at time $t_{Tc-99m-MDP}$ after the injection, the time required for the same percentage uptake of Sr-89 by the same bone region, t_{Sr-89}, can be calculated. By making the assumption that Equation 1 applies at regions of osseous metastases as well as normal bone, the metastasis's uptake of Sr-89 can be determined at different time intervals after the administration of the radiopharmaceutical and an estimation of the tumor absorbed dose can be made. Equation 1 was considered to be age-independent for ages grater than 50 years [5,8].

For the purpose of the calculation of the absorbed dose three patients with extensive metastatic prostate carcinoma were given a single injection of 740 ± 74 MBq of Tc-99m-MDP, two days prior to the administration of Sr-89. A number of sequential quantitative images obtained over the first 24 hours (Figure 1) after the Tc-99m-MDP injection provided data on the Tc-99m-MDP tumor uptake and Equation 1 was used in order to derive the strontium retention curve. Data were treated by conjugate view techniques [9] and the adsorbed dose calculation was based on the dosimetric method of ICRP Publication 30 [10]. The mass of the metastatic focus was determined by measuring the size of the lesion on standard bone radiographs. The density of bony metastases was assumed to be 1.5 gr/cm^3 while a density of 2 gr/cm^3 was assumed for normal bone [11].

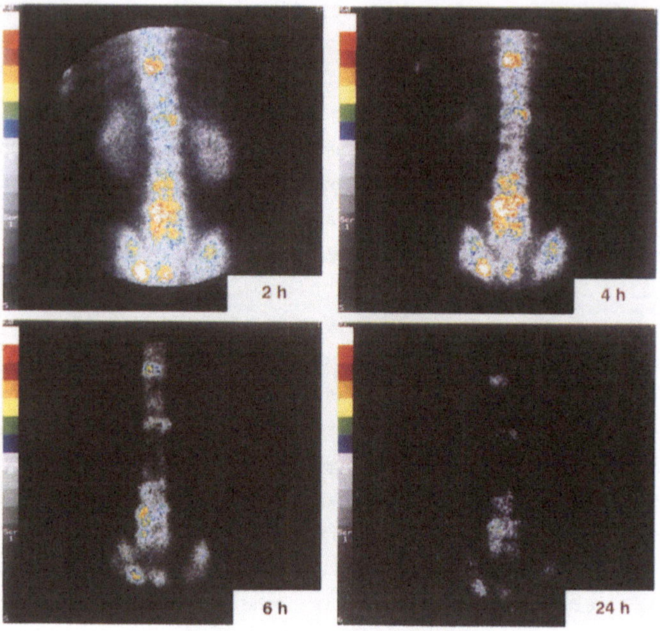

RESULTS

The measured values of the parameters involved in the dose calculation are summarized in Table 1, along with the estimated values of the absorbed dose. Equation 1 is valid for $t_{Tc-99m-MDP}$ less than 8 hours, which corresponds to t_{Sr-89} of approximately 10 days. Therefore the tumor absorbed dose from Sr-89 over the period of the first 10 days following administration can be estimated.

Patients with prostate cancer usually present reduced renal plasma clearance which results to prolonged retention of Sr-89 in the metastatic sites [3,12]. Strontium renal plasma clearance values for the patients involved in the present study were found to vary between 2.2 and 5.1 l/day; the normal value being 8.3 l/day [7]. An estimation of the tumor absorbed dose for infinite time after the Sr-89 injection was also performed, by making the assumption that the fraction of the administrated activity present at the tumor site on the 10th day after the injection remained there until physically decayed.

DISCUSSION

Tumor absorbed dose is a critical factor for the success of treatment with Sr-89 when it is used for the palliation of pain in patients with osseous metastases. The fact that Sr-89 does not emit gamma rays prohibits any kind of pretherapy dosimetry estimates; thus treatment with this radionuclide (regarding the administrated activity) must be conducted empirically.

TABLE 1. Estimated absorbed dose to bony metastases and normal bone following Sr-89 therapy. Normal and metastatic vertebrals in both cases are of the same volume.

	Administrated activity (MBq)	Mass (gr)	Dose in 10 days (cGy)	Dose over infinite time (cGy)
CASE 1	100			
Vertebral metastasis		150	63	270
Normal vertebral		200	24	84
CASE 2	105			
Vertebral metastasis		80	74	344
Normal vertebral		107	37	188
Pelvis metastasis		250	75	420
CASE 3	100			
Vertebral metastasis		70	102	437
Normal vertebral		120	43	183

The proposed method for the estimation of the tumor absorbed dose from Sr-89 through Tc-99m-MDP scintigraphy is based on data for normal bone and Equation 1 can only used to predict uptake values over the period of the first 10 days after the injection. Furthermore the retention of Sr-89 and Tc-99m-MDP which are known to be similar, were assumed to be the same. All these assumptions suggest that the proposed technique can only lead to an approximation of the absorbed dose.

However, even an indication of the absorbed dose prior to treatment, is a useful tool for the clinical doctor. It helps him decide on the administrated activity necessary for the adequate irradiation of the metastases.

Tc-99m-MDP is an inexpensive, routinely used radiopharmaceutical and the suggested method requires a single visit of the patient to the hospital prior to treatment. On the other hand, Sr-85 which can be alternatively used for the estimation of the absorbed dose delivered from Sr-89, is an expensive and hardly available radiopharmaceutical. When it is used for dosimetric purposes, regular visits of the patient to the hospital are required over a long period of time after the Sr-89 administration. The absorbed dose can only be calculated at the end of the treatment course.

Taking into consideration the advantages as well as any kind of inaccuracies introduced by the proposed method we believe that it can successfully serve its purpose: to provide a first order approximation of the tumor absorbed dose prior to treatment with Sr-89.

REFERENCES

1. Limouris GS, Toubanakis N, Shukla SK, Manetou A, Stauraka A, Vlahos L. In: Clinical Medicine and Research XXII. H.Bergamann, A. Kroiss and H.Sinzinger, editors. Birkhauser Verlag Basel/Switzerland, 1997:307-311.
2. Kloiber R, Molnar C, Barnes M. Sr-89 therapy for metastatic bone disease: Scintigraphic and radiographic follow-up. Radiol 1987;163:719-723
3. Blake G, Zivanovic M, McEwan A, Ackery D. Sr-89 therapy: strontium kinetics in disseminated carcinoma of the prostate. Eur J Nucl Med, 1986;12:447-454
4. Edawrds K, Santoro J, taylor A. Use of bone scintigraphy to select patients with multiple myeloma for treatment with strontium-89. J Nucl Med 1994;35(12):1992-1993
5. Leggett RW, Eckerman KF, Williams LR. Strontium-90 in bone:A case study in age-dependent dosimetric modeling. Health Phys, 1982;43(3):307-322
6. Mele M, Conte E, Fratello A, Pasculli D, Pieralice M, D'Addabbo A. Computer analysis of Tc-99m-DPD and Tc-99m-MDP kinetics in human: Cosice communication. J Nucl Med 1983;24:334-338

7. ICRP:Alkaline earth metabolism in adult man. In: ICRP Publication 20. 1972:135-143
8. Newton D, Harrison GE, Rundo J, Kang C, Warner AJ. Metabolism of Ca and Sr in late adult life. Health Phys, 1990;59(4):433-442
9. Fleming J. A technique for the absolute measurement of activity using a gamma camera and computer. Phys Med Biol 1979;24:176-180
10. ICRP:Dosimetric model for bone. In: ICRP Publication 30:Limits for intakes of radionuclides by workers. Part 1. Oxford:Pergamon Press 1979:35-46
11. Blake G, Zivanovic M, McEwan A, Cordon B, Ackery D. Sr-89 therapy: strontium kinetics and dosimetry in two patients treated for metastasising osteosarcoma. The Br J Rad 1987;60:253-259
12. Blake G, Zivanovic M, Lewington V. Measurements of the plasma clearance rate in patients receiving Sr-89 radionuclide therapy. Eur J Nucl Med, 1989;15:780-783

Radioactive Isotopes in
Clinical Medicine and Research XXIII
ed. by H. Bergmann, H. Köhn and H. Sinzinger

RHENIUM-186-HEDP AND STRONTIUM-89-CHLORIDE IN TREATMENT OF METASTATIC BONE PAIN

K. Liepe, W.G. Franke, R. Hliscs, A. Kühne, J. Kropp

Department of Nuclear Medicine, University Hospital, Dresden University of Technlogy, Fetscherstr. 74, 01307 Dresden, Germany

SUMMARY: In 25 patients we investigated the influence of Re-186 or Sr-89 on pain relief, reduction of analgesic consumption, and impairment of bone marrow function. We calculated the blood clearance, the excretion rate in urine and the accumulation in the bone. Blood samples were drawn weekly for 6 weeks and counted. 66% of the patients were able to reduce their analgesic intake. 66% of the patients had a significant, 17% a minor improvement of life quality. No differences were observed between the results of Sr-89 and Re-186-therapy. The excretion rate of Re-186 in the urine was 59% of the administered activity within 48h. Platelets decreased to 134.000 $\pm$ 68.000//mm^3 and leucocytes to 4.300 $\pm$ 2.000/mm^3. The bone accumulation of Re-186 was 36 $\pm$ 6%, with 17 $\pm$ 4% in the metastases as an average.

Introduction

Bone is a frequent and common site of metastatic disease by breast and prostate cancer. However, other tumors also show bone metastases, e.g. lung and bladder carcinoma as well as B-cell-lymphoma. Metastatic bone pain is the most serious problem for the patient concerning quality of life and requires an effective treatment (1).

The external-beam radiotherapy is suitable for single bone metastases. The systemic radionuclide therapy represents the better possibility for palliation of multiple metastases.

Rhenium-186 and Strontium-89 (Metastron®) are preferentially used radiopharmaceuticals for this purpose in Germany.

Rhenium-186 is a β-emitting radionuclide with a maximum energy of 1.07 MeV and a physical half life of 89,3 hours. The gamma emission of 137 keV allows imaging with a gamma camera to control the intracorporal distribution of the radionuclide. Rhenium is complexed to hydroxyethylidendiphosphonate (HEDP) which localizes in bone by bridging the hydroxyapatite.

The calcium analogue Strontium-89 (Metastron®) is a pure beta emitter with a maximum energy of 1,49MeV and a physical half-life of 50.5 days (2).

MATERIALS AND METHODS

In this study we evaluated the influence of Rhenium-186 (Re) and Strontium-89 (Sr) on pain relief, reduction of analgesic intake and impairment of bone marrow function. In addition we calculated the blood clearance, the excretion rate in urine and the accumulation in the bone.

We investigated 25 patients (mean age: 59 years, range: 34-74 years) with in total 30 treatments. The group of patients was made up of 4 female and 21 male patients (pts). Bone metastases orginated from breast- (4 pts), prostate- (16 pts), bladder- and in one case each from lung-, pancreatic- carcinoma and B-cell-lymphoma.

Entry criteria into the study was a positive ^{99m}Tc- HMDP bone scan consistent with a mininum of three metastases and an obvious pain symptomes, in addition a sufficient hematologic status with leukocyte count $\geq 3000/mm^3$, hemoglobin $\geq$ 6.000mmo/l, platelet count $\geq 100000/mm^3$. Chemotherapy and biphosphonate-therapy was discontinued 4 weeks before injection of the radiopharmaceutical. Patients who had pathological bone fractures, spinal cord compression or an unstable spine were rejected from the therapy.

Treatment

18 patients (pts) were treated with Rhenium-186-HEDP (doses between 1050 MBq and 1563 MBq) and 7 pts with Strontium-89 (doses between 100 and 153 MBq).
Between 3 to 11 month after the first application 5 pts received a second treatment with the same radionuclide as the preceding therapy (one with Sr-89; four with Re-186).

The pts were hospitalized two days for the Re-186-therapy. Following the administration of the radioisotope three blood samples within the first three hours were drawn and urine was collected during 48 hours after therapy, divided in 6 periods to determine the excretion rate. Four hours after injection of Rhenium the pts underwent gamma camera imaging to determine the radionuclide accumulation in the bone metastases.

The Sr-89-therapy was to treat as an outpatient. After therapy the pts were contained for 6 hr within the department.

All patients underwent a ^{99m}Tc-HMDP bone scan within 5 weeks before and 6 weeks after treatment.

Before and 6 weeks after the therapy an extended interview with a standardized package of questions concerning pain relief, analgesic intake and Karnofsky index was realized.

Blood counts were taken weekly for 6 weeks to observe the bone marrow function.

Results

The excretion rate of Re-186 in the urine was 59% of the total injected activity as an average (range: 25,6%-77,4%) during the first 48 hours. The excretion rate in the first eight hours was 36% as an average of the total injected activity (range: 17% to 59%). In the 8 to 16 hour period it decreased to 8% and from the 40th to 48th hour period to 2% [Fig.1].

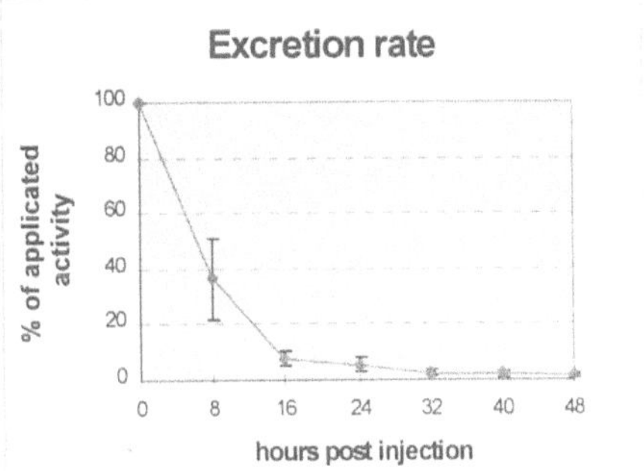

Fig. 1

The decrease of blood activity in the second hour after application was 53% (range 29% to 81%) and in the second and third hour 67% (range 40% to 97%). We could not establish a correlation between excretion rate and the slope of the blood clearance curve. These measurements were not feasible with Sr-89 due to the pure beta-emission.

Two pts with a second therapy and two other pts with only a single thearpy died during 6 weeks after treatment and four pts were lost for the follow-up, resulting in 22 complete observations periods of 6 weeks which could be evaluated.

Hematological toxicity was limited to thrombo- and leucopenia. The decline in the blood count was reversible in all the pts and no critical margin was observed.

The platelets decreased to 134.000 $\pm$ 68.000/mm^3 as an average (max. to 72.000/mm^3) during the 6 weeks and in one case only below 100.000/ mm^3 [Fig.2]. The leukocytes decreased to 4.300 $\pm$ 2.000/mm^3 as an average (max. to 2.400/ mm^3) [Fig.3]. The nadir occured between the third and the sixth week.

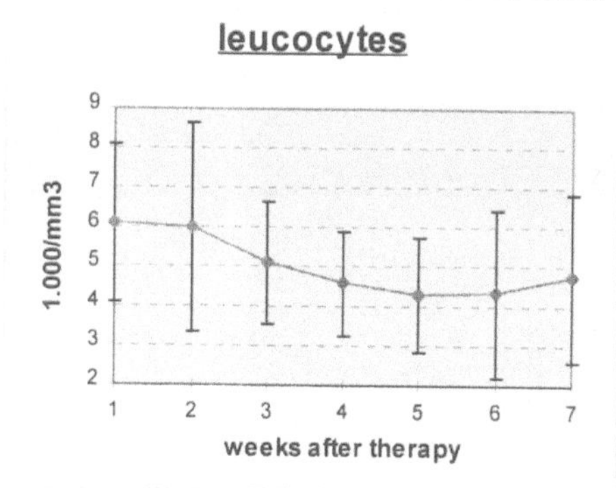

Fig. 2

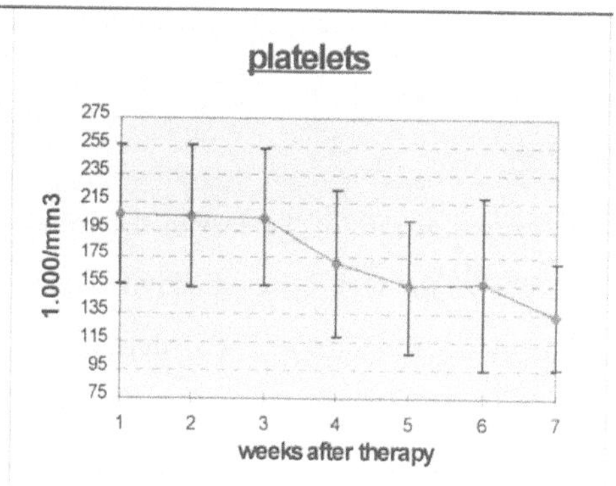

Fig. 3

The analgesic intake was able to reduce in 66% of the patients. 66% of the pts reported a considerable and 17% a minor pain relief. 77% of patients described an improvement of their life quality. We could see a raise of the Karnofsky index from 68% to 75% as an average (range: from 53 to 87% before therapy) (range: from 55% to 98% six weeks after therapy). No difference was observed between Sr- and Re-therapy.

The Tc-99-HMDP bone scan showed no major reduction of bone metastases 6 weeks after therapy in comparison to the bone scan before the therapy. In one patient we could see a reduction of bone metastases one year after the therapy. In this time the patient had not chemotherapy or radiation. The bone scan index was 42,5 before the therapy and 12,5 points one year after therapy.

The patient suffering from lymphoma had in the Re-186 scan 4 hours after application only a faint accumulation of the radiopharmaceutical in the metastases and no pain relief. The other cases showed an identical accumulation between the Re-186 scan and Tc-99m-HMDP bone scan. The bone accumulation of Re-186 was 36% in the whole body of the applied activity, with 17% in metastases as an average four hours after therapy.

Discussion

Studies form other clinics with Re-186 and Sr-89 showed an improvement of life quality in 80% of patients treated with a single injection (3,4), comparable with our results.
Thrombocytopenia proved to be the dose-limiting toxic effect, while leucopenia played a minor role (5). Our patient with a platelet decrease to 72.000/mm^3 was treated with 150 MBq of Sr-89 and had a superscan in the bone scan. The other patients showed no decrease of the platelets below 100.000/mm^3. It is describe a reversible decline in the total number of thrombocytes and leucocytes, typically with nadir at 4 to 6 weeks (5). In our study the nadir occured between the third to the sixth week. A dangerous bone marrow suppression was described in patients receiving doses up to 3515 MBq Re-186 (6). Because we applied only doses of the Re-186 between 1050 to 1563 MBq, such an obvious suppression effect is improable.

Our investigation showed, that radionuclide therapy is also useful in patients with metastases from various tumors, e.g lung carcinoma.

The relatively short physical half life of Re-186 allows higher doses compared to the long living radionuclides like Sr-89. The possibility to treat as an outpatient with Sr-89 is useful for the patients. The majority of our patients was treated with Re-186, which allows a higher dose than Sr-89.

In conclusion with this therapy regime most of our patients experienced a pain relief and an improvement of life quality without induction of serious bone marrow reduction. The radionuclide therapy is not only useful for bone metastases from prostate- and breast- cancer and also applicable for example lung-cancer. We could not establish a difference between Re-186 and Sr-89 concerning the therapy effects and a high initial urine excretion rate is no hindrance for significant pain relief.

REFERENCES

1. Campa JA, Payne R. The managment of intractable bone pain: a clinician`s perspective. Sem. Nucl. Med. 1992; No. 1: 3-10

2. Hosain F, Spencer RP. Radiopharmaceutical for pallation of metastatic osseous lessions: biologic and physical background. Sem. Nucl. Med. 1992; No. 1: 11-16

3. Maxon H, Schroder L, Hertzberg V, Thomas S, Englaro E. Rhenium-186 HEDP for treatment of painful metastases. J. Nucl. Med. 1991; 32: 1877-1881

4. Quility P, Kirk D, Bolger J, Dearnaly D. A comparison of the palliative effects of Strontium and external radiotherapy in metastatic prostata cancer. Radiother. Oncol. 1994; 33-40

5. Klerk J, Zonnenberg B, Schip A, Dijk A, Han S. Dose escalation study of Rhenium 186 HEDP in patients with metastatic prostata cancer. Eur. J. Nucl. Med. (1994) 21: 1113-1110

6. Klerk J, Schip A, Zonnenberg B, Dijk A. Evaluation of thrombocytopenia in patients treated with Rhenium-186-HEDP. J. Nucl. Med. (1994) 35: 1423-28

Radioactive Isotopes in
Clinical Medicine and Research XXIII
ed. by H. Bergmann, H. Köhn and H. Sinzinger

THE DEVELOPMENT OF CHROMATOGRAPHIC $^{188}W/^{188}Re$ GENERATORS FOR THERAPY

V.V. Basmanov, O.V. Kolesnik and N.P. Lisichkina

State Scientific Center of Russian Federation - Institute of Physics and Power Engineering, 1, Bondarenko sq, Obninsk, 249020, RUSSIA

SUMMARY: The static and dynamic adsorption processes using alumina, oxides of zirconium(IV), yttrium(III), tin(IV) and solutions of tungsten (C_W=50-1000 µg/ml) have been investigated. The obtained values of capacity varied from 1,5 to 75 mg/g adsorbent. Several rhenium-188 generators based on alumina and zirconium(IV) oxide were loaded with 370-1110 MBq high specific activity ^{188}W. Carrier-free ^{188}Re was eluted as sodium perrhenate with normal saline (3-17 ml). Tested $^{188}W/^{188}Re$ generators showed high technical performance and reliability. The next step is the development of "full-scale" clinical generators and their testing using animals.

INTRODUCTION

Rhenium-188 generator is based on tungsten-188/rhenium-188 radionuclide couple. These radionuclides have convenient nuclear and physical properties for prospective therapeutic application of ^{188}Re-based radiopharmaceuticals during several months ($T_{1/2}(^{188}W)$ = 69,4 days, $T_{1/2}(^{188}Re)$ = 16,98 hours; rhenium-188 has mixed radioactive emission - corpuscular [E_β(max)=2,1 MeV] and γ-ray [E = 155 keV] - which are applicable for therapy and simultaneous visualization of biodistribution of daughter radionuclide). The most preferable potential source of carrier-free rhenium-188 in clinics is chromatographic generator.

Mainly two different types of rhenium-188 experimental chromatographic generators are described in literature. The first type is based on adsorbents or ion-exchange resins (preferably hydrated alumina (1-5), rarely zirconium oxide (5-7), Dowex 1x8 (8) and others).The usual quantity of alumina in columns varies from 3 g (4) to 7 g (3). The dimensions of glass columns are 7-18 mm (inner diameter) and 25-100 mm (height) (2-4). However, it is necessary to use raw tungsten-188 with high specific activity (usually 3-5 Ci per g) which can be produced only in not numerous high-flux reactors for preparing the generators with clinical acceptable levels of daughter radionuclide specific concentration (no less than several mCi per ml of eluate). The second type is so called «gel» generator which includes an insoluble porous matrix - gel or salt (some chemical compounds of low specific activity tungsten-188, for example, zirconyl (9) or aluminium (10) tungstate). Both of abovementioned types of generators are usually eluted with normal saline (the volume is 10-20 ml (2-4, 9)). The activity of loaded tungsten-188 in prepared experimental generators varied from 1 to 1000 mCi (2-5, 9, 10). The performance of alumina based chromatographic generators are rather high: ^{188}Re yield is 70-80 %, radiochemical purity (the content of perrhenate-ions in the eluate) is more than 99 %, the parent breakthrough is 10^{-3} - 10^{-4} % and even less, the contents of stable impurities are at μg level.

The primary aim of this study was to develop the basis of the method of rhenium-188 generator production at IPPE. Initially there were researched the adsorption capabilities of hydrous oxides of different elements at the concentration range of tungsten aqueous solution from 50 to 1000 μg/ml in static and dynamic conditions. Then there were prepared several experimental rhenium-188 generators using ^{188}W with high specific activity and tested during their useful shelf-life.

MATERIALS AND METHODS

Adsorption experiments. Alumina for chromatography and hydrated oxide of zirconium(IV) in neutral and acidic forms, hydrated oxides of tin(IV) and yttrium(III) in acidic form were used as adsorbents. All adsorbents were the commercial products and used without any additional treatment. Particle size was about 10-30 μm. Stock aqueous solution of tungsten was prepared by tungsten(VI) oxide dissolving in excess of concentrated sodium hydroxide at heating. Tungsten concentration (C_W) was 20 mg/ml. Solutions used in adsorption experiments were prepared by diluting of the stock solution with distilled water. pH value of diluted solutions was changed by adding of HCl or HNO_3. All the reagents were chemically pure or spectral grade. Bath technique with shaking of reaction vessels (120 min^{-1}) was used for carrying out the static adsorption experiments (adsorbent : solution ratio was 1 g : 50 ml). Dynamic adsorption was researched by using a peristaltic pump which controlled the rate of solution flow and automated sampler «Yargo». The quantity of adsorbents varied from 0,5 to 4,3 g. The content of tungsten in aqueous solutions was determined photocolorimeterically with detection limit about 1 μg/ml.

Preparing and testing of rhenium-188 generators. The loading process was similar to the dynamic adsorption experiments. The construction of the generators included two consecutively connected («work» and «guard») columns which can be washed separately. The dimensions of used glass columns were 8 mm (inner diameter) and 75 mm (height). Radiation protection was ensured by using the shielded containers of indium-113m generators (GI-1 model). Tungsten-188 with high specific activity (3,7 Ci/g) was obtained from Research Institute of Atomic Reactors (Russia) in chemical form of sodium tungstate. The main radionuclide impurities were osmium-191 (0,2 %) and iridium-192 (0,01 %). The preparation of loading solution (C_W = 60-240 µg/ml) and correction of pH value were similar to described above procedures. Analyses were carried out as follows: radioactivity (^{188}W, ^{188}Re, ^{191}Os, ^{192}Ir)- using high resolution γ-spectrometry with Ge/Li detector; it was possible to detect the contents of ^{188}W, ^{192}Ir or ^{191}Os in eluates only after two or more weeks delay for complete decaying of rhenium-188; content of tungsten in aqueous solutions - by polarography; stable impurities in solutions and eluates - using atomic-absorption spectroscopy; pH - by potentiometry; radiochemical purity of sodium perrhenate (^{188}Re) - using paper chromatography. Normal saline (0,15 M NaCl) was used as eluent. The prepared generators were being eluted twice a week on regular basis during 5-9 months.

RESULTS AND DISCUSSION

Adsorption experiments. The research of tungsten hydrolysis in strong alkaline (pH 14) and acid (pH 1) solutions and neutral (pH 7) solution has shown that the stability of solutions greatly decreases at the change from alkaline to acid media. This phenomenon directly connected with polymerization of tungsten monomers in acid media (11) and formation of polytungstates at concentration levels up to about thousands µg/ml and higher. The stability of acid solutions was practically unlimited at C_W up to 200-300 µg/ml. When C_W has been increased from 300 to 2000 µg/ml the stability was observed during only approximately one-two days. So the upper concentration limit in acid solution is about 100-2000 µg/ml, in neutral and alkaline media this limit is higher (about one or two orders of magnitude).

Static adsorption experiments with chromatographic alumina, hydrous oxides of zirconium(IV), yttrium(III) and tin(IV) has shown that the capacity varied from about 1500 µg/g (Y_2O_3) and 3000-5000 µg/g (SnO_2) up to 10000-11000 µg/g

(Al_2O_3 and ZrO_2). The adsorption equilibrium with all adsorbents except tin(IV) oxide was reached in 30-60 min after the beginning of the process. In the case of SnO_2 kinetics of adsorption process was slow and within 180 min the evident equilibrium was not noted. According to the results of experiments at different temperatures (20-80 °C) it can be assumed that the adsorption mechanism for all adsorbents is limited by both diffusion and chemical factors and the first factor is predominant.

Subsequent dynamic adsorption studies were carried out using only the most prospective adsorbents - Al_2O_3 and ZrO_2. The summary of obtained results is presented in the Table 1.

Table 1. Dynamic adsorption capacity of chromatographic alumina and hydrous zirconium(IV) oxide at room temperature

Adsorbent	C_W, μg/ml	pH of solution	Capacity, μg/g
ZrO_2 (neutral)	240	8,3	5500 ± 500
ZrO_2 (acidic)	132	2,4	3700 ± 400
	500	2,3	5400 ± 500
	1000	3	5200 ± 500
Al_2O_3 (neutral)	240	8,3	1300 ± 100
Al_2O_3 (acidic)	500	3	62000 ± 2000
	1000	3	75000 ± 2000

According to the given data acidic alumina is more preferable for the generators preparation than zirconium(IV) oxide. Discrepancy between the values of static and dynamic adsorption found for alumina is explained by the difference in initial concentration of tungsten solutions used in those studies.

Preparing and testing of rhenium-188 generators. Al_2O_3 and ZrO_2 in neutral and acidic forms only were used for manufacturing the experimental rhenium-188 generators. The general information about prepared generators is collected in the Table 2.

Table 2. Several characteristics of experimental rhenium-188 generators

N	Adsorbent of «work» column; quantity, g	Adsorbent of «guard» column; quantity, g	Activity of adsorbed tungsten, mCi	Structure of tungsten adsorption zone in «work» column
1	ZrO_2 (neutral); 2,7	ZrO_2 (neutral); 2,2	28	full length
2	ZrO_2 (acidic); 4,3	ZrO_2 (acidic); 3,6	24	full length
3	Al_2O_3 (neutral); 2,6	Al_2O_3 (neutral); 2,1	17	full length
4	Al_2O_3 (acidic); 2,5	Al_2O_3 (acidic); 2,0	22	initial section
5	Al_2O_3 (acidic); 2,1	Al_2O_3 (acidic); 2,0	12	initial section

All prepared generators demonstrated good technical performance. Elution processes using evacuated vials and technical maintenance were very easy and simple.

Several important parameters of quality registered during period of 5-9 months are summarized in the Table 3.

Table 3. Yield of ^{188}Re and contents of main radionuclide impurities in rhenium-188 generators

N	Yield of ^{188}Re		Content of ^{188}W		Content of ^{192}Ir	
	«work»[a]	tandem[b]	«work»	tandem	«work»	tandem
1	64-71	51-60	$(8\div20)\cdot10^{-3}$	$(5\div80)\cdot10^{-6}$	$(2\div3)\cdot10^{-4}$	$(2\div5)\cdot10^{-5}$
2	85-95	85-90	$(2\div40)\cdot10^{-3}$	$(8\div30)\cdot10^{-6}$	$(4\div20)\cdot10^{-4}$	$(8\div20)\cdot10^{-6}$
3	64-68	55-60	$(7\div76)\cdot10^{-2}$	$(5\div40)\cdot10^{-5}$	$(2\div4)\cdot10^{-3}$	$(3\div9)\cdot10^{-4}$
4	85-95	80-90	$(2\div10)\cdot10^{-4}$	$(2\div70)\cdot10^{-6}$	$(3\div8)\cdot10^{-4}$	$(4\div10)\cdot10^{-5}$
5	85-95	80-90	$(8\div20)\cdot10^{-4}$	$(3\div10)\cdot10^{-5}$	$(2\div4)\cdot10^{-3}$	$(2\div8)\cdot10^{-4}$

a - elution of the «work» column only
b - elution of the «work» and «guard» columns consecutively connected

The radiochemical purity was more than 99 %, values of pH were 2,5-4,7 for acidic adsorbents and 4,4-8,0 for neutral ones. The contents of stable impurities were as follows: Al ≤ 5-10 μg/ml (acidic) or ≤ 2,5 μg/ml (neutral); Zr ≤ 0,5 μg/ml and W ≤ 2,5 μg/ml after a month of eluting, Fe ≤ 1-2,5 μg/ml. The generators 1-3 can be completely eluted with 3 ml saline («work») or 8-10 ml (tandem) while the same parameters for the generators 4 and 5 were 7 and 17 ml correspondingly. The yield of ^{188}Re was 15-25 % higher for acidic adsorbents and slightly decreased when the «guard» columns had been connected (at 5-10 %). The efficiency of ZrO_2 as the «guard» adsorbent was better than Al_2O_3.

CONCLUSION

As the results of developed research the main dependence of rhenium-188 generators preparation has been clarified. Data of adsorption processes helped to fabricate several experimental generators which showed quite high technical performance and quality of eluates during 5-9 months. The present study information obtained will allow to prepare soon «full-scale» clinical generators and to begin the tests with animals

REFERENCES

1. Klofutar C, Krasovec F, Kodre A. Radiochemical separation of rhenium(VII) from tungsten(VI). J Radioanal Chem 1970; 5: 3-10.

2. Gureev E, Brodskaya G, Islamov T. The method of production of rhenium-188 generator. The USSR invent. certif. [1] 1665826, Int. Cl. G21G 4/00, date of filling Jan.15 1987. (In Russian).

3. Brodskaya G, Gureev E, Gapurova O. The method of production of rhenium-188 generator. Patent of the USSR [1] 1824011, Int. Cl. G21G 4/04, date of filling Dec.14 1989. (In Russian).

4. Callahan AP, Rice DE, Knapp FF Jr. Rhenium-188 for therapeutic applications from an alumina based tungsten-188/^{188}Re radionuclide generator. NucCompact-Eur/Am Commun Nucl Med 1989; 20: 3-6.

5. Knapp FF Jr, Mirzadeh S. The continuing important role of radionuclide generator systems for nuclear medicine. Eur J Nucl Med 1994; 20: 1151-1165.

6. Plotnikov V, Kochetkov V. About the process of separation of little quantity of tungsten and rhenium with using of zirconium hydroxide. J Anal Chem (Russ.) 1966; 11: 1260-1261 (In Russian).

7. Callahan AP, Rice DE, Knapp FF Jr. Availability of ^{188}Re from a tungsten-188/^{188}Re radionuclide generator system for therapeutic applications [abstract]. J Nucl Med 1987; 28: 657.

8. Blachot J, Herment J, Moussa A. Un generateur de ^{188}Re a partir de ^{188}W. Int J Appl Radiat and Isot 1969; 20: 467-471.

9. Ehrhardt G, Ketring A, Turpin T, Razavi M, Vanderheyden J-L, Fu S-M, Fritzberg A. A convenient tungsten-188/rhenium-188 generator for radio-therapeutic applications using low specific activity tungsten-188. In: Technetium and rhenium in chemistry and nuclear medicine 3. Nicolini M, Brandoli G. editors. New York: Corina International-Raven Press, 1990: 631-634.

10. Vanderheyden J-L, Fu-Min Su. Radionuclide generator system and method for its preparation and use. Pat US N 4990787, Int. Cl. C01G 47/00, date of filling Sep.29 1989.

11. Tytko K-H, Glemster O. Isopolymolybdates and isopolytungstates. Adv Inorg Chem Radiochem 1976; 19: 239-315.

RADIOPHARMACOLOGY

Radioactive Isotopes in
Clinical Medicine and Research XXIII
ed. by H. Bergmann, H. Köhn and H. Sinzinger

EVALUATION OF mRNA TARGETING BY LABELED OLIGONUCLEOTIDES FOR TUMOR-DIAGNOSIS

J. Muth, H. Schirrmeister, B. Römer, I. Buchmann, S.N. Reske

Department of Nuclear Medicine
89081 Ulm Germany

SUMMARY: Synthetic antisense oligonucleotides which are labeled with radioactive isotopes may offer the possibility of specific *in vivo* detection of cancer associated mRNA based on Watson-Crick base pairing. As cancer model for follicular non-Hodgkin lymphomas an adjustable Bcl-2 expression system, which can produce Bcl-2 mRNA in high amounts, was chosen. A series of oligonucleotides was evaluated with this test cell line.

INTRODUCTION

Radiolabeled antisense oligonucleotides may offer the possibility of specific *in vivo* detection of cancer associated mRNA based on Watson-Crick base pairing. For this purpose a series of oligonucleotides containing phosphate modifications like phosphorothioates and normal internucleotide linkages was synthesized according to the phosphoramidite procedure. The substitution of oxygen against sulfur and phenyl-groups results in properties such as higher stability against nucleases, enhanced cell membrane permeability and higher stability compared to methylphosphonates. For this purpose a new class of phosphoramidites was synthesized. As cancer model for follicular non-Hodgkin lymphomas an adjustable Bcl-2 expression system, which can produce Bcl-2 mRNA in high amounts, was chosen. Our goal of this work was to investigate the interaction of oligonucleotides with complementary mRNA in this Bcl-2 adjustable system.

MATERIALS

For our purpose a series of ODN containing unmodified internucleotide linkages, phosphorothioates and phenylphosponate linkages were synthesized according the phosphoramidite method (1 μmole scale, Table 1). This include unmodified ODNs (**1**, **2**), ODNs (**10-12**) which are endcapped with one phosphorothioate linkages at the 3′ and 5′-end position (**PS**), ODNs modified a primary amino-group (**Amino**) *via* a special phosphoramidite (**3-9**) (PerSeptive) or a special CPG-support (**13-15**) (Clontech). To enhance the membrane permeability some oligodeoxynucleotides were synthesized with alternating phenylphosphonate linkages (**Ph**). As target site within the sequence of Bcl-2 we used the translation start site (ATG-codon, 18-20 nt, Cotter 1994). All oligodeoxynucleotides were purified with RP-HPLC. Buffers for RP HPLC were 0.1 M triethylammonium acetate (pH 7.25) containing 5-25 % CH_3CN in 40 minutes (ODN **1**, **2** **10-15**) or 0-50 % CH_3CN in 30 minutes (**3-9**). To obtain the phenylphosphoramidites the protected nucleosides of A, C, T, G were phosphitilated with 3 eq. for 3 days with a new synthesized phosphitilation reagent. After HPLC purification the oligonucleotides were labeled with ^{32}P and ^{125}I.

No	Sequence	Typ
1	5′-TAC-CGC-GTG-CGA-CCC-TCT-3′	(Inverse)
2	5′-TCT-CCC AGC GTG CGC-CAT-3′	(Antisense)
3	5′-**Amino**-TAC-CGC-GTG-CGA-CCC-T$_{Ph}$C$_{Ph}$T-3′	(Inverse)
4	5′-**Amino**-TGC ACT CAC GCT CGG C$_{Ph}$C$_{Ph}$T	(Scramble)
5	5′-**Amino**- TCT-CCC AGC GTG CGC-C$_{Ph}$A$_{Ph}$T	(Antisense)
6	5′-**Amino**-TGC A$_{Ph}$CT CA$_{Ph}$C GCT$_{Ph}$ CGG CC$_{Ph}$T	(Scramble)
7	5′-**Amino**- TCT$_{Ph}$-CCC A$_{Ph}$GC GTG C$_{Ph}$GC-CA$_{Ph}$T	(Antisense)
8	5′-**Amino**- TCT$_{Ph}$-CCC A$_{Ph}$GC GT$_{Ph}$G C$_{Ph}$GC-CA$_{Ph}$T	(Antisense)
9	5′-**Amino**-TAC-C$_{Ph}$GC-GT$_{Ph}$G-CG$_{Ph}$-CCC-TC$_{Ph}$T-3′	(Inverse)
10	5′-A$_{ps}$TG GCC CAC GCT-GGG-AGA-A$_{ps}$C-3′	(Sense)
11	5′-T$_{ps}$AC-CGT-GTG-CGA-CCC-TCT-T$_{ps}$G-3′	(Scramble)
12	5′-G$_{ps}$TTCT-CCC AGC GTG CGC-CA$_{ps}$T-3′	(Antisense)
13	5′-A$_{ps}$TG GCC CAC GCT-GGG-AGA-A$_{ps}$C-**Amino**-3′	(Sense)
14	5′-T$_{ps}$AC-CGT-GTG-CGA-CCC-TCT-T$_{ps}$G- **Amino**-3′	(Scramble)
15	5′-G$_{ps}$TTCT-CCC AGC GTG CGC-CA$_{ps}$T- **Amino** -3′	(Antisense

Table 1: Synthesized oligodeoxynucleotides

The labeling reaction was performed in 20 μL reaction volume containing 10 units Polynucleotidekinase, 2 μL of oligonucleotide with free 5′ hydroxylgroup (20 picomoles), 2 μL Phosphorylation buffer (10x) puffer 5 μL γ-^{32}P-ATP-(≈50 μCi) and 10 μL H_2O. After incubation for 1 h at 37 °C the reaction mixture was purified by spin column purification (Sephadex G-25). Oligonucleotides which are modified with a primary amino group at the 3′-or 5′-end are suitable for labeling *via* a ^{125}I-labeled derivate of hyaluronic acid. For this purpose 1 A_{260} U of the modified oligonucleotide (**8**, **9**, **13**, **14**, **15**) was incubated under stirring for 4 hours with 30 µL of Bolton-Hunter reagent (80-160 µCi, Amersham, ICN) in Borate Buffer (pH 9) at 4 °C. After cleaning up by spin column purification the labeled oligonucleotide was used for *in vivo* studies.

In vitro transcription of Bcl-2 Sense mRNA.: Plasmid pB4 (ATCC: 798051) was opened with restriction enzyme *Eco*RI. One cDNA insert (932 bp,) which carries a part of Bcl-2 DNA was cloned into the opened plasmid (pSPT 18). The orientation of this integrated insert was checked by a double digest with *Pvu*II and *Bam* HI) on an agarose gel (1 %). This new plasmid carries both promotors SP6 and T7 and can generate RNA transcripts in sense or antisense orientation. After linearization with *Pvu* II (10 units) the RNA transcription was performed in 20 µL volume containing 1 µL T7 RNA polymerase (10 units), 11 µL H_2O, 2 µL reaction buffer (10x), 4 µL nucleotide triphosphates (10 mM A, G, C, U triphosphates), 1 µL RNase (20 units) inhibitor. After incubation for 1 hour at 37 °C and DNase I digestion at 37 °C for 45 minutes the mixture was cleaned up by spin column purification (Sephadex G-50) and precipitated in sodium acetate and ethanol. 1 µg of the RNA was incubated -in buffer containing 100 mM NaCl, 10 mM TrisHCl (pH 7.5) separately for 1 hour at 37 °C with each labeled oligonucleotide (antisense ODN **2** and control-ODN **1**). The reaction mixture was analyzed on a 20 % PAA gel.

mRNA isolation with Oligo dT 25 -Beads (Dynal): 5-8 x 10^6 cells of BH2-HeLa (Tet off™) cells were cultivated in DME-media at 37 °C (5 % CO_2) overnight. After removing the media the cells were washed with PBS-solution and harvested with 10 mL TEN-solution. After centrifugation for 5 minutes at 1800 rpm the pellet was treated with Lysis-Binding buffer and was given to 80 µL (0.4 mg) of the Oligo dT25-Beads solution. The beads were washed (2 x) with LiDS/washing buffer and (1x) with washing buffer. The bounded RNA was eluted after incubation with elution buffer at 65 °C for 2 minutes. The RNA was analyzed on 5 % PAA-gel.

Oligonucleotide-uptake: 5-8x 10^6 cells BH2 HeLa (Tet off™) cells were cultivated in the presence with the labeled oligodeoxynucleotides (**1**, **2**, **6**, **8**, **9** **10-15**, antisense-ODNs, control-ODNs, labeled with ^{32}P or ^{125}I) overnight. The cells were washed with PBS-solution (three times. harvested and lysed with 1.3 mL TRIzol® GIBCO (3x 100 µL of this solution was counted). 200 µL chloroform was added and mixture was centrifuged for 10 min (13000 rpm). The upper phase was mixed again with 200 µL chloroform and the separation was repeated. The RNA in the water phase was precipitated with 500 µL isopropanol at -20 °C for 1 hour. After centrifugation for 20 minutes (13000 rpm) the RNA pellet was washed with 1 mL ice cold ethanol and dried and counted. The phenol phase was centrifuged with 1 mL ethanol for 5 minutes (7000 rpm). The protein phase (upper phase) was separated and precipitated with 500 μL isopropanol. After incubation at RT for 10 minutes the mixture was centrifuged for 5 minutes (10000 rpm). The protein pellet was washed three times for 20 minutes with 0.3 M guanidinium HCl /95 % ethanol and dried. The DNA pellet was washed two times with 0.1 M sodiumcitrate/10 % ethanol for 30 minutes. After washing with ethanol the pellet was centrifuged and dried. Note all solutions which we have used were counted by a γ-Counter (^{125}I, Packard) or β-Counter (^{32}P, LKB). The recovery of the used activity was recalculated (Table 2).

RESULTS AND DISCUSSION

Finally the modified oligonucleotides could be synthesizesed on a 1 μmole scale with coupling average higher 98 % by using the phenylamidites of A, C and T. The phenylphosphon-amidites for the modified probes were obtained by functionalization of the 3′OH group of the protected nucleosides with a new Phenyl-phosphitylation reagent, yielding the phenyldiisopropyl phosphoramidites (A,C,T;>60%, ^{31}P-NMR >95%). The synthesis of the amidite of G failed caused by a side reaction at the O^6 position of G. To evaluate the RNA target site a RNA fragment was produced by *in vitro* transcription with T7 polymerase. The RNA fragments were hybridized with a ^{32}P labeled oligo-probes (antisense ODN **2** and a control ODN **1**)

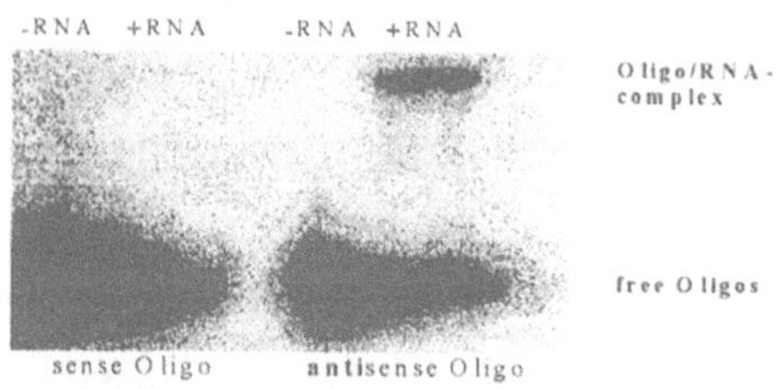

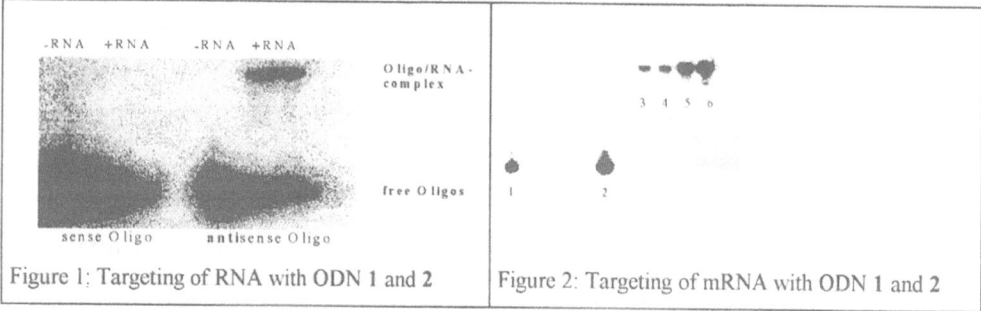

Figure 1: Targeting of RNA with ODN 1 and 2

Figure 2: Targeting of mRNA with ODN 1 and 2

After 1 hour incubation time the mixture was analyzed on a 20 % PAA gel. In Figure **1** lane 2 shows that no interaction of a control ODN **1** with the target RNA occured. lane 4 cleary demonstrate the high specifity of the antisense ODN **2** with the target RNA transcript. Note in lane 4 the excess of probes can be seen at at the bottom of the gel. lane 1 and 3 represent both ^{32}P labeled ODNs (**1**, **2**). A series of experiments were conducted to demonstrate the interaction between labeled probes *in vivo* mRNA (Figure 2). For this purpose we isolated the Bcl-2 mRNA from cells which were cultivated in presence of doxicyclin in the media. Both labeled probes (**1, 2,** ^{32}P; lane 1, 2) were hybridized with the bound mRNA. The antisense probe shows in this *in vitro* experiment high affinity (more than 8 times, lane 6) to target mRNA of the Bcl-2 overexpression system compared to control cells without induced Bcl-2 expression (lane 4). We obtained similar results by incubating the probes overnight (16 h) with the cells. In case of the control probe **1** we got comparable results with the antisense probe **2** (lane 5 and 3) and we believe that this can be caused caused by the high G/C content of the mRNA (66 %). The experiments with the unmodified oligonucleotides **1** and **2** and both cell typs no significant hybridization with the RNA was observable. (5 %) In the case of the endcapped probes ODN **10-11** the ratio between Bcl-2 producing cells and controls the amount of bounded activity on the RNA increased dramatically dependent on the modification. So the activity in the RNA -fraction increasesed from ≈6 (5) % ODN **1-2**) to ≈12 (23 %,ODN **10-12**) for low(high) Bcl-2 expression. In the case of high Bcl-2

ODN	RNA %	DNA %	Protein %	Uptake%	Recovery%	
1	6.9 (5.2)	22.3 (23.1)	0.5 (0.3)	28.7 (26.2)	84.7 (82.7)	
2	7.5 (5.3)	18.0 (21.9)	0.7 (0.4)	31.7 (31.7)	85.5 (84.7)	
10	12.2 (25.5)	5.4 (11.6)	0.3 (0.1)	16 (24.5)	85 (84.5)	
11	13.4 (23.6)	4.2 (22.7)	0.4 (0.2)	15 (20)	94.5 (92.5)	
12	14.5 (23.2)	5.5 (11.8)	0.6 (0.2)	17.5 (22.5)	90 (81)	
13	49.5 (60.4)	12 (14.4)	2.6 (0.5)	4 (13.5)	86.5 (77.5)	
	6.9 (3.7)*	2.9 (3.2)*	5.3 (5.0)*	1 (<1)	125 (101.5)	
	3.5 (0.26)*		3.1 (2.17)*	1 (<1)	118 (100)	
14	26.6 (63.8)	20.5 (40.6)	0.2 (0.1)	6 (11.5)	88.5 (84.5)	
	13.1 (1.8)*	1.9 (1.37)*	2.3 (2.8)*	2.5 (1)	109 (84.5)	
	10.0 (4.3)*		5.9 (6.9)*	1 (1)	114 (102)	
15	31.5 (64.0)	4.9 (15.3)	1.4 (0.1)	4 (12.5)	88 (92.5)	
	11.0 (4.1)*	12.2 (10.1)*	17.1 (19.7)*	2 (1)	109 (99)	
	5.6 (0.8)*		1.4 (12.4)*	2.5 (<1) *	110 (94) *	
8	0.8 (0.6)*	11.3 (8.2)*	15.9 (6.2)*	2 (2) *	nd	
9	1.2 (0.4)*	7.2 (3.8)*	25.8 (6.6)*	1.5 (2) *	104 (106)*	*labeled mit ^{125}I
						( ) Bcl-2 +

Table 2: Cellular uptake and distribution into RNA, DNA, protein

expression the activity reached a level of until ≈60 % for the high stabilized amino-modified ODN (**13-15**). This effect can be explained by a different metabolish rate of free phosphate dependent of the 3′-modification. Only a minor amount could be measured in the protein fraction. After labeling *via* Bolton Hunter the uptake of the oligonucleotides decreased (similar to FDG), this can be caused by the steric modification of the 3′-termius. The lipophilicity of the phenylphosphonate modified oligonucleotides (ODN **8**, **9**) was extremly enhanced which caused difficulties during the separation procedure.

CONCLUSION

1.) Phosphorothioates, Phenyl -and amino-modified ODN′s were synthesized with high chemical yields. 2.) Published biological active ODN′s directed against Bcl-2 sequence may possess a high degree of unspecific Bcl-2 hybridization. 3.) Cellular uptake and distribution into RNA, DNA, protein and supernatant is dependant on: radioactive label, ODN-modification, Bcl-2 expression, possibly metabolic dephosphorylation and ^{32}P utlilization and not dependant on sequence specifity of the ODN. 4.) ^{32}P radiolabel is not useful for uptake and distribution studies. 5.) More specific target sequence of Bcl-2 is needed.

ACKNOWLEDGEMENTS

We would like to acknowledge the BMFT (D.0602) for support of this research. We would like to thank Dr. S Cunningham (Clontech) for the donation of the BH2 cells.

REFERENCES

1. Yin D., Schimke R.(1995) Cancer Research 55 4922-4928
2. Cotter F., Johnson P.,Hall P., Pocock C. (1994), Oncogene 9 (10) 3049-3055

Radioactive Isotopes in
Clinical Medicine and Research XXIII
ed. by H. Bergmann, H. Köhn and H. Sinzinger

SYNTHESIS AND EVALUATION OF [^{123}I]IODOAMINOGLUTETHIMIDE, A LIGAND FOR VISUALIZATION OF THE AROMATASE ENZYME BY SPECT

F. De Vos, G. Slegers, C. Van de Wiele and R.A. Dierckx

Department of Radiopharmacy, University of Ghent; Harelbekestraat 72, B-9000 Ghent, Belgium and Department of Nuclear Medecin, University Hospital, De Pintelaan 185, B-9000 Ghent, Belgium

SUMMARY: The radiosynthesis of [^{123}]iodaminoglutethimide (I-123 IAG), an analogue of aminoglutethmide, and possible tracer for visualization of the aromatase enzyme complex by SPECT is described. I-123 IAG was synthesized by electrophilic substitution of aminoglutethimide with n.c.a. [^{123}I]NaI. High specific activities were obtained (315 Gbq/mg - 8.5Ci/mg). Biodistribution studies with female NMRI mice were undertaken. High accumulation of radioactivity in liver and intestines were observed, indicating the important biliary clearance of the radioligand. The high gonades to blood and muscle ratios reflected the high aromatase activities in these organs.

INTRODUCTION

Estrogens are produced by the conversion of androgens by the aromatase complex, an enzyme complex situated in the endoplasmic reticulum. In premenopausal women the ovarian follicle is mainly responsible for the production of estrogens by stimulation of LH and FSH (1). In postmenopausal women the synthesis of estrogens takes mainly place in adipose tissue but also in liver and muscle (2).

Different studies found aromatase activity in cancerous and normal glandular breast, the former 8 times higher than in normal tissue (3-4). Furthermore, clinical studies suggest that breast cancers with high aromatase activity respond better to treatment with aromatase inhibitors such as aminoglutethimide, than tumors with undetectable aromatase activity. Thus theoretically the visualization of intratumoral aromatase activity might allow prediction of respons to therapy in aminoglutethimide treated breast carcinoma patients. In order to provide imaging agents for the aromatase complex, the authors have developed [^{123}I]iodoaminoglutethimide (I-123 IAG) as possible ligand for the aromatase complex. I-123 IAG has been prepared for in vivo characterisation of aromatase positive breast carcinomas and for the prediciton of the efficiency of future aminoglutethimide therapy in patients.

MATERIAL AND METHODS

The synthesis of I-123 IAG is shown in Fig. 1. 74 Mbq (2 mCi) n.c.a. [^{123}I]NaI was added to a mixture of 0.8 μmol aminoglutethimde and 30 μl 0.25M phosphate buffer pH 2.5. Then 1.6 μmol chloramine-T dissolved in 10μl acetone was addded to the solution. The reaction proceeded at room temperature for 2 min and was subsequently stopped by the addition of 10 μl 1M sodiummetabisulphite. The pH was set at 7.0 with 1 M NaOH and the reaction mixture was diluted with water to 100 μl. Purification was done by HPLC on a RP C-18 nucleosphere column (150 mm x 4.6 mm, 3 μm particle size) while UV absorption was measured at 242 nm (2.0 A.U.) and radioactivity by gamma counting with NaI(Tl). The eluent consisted of 0.01M phosphate buffer pH 6.8 and ethanol (30/70 v/v). The radioactivity fraction corresponding to I-123 IAG was collected and sterilised by filtration (0.22 μm).

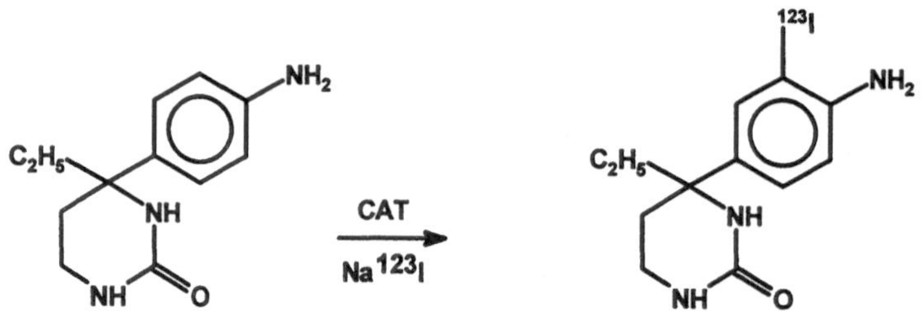

Fig. 1.: Radiosynthesis of I-123 IAG

Chemical and radiochemical purity was determined by HPLC. The mobile phase consisted of a mixture of acetonitrile and 0.01M phosphate buffer pH 6.8 (48/52 v/v). Detection was done by UV at 242 nm (range 0.010 A.U.) and by NaI(Tl).

Twenty-seven female mice (n=3 per time point, strain NMRI, 20-25 g body weight) were injected intravenously (i.v.) via tail vein with 185 Kbq (5μCi) of I-123IAG, dissolved in

100µl phosphate buffer pH 6.8, containing 5% of ethanol. The animals were anesthesized and killed by decapitation at preset time points (Table 1) after administration of the tracer. The blood was collected. The organs were rapdily removed, washed with 0.9% saline, and weighed. Radioactivity was counted and corrected for physcial decay and geometry. Results are expressed as percent injected dose per gran tissue (% ID/g). For the excretion percent injected dose (% ID) values are used.

RESULTS AND DISCUSSION

The reaction between aminoglutethimide and n.c.a. [^{123}I]NaI led to I-123 IAG. The radiosynthesis was realized by an electrophilic substitution of aminoglutethimide with ^{123}I, using chloramine-T as oxidizing agent and a water/acetone mixture as reaction solvent (Fig. 1). The presence of an amino function, which promotes electrophilic substitution in ortho and para position, makes direct iodination the method of choice for the production of I-123 IAG. As the para position to the amino functional group in aminoglutethimide is already occupied, the ortho substituted iodo analogue of aminoglutethimide was the only product formed. The reaction proceeded very fast at room temperature and radiochemical yields of 85% within 2 min were obtained under the described conditions. The small reaction volume (< 100 µl) made purification on an analytical column possible. HPLC purification gave pure I-123 IAG. I-123 IAG (Rt = 11.5 min) was separated from aminoglutethimide (Rt = 4.3 min) and the other reagents in the reaction mixture (Rt < 6 min).

Radiochemical purity was higher than 99%. Carrier iodoaminoglutethimide was lower than the detection limit (100 ng/ml). Starting from 74 Mbq N.c.a. [^{123}I]NaI specific activities of at least 315 Gbq/mg (8.5Ci/mg) were obtained.

The distribution of ^{123}I activity in mice in the various organs is shown in Table 1. From these results it is clear that the radioactivity was rapidly distributed in the body. Five minutes post injection only 4.14% ID/g remained in the blood compartment. This was reflected by a rapid and high uptake in liver (up to 27.01% ID/g at 5 min p.i.), and a rapid decline in heart,

Table 1. Biodistribution of radioactivity in mice after i.v. injection with 185kbq (5μCi) of I-123 IAG*.

	Time (min)								
	5	15	30	60	120	180	360	720	1440
Blood	4.14	3.37	2.12	1.68	1.31	0.70	0.23	0.29	0.02
Liver	27.0	22.4	15.4	11.3	8.49	4.96	1.66	1.45	0.10
Small intestine	10.6	9.95	29.0	67.2	45.1	11.8	6.90	3.13	0.11
Large intestine	5.95	4.29	3.13	1.81	11.7	15.4	5.85	3.13	0.15
Lungs	8.47	7.15	5.14	3.03	2.27	0.91	0.22	0.22	0.03
Heart	8.36	5.89	3.96	1.90	1.50	0.73	0.19	0.13	0.03
Gonades	10.2	7.92	4.80	4.16	2.19	0.83	0.27	0.34	0.06
Muscle	4.49	4.59	2.23	1.75	1.10	0.50	0.18	0.21	0.03
Excretion	0	1.30	11.1	12.8	15.6	52.6	75.5	89.7	98.5

*Results for the various organs are expressed as % injected dose/g tissue (%ID/g). Units for excretion are % injected dose (%ID). The values are corrected for physical decay and geometry.

lungs and kidney activities. The uptake in the liver was followed by a moderate decrease, while the activity in the intestines increased up to 67.22% ID/g for the small intestine at 1h p.i. This typical profile of high accumulation in the liver followed by a transit through the small intestine and large intestine, suggests the major importance of biliary excretion. The high gonades (uterus and ovaria) to blood and muscle ratios (2.27 to 2.48) are a reflection of the high concentrations of the aromatase enzyme in these organs. The low accumulation in the heart and lungs, (< than 2.18% ID/g at 60 min p.i.) are promising for the detection of the aromatase enzyme in breast carcinoma by SPECT. The radioactivity was rapidly cleared from the body. At 12h and 24h, respectively 89.7% ID and 98.5% ID were excreted by urinary and fecal excretion. No accumulation was observed in any tissue.

CONCLUSION

We have developed a radiosynthesis for the production of I-123 IAG, a possible ligand for visualization of the aromatase compex by SPECT. Further experiments in nude mice, bearing aromatase positive and negative tumors will prove the specificity of I-123 IAG and its potential as imaging agent for the aromatase complex in vivo by SPECT

REFERENCES

1. Sasano H, Okamoto M, Mason JI, Sipson ER, Mendelson Cr, Sasano N, Silverberg SC. Immunolocalization of aromatase, 17α-hydroxlase and side-chain cleavage cytochromes P-450 in human ovary. J reprod Fertil 1989; 85:163-169.

2. Santen RJ. Potential clincial use of new aromatase inhibitors. Steroids 1987; 50:575-583.

3. Vermeulen A, Delsypere JP, Paridaens R, Leclercq G, Roy F, Heuson JC. Aromatase 17β-hydroxysteroid dehydrogenase and intratissular sex hormone concentrations in cancerous and normal glandular breast tissue in postmenopausal women. Eur J Cancer Clin Oncol 1986; 22:515-525.

4. Miller Wr, O'Neil J. The significance of steroid metabolism in human cancer. J Steroid Biochem Mol Biol. 1990;37:317-325.

Radioactive Isotopes in
Clinical Medicine and Research XXIII
ed. by H. Bergmann, H. Köhn and H. Sinzinger

COMPARATIVE ANALYSIS OF KINETIC MODELS TO STUDY GLUCOSE METABOLISM OF THE BRAIN

Z.T. Krasznai, L. Balkay, T. Márián, M. Emri, F. Németh and L. Trón

PET Centre, University Medical School Debrecen, and PET Study Group of the Hungarian Academy of Sciences, Poroszlay u 6, Debrecen, 4026, Hungary

SUMMARY: In vivo glucose metabolism of the brain was examined using the [^{18}F] fluoro-deoxy-D-glucose (FDG) analogue of the glucose. A relatively high number (20-25) of volumes of interest (VOI) were defined on the PET images. Data of the kinetic studies belonging to these VOI-s were evaluated using the standard uptake value (SUV) method, or calculating glucose metabolic rate (GMR) applying Patlak analysis (PA); and three-compartment model with nonlinear regression (TCM). Correlation of data for all pairs of calculated parameters showed that accurate determination of glucose utilisation in anatomic regions of white matter and those located next to large blood vessels require application of the three-compartment tracer kinetic model calculations with no simplifying assumptions.

INTRODUCTION

A unique feature of PET is the possibility for the in vivo quantification of tissue radioactivity converting these data into quantitized parameters of biochemical or physiological processes. The majority of methods allowing quantification require a dynamic set of tomographic images accurately corrected for tissue attenuation. The quantitation methods used in the different laboratories differ from each other. Using kinetic modell calculations there are still alternative procedures available. It has been proposed that the assumption on a negligible FDG dephosphorylation rate cannot be consistent with a correct quantitation of experimental data(1). Similarly, it was also suggested that the contribution of the activity in the vascular compartment to that measured tissue activity has to be taken into account. Here we present the results of a detailed analysis of the same set of experimental data using different quantitation methods. A detailed analysis of the same set of experimental data using different quantitation methods. A systematic comparison of results obtained by quantitation of the same primary data using different methods can be instrumental in choosing the most appropriate procedure.

MATERIALS AND METHODS

The quantitative PET measurements were made on a GE 4096 Plus whole body positron camera with 5mm in-plane resolution and 6.5mm inter-slice distance. The axial field of view of the camera is 103mm. The camera produced 15 transaxial slices of the brain. The PET investigation was performed on three healthy elderly subjects with no signes of structural or functional brain lesions. 18F-deoxy-D-glucose (FDG) was used as tracer, which was given as a bolus injection (10 sec) in the right or left cubital vein (administered activity: 0.15 mCi/kg in 5 ml physiological salt solution). Data acquisition with PET camera and blood sampling started parallel with the bolus injection. The PET images were reconstructed with a Hanning filter (width=4.5 mm) using attenuation correction obtained from a separate transmission scan. We have defined approximately 130 ROI's on the 15 slices of each PET image, but since anatomic structures appear on more than a single slice, finally 20-25 volumes of interests (VOI) per person have been used according to the major anatomic structures of the brain.

SUV values (2) were calculated as the ratio of the activity concentration within a defined VOI accumulated during a set time interval and the injected dose per body weight of the subject. Accordingly, SUV (40-60) refers to a SUV value calculated from the counts acquired between 40 min and 60 min following the injection of the tracer.

Glucose metabolic rate (GMR) calculations based on the three-compartment (3,4) model (TCM) were carried out using MATLAB to solve the set of differential equations describing the transport of FDG between the intravasal, the exchangeable intracellular (and intracellular) and the metabolic compartments using the appropriate kinetic constants k_1, k_2, k_3, and k_4. Contributions to the measured tissue activity concentration are described by three additive terms: activity concentration in the exchangeable and metabolic compartments and the product of the activity concentration measured in the intravasal compartment and V_0, a localization dependent proportionality factor (5).

A fairly rapid calculation of GMR (Patlak method) can be applied if one is not interested in numerical values of the rate constants and if $k_4=0$ may be assumed according to (6).

RESULTS AND DISCUSSION

Numerical value of the SUV was calculated for all VOI using acquisition times 40 to 50 min, 40 to 60 min, 45 to 55 min, 45 to 60 min and 50 to 60 min. Correlation of any two out of this five SUV parameters were found to be linear with a very high correlation coefficient ($R^2>0.99$

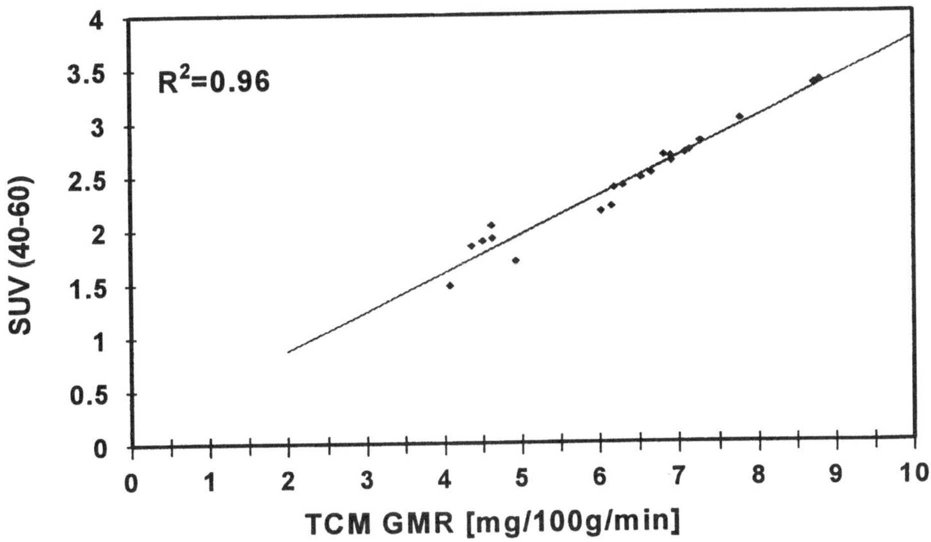

Figure 1. A representative correlation of GMR data calculated by the TCM and SUV data

for each cases). In addition, all regression lines had a zero intercept. Thus, for relative measurements all kind of SUV parameters, e.g. SUV(40-50) or SUV(45-60), are equivalent as they give the same ratio of SUV values for different VOI's.

SUV(40-60) data are plotted vs GMR data calculated by TCM on Fig. 1. Correlation of these variables is also linear ($R^2=0.96$) with a nonzero intercept. It is interesting that fitting the experimental points belonging to higher GMR values is significantly better than that at lower variables (data not shown). Regression analysis of Patlak GMR and GMR by TCM yielded similar results with R^2=0.92. and again with nonzero intercept (Fig.2.). Quite similarly to the remark to Fig. 1. the correlation of data belonging to low GMR regions is relatively loose. These distinguished regions are the pons, the corpus callosum, the right and left capsula internas,

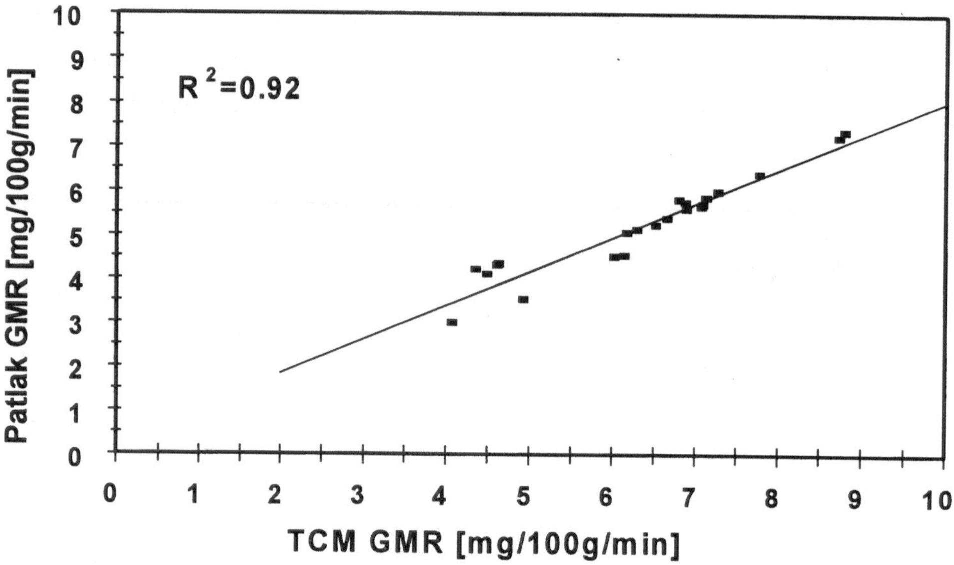

Figure 2. A representative correlation of GMR data calculated by the TCM and Patlak GMR data

the right and left olfactory gyri and the two hemispheres of the cerebellum. These data belong in both cases either to white matter VOI's or to VOI's situated close to large blood vessels. The measured tissue accumulation in the regions of the pons and the olfactory gyri could be affected by the FDG present in the large arterial vessels at the basis of the brain.

The basic difference between the quantification based on TCM calculations and that according to Patlak is in the assumption relating to the value of k_4. Thus it is of interest to plot the difference between these data as a function of this kinetic constant (Fig.3.). In accord with the expectation the difference is growing as the numerical value of k_4 increases. Interestingly, there is a substantial deviation of these parameters also at very low k_4 values or even at k_4=0. The possible explanation for this residual difference is that in contrast to the Patlak method, the TCM procedure takes the contribution of the activity concentration in the vascular compartment into account.

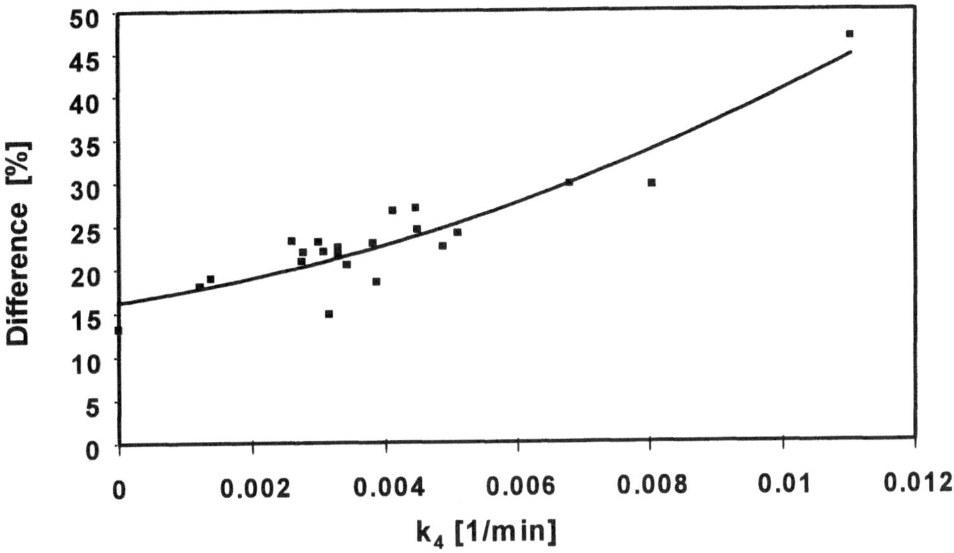

Figure 3. Deviation of GMR values calculated by the TCM and the Patlak analysis expressed as percentage of the former vs numerical value of FDG dephosphorylation rate

CONCLUSION

Comparison of indexes of glucose metabolic activity (SUV values, rendered to different data acquisition times, Patlak GMR data and GMR data calculated according to TCM. showed that any two out of these parameters are linearly related. However, these quantified data will not provide identical results even on a relative scale because of the non-zero intercepts of appropriate regression lines. Analysis of the deviations between the calculated entities proved that the accurate determination of glucose utilization in anatomic regions of white matter and those being close to large blood vessels require application of the three compartment tracer kinetic calculations without any simplifying assumptions.

ACKNOWLEDGEMENT

This study was supported by OTKA grants T 16150 and F 16504 and ETT grants 349/96 and 362/96.

REFERENCES

1. Hawkins, R.A., Phelps, M.E., Huang, S.C. Effect of temporal sampling, glucose metabolic rates, and disruptions of the blood-brain barrier on the FDG. Model with and without a vascular compartment: studies in human brain tumors with PET. *J. Cereb Blood Flow Metab* **6**,170-1832.

2. Hoh, C.K., Dahlbom, M., Hawkins, R.A., et al (1994) Basic principles of positron emission tomography in oncology: quantification and whole body techniques. *Wien Klin Wochenschr* **106/15**, 496-504

3. Phelps, M.E., Huang, S.C., Hoffman, E.J., at al (1979) Tomographic measurement of local cerebral glucose metabolic rate in humans with 2-[F-18]fluoro-2-deoxy-D-glucose: validation of method. *Ann Neurol* **6**, 371-388

4. Huang, S.C., Phelps, M.E., Hoffman, E.J., at al (1980) Noninvasive determination of local cerebral glucose metabolic rate in man. *Am. J. Physiol* **238**, E69-E82

5. Evans, A.C., Diksic, M., Yamamoto, Y.L. et al (1986) Effect of vascular activity in the determination of rate constants for the uptake of F^{18} -labeled 2-Fluoro-2-deoxy-D-glucose: error analysis and normal values in older subjects. (1986) *J. Cereb Blood Flow Metab* **6**,724-738

6. Patlak, C.S., Blasberg, R.G. (1985) Graphical evaluation of blood to brain transfer constants from multiple time uptake data. Generalizations. *J. Cereb Blood Flow Metab* **5**, 584-590

Radioactive Isotopes in
Clinical Medicine and Research XXIII
ed. by H. Bergmann, H. Köhn and H. Sinzinger

BONE SCINTIGRAPHY AND PALLIATIVE THERAPY WITH MULTIBONE KIT

J. Kőrnyei*, J. Törkő*, E. Lőrinczy, I. Szilvási, I. Balogh, I. Földes, J. Palatka, L. Duffek

* Institute of Isotopes Co. Ltd,
Konkoly Thege street 29-33, Budapest, H-1121, Hungary

SUMMARY: Special cold kit formulation, MULTIBONE, was recently elaborated which can provide easy and fast labelling of EDTMP with Tc-99m, Y-90 (or even Sm-153). Clinical trial of MULTIBONE is an ongoing project in Hungary both for follow up and palliative therapy of painful bone metastases of prostate, breast or some other cancers. Tc-99m MULTIBONE was compared with Tc-99m MDP in 20 patients, while palliative treatments with Y-90 MULTIBONE were carried out in 25 cases. Results obtained confirm that MULTIBONE kit can become a useful tool in diagnostic bone scintigraphy and radionuclide therapy.

INTRODUCTION

Tc-99m diphosphonates are known as bone seeking agents for long time due to their in vivo chemisorption on the inorganic bone matrix, on the hydroxyapatite. The increased blood perfusion and the increased osteoblastic activity results in higher bone uptake so the lesion to normal bone ratio exceeds the value of 1, except such cases when lesions caused by increased osteoclastic activity. On the other hand the accumulation of Tc-99m diphosphonates in lesions depends on other functional groups being present in the molecule, for example it is observed that hydroxy ethyliden diphosphonate (HEDP) showes higher lesion to normal bone ratio than methylene diphosphonate (MDP). Further from diphosphonates, aminophosphonates such as ethylene diamine tetramethylene phosphonate (EDTMP) is taken up much more in the bone lesions than in the healthy bone and an extremely high lesion to normal bone ratio (16 : 1) was observed in case of Sm-153 EDTMP[(1)]. Thus EDTMP seems to be one of the most promising agent for both follow up and palliative therapy of bone metastases.

The aim of the present work is
- to utilize the excellent biodistribution properties of EDTMP in the follow up of bone metastases, using Tc-99m labelling,
- to introduce Y-90, a beta-emitter of higher energy than Sm-153, in order to increase the therapeutic effect.

For these purposes a single vial kit, MULTIBONE, was elaborated for labelling with different radionuclides such as Tc-99m, Y-90 or even Sm-153. In this manner both the follow up and therapy of bone metastases can be performed by using the same agent labelled with the proper radionuclide.

MATERIALS AND METHODS

EDTMP was sythetized from ethylene diamine via a reaction with formaldehyde and phosphorous acid[2]. Compound obtained was purified by recrystallization and identified by elemental analysis, IR and NMR spectra. Kit formulation was elaborated in order to find the optimal EDTMP / tin(II) ratio which can ensure stable labelling with all interesting radionuclides (Tc-99m, Y-90, Sm-153).

Labelling of MULTIBONE kit is simple: in case of Tc-99m only the pertechnetate solution should be injected into it. Labelling with Y-90 or Sm-153 requires dissolution of the kit in 2.0 ml saline followed by adding the sterile yttrium or samarium chloride of high specific activity (> 500 GBq/g) in max. 1.0 ml volume (pH= 2.5 - 3.5). Labelling is completed by incubation at room temperature for 10-15 min. The pH value of the labelled radiopharmaceuticals is 5 - 8 due to the optimal buffer capacity of MULTIBONE kit. Radiochemical purity was always found higher than 98 % in case of each above mentioned radionuclides.

Clinical trial of Tc-99m MULTIBONE was carried out in 20 patients. Each patient suffers from metastatic prostate or breast cancer identified by hystological studies as well as by bone scintigraphy with Tc-99m MDP. The shortest time between Tc-99m MDP and MULTIBONE studies was 2 weeks, while the longest period was 6 weeks. In this manner the state of the patients could be considered identical when the scintigrams were prepared by administering 370 - 740 MBq Tc-99m MDP or MULTIBONE. In this comparative study the number of metastases identified and the imaging quality were in the focus of interest.

Evaluation of the bone scans was performed by using ROI method. The activity of normal bone in % was calculated if the activity of the lesion was considered as 100 %. Thus the less normal bone % corresponds to the better contrast i.e. higher imaging quality.

Palliative treatment of 25 patients was performed with Y-90 MULTIBONE. In each case the bone metastases were proved by hystological studies and patients suffer from strong bone pain. At the same time any other anodyne was uneffective to these patients. 110 - 370 MBq Y-90 MULTIBONE was administered as single injection. Haematological studies (determination of red blood cells, white blood cells, platelets) as well as scoring of the pain were carried out on the 1st, 3rd, 5th, 7th, 9th, 12th and 15th weeks after injection. For pain scoring a 9 degree scale was used as follows: 0 = painless state, 1, 2, 3 = significantly decreased pain, 4, 5, 6 = decreased pain, 7, 8 = slightly decreased pain, 9 = no palliative effect.

RESULTS AND DISCUSSION

Tc-99m MULTIBONE and MDP scintigrams showed that several bone metastases were observed in the 20 patients included in this comparative study. The number of metastases identified are summed up in Table 1.

Table 1.
Bone metastases identified by Tc-99m MULTIBONE and MDP.

Patient No.	Multibone	MDP
I/1.	4	4
I/2.	3	3
I/3.	4	4
I/4.	1	1
I/5.	17	17
II/1.	18	18
II/2.	30	30
II/3.	19	16
II/4.	9	9
II/5.	19	19

Patient No.	Multibone	MDP
III/1.	18	11
III/2	4	4
III/3	2	2
III/4	17	18
III/5.	4	5
IV/1.	6	6
IV/2.	20	20
IV/3.	1	1
IV/4.	20	20
IV/5.	2	2

In sum 216 and 210 bone metastases have been identified by Tc-99m MULTIBONE and MDP, respectively. Concerning the imaging quality, the normal bone ROI-s were expressed as % of lesions in case of both radiopharmaceuticals. The evaluation of imaging quality data can be seen in Table 2.

Table 2.
Comparison of imaging quality with Tc-99m MULTIBONE and MDP.

Difference in % normal ROI-s, (MDP) - (MULTIBONE)	Imaging quality	Patients	%
> 0	Better imaging with MULTIBONE	13	65
= 0	MULTIBONE is equal to MDP	5	20
< 0	MULTIBONE is worse than MDP	2	15

On the other hand activity ratios between leison and normal bone ROI-s have been calculated. Data are shown in Table 3.

Table 3.
Lesion to normal bone ratios

lesion / normal bone ratios	MULTIBONE	MDP
average	5.55 +/- 2.78	2.60 +/- 1.36
maxium	8.33	3.86

Based on the data obtained it can be seen that both Tc-99m MULTIBONE and MDP are suitable to localize bone metastases and in 80 % of the cases the number of lesions identified is identical. In 10 % MULTIBONE, in further 10 % MDP seems to be more sensitive in imaging of bone lesions. On the other hand the relative accumulation of MULTIBONE is higher in 65 % of the patients while in 15 % MDP uptake seemed to be more intensive. In 20 % the relative uptake of Tc-99m MULTIBONE was equal to that of Tc-99m MDP. The imaging quality depends very much on lesion to normal bone ratio which is much higher in case of MULTIBONE (average: 5.55, maximal: 8.33) in comparison with MDP (average 2.60, maximal: 3.86). The relatively low normal bone uptake of MULTIBONE ensures an extremely low radiation dose to healthy tissues even in case of diagnostic imaging. During the trial no adverse reaction was observed at all. Thus Tc-99m MULTIBONE seems to be a very promising agent in follow up of bone metastases.

Y-90 MULTIBONE therapeutic treatments showed tolerable damage in haematological state of the patients i.e. the concentrations of red blood cells, white blood cells as well as platelets. Pain score data of every patient, as a function of time after treatment, are summed up in Table 4.

Table 4.
Pain score data of patients treated with Y-90 MULTIBONE

Pts	Pain score data on the 5th week after injection	7th	9th	12th	15th	Pts	Pain score data on the 5th week after injection	7th	9th	12th	15th
I.	5	3	6	7	7	XIV.	6	6	6	6	6
II.	6	4	5	5	7	XV	1	0	0	0	0
III.	5	8	6	4	5	XVI.	1	0	0	0	0
IV.	1	2	4	3	5	XVII	6	3	3	3	3
V.	3	2	3	3	5	XVIII.	5	3	5	5	6
VI.	5	4	4	3	3	XIX.	6	5	6	5	6
VII.	3	3	3	5	6	XX.	7	9	6	6	6
VIII	5	0	1	2	8	XXI.	8	8	7	7	6
IX.	4	3	3	3	4	XXII.	9	8	8	7	7
X	6	4	5	8	9	XXIII.	3	3	3	3	3
XI.	3	4	3	8	8	XXIV.	2	2	2	2	2
XII	6	3	0	0	0	XXV.	3	3	2	2	2
XIII	9	9	3	3	3						

Notes: score = 0 corresponds to the painless state while 9 = no palliative effect.
score = 1,2,3: significantly decreased pain, 4,5,6: decreased pain, 7,8: slightly decreased pain.

Evaluation of pain score data leads to the following results presented is Table 5.

Table 5.
Evaluation of pain score data

Cases	Number of patients	%
A.) Palliative effect at all (at least some scores < 9)	25	100
B.) Significantly decreased pain at least in one period (scores < 4)	17	68
C.) Significantly decreased pain in three subsequent checking time (scores < 4)	12	48
D.) Painless state attained (score = 0)	3	12

Based on the data in Table 5. it can be emphasized that some palliative effect can be observed in every case and cca. 2/3 part of the patients felt significantly decreased pain at least in one period investigated. On the other hand in case of 11 patients the pain started to increase again till the 15th week after injection but scores remained below 9, except one case.

CONCLUSION

The recently elaborated MULTIBONE kit, when labelled with Tc-99m, can be considered as a useful tool in diagnostic imaging of bone metastases of different tumours (primarly prostate and breast cancers). The high lesion to normal bone ratios ensure excellent imaging quality and the relatively low uptake in normal bone causes low radiation in normal tissues even in case of follow up studies.

The Y-90 MULTIBONE injection showed palliative effect in every patients treated and in 68 and 12 % of the cases the pain was significantly decreased and completely ceased, respectively. The physical properties of Y-90 (i.e. high beta energy) and the excellent biodistribution properties of EDTMP can be combined and utilized for successful palliative therapy by using MULTIBONE kit.

REFERENCES

1. Lattimer JC, Corwin LA, Stapleton JRJ, Volkert VA. Clinical and clinopathological effects of Sm-153 EDTMP administered intravenously to normal beagle dogs. J. Nucl. Med 1990; 31(5): 586-593

2. Moedritzer K, Irani RR. The direct synthesis of alpha-aminomethyl phosphonic acids. Mannich-type reactions with orthophosphorous acid. J. Organic Chem 1966; 31: 1603-1607

Radioactive Isotopes in
Clinical Medicine and Research XXIII
ed. by H. Bergmann, H. Köhn and H. Sinzinger

PHARMACOSCINTIGRAPHIC STUDY OF LOCALIZATION IN THE G.I. TRACT OF CONTROLLED RELEASE TABLETS USING ^{153}Sm AS MARKER.

R. Palumbo, B. Palumbo, L. Cardinali, S. Bonaca, J. Hartwig*, C. Rastelli* – Chair of Nuclear Medicine, University of Perugia, Italy. – *Innopharma srl. Cinisello B. mo (Milano – Italy)

Summary

The aims of this preliminary pilot study were: to validate the gammascintigraphic method (pharmacoscintigraphy) with the new formulation; to generate some preliminary data regarding the transit time and disintegration behaviour of the new oral delivery placebo-tablets. Four volunteers received 2 mg of $^{153}Sm_2O_3$ by oral route, in one mesalazine placebo tablet. ^{153}Sm oxide, obtained by means of neutron irradiation after a normal manifacturing procedure, is a γ-emitter of E-103 Kev, with t1/2 of 46,8 h, not adsorbed from G.I tract. ^{153}Sm – SCAN was performed at 5,30 min. and 1, 1,5, 2,5, 3, 4, 5, 5, 7, 8, 10, 24 h after the dose. Time of disintegration in the colon varied from 5 to 8 h. Excellent imaging was obtained with very low radioactivity exposure (50 mRad). The "clock" release formulation achieved its target in most of subjects.

INTRODUCTION

The development of new oral delivery systems that enable controlled or time release of a drug, thereby ensuring an improved therapeutic index by increasing efficacy while reducing side-effects, is one of the main objectives of pharmaceutical research at present.

For this reason new evaluation methods are required with the aim of proving the real advantages of these modified release systems versus conventional formulations. Amongst various new evaluation methods, gamma-scintigraphy appears as the more suitable non-invasive means of acquiring information regarding the gastrointestinal tract under normal physiological conditions (1) (2).

5-amino-salycilic-acid, 5-ASA, is the therapeutically active moiety of sulphasalazine, a well known treatment for inflammatory bowel disease i.e. ulcerative colitis and Crohn's disease. Although its mechanism of action has not been completely elucidated, it is clear that therapeutic effect is exerted locally. Following the oral administration of conventional formulations mesalazine is absorbed from the small intestine quickly and may not reach the colon in sufficient amounts to be effective (3).

Recent research has focused on the development of oral delivery systems capable of releasing the active principle at the site of action – the colon – thus avoiding small intestine absorption. This kind of formulation would also avoid the problem of gastric intolerance (3-6).

A new tablet formulation has been designed to release an active principle after a pre-established time-lag (approx. 6-8 h).

The validity of this kind of formulation in obtaining release at the site of the colon rests on the reported regularity in transit time through the small intestine (7).

MATERIALS AND METHODS

Subjects

Four male, caucasian healthy volunteers from 29-32 years were recruited for the study.

None of them took any medication during the two weeks preceeding the study.

Dosimetry estimate of radiation dose

The radiation dose to be received by the whole body and vital organs were determined prior to dosing according to the guidelines provided by the International Committee of Radio Protection (10), the World Health Organization (11) and from the available literature (12).

Radioactive marker

Samarium (^{153}Sm) is a γ-emitter with an useful energy for imaging (28%) of 103 KeV and a 46.8 h half-life, while Sm oxide is a compound not absorbed by oral route. ^{153}Sm oxide was given orally contained into a tablet.

No active principle was included in the inner core, but ^{153}Sm oxide was included amongst the excipients in order to have a radiolabelled marker (^{153}Sm) for gamma-scintigraphy after neutron irradiation in a nuclear reactor.

^{153}Sm oxide was preferred to other radioactive tracers since, besides being suitable for scintigraphy, it is not absorbed from the G.I tract (8) and has a decay half-life (46.8 h) long enough to guarantee sufficient activity over the whole observation time. Furthermore, the procedure forseeing radioactivation after manufacturing by means of neutron irradiation avoids practical manufacturing problems, does not alter the release behaviour of the preparation, nor drug stability and minimises the radiation risks (9).

As far as radiotoxicity is concerned, ^{153}Sm is an isotope classified by the radio-protection Agency ICRP into a low radio-toxicity Group, i.e. III, which ensures a low degree of risk for the volunteer (10,11).

Tablet irradiation

The radioactivity of each of the 4 placebo tablets immediately after irradiation was 1 MBq. The tablets were subsequently transported from Pavia to Perugia in 48 h and left in deposit until initiation of the study was approx. 90 h. Upon initiation of the study the radiation measured was about 0.25 MBq. This means that the Radiation Dose received was actually equivalent to only approx. 50mRad.

Anatomical regions

With the aim of establishing the transit-time and the position of tablet opening, a schematic anatomical representation of the whole gastro-intestinal route was drawn indicating the areas of interest, namely: stomach, duodenum, jejunum, ileum, cecum, ascending colon, transverse colon, descending colon, sigmoid colon and rectum.

These regions of interest were identified in advance and scanned as a template to each of the acquired scintigrams. Xiphoid and umbilical marker were used for alignement.

Gamma camera recording

Subjects were placed supine under the collimator of a computerized Gamma-Camera and ^{153}Sm radiations were recorded at different time intervals. Starting from the time of administration, images, 2 min. in duration, were obtained after 5 and 30 min. and 1, 1.5, 2, 2.5, 3, 4, 5, 6, 7, 8, 10, and 24 h.

The study was divided into two periods:

1. Run-in (Period I: days −4 to −1)

The run-in period was needed to standardize bowel contents by placing subjects on a strict diet for 3 days before the labelled tablet administration.

Volunteers followed a balanced, regimented solid diet containing 20 g of dietary fiber and based on the subjects' normal nutritional requirements. In addition on the evening of day −1, dinner consisted in a nutritionally complete liquid food ensuring the necessary caloric intake.

2. ^{153}Sm oxide labelled tablet administration (Period II: days 1 to 3)

The volunteers received (day 1, at 8.00 a.m.) 2 ^{153}Sm oxide by oral route, in one mesalazine placebo-tablet. They were allowed to take breakfast 2 h (10.00 a.m.) after dosing and to have a standardized lunch 3 h later (1.00 p.m.). Gamma-camera images recorded in ANT-POST at frequent intervals (13 times) within the 24 h following administration.

RESULTS

Tablet G.I. transit time

The tablet was well visible starting from 5' after injection until complete disintegration.

The behaviour of the tablet was fairly similar in three volunteers, i.e. n°1, 3 and 4 (fig 1). In these subjects gastric residence time varied from 0.5 to 2 h. Time to initiation of disintegration varied from 5 to 8 h, disintegration taking place in the colon.

Radioactivity was still detectable at 10 h, but not at 24 h in volunteer n° 1, whereas it was still detectable at 24 h in the other two (n° 3 and 4).

Regarding the remaining volunteer (n° 2), gastric transit time was similar, but permanence in the small intestine was unusually long, the undesintegrated tablet being still detectable there 28 h after administration. Unfortunately evacuation took place and radioactivity was not detectable at 34 h, when a gamma camera recording was repeated.

The individual data is summarized in table 1.

G.I. transit of the tablets and their disintegration can be followed visually in a video recording that provides more detailed information of higher quality.

TABLE 1. G.I. transit and disintegration times of the placebo tablets

Parameter (min)	Volunteer 1	Volunteer 2	Volunteer 3	Volunteer 4
Tablet gastric residence time	60	120	30	30
Tablet colon arrival time	480	---	210	300
Tablet initiation disintegration time	480	---	300	360
Tablet total G.I. transit time	>10h <24h	>28h <34h	>24h	>24h

Safety

The subjects' vital signs were measured on day −3 and day 4 at the end of the study.

Values 10% above or below the normal range were considered abnormal. The only abnormal values observed were some minor differences in the WBC differential count of no clinical significance and an increase in both transaminase values in volunteer n° 3. This subject is being followed up until resolution one week later when the laboratory tests were repeated; the abnormal laboratory tests were not associated with any symptoms. The subject seemed to be in excellent health throughout the study and during the follow-up. As the test tablet contained placebo, it is difficult to attribute the increase in transaminase to participation in the study.

CONCLUSIONS

The **first objective** was to validate the pharmacoscintigraphic evaluation procedure for a new controlled release tablet formulation. Excellent imaging was obtained with a relatively low radioactivity level (0.25 Mbq), that allowed radioactivity exposure to be reduced to approx. 50 mRad.

This level of exposure is lower than that recommended by the Euratom directive regarding the use of radioactive material. The photographic can be gleaned from video-recording.

The **second objective** of this study was the generation of preliminary data regarding the transit and release behaviour of the new tablet formulation designed to release its contents in the G.I. tract after a pre-established time –lag (i.e. approx. 6-8 h), in a small group of volunteers. The results show that this "clock" release formulation achieved its target in 3 out of 4 subjects.

There is no immediate explanation for the anomalous behaviour of the tablet in the fourth volunteer other than the fact that G.I. transit time was unusually long and may have interfered with tablet disintegration in some way.

Regarding the documentation of **safety**, the tests were carried out to document the safety of the tablet coating and of the procedure itself. Only one significant abnormality was found – an increase in transaminases in one volunteer. There is no apparent reason why the tablet coating of the formulation and/or the procedure itself should cause this adverse effect, which could be due to a number of causes other than liver parenchymal abnormalities (i.e. muscular damage).

In summary, the procedure was validated both as far as radioactivity dosimetry and gamma camera imaging was concerned, whilst provision needs to be made for improved visual documentation. Preliminary data regarding transit and release behaviour of the new tablet formulation were generated that are very encouraging.

REFERENCES

1. **Wilding I.R.** et al. The role of gamma-scintigraphy in oral drug delivery. Adv. Drug Del. Rev. 7, 87-117 (1991).
2. **Davis S.S.** et al. Gamma-scintigraphy in the evaluation of pharmaceutical dosage forms. Eur. J. Nucl. Med. 19, 971-986 (1992).
3. **Brodgen R.N. and Sorkin E.M.** Mesalazine – A Review of its Pharmacodynamic and Pharmacokinetic Properties and Therapeutic Potential in Chronic Inflammatory Bowel Disease. Drugs 38(4): 500-523, 1989.
4. **Hardy J.D.** et al. Evaluation of an enteric-coated delayed release 5-ASA tablet in patients with inflammatory bowel disease. Aliment. Pharmacol. Therap. 60, 273-280 (1987).
5. **Haley J.N.C.** Gastrointestinal transit and release of mesalazine tablet in patients with inflammatory bowel disease, Scan. J. Gastroenterology, 25, 47-51 (1990).
6. **Hardy J.G.** et al. Localization of drug release sites from an oral sustained release formulation of 5-ASA (pentasa) in the G.I. tract using gamma-scintigraphy. J. Clin. Pharmacol. 33, 712-718 (1993).
7. **Davis S.S.** et al. Transit of pharmaceutical dosage forms through the small intestine. Gut 27: 886, 1986.
8. **Hardy J.G.** et al. Evaluation of an enteric coated naproxen pellet formulation Aliment. Pharmacol. Therap. 5, 69-75, 1991.
9. **Wilding I.R.** Pharmaco-scintigraphic evaluation of oral delivery systems: Part I Pharmac. Technolo. Eur. 19-26 (April 1994).
10. ICPR publication 26. Recommendations of the International Commission on Radiological Protection: Pergamon Press, Oxford, 1977.
11. World Health Organisation. Report of a WHO Expert Committee on the use of ionising radiations and radionucleides on human beings for medical researches, training and non-medical purposes. Tech. Rep. Serie, WHO, Geneva, 611, 1977.
12. **Siegel J.A.** et al. Radiation dose estimates for oral agents used in upper gastro-intestinal disease. Nucl. Med. 24, 835-837 (1983).

ENDOCRINOLOGY, THYROID

Radioactive Isotopes in
Clinical Medicine and Research XXIII
ed. by H. Bergmann, H. Köhn and H. Sinzinger

ON THE USE OF ROUTINE PREOPERATIVE SCINTIGRAPHY IN THYROID CARCINOMA PATIENTS

Als C*•, Gedeon P*•, Netzer P°, Kinser J*, Markwalder R•, Laissue J•, Rösler H*.
Dept. of Nuclear Medicine*, Institute of Pathology•, Dept. of Gastroenterology°, Inselspital, University of Bern, CH-3010 Bern, Switzerland

Summary

Preoperative (PO) thyroid (T) scintigraphy (S) in 924 case histories of thyroid carcinoma (TC) was evaluated in a former goiter-endemic Pre-Alpine region. From 1971-1996, POTS was omitted in 178 (22.2%) of 802 TC. There were 92 papillary, 58 follicular, 11 oncocytic, 6 anaplastic, 4 medullary TC and 7 other C. Incomplete diagnosis of T disease by omission of POTS prior to surgery has immediate and delayed consequences. POTS prevents unnecessary surgery. It is an *epidemiologic* monitoring tool of hyperthyroidism (HT). It *therapeutically* and *functionally* influences the extent of T resection, thereby preventing late HT. Moreover, POTS *prognostically* influences the total activity of therapeutic 131-I on the ALARA basis (as low as reasonably achievable).

Introduction

The use of several complementary diagnostic or therapeutic methods in medicine is decided on the basis of technical feasibility, reliability and cost-benefit considerations. The clinical demand for a technique is guided by the knowledge of the possible benefit at any moment of disease evolution. This benefit can be immediate as well as delayed. Functional thyroid scintigraphy with rectolinear scanners was the unique possibility for rendering a thyroid 'image' after World War II. The image quality continuously improved using gamma cameras and quantitation techniques. Complementary morphologic information became available by ultrasound in the 1970's. As ultrasound can be performed easily in any physicians private practice and as no radiation burden is involved, the demand for thyroid ultrasound has been increasing while the demand for thyroid scintigraphy has decreased.

Political pressure in view of reducing medical expenses and some competitive behaviour among medical specialists have influenced new diagnostic algorithms. In fact, clinicians rely more and more on TSH and thyroid hormone levels, novel thyroid antibody assays, as well as on high resolution ultrasound and cytology alone. But this approach weights regional morphologic rather than functional information. Thus, independent of the TSH level, the search for information on the existence, localization and etiology of possible functional anomalies within the thyroid tissue is omitted. What are the causes and the possible impact of omission of preoperative thyroid scintigraphy (POTS) on therapeutic, epidemiologic and prognostic outcomes, especially in the case of thyroid carcinoma?

Materials and Methods

In the course of a retrospective global work-up of thyroid carcinoma in the Department of Nuclear Medicine, all patients with a thyroid malignancy diagnosed between 1945 and December 31, 1996, were reevaluated. Additional records of patients with thyroid carcinoma were found in the Department of Surgery (see Table 1). Postoperative information on the histologic type of thyroid carcinoma (1) were compared with available preoperative scintigrams. Histologic classifications of TC were subdivided as papillary, follicular (including oncocytic), anaplastic and others (including medullary TC, lymphomas, sarcomas, metastases).

Depending on the clinical situation, preoperative thyroid scintigraphy was performed with 99m-Tc (100 MBq intravenously), 123-I (7.4 MBq orally) or, exceptionally 131-I (1.85 MBq orally). Since 1991, an additional thyroid scintigraphy with 99mTc-MIBI (methoxy-isobutyle-isonitrile) has been performed as an experimental double-tracer technique on a Transcam gamma camera (2,3). The baseline scintigraphy was performed on a Siemens Scintimat rectolinear scanner up to 1992, later on on a MSE Polyscan. As the diagnostic scintigraphic procedures were standardized up to the end of 1970, only the cases from 1971 to 1996 are considered hereafter (Fig 1).

Results

A total of 924 case records of patients with TC from the Departments of Nuclear Medicine (n=875) and Surgery (n= 49) were reevaluated. The frequency distribution of the histologies of the resected thyroid carcinomas is listed in Table 1. Over the period 1945-1996, a total of 270 patients (29.2%) had not been examined by TS preoperatively. From 1971 to 1996, when most TC were diagnosed, 178 out of 802 patients (22.2%) had no preoperative scintigraphy (Fig 1). Out of these 178 patients, 92 had papillary TC, 58 follicular TC, 11 oncocytic TC, 6 anaplastic TC, 4 medullary TC and 7 diverse C. Table 1 shows that the frequency distribution of the histologic subtypes of all 924 TC and of the 178 TC without POTS were not significantly different ($p>0.05$). Figure 1 shows these 178 patients as a percentage of the total number of patients with differentiated and undifferentiated TC diagnosed per year up to 1996. There was a minimal frequency of POTS at the beginning of the 1970es (51%), with a sudden increase in 1977 up to 93%, oscillating from then on between 67% and 94% (Fig 1).

Table 1: % of histologic subtypes in all 924 TC and in 178 TC without POTS (s) = subgroup

period	TC (n)	no POTS	pap	follic	anapl	others
1945-1996	924	270	437	408	38	41
		(29.2%)	*47.5%*	*44.3%*	*4%*	*4.2%*
1971-1996(s)	822	178	92	69	6	11
		(22.2%)	*52.4%*	*38.4%*	*3.1%*	*6.1%*

Figure 1: % of patients with TC without POTS from 1971-1996.

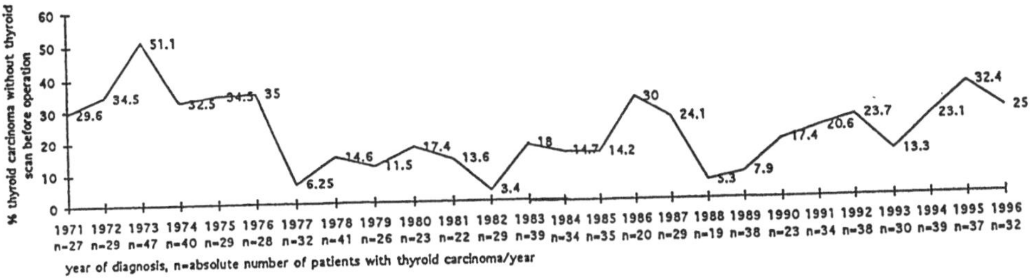

Discussion

Scintigraphy is a useful tool for outlining the totality of the thyroid gland, for localizing any palpable or painful area or nodule within or without, for differentiating between cold or warm nodules and for giving an etiologic diagnosis of hyperthyroidism in conjunction with clinical findings, blood hormone levels and antibody tests (2,3,4). What was the reason for the omission of POTS in 22.2% of the 822 TC patients and what are the clinical implications of thyroid scintigraphy in general? Of the reasons why POTS was not performed, technical feasibility, rapidity, safety and reliability were not the problems. Some learning and information were necessary in the 1970's, before clinicians were aware of the immediate advantages of POTS (Fig. 1). After 1977, any new surgeon starting to work in the hospital influenced the patient-referral scheme. Cost-benefit considerations emerged in the 1980's, especially with the upcoming of alternative techniques as CT and MRI. Competition problems shall not be detailed here. But above all, some medical doctors, especially if referring from peripheral hospitals, might have been unaware of immediate and long-term clinical implications.

1) The first argument in favor of thyroid scintigraphy is the *morphological information* of a nodule in respect to the thyroid gland. A mechanical compression of the trachea is related to a thyroid anomaly. In this respect, the local compression due to inflammatory disease such as

subacute and chronic, localized thyroiditis is diagnosed by characteristic scintigrams. Moreover, if combined with double-tracer MIBI scintigraphy, echography and clinical findings, the initial scintigraphic characterization - thanks to a specific diagnosis, hence treatment - leads to a more cost-efficient use of complementary diagnostic methods.

2) 'Radical' surgery, based on concepts of molecular biology, was introduced in Bern in 1990 (11). For nodular thyroids, this implies that at least a hemithyroidectomy, with eventually a subtotal resection of the heterolateral lobe, is routinely performed. The remaining 4 g of thyroid remnants do as a rule not contain a relevant volume of functionally autonomous tissue. The 'radical' concept has now become the modern standard of thyroid surgery in many centres. However, other hospitals do resect thyroids less radically. Moreover, most of the patients reported here were operated before 1990.

Under the two conditions cited above, POTS has *functional and therapeutic* implications. In case a surgical resection of the thyroid gland has been planned on the basis of clinical, echographic and cytologic evidence, a scintigraphy of the thyroid gland still has *therapeutic* implications. Indeed, in a (former) goiter-endemic region, the surgeon will easily palpate any intrathyroidal nodule intra-operatively that will guide the extent of resection (5). But without a POTS, he will not be aware of functionally autonomous areas that are frequent in goiter-endemic areas and become clinically relevant with age (6). They can be detected only by scintigraphy (4,7). The functional nature of the palpated nodule that is to be resected can be 'cold', 'warm' or 'hot', i.e., functionally hypo- or hyperavid for iodine, whatever the TSH level might be. No other in-vivo (Doppler ultrasound) or ex-vivo (cytology, histology) diagnostic modality is capable of reliably diagnosing regional functional autonomy (4,7). Even autoradiography, which depicts regional functional autonomy within the thyroid tissue but is too laborious for routine workups, does not correlate with the peripheral functional status (7). Thus, POTS will influence the extent of the surgical resection, thereby helping to prevent outcomes of delayed or recurrent hyperthyroidism. Hypothyroidism, which correlates with the extent of surgical thyroidectomy (5), is more easily stabilized by T4 supplementation than hyperthyroidism is stabilized by medical thyreostasis (6). Thus, preoperative scintigraphy of the thyroid gland does have *functional and therapeutic* implications. The improved insight into the functional behavior and into other non-malignant anomalies of a goiter that is to be operated on leads to the greatest possible impact on treatment and follow-up strategies. The benefit for the patient is obvious.

3) There are, moreover, *epidemiologic* reasons. Any population-based long-term follow-up of the frequencies of functional autonomous nodules is not possible without the routine use of thyroid scintigraphies before treatment (2,3). It has, moreover, been shown that the changing frequencies over time of hyperthyroidism due to solitary as well as multifocal, functionally autonomous nodules (sAFTN and mAFTN) are clinical markers of the iodine supply of a population (2,3,8,9). As a consequence of a successful iodination policy, the Bernese sAFTN/mAFTN ratio decreased from 2.6 to 0.9 between 1976 and 1982 ($p<0.005$) and down to 0.4 in 1991 (2). These epidemiologic frequencies can be easily established as long as thyroid scintigraphy is considered a base-line diagnostic tool. Renouncing the precise individual diagnosis of the nature of underlying thyroid disease before a definite treatment is applied leads to a deficiency of essential information and in effect hinders advances in thyroidology. Thus, thyroid scintigraphy is important as a long-term *epidemiological* monitoring tool of Plummer's disease directly and of iodine supply indirectly.

4) A fourth argument for performing POTS is the *prognostic significance for the individual*. The risk of late recurrent hyperthyroidism due to an insufficient thyroid gland resection in case of non-radical surgery is only the first argument in this respect. Further aspects are linked to the finding of a differentiated TC in the surgical resection specimen. In this case, the postoperative 131-I-ablation of the thyroid remnants is indicated. It has indeed been proven that this procedure does decrease morbidity due to late metastatic recurrences (1). The hyperavid remnant tissue is in competition with the less avid metastases for iodine. Only after destruction of the thyroid remnants by 131-I are the metastases more likely to become scintigraphically apparent (10). In this respect, the comparison of the pre- and postoperative scintigraphies is mandatory for interpreting persistent foci of 131-I uptake in the former thyroid bed. And it is precisely the knowledge of the proper delimitation of this thyroid bed which is dependent on the preoperative scintigraphy. The nuclear medicine specialist has to decide whether or not a 131-I therapy is necessary after ablation of the thyroid remnants. He is guided by the intent to administer the least reasonably achievable activity of 131-I in a patient's lifetime (ALARA), with the maximum security to keep him tumor-free. He will feel more secure with an adequate functional scintigraphic follow-up. As it is precisely the comparison of the pre- and postoperative functional thyroid areas that will help in deciding the total amount of 131-I required for therapy, it is understandable that preoperative TS has *prognostic* implications.

5) A fifth argument in favor of POTS is the confirmation of the *choice of therapy*. In the present work, we did not consider those patients with partial thyroidectomy, but without a prior POTS, for whom the histologic diagnosis later on revealed a benign disease that could potentially have been treated by another method than surgery. Thus, in case a subacute thyroiditis or a chronic, regionally dominant thyroiditis is treated by non-radical surgery, the causal disease and the clinical symptomatology can recur in the persistent thyroid lobe. Moreover, another diagnosis rests on clinical-scintigraphic evidence but cannot be made retrospectively by histology: it is a solitary, functionally autonomous thyroid nodule in an otherwise 'normal' thyroid (7). Those patients can safely and efficiently be cured by 131-I therapy.

In conclusion, the indications for POTS are influenced by surgical techniques, the local epidemiology of Plummer's disease and by iodine supply (3). POTS is an important tool for choosing an optimal treatment modality and for deciding on as low as reasonably achievable therapeutic 131-I amounts in case of TC. If one intends to improve morphologic, therapeutic, functional, diagnostic and epidemiologic information on thyroid disease in general, special importance ought to be given to a complete diagnostic work-up including scintigraphy.

References

1. Rösler, Birrer A, Lüscher D, Kinser J. Langzeitverläufe beim differenzierten Schilddrüsenkarzinom. *Schweiz Med Wochenschr 1992;122:1843-1857.*
2. Als C, Listewnik M, Rösler H, Bartkowiak E. Immunogenic and non-immunogenic hyperthyroidism: recent trends in prealpine Switzerland and in coastal poland. *Nucl. Med. 1995;34:92-99.*
3. Als C, H. Rösler. "Toxische Adenome der Schilddrüse werden seltener in Bern." *Schw. Med. Wschr. 1995, 31/32:1495-1499.*
4. Horst W., Rösler H., Schneider C., Labhart A. 306 cases of toxic adenoma: clinical aspects, findings in radioiodine diagnostics, radiochromatograph and histology; results of I-131 and surgical treatment. *J Nucl Med 1967; 8: 515-528.*
5. Seiler CA, Glaser C, Wagner H. Thyroid gland surgery in an endemic region. *World J Surg 1996;20:593-597.*
6. Als C, Baer HU, Glaser C, Rösler H. Zur Wahl der Therapie bei der unifokalen funktionellen Autonomie der Schilddrüse. Eine Übersicht. *Schweiz. Med. Wochenschr. 1997;127:891-898.*
7. Campbell WL, Santiago HE, Perzin KH, Johnson PM. The autonomous thyroid nodule: correlation of scan appearance and histopathology. *Radiology 1973;107:133-138.*
8. Als C, Lauber K, Brander L, Lüscher D, Rösler H. The instability of dietary iodine supply over time in an affluent society. *Experientia (Basel) 1995;6:623-633.*
9. Baltisberger BL, Minder ChE, Bürgi H. Decrease of incidence of toxic nodular goitre in a region of Switzerland after full correction of mild iodine deficiency. *Eur J Eondocrinol 1995;132:546-549.*
10. Wollman SH. Analysis of radioiodine therapy of metastatic tumors of the thyroid gland in man. *J Nat Cancer Inst* 1953;13:815-828.
11. Seiler CA, Glaser C, Wagner H. Thyroid gland surgery in an endemic region. *World J Surg* 1996;20:593-597.

Radioactive Isotopes in
Clinical Medicine and Research XXIII
ed. by H. Bergmann, H. Köhn and H. Sinzinger

THE VALUE OF HMPAO SPECT SCANNING IN PATIENTS WITH CONGENITAL HYPOTHYREOSIS

R. Junik, K. Łącka, I. Kubik, and M. Gembicki.

Dept. of Endocrinology, K. Marcinkowski University of Medical Sciences, Poznań, Poland

Summary: The aim of this study was to assess the value of SPECT scanning in patients with congenital hypothyreosis. Twenty-nine patients underwent neurological examination, the Intelligence Quotient (IQ) assessment and SPECT scans. Right to left asymmetries ranged within 11-25% in cortical regions and reduced rCBF were observed in 24/29 (83%) patients. In the group with photopenic foci, 8 of 24 subjects with significant perfusion defects had single lesions, 13 had two lesions, 2 had three, and 1 had four. There was significant difference of IQ in patients with hypothyreosis depending on numbers of rCBF lesions ($p=0.0068$). Conclusion: the rCBF is both reduced and asymmetric in patients with congenital hypothyreosis.

Introduction

It is well known from experimental and epidemiological studies that iodine is foundamental during fetal/neonatal life for the complete brain development (1). Hypothyroidism is associated with changes in cerebral metabolism and mental state. Thyroid hormone is essential for the development of the nervous system and its deficiency in the infants impairs permanently the activity of the brain (2). Cretinism is associated to congenital hypothyroidism (CH) and is characterized by three major features, deafmutism, mental retardation and motor disorders (3). Normal brain development can be restored only when replacement therapy is performed soon after birth. The thyroid hormone deficiency severely impairs the anatomy and connectivity of the brain. Ears (4) has shown that cretinism is essentially characterized by a hypoplastic neuropile i.e. a drastic decrease in connectivity. It has marked effects on axonal and dendritic outgrowth during the critical period of brain development and it impairs permanently the electrical activity and glucose utilization of the brain (5).

Review of published work indicates that despite early treatment many children with CH identified by neonatal screening still have some impairment of intellect, and that this is associated with severity of hypothyroidism prior to diagnosis (6). Retrospective reviews of outcome in CH prior to the introduction of screeninig indicated a mean Intelligence Quotient (IQ) deficit of 17-24 points with 30% of patients falling within the mental handicap range of ability. 10% of the hypothyroid children had an IQ more than 2 SD below the population mean (the traditional cut off for mental handicap), compared with 2% of the controls (6, 7).

SPECT (single photon emission computed tomography) offers a possibility of a functional imaging in cerebrovascular disease and other disorders concerning central nervous system.

Therefore the aim of this study was to assess the value of SPECT scanning in patients with congenital hypothyroidism.

Patients and Methods

Twenty-nine patients with congenital hypothyreosis (14 males and 15 females, mean age 34,9±8,2 yr, range from 17 to 58 yr) were studied. Patients underwent neurological examination and the Intelligence Quotient (IQ) assessment. Endocrinological work-up, including plasma levels of pituitary and thyroid gland hormones, was carried out. There was athyroidism in 8 patients, thyroid ectopy in 16, and disturbances in biosynthesis of thyroid hormones in 5 cases. All patients fulfilled the criteria of primary hypothyroidism. All others laboratory findings were within normal limits.

The diagnosis of CH had been made between 2 month and 12 year of age. Since that time only 8 patients were treated regularly. None of the patients had recived any medication except l-thyroxine prior to cerebral SPECT imaging. Other imaging techniques including CT and/or MRI were applied in all case in order to exclude morphological changes. All studies were performed with informed consent from the patients (or parents) after presenting a detailed explanation of the study.

SPECT imaging was performed after intravenous (i.v.) injection of 740 MBq 99mTc-HMPAO (hexamethyl-propyleneamine oxime). Radiotracer was injected according to manufacturer's instruction within 20 min of its preparation and imaging was begun 5-40 min after injection. Patients underwent examination in a quiet and dimly lit room.

Tomographic images were obtained using a rotating gamma camera equipped with a low-energy high-resolution collimator (Siemens, Diacam) connected to an ICON cumputer for three-dimensional reconstruction. Data were collected from 90 angular increments over 360 degrees in 64x64 matrices with an aquisition time of 20 s per view. The camera was set for elliptical rotation, with a 15% energy discrimination window centered at 140 keV. Transverse, sagittal and coronal slices were generated by filtered backprojection using a Butterworth filter (cutoff frequency 0.45, order 7). The reconstructed images were corrected for attenuation with the Chang's method with an attenuation coefficient equal to 0.12 cm^{-1}.

Semiquantitative analysis of the cortical 99mTc-HMPAO uptake was performed. Regions of interest (ROIs) were drawn in the bilateral frontal, temporal, parietal, occipital and cerebellar areas on transverse slices with reference to an anatomical map. The counts per pixel in each ROI were calculated and the ratios of the counts per pixel in the cerebral cortical ROIs to those in the cerebellar or whole brain ROIs were obtained. The relative rCBF (regional cerebral blood flow) was expressed as the ratio between regional and cerebellar or whole brain activity. Inter-hemispheric side-to-side asymmetry indices for mirrored sets of predefined ROIs were calculated. Regional asymmetries of 10% or more were considered significant.

Statistical analysis: Statistical analysis of the data was performed using the Mann-Whitney U test, Kruskal - Wallis ANOVA nonparametric test and Spearman correlation. Associations with P values < 0.05 were considered significant. The results are given as the mean (± 1 standard deviation, S.D.).

Results and Discussion

The abnormalities of rCBF and right to left asymmetries in cortical regions in patients with CH are showed in table 1.

Table 1. The rCBF changes and right to left asymmetries in patients with CH, range 11-25%.

No of lesions	0	1	2	3	4
No of patients	5	8	13	2	1
Percentage (%)	17	28	45	7	3

Five patients (17%) showed homogenous distribution over all cortical regions but 2 of them revealed decreased tracer uptake. According to rCBF deficits patients were subdivided into 3 groups: I - without fotopenic foci, II - with single fotopenic focus, and III - with more than one lesion.

The mean IQ score was 78 ± 13, range 65-100. There was significant difference of IQ in patients with hypothyreosis depending on numbers of rCBF lesions. Patients with 1 lesion revealed IQ 82.3 ± 14.8, and those with 2-4 lesions 78.7 ± 11.9, respectively ($p=0.0068$). However, level of IQ in a particular patient did not completly separate patients from both groups.

The anatomical distribution of hypoperfused areas is given in table 2.

Table 2. Localization of the foci of decreased perfusion in patients with CH.

	Right hemisphere				Left hemisphere			
Lobes	temporal	parietal	frontal	occipital	temporal	parietal	frontal	occipital
Group 2	2	-	-	-	9	5	1	2
Group 3	4	2	2	-	8	3	4	1

There was no significant difference in rCBF lesions between groups of patients with respect to cause of hypothyroidism, duration and treatment of disease, age or gender, blood serum concentration of TSH, T4, T3.

CH patients revealed marked focal changes in the brain tissue perfusion. The mechanism of reduction of rCBF is uncertain but perhaps can be explained by a disturbances in cerebrovascular circulation in immature brain. The hypothyroid brain remains immature for a longer period of time during the critical period of neuronal differentiation, i.e. when cerebral connectivity is established. Because thyroid hormone is required during a short postnatal period, a change in timing of neuronal differentiation might desynchronize the program of differentiation leading to the permanent poor connectivity seen in adulthood (2). Probably there are similar disturbances in developing of precapillary and capillary vessels in brain circulation in CH patients.

There were no significant differences in rCBF between the males and females CH patients. This would suggest no difference in the aging process of male and female brains. These findings are consistent with previous PET findings reported by Duara (8). According to our findings differences are probably due to severity of the disease in patients who had more severe perfusion deficits.

Normal patterns of rCBF were observed only in 5 patients. The highest deficits of perfusion were seen in the temporal regions, followed by parietal regions. This is probably due to severe impaired whole mental function in some patients. In our patients mental impairment was varied, mild, moderate and severe. It seems to be an explanaition of perfusion deficits visible in different regions and amounts.

A collaborative European study on 790 hypothyroid children diagnosed by screening suggested that very early therapy is associated with better outcome. Taking a subgroup of 116 children shown to have agenesis of the thyroid on isotope scan, a negative correlation was found between age at start of treatment and psychometric score, and all the cases starting treatment after 50 days had developmental scores below the mean (9). One of the early findings in the New England study was an association between impaired outcome and poor compliance with treatment, and subsequent analysis indicated that inadequate therapy was the only significant factor determining IQ at 3-5 years of age (10). Other results also indicate that quality of treatment may have an effect on outcome (11). It has been suggested that the better results reported in the New England patients, compared with other studies, might be related to more rapid correction of plasma T4 level, particulary in infants with more severe hypothyroidism (6).

The commence of l-thyroxine replacement therapy varied in our patients from 2 month to 12 years of age. Outcome measured as IQ score was lower comparing to patients from neonatal screening. Mean IQ score in CH patients was 78 ± 13 (range within 65-100), probably due to very late beginning of therapy. That might be an explanation of some differences between our findings and those obtained by others. No significant correlations were seen between SPECT lesions or IQ values and thyroid hormones level. Our results are similar to those obtained by Peter (12). According to him, there is no correlation between individual IQ and T3 or/andT4 levels. The correlation was observed between the IQ values and serum Tg levels. The mean TSH and T4 levels during the first and second year were also analyzed in respect of IQ without significant difference (12). Normal distribution of IQ values was found in groups of hypothyroid children detected by neonatal sreening. The mean IQ level was 103 comparing the values 92 of patiens diagnosed before the screeninig programme (12).

Conclusion: The rCBF is both reduced and asymmetric in patients with congenital hypothyroidism. However, the mechanism of disorders in CH cannot be determined on the basis of rCBF study. Present results show that there is not distinctive pattern of HMPAO uptake in patients with CH. The interpretation of the rCBF deficits should be done with the knowledge of the stage of the disease and specific nature of mental deficits.

References

1. Vitti P, Lombardi FA, Antonangeli L, Rago T, Chiovato L, Pinchera A, Marcheschi M, Bargagna S, Bertucelli B, Ferretti G, Sbrana B. Mild iodine deficiency in fetal/neonatal life and neuropsychological performances. AMA 1992;19:57-59.
2. Nunez J, Couchie D, Aniello F, Bridoux AM. Thyroid hormone effects on neuronal differentiation during brain development. AMA (Acta Medica Austriaca) 1992;19:36-39.
3. Delong GR. Observations on the neurology of endemic cretinism. In: Delong GR, Robbins J, Condliffe PG (eds): Iodine and the brain. New York, Plenum Press, 1988, pp 211-238.
4. Eayrs JT. Thyroid and developing brain: anatomical and behavioural effects. In: Hamburgh M, Barrington EJW (eds). Hormones and Development. New York, Appleton Century Crofts, 1971, pp 345-355.
5. Nunez J. Thyroid hormones. In: Lajta A (ed), Handbook of Neurochemistry. New York, Plenum Press, 1986, pp 1-29.
6. Grant DB, Fuggle P, Tokar S, Smith I. Psychomotor development in infants with congenital hypothyroidism diagnosed by neonatal screening. AMA 1992;19:54-56.
7. Glorieux J, Desjardins M, Letarte J, Morisette J, Dussault JH. Useful parameters to predict the eventual mental outcome of hypothyroid children. Ped Res 1988;24:6-8.
8. Duara R, Barker W, Chang J. Age and sex differences in cerebral glucose consumption measured by PET using [18-F] fluoroglucose (FDG). J. Nucl. Med., 1985, 26:68 (abs.).
9. Illig R, Largo RH, Qin Q, Torresani T, Rochiccioli P, Larson A. Mental development in congenital hypothyroidism after neonatal screening. Arch Dis Childch 1987;62:1050-1055.
10. New England congenital hypothyroidism Collaborative: Neonatal hypothyroidism screening: status of patients at 6 years of age. J Pediatrics 1985;107:915-918.
11. Heyerdahl S, Kase BF, Lie SO. Intellectual development in children with congenital hypothyroidism in relation to recommended thyroxine treatment. J Pediatrics 1991;118:850-857.
12. Peter F, Muszsnai A, Szigetvari A. Intellectual assessment of hypothyroid children detected by screening. AMA 1992;19:60-61.

Radioactive Isotopes in
Clinical Medicine and Research XXIII
ed. by H. Bergmann, H. Köhn and H. Sinzinger

ADVANCED STAGE THYROID CANCER - TREATMENT WITH ISOTRETINOIN

A.R.Börner, D.Simon, M.Weckesser, K.-J.Langen, H.-D.Röher, H.-W.Müller-Gärtner
Inst.of Medicine, Research Centre Jülich, Dept. of Nuclear Medicine and Dept. of General and Trauma Surgery, University Düsseldorf, Germany

SUMMARY
Isotretinoin has been successfully applied in a variety of malignant tumours displaying growth inhibiting and differentiation enhancing effects. As cell culture studies have proposed positive responses to Isotretinoin in differentiated thyroid cancer we applied the vitamin A derivative to 15 patients with advanced metastatic thyroid cancer. 14 patients showed at least a partial response in Tg, FDG PET or radioiodine measurements. In conclusion, Isotretinoin is useful in advanced thyroid cancer.

INTRODUCTION
13-cis-retinoic acid (Isotretinoin) is a vitamin A derivative and has shown differentiation enhancing and growth inhibiting proberties in many tumour entities (1). In promyelocytic leukemia it is known to cure the disease (2). In breast cancer it has been used to reduce tumour angiogenesis and tumour growth. In a follicular thyroid cancer cell line Isotretinoin was able to reduce cell numbers and H-3-thymidine uptake while enhancing iodine metabolism, binding of EGF and TSH significantly (3). This study evaluates the effects of Isotretinoin on otherwise intractable disease in advanced differentiated thyroid cancer.

MATERIAL AND METHODS
Up to now fifteen patients were enrolled in a study of Isotretinoin action in advanced and metastatic differentiated thyroid cancer. Six patients suffered from papillary, 7 from follicular and 2 from mostly oxyphilic thyroid cancer. Mean age was 68 years (24-76). No further therapeutic option was available to those patients by surgery, radioiodine therapy or external

radiation therapy. All patients showed progressive disease and were treated with 1-1.5 mg Isotretinoin per day. Tg was measured every 4-6 weeks together with liver enzymes, cholesterol and triglycerides, red and white blood cell count and electrolytes. Measurements of radioiodine accumulation and glucose metabolism of the metastases or recurrences (3) were performed before, during and after Isotretinoin treatment. Iodine metabolism was measured in hypothyroidism using I-131-NaI scintigraphy. Glucose metabolism was evaluated as standard uptake value (SUV) by F-18-FDG PET. No server or life threatening side effects of Isotretinoin were observed. All patients developed dry skin and mouth and mild cheilitis. Patients were treated for a mean time of 380 days. Then treatment was stopped and restarted after a mean interval of 68 days in 8 patients.

RESULTS

Tumour response was judged positive (+), slightly positive (x) or negative (-). If the measurements were not performed or non-diagnostic, a 0 is given.

Patient	Tumour	Iodine accumulation	TG	F-18-FDG
1. W.W.	Oxy.	-	+	+
2. P.G.	Foll.	-	-	-
3. T.F.	Pap.	+	+	0
4. M.H.	Pap.	-	(x)	+
5. W.M.	Oxy.	-	(x)	(x)
6. K.W.	Pap.	+	+	0
7. S.A.	Foll.	(x)	(x)	(x)
8. K.H.	Foll.	(x)	+	(x)
9. Z.I.	Foll.	(x)	-	-
10. H.D.	Pap.	-	(x)	(x)
11. T.R.	Foll.	-	(x)	+
12. P.J.	Foll.	-	+	0
13. K.G.	Pap.	-	(x)	0
14. K.A.	Foll.	-	(x)	(x)
15. G.B.	Pap.	-	+	0

3 Patients showed Tg-decreases while 10 patients developed a reduction in Tg increses over time. In one patient Tg-levels remained stable during Isotretinoin therapy. Only one patients revealed unchanged increases in Tg-levels. An example is given in figure 1.

Figure 1

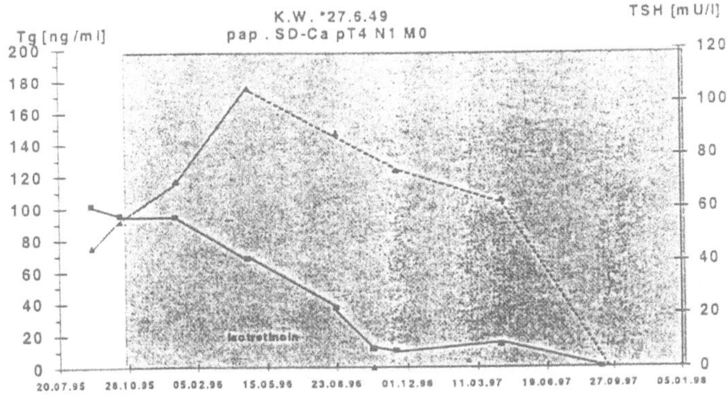

Figure 2: SUVs before (black), during (white) and after (grey) Isotretinoin therapy

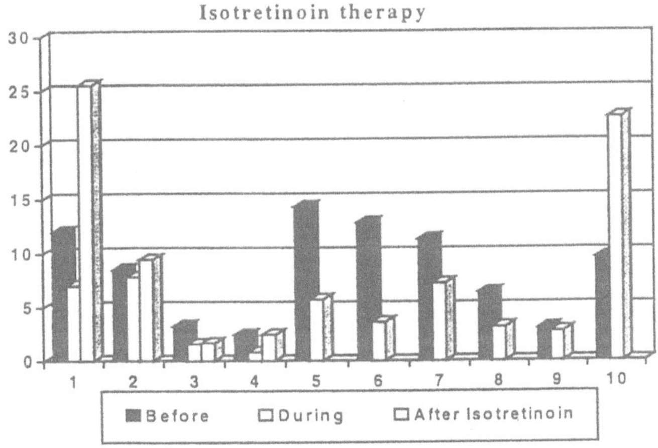

Before and during Isotretinoin therapy, tumour glucose hypermetabolism was measurable in 10 to 15 patients using F-18-FDG PET. Four patients showed dramatically reduced, another 5 patients slightly reduced glucose hypermetabolism during Isotretinoin therapy (Fig.2). In the 4 patients who stopped Isotretinoin this effect was reversed after withdrawal. Only one patient showed increased glucose hypermetabolism consistent with volume increases in lung metastases during Isotretinoin therapy. Radioiodine accumulation was improved in 5/15 patients but dosimetry revealed improved therapeutic use only in two patients both with pre-existing residual iodine metabolism in their metastases. No measurable accumulation of radioiodine with planar imaging or SPECT was found in 10/15 patients during Isotretinoin therapy as well as before. All patients with shortness of breath were relieved regardless of tumour response to Isotretinoin therapy.

DISCUSSION

The retinoid Isotretinoin is assumed to show growth antagonising effects, anti-angiogenesis and induction of apoptosis in a large range of tissues (4,2). Previous studies have shown that Isotretinoin is a therapeutical option if surgery, radioiodine therapy and external radiation therapy are no longer possible in advanced thyroid cancer (5,6,7). These first clinical long-term results give evidence for a growth inhibiting and differentiation enhancing effect of Isotretionoin in recurrence or metastases of differentiated thyroid cancer. Up to now 14/15 patients treated with Isotretinoin have shown at least a partial response to this therapy regimen either in terms of Tg, F-18-FDG or radioiodine measurements. In one third of patients iodine metabolism was induced. These results correspond well to cell culture studies in thyroid cancer cell lines (2,8,9). Isotretinoin in dosage already used in dermatology and oncology is able to induce stagnation of recurrence or metastases in otherwise intractable thyroid cancer.

REFERENCES

1. Bollag W, Holdener EE. Retinoids in Cancer Prevention and Therapy. Ann Oncol 1992; 3:513-526
2. Degos L. Retinoic acid in promyelocytic leukemia. A model for differentiation therapy. Curr Opin Oncol 1992; 4:42-52
3. Van Herle AJ, Agatep M, Padua DN III, van Herle HML, Juillard GJF. Effects of 13-cis-retinoic acid on growth and differentiation of human follicular carcinoma cells (UCLA RO 82 W-1) in vitro. J Clin Endocrinol Metab 1990; 71:755-76
4. Börner AR, Müller-Gärtner HW. Radiojodtherapie und Radiojodnachsorge bei differenzierten Schilddrüsenkarzinomen. Zentralblatt für Chirurgie 1997; 122:274-285
5. Börner AR, Simon D, Müller-Gärtner HW. Isotretinoin therapy in oxyphilic follicular thyroid cancer. Ann Int Med 1997; 127:146
6. Schmutzler C, Brtko J, Bienert K, Köhrle J. Effects of retinoids and role of retinoic acid receptors in human thyroid carcinomas and cell lines derived therefrom. Exp Clin Endocrinol Diabetes 1996; 104:16-9

7. Simon D, Köhrle J, Schmutzler C, Mainz K, Reiners C, Röher HD. Redifferentiation therapy of differentiated thyroid carcinoma with retinoic acid: basics and first clinical results. Exp Clin Endocrinol Diabetes 1996; 104:13-15
8. Arai M, Tsushima T, Isozaki O, Shizume K, Emoto N, Demura H, Miykawa M, Onoda N. Effects of retinoids on iodine metabolism, thyroid peroxidase gene expression and deoxyribonucleic acid synthesis in porcine thyroid cells in culture. Endocrinology 1991; 129: 2827-2833
9. Köhrle J, Schreck R, Bienert K. Retinoids induce type I iodothyrosine 5′-dejodinase in human follicular thyroid carcinoma cell lines. Exp Clin Endocrinol 1994; 102:49

Radioactive Isotopes in
Clinical Medicine and Research XXIII
ed. by H. Bergmann, H. Köhn and H. Sinzinger

IS SPECT-TECHNIQUE NECESSARY FOR PREOPERATIVE DIAGNOSTIS OF PARATHYROID ADENOMA ?

D. Moka, E. Voth, M. Dietlein, K. Smolarz, A. Larena-Avellaneda and H. Schicha
Department of Nuclear Medicine, University of Cologne and Department of Surgery,
St. Katharinen-Hospital, Frechen, Germany

SUMMARY

To assess the value of the ^{99m}Tc-MIBI SPECT in preoperative localization of small parathyroid adenoma (PTA) 29 consecutive patients (10 male, 19 female, mean age 65 ± 12 years) with established diagnosis of pHPT and non-diagnostic ultrasonography were scanned preoperatively. Planar 99mTc-pertechnetate images, planar and SPECT ^{99m}Tc-MIBI-images were obtained using a 3 head gamma camera (Picker Prism 3000). All patients had small, solitary PTA (≤ 1g). Sensitivity in planar MIBI-scintigraphy was 72 %. Using MIBI SPECT there was an increase in sensitivity to 96 %. MIBI SPECT should therefore be performed in all cases when planar MIBI-scintigraphy is non-diagnostic.

INTRODUCTION

Primary hyperparathyroidism (pHPT) is mainly caused by a solitary parathyroid adenoma. Expert parathyroid surgeons are able to find this adenoma correctly in about 95 % of cases without prior preoperative localization imaging techniques. However, in hospitals where this operation is only infrequently performed (2), there has been an increase of morbidity and unsuccessful parathyroidectomy (12). A preoperative reliable localization technique like ^{99m}Tc-MIBI-scintigraphy can guide the surgeon during exploration (2).
The aim of this study was to show the value of ^{99m}Tc-MIBI-scintigraphy for preoperative localization of small parathyroid adenomas. To attain sufficient resolution, especially in small parathyroid adenomas, ^{99m}Tc-MIBI-scintigraphy was performed in conjunction with single photon emission computer tomography (SPECT) (6) using a modern 3 head gamma camera. 3D-displays (volume-rendered reprojection) were used for better visualization of the adenoma site.

PATIENTS AND METHODS

29 consecutive patients (10 male, 19 female, mean age 65 ± 12 years) with established diagnosis of pHPT prior to a sheduled bilateral neck exploration were included in this study. All patients had elevated levels of serum calcium (2,98 ± 0,22 mmol/l; normal range: 2,20 -

2,65 mmol/l) and parathormone (275 ± 77 ng/l; normal range: 12 - 72 ng/l)) and in all patients cervical ultrasonography (7.5 MHz linear array) was non-diagnostic.

After performing a thyroid examination including determination of the serum - fT_3-, - fT_4- and - TSH-levels and ultrasonography, a planar ^{99m}Tc scintigraphy of the thyroid was performed to localize radionuclide accumulating thyroid lesions. Following the protocol of *Taillefer et. al.* (10), planar and tomographic cervico-thoracic images were taken 15 min. and 120 min. after i.v. injection of 740 MBq ^{99m}Tc-MIBI (Cardiolite®, Du Pont Pharma, FRG). Additional subtraction images (^{99m}Tc-MIBI- minus ^{99m}Tc-pertechnetate-planar-images) were determined to check for radionuclide accumulating thyroid lesions.

Patients were examined in supine position without hyperextension of the neck. Both planar images and SPECT were assessed using a 3-head gamma camera (Picker Prism 3000) with a high resolution collimator and an evaluation technique described recently (5).

Positive adenoma location was indicated by an abnormal radionuclide focus in the neck region or mediastinum. Normal parathyroid glands (a histopathologic correlation was obtained in every patient) were considered as true negatives for the calculation of specificity.

RESULTS

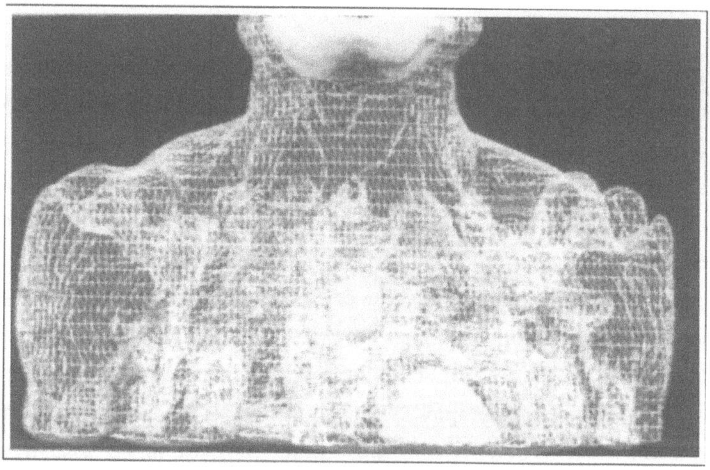

Fig. 1 ^{99m}Tc-MIBI-SPECT (anterior 3D-display), delineating a mediastinal parathyroid adenoma (3600 mg) in a 72 years old female patient with pHPT.

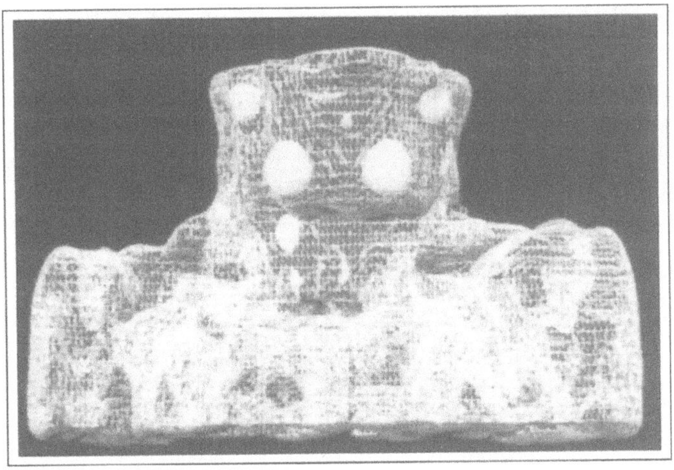

Fig. 2 ^{99m}Tc-MIBI-SPECT (anterior 3D-display), delineating two parathyroid adenomas (760 mg and 170 mg) in a 53 years old male patient prior to surgical exploration.

A hyperplastic gland or carcinoma was detected in none of the patients. The weight of the histologically confirmed solitary adenomas varied from 170 mg to 1000 mg (mean weight of 670 ± 310 mg). Serum calcium and parathyroid hormone returned to normal values postoperatively.

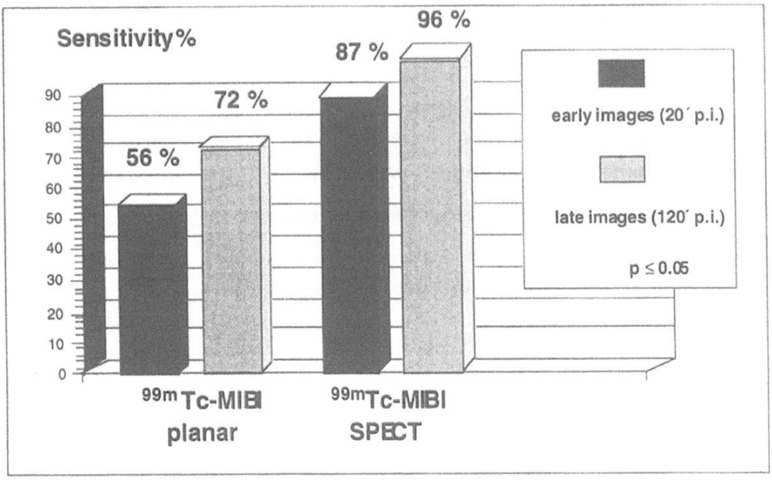

Fig. 3 Comparison of planar and SPECT sensitivity in all patients.

Using ^{99m}Tc-MIBI-parathyroid planar images parathyroid adenomas were correctly identified and precisely localized in 21 of 29 patients (72 %). Sensitivity increased up to 96 % using SPECT and the 3D-display in cine mode (volume-rendered reprojection; fig. 1)).

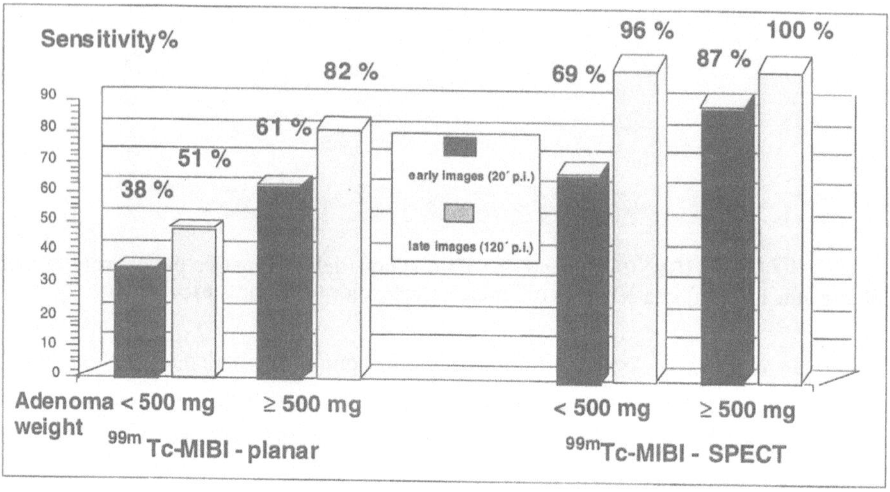

Fig. 4 Comparison of sensitivities of planar images and SPECT in relation to adenoma weight (< 500 mg and 500 to 1000 mg).

All results show that there is an increase in sensitivity between early and delayed images especially in small parathyroid adenomas. With adenoma weights higher than 500 mg good sensitivity is achieved with planar scintigraphy too. However reliable sensitivity can only be ensured using SPECT.

Specificity of ^{99m}Tc-MIBI-parathyroid scintigraphy was 100 %, none of the normal parathyroid glands being visualized.

DISCUSSION

Standard imaging methods (ultrasonography, CT, MRI, ^{201}Tl/^{99m}Tc-subtraction scintigraphy) have only a limited value in preoperative localization of parathyroid adenomas because of their low sensitivities in detection of small lesions (12). ^{99m}Tc-MIBI parathyroid scintigraphy is already known to be higher effective for the localization of enlarged glands (> 1g) (4). However, these adenomas do not present a challenge to an experienced parathyroid surgeon. Our study showed, that small adenomas (≤ 1g) could also be localized reliable. In contrast to planar scintigraphy the sensitivity of site localization by MIBI SPECT was comparable to that normally achieved by expert surgeons in primary bilateral neck exploration. Furthermore, this imaging method also revealed multiple or ectopic adenomas (Fig. 2).

Normally, in cases of reoperation and in surgical high-risk patients with serious co-morbid diseases there is an increase in morbidity (8). A preoperatively exact adenoma localization can improve operation success rates even of less experienced surgeons. Because MIBI-SPECT is highly specific (100 % in our study, 92 - 100 % in other studies) a single focus in pHPT represents the adenoma and a scan-directed operation can be carried out (2). Retrospectively, therefore, the surgeons in our study would have been able to perform a scan-guided unilateral parathyroidectomy. This procedure would have reduced operation time significantly (between 30 and 60 % (1, 3, 11)) and operation costs would have been cut down to to 20 % (7). A mediastinal or bilateral neck exploration remains only mandatory when despite the use of tomographic ^{99m}Tc-MIBI parathyroid scintigraphy, the adenoma could still not be localized, e.g. in cases of multiple foci or when concomitant thyroid diseases hamper detection (9).

CONCLUSION

Although, for solitary adenomas, accurate, preoperative adenoma localization can render extensive bilateral exploration unnecessary, a general preoperative MIBI SPECT cannot be recommended in all patients with pHPT, especially if the operation is to be performed by an expert parathyroid surgeon. Nevertheless, a preoperative diagnostic of abnormal glands using ^{99m}Tc-MIBI SPECT is appropriate:

a. in patients where preoperative ultrasonography was non-diagnostic
b. in patients with persistant or recurrent pHPT
c. in patients with suspected ectopic or mediastinal adenomas
d. in patients after prior large-scale neck surgery
e. in surgically high-risk patients with serious co-morbid diseases
f. in hospitals where parathyroidectomy is infrequently performed.

In those cases ^{99m}Tc-MIBI parathyroid SPECT with 3D-display can help to prevent extensive dissection of the neck and mediastinum and therefore decrease the ratio of postoperative morbidity (injuries to the laryngeal nerve and hypoparathyroidism).

Because planar ^{99m}Tc-MIBI scintigraphy can reliably detect only larger adenomas (> 500 mg), ^{99m}Tc-MIBI SPECT should be performed in all cases where planar scintigraphy is non-diagnostic.

REFERENCES

1. Casas AT, Burke GJ, Mansberger AJ and Wei JP. Impact of technetium-99m-sestamibi localization on operative time and success of operations for primary hyperparathyroidism. Am Surg 1994; 60: 12-16.
2. Harness JK, Organ CH and Thompson NW. Operative experience of U.S. general surgery residents in thyroid and parathyroid disease. Surgery 1995; 118: 1063-1070.
3. Irvin III G, Prudhomme DL, Deriso GT, Sfakianakis G and Chandarlapaty SK. A new approach to parathyroidectomy. Ann Surg 1994; 219: 574-579.
4 McBiles M, Lambert AT, Cote MC and Kim SY. Sestamibi parathyroid imaging. Sem Nucl Med 1995; 25/3: 221-234.
5. Moka D, Voth E, Larena-Avellaneda A, Schicha H. 99mTc-MIBI-SPECT for the location of small parathyroid adenoma. Nuklearmedizin 1997; 36: 240-244.
6. Perez-Monte JE, Brown ML, Shah AN, Ranger NT, Watson CG, Carty SE and Clarke MR. Parathyroid adenomas: Accurate detection and localization with Tc-99m Sestamibi SPECT. Radiology 1996; 201: 85-91.
7. Petti GJ, Chonkich GD and Morgan JW. Unilateral parathyroidectomy: the value of the localizing scan. J Otolaryngol 1993; 22: 307-310.
8. Shaha AR, LaRosa CA and Jaffe BM. Parathyroid localization prior to primary exploration. Am J Surg 1993; 166: 289-293.
9. Staudenherz A, Abela C, Niederle B, Steiner E, Helbrich T, Puig S, Kaserer K, Becherer A, Leitha T and Kletter K. Comparison and histopathological correlation of three parathyroid imaging methods in a population with a high prevalence of concomitant thyroid diseases. Eur. J. Nucl. Med. 1997; 24: 143-149.
10. Taillefer R, Boucher Y, Potvin C and Lambert R. Detection and localization of parathyroid adenomas in patients with hyperparathyroidism using a single radionuclide imaging procedure with technetium-99m-sestamibi (double-phase study). J Nucl Med 1992; 33: 1801-1807.
11. Uden P, Aspelin P, Berglund J, Lilja B, Nyman U, Olsson LE and Zederfeldt B. Preoperative localization in unilateral parathyroid surgery. A cost-benefit study on ultrasound, computed tomography and scintigraphy. Acta Chir Scand 1990; 156: 29-35.
12. Wen S, Düren M, Morita E, Higgins C, Bum Q, Siperstein A and Clark O. Reoperation for persistent or recurrent primary hyperparathyroidism. Arch Surg 1996; 131: 861-869.

ONCOLOGY, HAEMATOLOGY

Radioactive Isotopes in
Clinical Medicine and Research XXIII
ed. by H. Bergmann, H. Köhn and H. Sinzinger

COMPARISON OF INTERLESIONALLY AND SYSTEMICALLY ADMINISTERED RADIOLABELLED MONOCLONAL ANTIBODIES IN IMPLANTED TUMOURS.

Robert Thomas, Paul Carnochan, Susan A Eccles, Michael Brada

The Institute of Cancer Research and Royal Marsden NHS trust, Sutton, Surrey, SM2 5PT.

SUMMARY: In this experimental tumour system, intralesional administration (ILA) of ^{125}I labelled MAb increased uptake by a factor of three over systemic administration. Although there was an element of non-specific entrapment following ILA there was a 2.5 times greater uptake using a specific MAb (ALN/11/53) compared to a nonspecific control MAb (ICR-2). The areas of activity were demonstrated by autoradiography. After 24 hours, at the tumour muscle junction, activity tended to conform to the shape of the tumour. This suggests a potential advantage over conventional brachytherapy, however, a number of significant adverse features were encountered. In particular, there was significant leakage of radioactivity in the first 24 hours by backtracking along the needle and the volume of activity was small (< 1/3rd of the tumour). Substantially more work is required to investigate methods to increase the distribution of activity throughout the whole tumour, reduce backtracking and measure its extent in larger tumours.

INTRODUCTION

Targeting tumours with radiolabelled MAb is now achieving high specificities. For example, Zalutsky et al (1) demonstrated tumour to normal tissues enhancement ratios as high a 200:1 following intravenous administration (IVA). The barrier to therapeutic success, however, is the extremely low percentage of the injected activity remaining in tumour (0.001 - 0.01%/g) (2,3). Therapeutic doses are consequently difficult to achieve without potential toxicity to systemic organs (4). One cause of this low uptake may arise from the fact that interstitial pressure within tumours is usually higher than the surrounding circulation (5,6). This physical pressure counter balances the MAb concentration gradient and together with their large size compounds are not able to penetrate into the tumour. Direct administration, into the solid component of tumour may circumvent this problem and improve local tumour uptake.

This study used an experimental tumour model to evaluate intralesionally administered (ILA) radiolabelled MAb. The retention and distribution of labelled MAb within the tumour, surrounding normal tissues and systemic organs were compared with those achieved following intravenous administration. In addition, the uptake of a non-specific, control, MAb were compared to determine the importance of antibody specificity for this route of administration.

METHODS

The experimental tumour used in this study was a highly metastatic transplantable rat fibrosarcoma HSN (8) . Tumour cells were passaged in-vitro then suspended at a concentration of $5x10^6$/ml in phostate buffered saline. 1 x 10^6 cells in 0.2ml were implanted into the lateral thigh of male CBH/cbi rats by deep muscular injection. Experiments were performed at 14 days when the tumours had reached a mean size of 1.5cm (Range 1.1-2.2 cm). All animals were managed in compliance with UKCCCR guidelines (9). Ethical approval was granted from the Institute of Cancer Research ethics committee.

ALN\11\53, a rat IgG2a MAb, was raised against a 180KD surface protein specifically expressed on HSN tumour cells (10). The control MAb (ICR-2), had no specificity for this tumour. MAbs were radiolabelled with ^{125}I (ICN Ltd, UK) using the iodogen method. Radiochemical purification was achieved using gel filtration (PD-10 Column - Pharmacia, UK) and checked using thin layer chromatography (10% trichloroacetic acid, Whatman 31-ET paper). Radiochemical purity was greater than 98% at the time of use.

Adult male rats (mean weight = 320 g) were anaesthetized using a Halothane and Oxygen mixture. The tumour dimensions were recorded with callipers. Six rats were injected intravenously using the right external jugular vein. Twenty nine further rats had ^{125}I labelled MAb infused directly into the centre of the tumour (14 ALN/11/53, 15 ICR-2) using a 27 gauge needle microtubing (*28 x 0.61 mm id x od, polythene; Portex Ltd*) and a harvard syringe pump **[Plate.1- right]**. Approximately 25 µl of ^{125}I-MAb was drawn up into the tubing, followed by 1 mm of air, 0.5cm of methylene blue and a further 1 mm of air. The air prevented mixing of the dye and ^{125}I-MAb. The infused volume (~25µl) and rate (50 µl/hr) were kept constant on each occasion but the delivered activity was also derived by subtracting the retained tube activity from the initial tube activity.

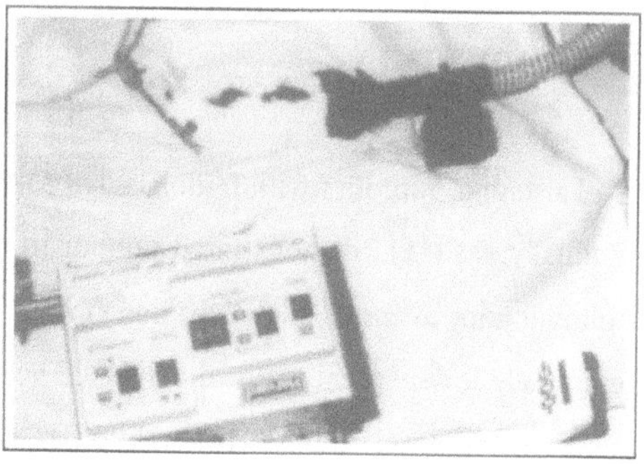

The rats undergoing ILA were killed at specified times following administration, the rats injected systemically were all killed at 48hrs. The tumours, adjacent tissues and systemic organs were dissected out. Tissues were weighed and then gamma counted separately using an EG&G ORTEC GMX-102000 system fitted with a germanium detector. Uptake of radiotracer was expressed as % injected dose (%ID) and % injected dose/gram of tissue (%ID/G). The intratumoural distribution of radioactivity was assessed by autoradiography. Each tumour was cryostat sectioned in planes perpendicular to the infusion needle trajectory. The thickness of each slice was 20 μm and separation between each slice initially 1mm **[Plate.2 - right]**. When the methylene blue was seen, indicating the level of MAb infusion, the slice separations were then reduced to 0.5mm. An average of 16 duplicate sets of slides were made per tumour. One set was used for autoradiography and the other stained with H&E. The proportion of tumour or adjacent tissue containing levels of activity above background was measured by overlying the two slides onto graph paper and counting the 1mm squares.

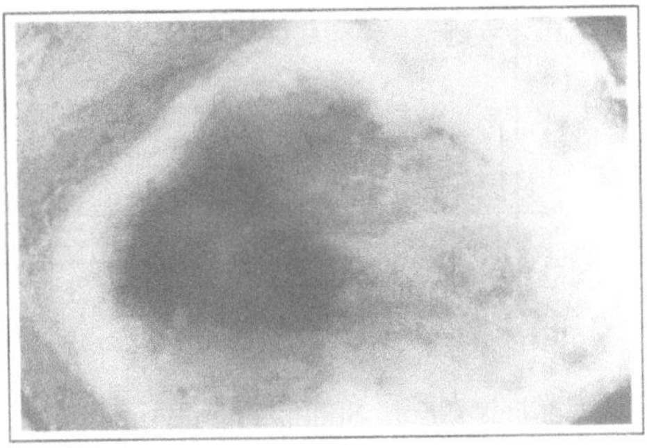

RESULTS & DISCUSSION

Tumour uptake. The radioactive uptake in tumour following ILA was significantly greater than via IVA. At the 48 hours following administration this was 6.8% v 4.2% using ALN/11/53 **[Fig.1- left]** and this difference was significant (student's t-test, 2 tailed probability p=0.01). This magnitude of improved uptake following ILA administration may not seem impressive considering that the IV injection is diluted in the animals entire blood volume. However, the ILA was given with a single needle which produced activity in less than a third of the tumour **[Plate.3 - below]**.

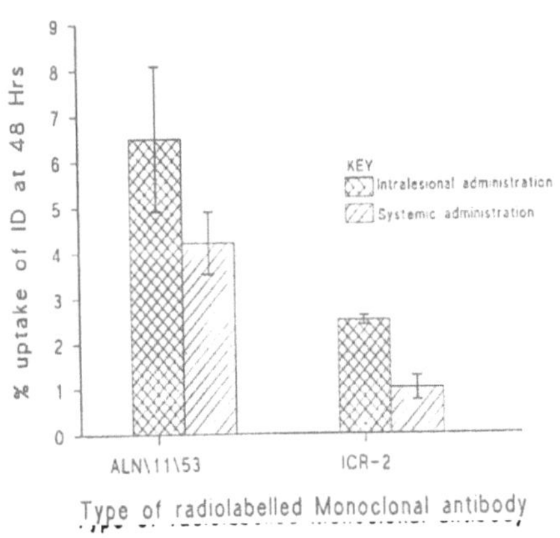

An element of this increased uptake is attributed to non-specific entrapment, as there was also an increased percentage uptake with ILA versus IVA using non specific MAb, albeit to a lesser extent. (2.5% v 1.1%). This phenomenon is consistent with previous reports in the literature which attributed this entrapment to the disturbed vascular flow within tumours (11,12). This non specific entrapment was not, however, the complete picture in this study, as following ILA there was a significantly greater uptake with specific versus non specific MAb (6.8% v 2.5%). **Figure.2 (left)** also demonstrates this superior uptake at all time points up to 72 hours post administration. Summating all time points, ALN\11\53 was superior to ICR-2 by ratios of 1:2.5. Using the students t-test, the 2 tailed probability of a difference was p = 0.04. This graph also clearly demonstrates a sharp fall off of activity up to 24 hours for both MAbs. This was caused by rapid leakage of unbound MAb. This leakage occured mainly by backtracking along the needle path as demostarted in the autoradiographs below **[Plate.3]**. In a previous study, using this model, backtracking was also noted but a correlation between infusion rate and backtracking was also demonstrated (unpublished data P Carnochan). However, even with the 50 μl/hr used in this study this was still clearly a significant effect, with backtracking occuring probabally after withdrawl of the needle. This presents a major drawback with this technique, in this model, and further work is required to reduce leakage by using manoevres such tissue glues. On the other hand, this has not been found to be such a problem in the clinical studies published so far. One factor could be the longer path length in larger tumours (13,14), a factor which also requires further investigation.

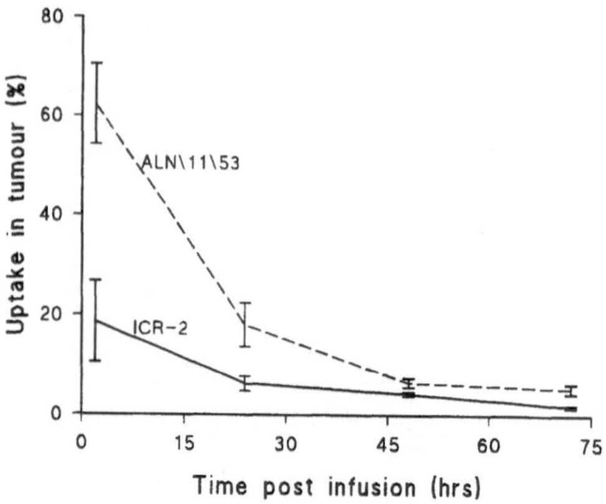

The normal tissue uptakes following intralesional administration of specific and nonspecific MAb were low (0.1- 0.6%/g of the injected activity) and there was no significant difference between the two antibodies for any tissue (liver, kidneys, overlying and adjacent muscle and equivalent muscle groups on the opposite leg). The low levels in this experimental system are consistent with the normal tissue levels seen in clinical studies. For example, following intralesional or intracystic labelled MAb in patients with glioma (13,14,15).

The distribution of radioactivity within tumour and the adjacent normal tissue following IL administration was small - (average for ALN\11\53 = 335 mm^3 , ICR-2 = 277 mm^3). For both MAb up to 24 hours, over half the volume of activity was present in the surrounding muscle compartments. At 24 hours the leaked volume of activity had cleared leaving most of the activity within tumour again for both MAb. This most likely represented greater non-specific clearing of the MAbs from muscle rather than the denser parenchyma of the tumour. From 48 to 72 hours the volume of activity within tumour for ALN\11\53 remained high whereas for ICR-2 it dropped. Representative examples of the characteristic patterns of radioactive distribution at different time points post infusion are illustrated **(Plate.3- above)**. At the tumour to muscle junction, from 24 hours, the radioactivity cut off sharply creating the tendancy for the radioactivity to conform to the shape of the tumour. This feature, if confirmed in objective quantitative studies, would represent a significant advantage over conventional brachytherapy which irradiates spheres irrespective of the local anatomy.

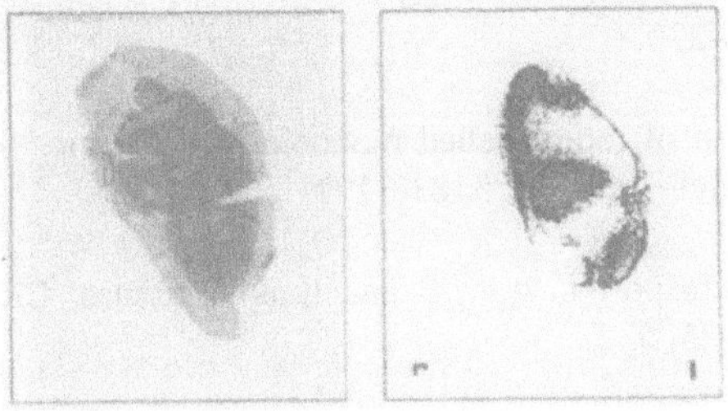

6 hours post infusion

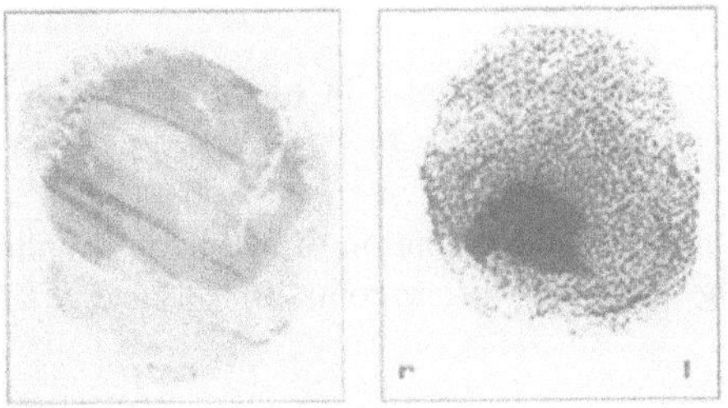

48 hours post infusion

In this experimental study, intralesional RIT resulted in higher uptake than systemic administration and using a specific MAb improved uptake and specificity. Direct infusion of radiolbelled MAb may allow radiotherapy dose escalation in tumours such as glioma, sarcoma and prostate where local control is still a significant problem. Substantial further work is required to enhance tumour retention, reduce the degree of backtracking whilst at the same time improving intratumoral activity distribution.

REFERENCES

1. Zalutsky MR, Moseley RP, Bigner D. Pharmacokinetics and tumour localisation of ^{131}I labelled anti-tenascin monoclonal anti body 81C6 in patients with gliomas and other intracranial malignancies. Cancer research 1989; 49: 2807-2813.

2. Epenetos AA, Courtenay-luck N, Pickering D. Antibody guided irradiation of brain glioma by arterial infusion of radioactive Mab against EGFR and Blood group A antigen. British Med Journal 1985; 290: 1463-1466.

3. Brady LW, Miyamoto C, Woo D V. Malignant astrocytomas treated with iodine-125 labelled monoclonal antibody 425 against epidermal growth factor receptor: A phase 2 trial. Int. J. Radiat Oncol., Biol. Phys 1991; 22: 225-230.

4. Epenetos AA, Snook D, Durbin H. Limitation of radiolabelled monoclonal antibodies for localisation of human neoplasms. Cancer research 1986; 46: 3183-3191.

5. Jain RK and Gerlowski LE. Extravascular transport in normal and tumour tissues. CRC Critical Reviews in Oncology/Haematology 1975; 5: 2.

6. Fleischman GJ, Secomb TW, Gross JF. Effects of extravascular pressure gradients of capillary fliud exchange. Math. Biosci. 1986; 81: 145-164.

7. Baxter LT and Jain KR. Transport of fluid and macromolecules in tumours. 1. Role of interstitial pressure and convection. Microvascular res. 1989; 37: 77-104.

8. Currie A and Cage JO. Influence of tumour growth in the evolution of cytotoxic lymphoid cells in rats bearing a spontaneously metasasing syngeneic fibrosarcoma. Br J Cancer 1973; 28: 136-146.

9. UKCCCR Guidelines for the welfare of animals in experimental neoplasia. UKCCCR, 20 Park Cresent, London, 1988.

10. Dean CJ, Styles J, Gyure L, Peppard J, Hobbs S, Jackson E, Hall J. The production of hybridomas from the gut-associated lymphoid tissue of tumour bearing rats. Clin Exp Immunol 1984; 57: 358-64.

11. Goldberg DM, Preston DF, Primus FJ, Hansen HJ. Photoscan localisation of GW-39 tumours in hampsters using radiolabelled anticarcinoenbryonic antigen immunoglobulin G. Cancer Res. 1974; 34: 1.

12. Primus FJ, MacDonald R, Goldberg DM, Hansen HJ. Tumour detection and localisation with purified antibodies to carcinoembryonic antigen. Cancer Res.1977 37: 1544-1547.

13. Thomas R, Flux G, Chittenden S, Hall A, Kitchen N, Thomas DGT, Bigner D, Zalutsky, Brada M. Intralesional 131-I labelled Mab therapy in patients with recurrent high grade gliomas [Abstract]. B J Cancer 1994. 70. Supplement XX11, 20.

14.Riva P, Arista A, Turiale G. Treatment of intracranial Human glioblastoma by Direct Intratumoural Administration of I^{131} labelled anti-tenascin monoclonal antibody BC-2. Int. J. Cancer 1992. 51: 7-13.

15.Hopkins K, Chandler C, Bullimore J, Sandeman D, Coakham H, Kemshead JT (1995). A pilot study of the treatment of patients with recurrent malignant gliomas with intratumoural yttrium-90 radioimmunoconjugates. Radiotherapy & Oncology 1995; 34: 121-131.

Radioactive Isotopes in
Clinical Medicine and Research XXIII
ed. by H. Bergmann, H. Köhn and H. Sinzinger

COMPARISON OF MRI AND SOMATOSTATIN RECEPTOR SCINTIGRAPHY (SRS) IN POSTSURGICAL FOLLOW-UP OF MENINGIOMA

S. Klutmann, A. Behnke, K.H. Bohuslavizki, N. Tietje, W. Brenner, H.-H. Hugo, H.M. Mehdorn, E. Henze

Clinics of Nuclear Medicine and Neurosurgery, Christian-Albrechts-Universitiy, Arnold-Heller-Str. 9, 24105 Kiel, Germany

SUMMARY: In this study SRS and MRI were compared in postsurgical follow-up of meningioma. Prior to and 2-3 months after surgery 27 patients received standard MRI as well as SRS after i.v. injection of 200 MBq In-111-octreotide. Planar whole-body images were obtained at 10 min, 1, 4, and 24 hrs. p.i., and SPECT was performed at 4 and 24 hrs p.i. Final diagnosis was proven histologically in all patients. Prior to surgery MRI showed focal contrast enhancement in all patients, and SRS revealed focal accumulation of In-111-octreotide in 27 patients. Thus, preoperative MRI and SRS yielded comparable results. After surgery MRI showed diffuse contrast enhancement in all patients. Thus, MRI did not allow to differentiate between tumor tissue and unspecific hyperperfusion. In contrast, SRS revealed focal accumulation of In-111-octreotide in 16 out of 27 patients indicating tumor remnants or relapse of meningioma. This resulted either in an operative revision or in more frequent follow-up examinations. In 11 out of 27 patients SRS was negative confirming total resection of meningioma. SRS has a significant impact in postsurgical follow-up in patients with meningioma.

INTRODUCTION

Surgery is the treatment of choice in patients with meningioma. However, the risk of local relapse is well-known. This holds especially true for meningioma located near the skull base since meninges at that site are attached very closely to the bones, thus rendering total resection of meningioma difficult [1-3]. Morphological imaging using MRI is well-established in the detection of meningioma. However, in the first 6 months following surgery MRI may fail to differentiate between tumor remnants or relapse of meningioma on the one hand and unspecific hyperperfusion on the other hand. Since meningioma were shown to express somatostatin receptors [4-10] the additional impact of functional imaging using SRS in postsurgical follow-up of patients with meningioma was studied.

MATERIALS AND METHODS

A total of 27 patients (20 females, 7 males) with suspected meningioma received MRI as well as SRS prior to and 2-3 months after surgery. The patients age ranged from 19 to 70 years. All patients underwent histological evaluation. Standard MRI (T1-, T2-wheighted) was performed on a 1.5 T machine including contrast enhancement with 0.1 mg/kg Gadolinium. Patients received 200 MBq In-111-octreotide i.v. Planar whole-body images were obtained simultaneously in anterior and posterior projection at 10 min, 1, 4, and 24 hrs using a large-field-of-view gamma-camera equipped with a medium-energy parallel hole collimator (Bodyscan, Siemens, Erlangen, Germany). In addition, SPECT was performed in a conventional manner at 4 and 24 hrs p.i. with a single head large-field-of-view gamma-camera equipped with a medium-energy parallel hole collimator (Diacam, Siemens, Erlangen, Germany). Tumor-to-background ratios were quantified by conventional ROI-technique. Results are given as mean ± one standard deviation.

RESULTS

Prior to surgery MRI showed focal contrast enhancement in all patients investigated. Accordingly, SRS demonstrated focal uptake of In-111-octreotide with an increase of tumor-to-background ratio with time (Table 1).

Two to three months after surgery MRI yielded diffuse contrast enhancement in the primary tumor site in all patients. Therefore, MRI failed to differentiate between unspecific hyperperfusion and tumor remnants or relapse of meningioma. Additional information was provided by SRS. In eleven out of 27 patients SRS was negative confirming total tumor resection, and no further interventions were performed so far (Fig. 1). In contrast, postsurgical SRS revealed focal accumulation of In-111-octreotide in 16 out of 27 patients showing an increase of tumor-to-background ratio with time (Table 1).

In nine out of these 16 patients total tumor resection was not feasible so that remnants were known. This was confirmed by positive SRS two to three months postsurgically (Fig. 2). In two out of the latter nine patients multilocular malignant meningioma was proven histologically. In five out of 16 patients positive SRS demonstrated meningioma tissue in the tumoral area despite assumed total tumor resection. These scintigraphic findings resulted in either operative revision (n=2) or more frequent follow-up examinations (n=3).

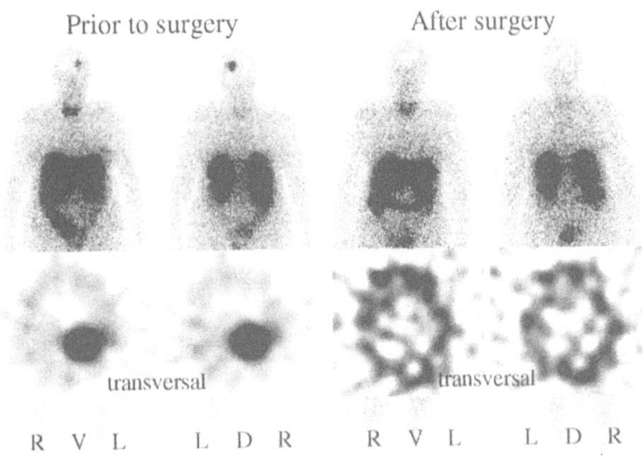

Fig 1: Planar SRS and transverse SPECT slices (inset) 24 hrs p.i. Preoperative transitionalcellular meningioma localized in the left lateral ventricle. Postoperative SRS-negative confirming total tumor resection.

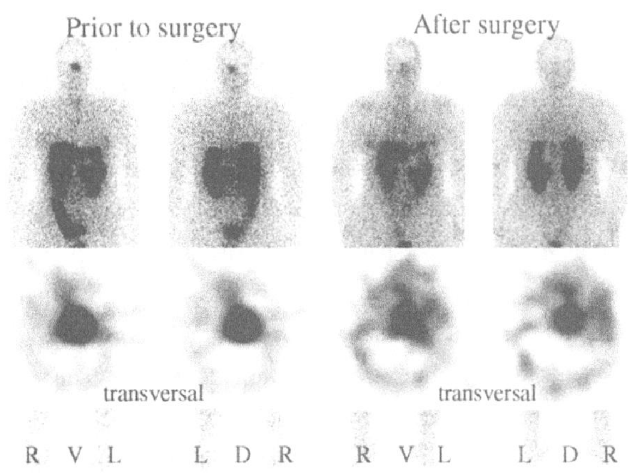

Fig 2: Planar SRS and transverse SPECT slices (inset) 24 hrs p.i. Preoperative menigotheliomatous meningioma localized in the left sphenoid bone area. Postoperative SRS-positive. Total tumor rsection was not feasible.

Table 1. Tumor-to-background ratio of 27 patients with meningioma with respect results of somatostatin receptor scintigraphy. Data represent mean ± one standard deviation.

	Prior to surgery	3 months after surgery	
	SRS positive	SRS positive	SRS negative
time p.i.	n=27	n=16	n=11
10 min	1.33 ± 0.10	1.39 ± 0.15	1.17 ± 0.03
1 h	1.46 ± 0.13	1.57 ± 0.13	1.20 ± 0.02
4 hrs	1.82 ± 0.19	1.82 ± 0.19	1.28 ± 0.03
24 hrs	2.85 ± 0.25	3.01 ± 0.25	1.49 ± 0.03

In the remaining two out of 16 SRS-positive patients focal accumulation of In-111-octreotide was detected at different localizations (right parietal area, right occiptal area) as compared to tracer accumulation observed prior to surgery (sellar region, right sphenoidal sinus).

DISCUSSION

Since meningioma were shown to express somatostatin receptors on their cell surface in near 100 % in votro [4, 5] as well as in vivo [6-10] SRS has proven helpful in the differential diagnosis of meningioma versus neurinoma when MRI failed [11, 12]. In this study the additional impact of SRS was compared to MRI in postsurgical follow-up of patients with meningioma.

Between 6/96 and 8/97 a total of 27 patients with suspected meningioma underwent SRS as well as MRI prior to and 2–3 months after surgery. Presurgically, MRI showed focal contrast enhancement indicating meningioma in all patients investigated. Accordingly, focal uptake of In-111-octreotide with an increase of tumor-to-background ratio was shown in all of them. Thus, positive SRS demonstrated the presence of somatostatin receptors, and final diagnosis of meningioma was proven histologically in all 27 patients. In summary, the diagnostic benefit of both SRS and MRI in the preoperative work-up of all patients investigated was comparable.

Two to three months after surgery MRI showed diffuse contrast enhancement in the primary tumor site in all 27 patients. Since the blood-brain-barrier is normally disrupted for several months after surgery, contrast enhancement allows in principle no discrimination between tumor remnants or relapse of meningioma and postoperative hyperperfusion. Therefore, morphological imaging such as MRI failed in postsurgical follow-up. In contrast, SRS provided additional information. Postoperative SRS was negative in 11 patients confirming total tumor resection, and no further interventions were performed so far.

In contrast, positive SRS was obtained in 16 patients following surgery. In nine out of these 16 patients total tumor resection was not feasible proven by focal accumulation of In-111-octreotide in the remaining meningioma tissue. However, in five out of 16 SRS-positive patients somatostatin receptors were detected whereas total tumor resection was assumed. In two out of these five patients scintigraphic findings resulted in an operative revision with histologically proven meninigioma tissue. The remaining three patients were referred to a more frequent follow-up pattern. Thus, in these five patients positive SRS directly influenced either treatment or postsurgical follow-up.

In the remaining two out of 16 postoperative SRS-positive patients localization of postoperative focal tracer accumulation was not consistent with localization of preoperative tracer uptake. One of these patients showed preoperative tracer accumulation in the right sphenoidal sinus area whereas postoperative SRS yielded a focus in the right occipital area, and SRS resulted in operative revision with resection of a second site meningioma.The second of these patients showed preoperative focal tracer uptake in the sellar region while postoperative tracer uptake was localized in the right parietal area, and the neurosurgeon ascertained total tumor resection. In this patient craniotomy and implantation of palacos was localized in the same region where an increase of In-111-octreotide was observed postsurgically. Therefore, SRS was primarily noted as false-positive, but turned out to be consistent with unspecific tracer accumulation probably due to an lymphocyte accumulation in the palacos area. This emphasizes the necessity to assess the results of SRS with a thorough knowledge of both complete history of the individual patient and the results of complementary imaging.

CONCLUSIONS

In conclusion, SRS is a highly specific functional imaging modality, which has a significant additional impact in postsurgical follow-up in patients with meningioma, thus, providing the basis to select those patients who need more frequent follow-up examinations or operative revision.

REFERENCES

1. Gokalp HZ, Arasil E, Erdogan A, Egemen N, Deda H, Cerci A. Tentorial menigiomas. Neurosurgery 1995; **36**: 46-51.
2. Risi P, Uske A, de Tribolet N. Meningiomas involving the anterior clinoid process. Br J Neurosurg 1994; **8:** 295-305.
3. DeMonte F. Surgery of skull base tumors. Curr Opin Oncol 1995; **7:** 201-206.
4. Reubi JC, Laissue J, Krenning EP, Lamberts SWJ. Somatostatin receptors in human cancer: incidence, characteristics, functional correlates and clinical implications. J Steroid Biochim Molec Biol 1992; **43:** 27–35.
5. Reubi JC, Kvols L, Krenning EP, Lamberts SWJ. In vitro and in vivo detection of somatostatin receptors in human malignant tissue. Acta Ocol 1991; **30:** 463–468.
6. Luyken C, Hildebrandt G, Scheidhauer K, Krisch B. Diagnostic value of somatostatin-receptor-scintigraphy in patients with intracranial tumours. Nuklearmediziner 1993; **16:** 317–324.
7. Scheidhauer K, Hildebrand G, Luyken C, Schomäcker K, Klug N, Schicha H. Somatostatin receptor scintigraphy in brain tumors and pituitary tumors: first experiences. Horm Metab Res 1993; **27:** 59–62.
8. Jochens R, Cordes M, Wolters A, Richter W, Amthauer H, Stoltenburg-Didinger G, Maier-Hauff K, Felix R. Untersuchungen von Hirntumoren und Hirnmetastasen mit [^{111}In-DTPA-D-Phe^{1}]-Octreotide-SPECT. Klin Neurorad 1995; **5:** 1–13.
9. Hildebrandt G, Scheidhauer K, Luyken C, Schicha H, Klug N, Dahms P, Krisch B. High sensitivity of the in vivo detection of somatostatin receptors by ^{111}Indium-[DTPA-octreotide]-scintigraphy in meningioma patients. Acta Neurochir Wien 1994; **126:** 63–71.
10. Maini CL, Tofani A, Sciuto R, Carapella C, Cioffi R, Crecco M. Scintigraphy visualization of somatostatin receptors in human meningiomas using 111-indium-DTPA-D-Phe-1-octreotide. Nucl Med Commun 1993; **14:** 505–508.
11. Reubi JC, Lang W, Maurer R, Koper JW, Lamberts SWJ. Distribution and biochemical characterization of somatostatin receptors in tumors of the human central nervous system. Cancer Res 1987; **47:** 5758–5764.
12. Bohuslavizki KH, Brenner W, Braunsdorf WEK, Behnke A, Tinnemeyer S, Hugo HH, Jahn N, Wolf H, Sippel C, Clausen M, Mehdorn HM, Henze E. Somatostatin receptor scintigraphy in the differential diagnosis of meningioma. Nucl Med Commun 1996; **17**: 302-310.

Radioactive Isotopes in
Clinical Medicine and Research XXIII
ed. by H. Bergmann, H. Köhn and H. Sinzinger

COMPARISON OF CONTRAST ENHANCED MRI, Tc-99m HYDROXY-METHYLENE DIPHOSPHONATE AND Tc-99m TETROFOSMIN SCINTI-MAMMOGRAPHY IN PATIENTS WITH SUSPICIOUS BREAST LESIONS

P. Lind*, W. Umschaden**; J. Oman***, E. Forsthuber****, K. Kerschbaumer****,
H.P. Dinges*****, O. Unterweger*, H.J Gallowitsch*, E. Kresnik*, P. Mikosch*, M. Molnar*.
Departments of Nuclear Medicine & Endocrinology*,
Radiology**, Surgery***, Gynecology**** and Institute of Pathology*****,
Landeskrankenhaus Klagenfurt, Austria

SUMMARY: In patients with suspicious breast lesions, scintimammography (SM) using Tc-99m tetrofosmin (TETRO) and hydroxymethylene-diphosphonate (HDP) and Gd-DTPA MRI were performed. For both TETRO and MRI sensitivity was 93% compared to 71% for HDP; specificity was lower for TETRO and HDP (71%) than for MRI (86%). This preliminary study shows that, in contrast to HDP, TETRO SM and Gd-DTPA MRI are of additional diagnostic value in diagnosing breast cancer.

INTRODUCTION

Mammography (MM) is a well established method to screen women for breast cancer (1). However, the problems of mammography in patients with dense breasts and the low specificity make further methods desirable. Additional techniques such as high frequency ultrasonography (US) have improved sensitivity but not specificity. Similar results were reported for MRI in early studies (2). From this point of view there is a need for further investigations that present detection of viable tumour tissue. Several radionuclide imaging techniques with different radiopharmaceuticals have been described in the last few years including monoclonal antibodies and nonspecific radionuclides and tracers (3-10). The purpose of this study was to compare scintimammography (SM) using Tc-99m tetrofosmin (TETRO), Tc-99m hydroxy-methylene diphosphonate (HDP) and dynamic Gd-DTPA enhanced MRI in patients with mammographically suspicious breast lesions.

MATERIAL AND METHODS

In 29 women (x:53 years; s:14 years; range: 28-81 years) with suspicious MM and/or US, further diagnostic work up (MRI, HDP and TETRO) was done within one week. Only those 21 patients who underwent surgery for histological clarification of the lesions were considered for further evaluation by MRI, HDP and TETRO SM. MRI imaging was performed using T2 TSE (TE 4000, TE 180), dynamic Gd-DTPA enhanced 3D FFE (TR15,TE 6.9, flip 30°) with subtraction and in some patients high resolution 3D FFE with SPIR and MTC (TR 49, TE 7, flip 50°). Planar SM in prone position, using a special wedge-shaped device to allow the breasts to be freely pendent, was performed five minutes after i.v. injection of 555 MBq Tc-99m TETRO and Tc-99m HDP respectively using a double-headed high-resolution gamma camera (Elscint Helix HR, LEHR collimator, Haifa, Israel). Planar prone TETRO SM was followed by supine SPECT imaging 20 minutes post injection. Most of the premenopausal women were imaged in the first part of the menstrual cycle. SM was evaluated as negative (-), equivocal (+: T/BG <1.2), probably (++: T/BG 1.2-1.5) and definitely (+++: T/BG >1.5) positive by two independent experienced nuclear medicine physicians of our department.

RESULTS

Histological evaluation of the 21 patients revealed breast cancer in 14 cases (6 pT1, 4 pT2, 4 pT4) and benign disease in seven of them (5 FCM, 2 FA). The following table shows the results of TETRO SM , HDP SM and Gd-DTPA MRI mammography:

	t.p.	f.n.	t.n	f.p	SENS	SPEC	NPV	PPV
TETRO PLANAR SM	12	2	6	1	86	86	75	92
TETRO SPECT SM	13	1	5	2	93	71	83	86
HDP SM	10	4	5	2	71	71	55	83
GD- DTPA MRI	13	1	6	1	93	86	86	93

Table 1: Results of planar (TETRO PLANAR SM) and SPECT (TETRO SPECT SM) Tc-99m Tetrofosmin scintimammography, planar Tc-99m Hydroxymethylene-diphosphonate scintimammography (HDP SM) and magnetic resonance imaging (Gd-DTPA MRI) in 21 patients with histologically proven benign and malignant breast lesions.

Eight of the 14 breast cancers demonstrated definitely positive TETRO uptake (FIG.1a,b), two probably positive and two equivocally positive uptake in the planar scan. TETRO SM failed to detect two small cancers, a medullary and an infiltrating ductal cancer pT1. The latter, located in the upper medial quadrant, could be demonstrated by TETRO SPECT SM. Out of the 14 breast cancers, only four showed definitely positive HDP uptake, three a probably positive, three equivocal and four no HDP uptake (Fig. 2a,b). One small (1cm) infiltrating ductal cancer, which demonstrated TETRO uptake, could not be detected by Gd-DTPA MRI mammography. Two fibroadenomas had probably or equivocally positive radiotracer uptake as well. TETRO SPECT SM and HDP SM showed more false positive results than MRI and TETRO PLANAR SM. Moreover, HDP SM was sometimes difficult to interpret because of symmetrically diffuse or spotted uptake of the tracer.

a

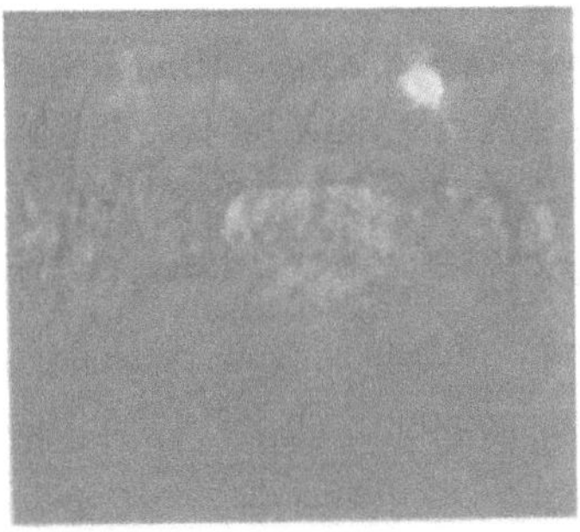

b

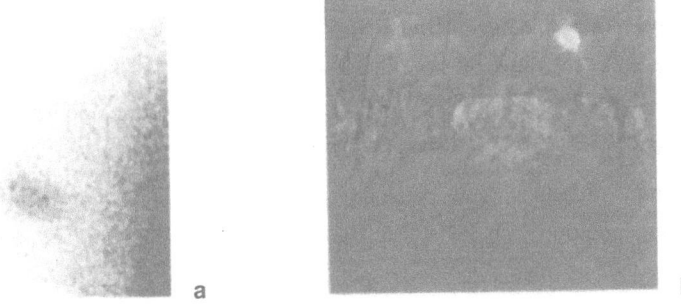

Figure 1: 57 year old woman with a palpable lesion in the left retromammilar area. MM: dense lesion with microcalcification; US: hypoechogenic lesion with a diameter of 2,5 cm; TETRO SM (a): clear uptake in the suspicious lesion ; MRI (b): lesion in the left breast with pathological Gd-DTPA contrast enhancement. HISTO: IDC pT4 (inflammatory component)

a

b

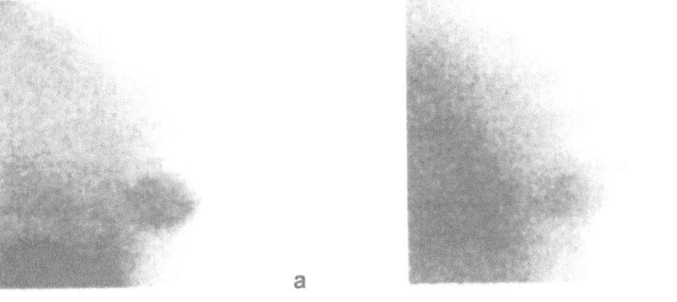

Figure 2: 75 year old woman with a palpable mass in the right breast. TETRO SM (A): Clear uptake in the palpable lesion; HDP SM (b): HDP SM shows only faint uptake in the lesion; HISTO: IDC pT4

DISCUSSION

Despite high sensitivity, mammography as a well accepted routine method has its limitations in dense breasts and due to low specificity. In order to improve the PPV of imaging procedures, several radionuclide imaging approaches have been studied in the last few years to detect breast cancer and to improve the low specificity of mammography. (3-10). The use of Tl-201 for breast cancer imaging was recently re-evaluated by Waxman et al. (3). Another re-evaluation was reported on Tc-99m-methylene diphosphonate, which is routinely used for bone scintigraphy, by Piccolo et al. (6). They found that 10-20 minutes p.i. of 740 MBq Tc-99m MDP 92% of patients with histologically proven breast cancer demonstrated focal MDP uptake. Tc-99m sestamibi, introduced for myocardial perfusion imaging, was also used for scintimammography. In several studies sensitivities between 80 and 95 % and especially the high negative predictive value of sestamibi scintimammography have shown that this new technique might be useful in complementing conventional mammography. Comparative studies between mammography, scintimammography and MRI performed by Palmedo et al. demonstrated comparable sensitivities (mammography: 95%, scintimammography: 91%, MRI: 91%) (7). In contrast, scintimammomgraphy showed the highest specificity (62%) compared to MRI (15%) and mammography (10%). In a similar study by Tilling et al. sensitivity and specificity for sestamibi scintimammograpy was 89% and 83% and 91% and 52% for MRI respectively (8).

In 1994 a new cationic complex tetrofosmin was introduced for myocardial perfusion scintigraphy. Similar to sestamibi, tetrofosmin was also used in oncology. In a study by Arbab et al. the authors conclude that cellular uptake of tetrofosmin and sestamibi are not completely identical. Tc-99m tetrofosmin uptake depends on both cell membrane and mitochondrial potential, while Tc-99m sestamibi accumulates inside the mitochondria (11). The first study on scintimammography using Tc-99m tetrofosmin in 33 patients was published by Mansi et al. in 1996 (9). He found a sensitivity of 93 % and a specificity of 100%. This high specificity might be due to a highly selected population of patients with a very small number of patients with benign disease. In our own first preliminary study on Tc-99m tetrofosmin scintimammography with 34 patients in 1996, we found a similar sensitivity of 91% but a much lower specificity (74%) due to positive tetrofosmin accumulation in some fibroadenomas (10).

In a larger following series on 137 patients, 84 of them with histological clarification, the high sensitivity of the early preliminary study could be confirmed. Also the specificity of about 80% was similar to the first series and remains in contrast to Mansi´s data. In the present study we compared Tc-99m tetrofosmin, Tc-99m hydroxymethylenediphosphonate scintimammography and Gd-DTPA magnetic resonance imaging in patients with mammographically suspicious breast lesions. According to Piccolo´s data on Tc-99m MDP, it should be of advantage to perform early soft tissue breast imaging before bone scintigraphy using Tc-99m diphosphonates in patients who are planned for breast surgery. However, the overall image quality of HDP SM was lower than that of TETRO SM. Only four out of 14 breast cancers demonstrated a definitely positive uptake with a T/BG ratio above 1.5. Moreover, some patients without breast cancer showed symmetrically diffuse or spotted uptake without evidence of pathology. Similar results are reported for Tc-99m DPD by Boubaker and Bischof Delaloye (12). In contrast to former studies dynamic Gd-DTPA MRI mammography with subtraction and high resolution 3-D FFE demonstrated high sensitivity as well as high specificity for breast cancer.

Conclusion: This preliminary study shows that both Tc-99m TETRO SM and Gd-DTPA MRI are of additional value in evaluating mammographically suspicious breast lesions. Because of the inferior image quality and the bad overall results of early soft tissue imaging using Tc-99m HDP before bone scanning, this tracer cannot be recommended for SM.

References

1. Kopans DB. Positive predictive value of mammography. AJR 1992; 158:521-526.
2. Heywang-Köbrunner SH. Contrast enhanced magnetic resonance imaging of the breast. Invest Radiol 1994;29:94-104
3. Waxman AD, Ramanna L, Memsic LD, Forster CE, Silberman AW, Gleischman SH, Brenner RJ, Brachman MB, Kuhar CJ, Yadegar J. Thallium scintigraphy in the evaluation of mass abnormalities of the breast. J Nucl Med 1993; 34:18-23
4. Lind P, Smola MG, Lechner P, Ratschek M, Klima G, Költringer P, Steindorfer P, Eber O. The immunoscintigraphic use of Tc-99m labelled monoclonal antibodies (BW 431/126) in patients with suspected primary, recurrent and metastatic breast cancer. Int J Cancer 1991; 47:865-869.

5. Lind P, Gallowitsch HJ, Mikosch P, Kresnik E, Gomez I, Oman J, Dinges HP, Boniface G. Radioimmunoscintigraphy with Tc-99m labeled monoclonal antibody 179H.82 in suspected primary, recurrent and metastatic breast cancer. Clin Nucl Med 1997; 22:30-34
6. Piccolo S, Lastoria S, Mainolfi C, Muto P, Bazzicalupo L, Salvatore M. Tc-99m Methylene diphosphonate scintimammography to image primary breast cancer. J Nucl Med 1995; 36:718-724.
7. Palmedo H, Grünwald F, Bender H, Schomburg A, Mallmann P, Krebs D, Biersack HJ. Scintimammography with technetium-99m methoxyisobutylisonitrile: comparison with mammography and magnetic resonance imaging. Eur J Nucl Med 1996:23:940-946.
8. Tiling R, Sommer H, Pechmann M, Moser R, Kress K, Pfluger T, Tatsch K, Hahn K. Comparison of technetium-99m sestamibi scintimammography with contrast enhanced MRI for diagnosis of breast cancer. J Nucl Med 1997:38:58-62.
9. Mansi L, Rambaldi PF, Proccacini E, Di Gregorio F, Laprovitera A, Pecori B, Del Vecchio W. Scintimammography with technetium 99m tetrofosmin in the diagnosis of breast cancer and lymph node metastases. Eur J Nucl Med1996;23:932-939.
10. Lind P, Gallowitsch HJ, Kogler D, Kresnik E, Mikosch P, Gomez I.Tc-99m tetrofosmin scintimammography: A prospective study in primary breast lesions. Nuklearmedizin 1996;35:225-229
11. Arbab AS, Koizumik K, Toyama K, Arki T. Uptake of technetium-99m tetrofosmin, technetium-99m MIBI and thallium-201in tumor cell lines. J Nucl Med 1996;37:1551-1556.
12. Boubaker A, Franzetti A, Pellanda A, Bischof Delaloye A. Reliability of Tc-99m Dicarboxypropane- Diphosphonate (DPD) for breast cancer imaging. J Nucl Med 1997; 38:21P

Corresponding address:
Peter Lind, M.D., Prof.
Department of Nuclear Medicine and Special Endocrinology
LKH Klagenfurt
St. Veiterstraße 47
9020 Klagenfurt
Tele: 0463-538-29103
Fax: 0463-538-23184
E-mail: peter. lind @ lkh-klg.co.at.

Radioactive Isotopes in
Clinical Medicine and Research XXIII
ed. by H. Bergmann, H. Köhn and H. Sinzinger

NEOADJUVANT TREATMENT OF PATIENTS WITH BREAST CANCER UNDER SURVEILLANCE OF 99m-Tc-TETROFOSMIN SCINTIGRAPHY

R. Obwegeser, Silvia Müllauer-Ertl, P Berghammer, E. Kubista, H. Sinzinger

Department of Nuclear Medicine and Special Gynecology, University Hospital Vienna, Austria

SUMMARY: A prospective trial was started to evaluate the efficacy of 99m-Tc-tetrofosmin scintigraphy for monitoring the clinical course of thirty-one patients getting neoadjuvant chemotherapy suffering from breast cancer. Clinical and imaging procedures were done at the beginning of treatment and just before surgery. Sensitivity for breast cancer was 69% for mammography, 85% for ultrasound and 96% for 99m-Tc-tetrofosmin scintigraphy. We discovered two cases of bone and two cases of lung metastases by means of 99m-Tc-tetrofosmin scintigraphy. Eight of ten detected suspicious thoracic areas were not confirmed by CT or clinical course.

These findings show that 99m-Tc-tetrofosmin scintigraphy is the most sensitive imaging technique to detect breast cancer. Preliminary data indicate that it might be also become the method of choice for monitoring treatment efficacy.

INTRODUCTION

In recent reports (1-4) 99m-Tc-tetrofosmin proofed to be a powerful agent in spotting breast cancer or its metastases. This is why we started a prospective trial to evaluate the efficacy of 99m-Tc-tetrofosmin scintigraphy in women suffering from breast cancer with a poor prognosis thus receiving preoperative chemotherapy. We monitored the clinical course of disease under neo adjuvant treatment by means of 99m-Tc-tetrofsomin scintigraphy compared to other imaging procedures.

MATERIALS AND METHODS

Thirty one patients aged 31 to 72 years suffering from 32 malignant palpable breast tumors were enrolled into this study taking place at the Vienna University Hospital. Histological diagnosis was obtained by fine needle biopsy (FNB). Neoadjuvant chemotherapy (cyclophosphamide, methotrexate and 5-fluoruracil; CMF) was started immediately upon completion of the staging of patients. CMF was given for 3-4 cycles after which surgery was performed to remove the tumor. In some cases, chemotherapy was changed to epirubicine and cyclophosphamide (EC) when CMF did not sufficiently diminish tumorsize. One woman with a large, inoperable tumor had a palliative irradiation of the breast. Tumor size was evaluated clinically, with ultrasound, mammography and 99m-Tc-tetrofosmin scintigraphy. This was done ad the beginning of therapy and was controlled immediately before surgery. Until now 22 patients already finished neoadjuvant therapy. Six patients are in progress (still undergoing neoadjuvant chemotherapy) and 3 women changed hospital and were lost to follow up.

RESULTS

Twenty-two patients with 23 breast cancers have undergone surgery, so far. Tumor size was 30±21 mm. Ten out of twenty-three tumors were multifocal. FIGO-stages and histology studies are given in table 1. 139 of 374 axillary lymph nodes examined showed metastatic spread. Five of these patients also had distant metastases (one liver, two bones and two lungs). Metastases in lungs and bones were seen on 99m-Tc-tetrofosmin films.

Table 1 Distribution of Figo-stages, type of histology and tumor grading (n=23)

FIGO-stage		Grading		Histology	
pT_1	8	G1	1	inv. ductal	11
pT_2	7	G2	7	inv. ductal NOS	8
pT_3	1	G3	15	inv. ducto-lobular clear cell	2
pT_4	7			inv. ducto-lobular	1
				inv. lobular	1

All the 26 breast tumors (including 3 patients that are lost of side) were clinically suspicious and well palpable. 99m-Tc-Tetrofosmin scintigraphy detected the malignancy in 25 cases and thus reach a sensitivity of 96% (table 2).

Table 2 Relevance of 26 palpable breast cancers using different imaging procedures

	Mammography	Ultrasound	Tetrofosmin scintigraphy
Ca detected	18	22	25
No tumor	3	2	1
Misinterpretation	5	2	0
Sensitivity	**69%**	**85%**	**96%**

In contrast, breast cancer was not detected by mammography in 3 patients. In one case MRI of the breast was negative. In 3 patients with breast cancer, mammography only visualized microcalcifications of benign structure without any tumor. Additionally, conventional imaging procedures (mammography and ultrasound) misinterpreted one tumor as mastitis and one as benign cyst. In another patient an impression of the bladder was found by 99m-Tc-tetrofosmin scintigraphy. Gynecologic examination revealed a tumor of the ovary that turned out to be ovarian cancer. In ten patients, a suspicious thoracic hot spot on 99m-Tc-tetrofosmin scintigraphy led to further examination. In eight of these patients, the hot spots on 99m-Tc-tetrofosmin films were not visible on CT scans. Two of these patients had lung metastases. Table 3 shows the effect of neoadjuvant therapy on breast tumors.

Table 3 Changes of breast tumors under therapy observed by different means

	Clinical aspect	MG/US	Tetrofosmin scintigraphy
Remission	18	11	15
Idem	5	6	5
Progression	0	1	2
"don't know"	0	5	1

DISCUSSION

In accordance with recent papers (5-7), we observed 99m-Tc-tetrofosmin scintigraphy to be a powerful means for detecting breast cancer and its metastases. Similar to Fenlon et al (7) we found a sensitivity of 99m-Tc-tetrofosmin scintigraphy of 96%. In contrast, the sensitivity of mammography is much lower in our patient compared to the patients in Fenlon's study (69% versus 81%, respectively). Perhaps there may be a reason in the a very special group of patients we examined. The 3 patients with a negative mammography were below 45 years of age and had a very dense breast tissue which can make mammography difficult. In one of this 3 patients even MRI of the breast did not show any suspicious area. Therefore, we suggest that 99m-Tc-tetrofosmin scintigraphy might be a powerful diagnostic procedure especially for young women with dense breast tissue that have a high risk for cancer (i.e. fast developing breast tumor of unknown origin, genetic disorders as BRCA 1 positive patients, etc.). As we could see sometimes a real discrepancy between clinical interpretation of tumor changes under chemotherapy and real tumor size in histology a challenge for a qualified imaging procedure is given. Similar to Berghammer et al (3) we also detected breast cancer metastases (2 lung and 2 bone) by 99m-Tc-tetrofosmin scintigraphy. Additionally, it was 99m-Tc-tetrofosmin whole-body-scintigraphy which guided us to find an ovarian carcinoma in one patient. Therefore, we suggest that 99m-Tc-tetrofosmin scintigraphy is a powerful means for the follow-up of breast cancer patients undergoing neoadjuvant chemotherapy.

REFERENCES

1. Adalet I, Demirkol MO, Müslümanoglu M, Bozfakioglu Y, Cantez S. $^{99}Tc^{m}$-tetrofosmin scintigraphy in the evaluation of palpable breast masses. Nucl Med Com 1997; 18:118-121.

2. Vieira MR, Weinholtz JHB. Technetium-99m tetrofosmin scintigraphy in the diagnosis of breast cancer. Eur J Surg Oncol 1996; 22:331-334.

3. Berghammer P, Wiltschke C, Sinzinger H, Zielinski CC. 99mTc-tetrofosmin soft tissue scanning and metastatic disease. Lancet 1996; 348:1169-1170.

4. Mansi L, Rambaldi PF, Procaccini E, DiGregorio F, Laprovitera A, Pecori B, Del Vecchio W. Scintimammography with technetium-99m tetrofosmin in the diagnosis of breast cancer and lymph node metastases. Eur J Nucl Med 1996; 23:932-939.

5. Lind P, Umschaden HW, Forsthuber E, Oman J, Kerschbaumer K, Gallowitsch HJ, Mikosch P, Kresnik E, Molnar M, Gomez I. Scintimammography using Tc-99m tetrofosmin. Acta Med Austriaca 1997; 24:50-54.

6. Batista JF, Solano ME, Oliva JP, Rodriguez JL, Gomez J, Stüsser RJ, Sanchez E. Usefulness of $^{99}Tc^{m}$-tetrofosmin scintimammography in palpable breast tumors. Nucl Med Comm 1997; 18:338-340.

7. Fenlon HM, Phelan NC, O'Sullivan P, Tierny S, Gorey T, Ennis JT. Benign versus malignant breast disease: comparison of contrast-enhanced MR imaging and Tc-99m tetrofsomin scintimammography. Radiology 1997; 205:214-220.

Radioactive Isotopes in
Clinical Medicine and Research XXIII
ed. by H. Bergmann, H. Köhn and H. Sinzinger

^{99m}Tc-FURIFOSMIN UPTAKE BY MELANOMA CELLS

Meghdadi Susan, Chehne F, Rodrigues Margarida, Karanikas G, Pehamberger H, Schlagbauer-Wadl Hermine, Sinzinger H
Departments of Nuclear Medicine and Dermatology, University of Vienna, Austria

SUMMARY Two melanoma cell lines, SK-MEL-28 and 518 A2 were incubated for different time intervals up to 180 minutes at 37°C. With ^{99m}Tc-furifosmin, an uptake of 2%-3% was achieved almost immediately without any significant further change thereafter for a total monitoring period of 180 minutes. In contrast, the ^{99m}Tc-tetrofosmin-uptake (about 3%) was comparable up to about 60 minutes showing thereafter a significant ($p<0.01$) increase. These findings indicate that the kinetics and uptake mechnisms of these two tracers might be different. Thus, it needs to be further elucidated whether the increased late uptake of ^{99m}Tc-tetrofosmin might be relevant to be considered for clinical imaging protocols.

INTRODUCTION

Melanoma shows by far the fastest growing prevalance for malignant tumors during the last decade in the Western hemisphere. Therefore, approaches to image the primary tumor and eventually recurrences are gaining central interest. In Nuclear Medicine there are several imaging approaches using unspecific or specific methods as well as specific antibodies or the respective fragments. Recently the cationic tracers thallium-201 chloride, technetium-99m-hexakis-2-methoxyisobutyl-isonitrile (^{99m}Tc-Sestamibi) and 1,2-bis[bis(2-ethoxyethyl)phosphino] ethene (^{99m}Tc-tetrofosmin) (1-4) have been shown to be imaging agents of outstanding promise achieving sensitivities of about 95% and specificities of around 80% for a great number of different tumors. For melanoma, however, there are insufficient data available yet. Furifosmin [technetium (III) -99m-Q12], [trans-(1,2-bis dihydro-2,2,5,5-tetramethyl-3 (2H) furanone - 4 - methyleneimino ethane bis tris(3-methoxy-1-propyl)-phosphine)] is the most recently discovered member of the family of cationic tracers which could eventually be used for imaging of melanoma. Before applying this tracer to melanoma patients we assessed the uptake behaviour in human melanoma cell lines comparing the data to ^{99m}Tc-tetrofosmin.

MATERIALS AND METHODS

Human malignant melanoma cell lines SK-MEL-28 and 518 A2 (5-7) were cultured in Dulbecco's Modified Eagle Medium (DMEM) (IL) (GIBCO BRL, Life Technologies Ldt, Paisley, UK) supplemented with 10% fetal calf serum (FES) (PAA Laboratories GmbH, Linz, Austria) in a humidified 5% CO_2, 95% ambient air atmosphere at 37° C. For the uptake experiments cells were trypsinized, washed once in medium containing FCS in order to remove the residual trypsin. Growth curves were generated after seeding $1x10^3$ cells/well from each melanoma cell line into 96 well plates. The cell numbers were determined from day 2 through day 8 (Coulter counter). For our study the cells were resuspended in DMEM/10%/FCS. They were incubated at a density of 1.10^6 /ml at 37°C for a time period of 10 - 180 minutes with 100 µCi /ml ^{99m}Tc- furifosmin or ^{99m}Tc-tetrofosmin. The cells were washed in buffer once and the cell bound activity was determined in a gamma counter.

STATISTICAL ANALYSIS

Values are presented as mean ±SD; calculation for significance was performed using analysis of variance.

RESULTS

Incubating 518 A2 cells with ^{99m}Tc-furifosmin results in an uptake at around 2%, which remains absolutely stable for 2-3 hours without any significant change. In contrast, the uptake of ^{99m}Tc-tetrofosmin was borderline to significantly higher at about 3% until 60 minutes incubation, while thereafter the ^{99m}Tc-tetrofosmin uptake increased significantly, reaching its maximum after 3 hours (fig.1). A quite similar behaviour can be monitored examining SK-MEL-28 cells. The ^{99m}Tc-furifosmin uptake at around 3% was stable for the entire observation period between 10-180 minutes, while the ^{99m}Tc-tetrofosmin-uptake was almost indentical until 40 minutes, thereafter showing a sharp increase resulting in a significantly higher uptake up to 180 minutes.

DISCUSSION

These findings indicate that for about 1 hour there is no relevant difference between ^{99m}Tc-furifosmin and ^{99m}Tc-tetrofosmin uptake by the two melanoma cell lines examined. However, prolonged incubation results in an increased ^{99m}Tc-tetrofosmin uptake indicating a different uptake mechanism. This different kinetic behaviour needs to be considered and the optimal imaging time needs to be elaborated from the in-vitro findings. At an immediate imaging these two tracers might behave comparably, while performing late images, ^{99m}Tc-tetrofosmin might have some advantage at late images. Considering also the enhanced blood clearance at this time, in-vivo imaging protocols have to assess the value of these in-vitro findings.

REFERENCES

1. Arbab AS, Koizumi K, Toyama K, Araki T. Uptake of technetium-99-tetrofosmin, technetium-99m-MIBI and thallium-201 in tumor cell lines. J Nucl Med 37: 1551-1556, 1996.
2. Ballinger JR, Bannerman J, Boxen I et al. Technetium-99m-tetrofosmin as a substrate for P-glycoprotein: in-vitro studies in multi-drug resistant breast tumor cells. J Nucl Med 37: 1578-1582, 1996.
3. Matnusnari I, Kinuya S, Nishikawa T et al. Technetium-99m-tetrofosmin uptake in lung cancer: comparison with thallium-201. Ann Nucl Med 10: 143-145, 1996.
4. Lind P, Gallowitsch HJ. The use of non-specific tracers in the follow-up of differentiated thyroid cancer: results with Tc-99m-tetrofosmin whole body scintigraphy. Acta Med Austriaca 23: 69-75, 1996.
5. Schrier PI, Versteeg R, Peltenburg LTC, Plomp AC, Van't Veer LJ, Kruse-Wolters KM. Sensitivity of melanoma cell lines to natural killer cells: a role for oncogene-modulated HLA class I expression? Semin Cancer Biol 2: 73-83, 1991.
6. Versteeg R, Peltenburg LTC, Plomp AC, Schrier PI. High expression of the c-myc oncogene renders melanoma cells prone to lysis by natural killer cells. J Immunol 143: 4331-4337, 1989.
7. Jansen B, Inou SA, Wadl H, Eichler HJ, Wolf K, Van Elsas A, Schrier P, Pehamberger H. N-ras oncogene expression changes the growth characteristics of human melanoma in two independent SCID-hu mouse models. Int J Cancer, 67: 821-825, 1996.

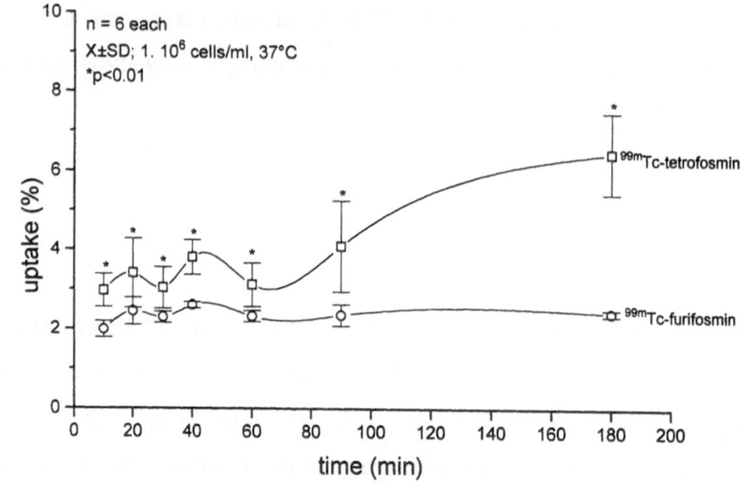

Fig.1
Uptake of Tc-99m-tetrofosmin and -furifosmin in 518 A2 cell-line:
Cellular uptake of Tc-99m-furifosmin reaches a maximum almost immediately without any further change thereafter, whereas the uptake of Tc-99m-tetrofosmin is comparable up to 60 minutes showing afterwards a significant increase.

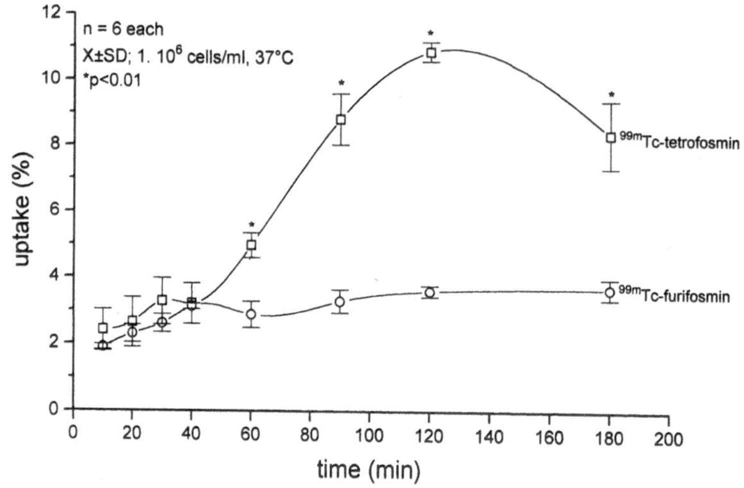

Fig.2
Uptake of Tc-99m-tetrofosmin and -furifosmin in SK-MEL 28:
Already at about 10 minutes incubation a constant uptake of Tc-99m-furifosmin is achieved, whereas Tc-99m-tetrofosmin increases significantly after 60 minutes incubation.

Radioactive Isotopes in
Clinical Medicine and Research XXIII
ed. by H. Bergmann, H. Köhn and H. Sinzinger

LYMPHOSCINTIGRAPHY IN TUMORS OF THE HEAD AND NECK USING A DOUBLE TRACER TECHNIQUE

S. Klutmann, K.H. Bohuslavizki, S. Kröger, S. Höft, J.A. Werner, W. Brenner, E. Henze

Clinics of Nuclear Medicine and and Otorhinolaryngology, Head and Neck Surgery, Christian-Albrechts-University, Arnold-Heller-Str. 9, 24105 Kiel, Germany

SUMMARY: Since knowledge of possible lymphatic drainage may facilitate preoperative planning a method of lymphoscintigraphy with exact correlation of lymphatic drainage to six known cervical compartments is presented. 78 patients with various tumors of the head and neck received 100 MBq Tc-99m-colloid in 3-4 peritumoral sites. 2 ml of perchlorate solution were given orally in order to block the thyroid. Patients received 50 MBq Tc-99m-pertechnetate i.v. for body-contouring 20 min p.i. Planar images were obtained over 5 min each at 30 min and 4-6 h after injection from anterior, right lateral and left lateral using a LFOV-gamma camera. The thyroid was seen in any of the patients. In 28/78=36 % of the patients the injection site was the only focal activity seen. In 50/78=64 % of the patients lymphatic drainage could be observed: 36/78=46 % showed unilateral, and 14/78=18 % exhibited bilateral lymphatic drainage. In all 50 patients showing lymphatic drainage lymph nodes could be easily assigned to the six cervical lymph node compartments described. Accurate correlation of lymphatic drainage and cervical compartments yields the basis for a re-evaluation of its impact in preoperative planning of different procedures of neck dissection.

INTRODUCTION

Lymphoscintigraphy has been used since the early sixties in order to proof lymphatic drainage of head and neck tumors [1-5], but was not convincing. With increasing impact of highly sophisticated procedures of neck dissection lymphoscintigraphy may increase in its diagnostic impact under the pre-requisite that lymphoscintigraphy enables an accurate correlation of lymphatic drainage with cervical lymph node compartments described [6]. Therefore, in this paper a method of lymphoscintigraphy in double tracer technique with simultaneous body-contouring is presented.

MATERIALS AND METHODS

Lymphoscintigraphy was performed pre/intraoperatively in 78 patients (7 female, 71 male) with various tumors of the head and neck. Patients received 100 MBq Tc-99m-colloid dissolved in 0.1-0.2 ml in 3-4 peritumoral sites. 2 ml of perchlorate solution were given orally in order to block the thyroid. Patients received 50 MBq Tc-99m-pertechnetate i.v. for body-contouring 20 min p.i. Planar images were obtained over 5 min each at 30 min and 4 h from anterior, right lateral and left lateral views using a LFOV-gamma camera equipped with a LEAP collimator (Gamma Diagnost Tomo, Philips, Hamburg).

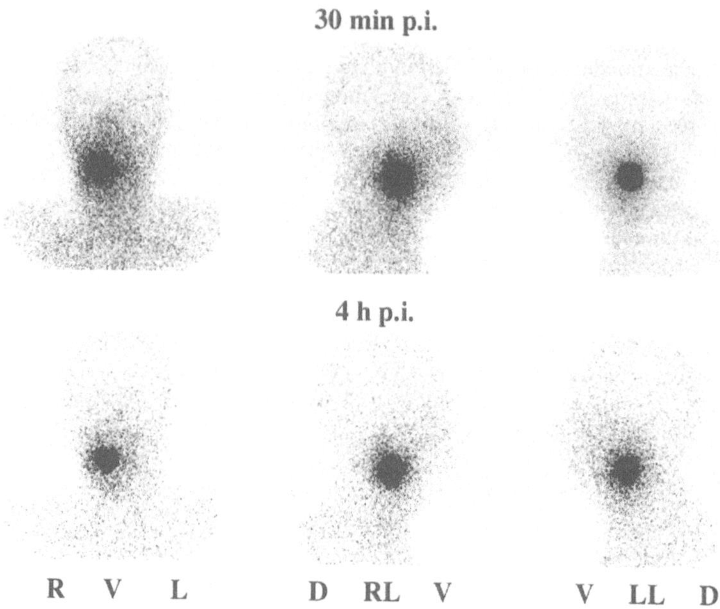

Fig 1: Planar images from anterior (R V L), right lateral (D RL V) and left lateral (V LL D) 30 min and 4 hrs p.i. 57-years old patient with carcinoma of the right hypopharynx. The injection site is the only focal activity seen. No lymphatic drainage was observed.

RESULTS

The thyroid was seen in any of the patients. In 28/78 = 36 % of the patients the injection site was the only focal activity seen, thus, no lymphatic drainage could be demonstrated at all (Fig. 1). In 50/78 = 64 % lymphatic drainage could be observed. 36/78 = 46 % of the patients showed unilateral (Fig. 2), and 14/78 = 18 % exhibited bilateral lymphatic drainage (Fig. 3). Although in 13 out of these 14 patients the primary tumor was localized unilateral, lymphatic drainage was observed on both sides of the neck. In all 50 patients showing lymphatic drainage involved lymph nodes could be easily assigned to the six cervical lymph node compartments described [6]. In one patient with bilateral lymphatic drainage scintigraphic findings resulted in a more extended bilateral neck dissection.

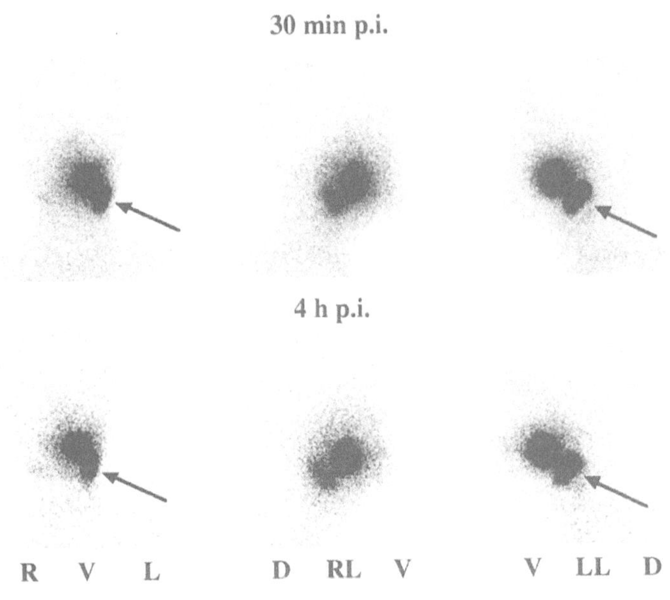

Fig 2: Planar images from anterior (R V L), right lateral (D RL V) and left lateral (V LL D) 30 min and 4 hrs p.i. 43-years old patient with carcinoma of the left palatine arc. Ipsilateral lymphatic drainage to the compartment II (arrow) was seen.

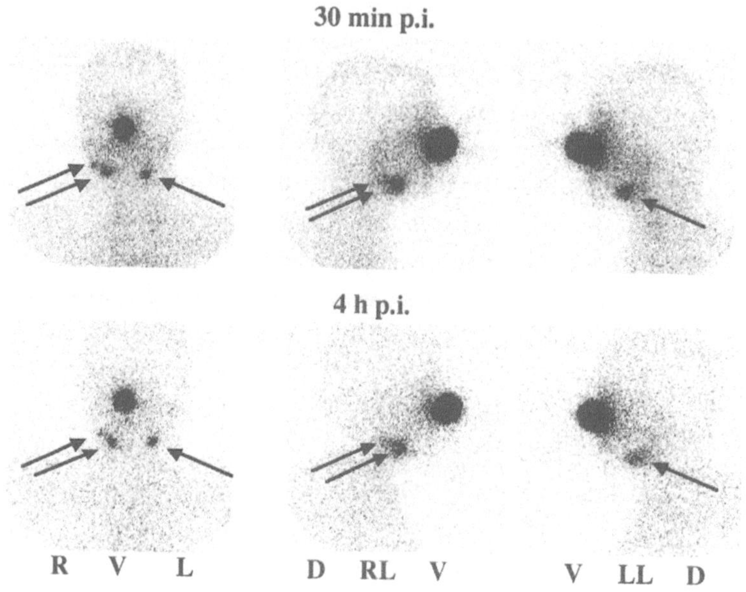

Fig 3: Planar images from anterior (R V L), right lateral (D RL V) and left lateral (V LL D) 30 min and 4 hrs p.i. 66-years old patient with squamous cell carcinoma of the right vestibule of nose. Ipsilateral and contralateral lymphatic drainage to both compartments II (arrows) was seen.

DISCUSSION

Perchlorate solution was given orally in order to block the thyroid, and, in fact, the thyroid was seen in any of the patients. Therefore, an overlap of thyroid gland and lymphatic drainage could be successfully avoided. Moreover, due to blockade of the thyroid an increase of renal excretion of Tc-99m-pertechnetate decreased the patients´ radiation burden [7].

For anatomical landmarking various methods have been commonly used: drawing of the patients´ body-contour after image acquisition is a simple technique but a rather inaccurate method of anatomical landmarking as well. In order to localize lymph nodes images can be obtained simultaneously with Co-58 markers positioned at the sternal notch or chin. However, this method of anatomical landmarking is inaccurate as well and, moreover, depends on detailed anatomical knowledge of the technical staff performing the study. In contrast, body-contouring by Tc-99m-pertechnetate applied intravenously is easy to perform and, moreover, allows an accurate correlation of anatomical structures to scintigraphically detected lymph nodes. Thus, in all 50 patients lymph nodes could be easily assigned to the six known cervical compartments [6].

In 28/78 patients the tumoral/peritumoral area was the only focal activity seen. Thus, no lymphatic drainage could be observed scintigraphically. This lack of lymphatic drainage may be due to normal anatomical variations when lymph nodes may be occasionally absent for no pathological reason at all. Furthermore, a lack of scintigraphic drainage may become manifest by tumor embolization of afferent lymph vessels and a radiocolloid hold-up proximal to this obstruction.

In contrast, in 50/78 patients lymphatic drainage could be observed. Thus, lymphoscintigraphy allows the clinician to identify potential routes for metastases of the malignoma. Visualization of lymph nodes draining the malignoma does not necessarily imply the presence of tumor cells within these nodes. Lymph node involvement can easier be identified by morphological imaging using MRI or B-ultrasound. The advantage which justifies continuing lymphoscintigraphy in oncological preoperative planning is the possibility to visualize lymphatic drainage in the individual patient [8-10]. These results may significantly alter the extent and type of surgery as was seen in one of fourteen patients with bilateral lymphatic drainage. This holds especially true in modern head and neck surgery performing a large variety of different types of neck dissections tailor-made to the individual necessity for the individual patients [11-14].

CONCLUSIONS

Lymphoscintigraphy with body-contouring using double tracer technique allows an accurate correlation of lymphatic drainage and cervical lymph node compartments. This yields the basis for a re-evaluation of its impact in preoperative planning of different procedures of neck-dissections.

REFERENCES

1. Schwab W, Scheer KE, zum Winkel K. Szintigraphie des cervikalen Lymphsystems. Arch Ohr-Nas- u Kehlk-Heilk 1964; **183:** 382-387.
2. Schwab W. Der lymphatische Transport von Radiokolloiden in die bestrahlte und unbestrahlte Halsregion (Szintigraphie des zervikalen Lymphsystems). Laryngol Rhinol Otol 1964; **43:** 230-234.
3. Schwab W, Scheer KE, zum Winkel K. Die Szintigraphie des zervikalen Lymphsystems nach radikaler Lymphknotenausräumung. Laryngol Rhinol Otol 1965; **44:** 326-330.

4. Schwab W, Scheer KE, zum Winkel K. Die Szintigraphie des zervikalen Lymphsystems nach strahelntherapeutischen und operativen Maßnahmen. Nucl Med 1965; **4:** 326-332.

5. Schwab W, zum Winkel K. Der gegenwärtige Stand der Szintigraphie des zervikalen Lymphsystems. Nucl Med 1967; **6:** 234-249.

6. Werner JA. Aktueller Stand der Versorgung des Lymphabflusses maligner Kopf-Hals-Tumoren. Eur Arch Otorhinolaryngol 1997; **Suppl. I:** 47-85.

7. Johansson L, Mattsson S, Nosslin B, Leide-Svegborn S. Effective dose from radiopharmaceuticals. Eur J Nucl Med 1992; **19:** 933-938.

8. Ege GN. Lymphoscintigraphy in oncology. In: Henkin RE, Boles MA, Dillehay GL, Halama JR, Karesh SM, Wagner RH, Zimmer AM (Editor). Nuclear medicine. Volume 2. Mosby, St. Louis 1996; 1504-1523.

9. Civantos FJ, Moffat FL, Duque C, Gulec SA. Current surgical techniques. Lymphoscintigraphy and sentinel node biopsy: a potential new approach in the management of the N0 neck. Curr Op Otolaryngol Head Neck Surg 1997; **5:** 99-104.

10. Bourgeois P. Lymphoscintigraphy in adult malignancy. In: Murray IPC, Ell PJ (Editor). Nuclear Medicine in Clinical Diagnosis and Treatment. Volume 2. Churchill Livingstone, Edinburgh 1994; 699-704.

11. Houck JR, Medina JE. Management of cervical lymph nodes in squamous carcinomas of the head and neck. Semin Surg Oncol 1995; **11:** 228-239.

12. Shah JP, Andersen PE. The impact of nodal metastasis on modifications of neck dissection. Ann Surg Oncol 1994; **1:** 521-532.

13. Shah JP, Andersen PE. Evolving role of modifications in neck dissection for oral squamous carcinoma. Br J Oral Maxillofac Surg 1995; **33:** 3-8.

14. De Campora E, Radici M, Camaioni A, Pianelli C. Clinical experiences with surgical therapy of cervical metastases from head and neck cancer. Eur Arch Otorhinolaryngol 1994; **251:** 335-341.

CLINICAL PET

Radioactive Isotopes in
Clinical Medicine and Research XXIII
ed. by H. Bergmann, H. Köhn and H. Sinzinger

CLINICAL APPLICATION OF ^{18}FDG-PET IN THE ASSESSMENT OF HEAD AND NECK TUMORS

H. Bender, H-J. Straehler-Pohl*, D. Linke, R. Rödel*, A. Schomburg, C. Ponath, and H-J. Biersack.

Departments of Nuclear Medicine and *Head-Neck-Surgery;
University of Bonn, Germany

SUMMARY: More than 150 patients were studied employing whole-body FDG-PET. Confirmed primary and recurrent tumors, lymph node and organ metastases showed high FDG-uptake comparable to cerebellum and markedly higher than mediastine or liver as reference organs. PET was most beneficial in the correct staging of local, distant lymph node and organ (lung, liver, bone) metastases as well as recurrences in the face of distorted anatomy. Sensitivities, specificities and accuracies were well above 90%, respectively. In CUP-syndrome, PET identified 24% prior undetected primary tumor sites.

INTRODUCTION

More than 5% of all newly diagnosed cancers are malignant tumors of the head and neck with roughly 85-90% being squamous cell carcinoma. Spread of tumor depends on the localization, size, and histology of the primary tumor, but complete local tumor resection, including lymph node (LN) metastases, renders cure in a high percentage. In addition, early detection of tumor recurrence and identification of the primary in CUP-syndrome (cancer of unknown primary) is associated with a much better prognosis.

Conventional staging methods include physical examination, ultrasound, computed tomography (CT) and magnetic resonance imaging (MRI). ^{18}Fluoro-deoxyglucose (FDG), shows a high accumulation in various malignant cells in vitro and in vivo (1-3). Several clinical studies have demonstrated the feasibility of FDG-PET in the detection of head-and-neck tumors (HNT) under study conditions (3-6). The aims of our investigation were to assess the utility of FDG-PET under clinical routine conditions, specifically to (a) establish tumor-typical FDG-uptake, and (b) specify eligibility criteria for patients.

PATIENTS, MATERIAL AND METHODS

In the pilot study, patients with large tumors (T≥2) or with palpable and cancer-suspicious cervical LN were included.

In the ongoing prospective study, patients with (a) suspected recurrence, (b) staging due to large, tumor-suspicious masses, or (c) cancer of unknown primary were enrolled. All patients were surgically treated and thus, PET findings could be confirmed by histology.

Patients fasted overnight (12-18 hrs), but were allowed to drink sugar-free liquids ad libitum. Blood-sugar was monitored prior to FDG-injection and was usually <130 mg%, with few exceptions.

PET-studies were performed on an ECAT Exact 921/47 scanner (Siemens/CTI) and consisted of a body-trunk (5-7 bed positions) transmission scan (7-10 min. per bed position), followed by an emission scan (10 min./bed position), 45-60 min. after injection of 185-300 MBq FDG. FDG was commercially obtained from the Nuclear Research Centers Karlsruhe (Germany) or Jülich (Germany).

Tomograms were reconstructed by filtered-backprojection (Hann filter, cut-off frequency 0.4 cycles/pixel, decay correction and x-y-z smoothing) and attenuation-corrected based on the measured transmission matrix. Primary image assessment (PET, CT/MRI etc.) was done without knowledge of the respective findings of the other imaging modalities..The final institutional dignosis (usually histology) was used as Gold-standard.

RESULTS

PILOT STUDY: A total of 50 patients were studied (21 females, 29 males; age: 27-78 years) with large tumors (T≥2; 37 primary and 9 recurrent tumors) or only with palpable, cancer-suspicious cervical LN (n=5). Primary tumor localizations were oropharynx (n=32), larynx (n=9), hypopharynx (n=5), and parotid gland (4). Histologically most cancers proved to be squamous cell carcinoma (n=44, 88%).

All known tumor masses (n=43) could be visualized and showed high FDG-uptake in viable tumor (n=39), but also pleomorphic adenoma (n=4) (sensitivity 100%). Necrotic areas exerted no or significantly less uptake. Palpable cervical LN (n=21) showed high FDG-uptake in 17 cases (histologically confirmed tumor) and moderate uptake in 4 cases (histologically inflammation). High uptake was associated with tumor invasion (n=16) and inflammation (n=1), while moderate uptake proved to be the results of non-malignant processes. Our data demonstrate a sensitivity, specificity and accuracy of 100%, 80% and 95%, respectively. Distant metastases (lung, liver, bone), with intense FDG-uptake, were correctly identified in 13 cases, which have not been known prior to the PET-study.

Qualitative comparison of FDG-uptake in tumors as compared to reference tissues (brain, mediastine, and liver) showed a FDG-accumulation in viable tumor comparable or exceeding brain-uptake (cerebellum) and was graded "tumor-typical". Moderate FDG-uptake was well below the activity in cerebellum, but above mediastine or liver and was graded "tumor-suspect". Uptake in the range of liver was usually found in less active/chronic inflammation and graded "unspecific". Uptake in morphologically identified lesions not exceeding background activity was graded "no evidence of disease".

PROSPECTIVE STUDY: In the ongoing prospective study, patients with (a) suspected recurrence (n=44), (b) staging due to large primary (n=33), or (c) cancer of unknown primary (n=25) were enrolled. The groups consisted of 45 females, and 57 males, age 20-83 years.

Primary tumor localizations were nasal cavity (n=9), nasopharynx (n=9), oral cavity (n=15) oropharynx (n=22), larynx (n=14), hypopharynx (n=6), parotid gland (2), and CUP (n=25). Histologically most cancers proved to be squamous cell carcinoma (n=87, 85%).

In patients with large, palpable tumors, FDG-PET was able to correctly identify 4/33 masses (15%) as non-malignant, 27/33 (82%) as malignant process, and was false-positive in 2 cases (6%). In addition, in 12 pts. (36%) only loco-regional LN metastases and in 13 pts (39%) distant metastases were found. The results demonstrate a sensitivity, specificity and accuracy of 96%, 67% and 91%, respectively. All tumors, including small LN metastases, showed intense FDG-uptake. All false-positive findings (n=2) were pleomorphic adenoma of the parotid gland.

In patients with suspected recurrence, local tumor recurrence without other tumor sites was found in 7/44 pts. (16%), whereas in 21/44 pts. (49%) regional LN, and in 11/44 pts. (25%)

distant metastases (mediastine n=4, lung n=5, liver n=1, bone n=1) could be established. No evidence of local recurrence but cervical LN or distant metastases were identified in 8/44 pts. (18%). In addition, 12/44 pts. (27%) were tumor-free. Two patients were false-negative. These data show a sensitivity, and accuracy of 95%, respectively. Tumors, including organ metastases, presented with intense FDG-uptake. Interestingly, most recurrences were associated with local LN metastases (49%) or distant metastases (25%), which underscores the need of more sensitive screening methods in the clinical follow-up.

In patients with CUP-syndrome (n=25), FDG-PET was able to identify 6/25 (24%) of prior unidentified primaries and correctly described further local metastases in 12/25 (48%), or distant metastases in 6/25 (24%) pts. Five (20%) had no evidence of disease and are currently followed-up.

Direct comparison of the diagnostic safety of FDG-PET versus CT/MRI shows a marked benefit of FDG-PET in the detection of local and distant LN metastases, and in the identification of reccurrence in the face of distorted anatomy. While FDG-PET is routinely used for whole-body or body-trunk scanning as compared to defined region-scanning in CT or MRI, more distant metastases were primarily identified in our patient group underscoring the screening potential of this method in selected patient groups.

DISCUSSION

We have investigated the clinical utility of FDG-PET in the staging of head-and-neck tumors (HNT) in selected patients under routine conditions. In the pilot study, our data demonstrated high FDG-uptake in viable primary and recurrent tumors as well as in LN and organ metastases. These data are in accordance with results previously published (3-6) indicating enhanced glucose-trapping in HNT.

Qualitative scoring of FDG-accumulation in histologically proven tumors compared to reference organs (cerebellum, mediastine, liver), suggested cerebellum-like glucose-utilization to be indicative for a malignant process (6). In contrast, inflammation showed usually an utilization comparable to liver or mediastine. Thus, metastases also in these regions presented with high contrast allowing tumor detection with high sensitivity and accuracy (3-8). In addition, qualitative image assessment using the above mentioned scoring system in high-risk patients (tumors T≥2, suspected recurrence) substantiated the high sensitivity and accuracy of FDG-PET in the functional assessment of tumor masses, morphological changes (scar vs.

recurrence) and the presence of LN and/or organ metastases. Our data clearly indicate, that FDG-PET, as compared to CT/MRI, has its main advantage (a) in the evaluation of LN involvement, (b) in the face of postsurgically distorted anatomy, and (c) whole-body scanning for distant metastases and/or in CUP-syndrome. Our findings are well in accordance with published data (6-10). A major limitation of CT/MRI in the assessment of normal sized or slightly enlarged LN is the lack of specificity, whereas FDG-PET primarily depends on the relative metabolic rate (3,4,11). The same is true in the case of postsurgical changes. Unless definite growth has been established, morphological imaging can not differentiate between scaring and recurrence. In contrast, FDG-PET allows early recurrence detection and/or functionally grade morphological structures (12), since FDG-trapping correlates well with the proliferation index (3,4), at least in HNT. Finally, FDG-PET is routinely used for whole-body scanning, which is not true in CT/MRI. Our data clearly indicate, that a high percentage of patients have a much more advanced state of disease, at least high-risk patients, underscoring the need for whole-body screening methods.

CONCLUSIONS

Our data substantiate, that FDG-PET is a sensitive and valuable diagnostic tool in the assessment of HNT mainly in (a) the primary staging of high-risk patients ($T \geq 2$), (b) CUP work-up, and (c) suspected recurrence. FDG-PET has a significant influence on the final staging in selected patient groups and its functional information complements morphological (e.g. CT, MRI) findings and vice versa.

REFERENCES

1. Minn H, Clavo AC, Grenman R, Wahl RL In vitro comparison of cell proliferation kinetics and uptake of tritiated fluorodeoxyglucose and L-methionine in squamous cell carcinoma of the head and neck. J. Nucl. Med. 1995, 36: 252-258.

2. Minn H, Clavo AC, Wahl RL Influence of hypoxia on tracer accumulation in squamous cell carcinoma: in vitro evaluation for PET imaging. Nucl. Med. Biol. 1996, 23: 941-946

3. Minn H, Joensu H, Ahonen A, Klemi P Fluorodeoxyglucose imaging: a method to assess the proliferative activity of human cancer in vivo. Comparison with DNA flow cytometry in head and neck tumors. Cancer 1988, 61: 1776-1781.

4. Haberkorn U, Strauss LG, Reisser C, Haag D, Dimitrakopoulou A, Ziegler S, Oberdorfer F, Rudat V, van Kaick G. Glucose uptake, perfusion, and cell proliferation in head and neck tumors: relation of positron emission tomography to flow cytometry J. Nucl. Med. 1991, 32: 1548-1555.

5. Bailet JW, Abemayor E, Jabour BA, Hawkins RA, Ho C, Ward PH. Positron emission tomography: a new, precise imaging modality for detection of primary head and neck tumors and assessment of cervical adenopathy. Laryngoscope 1992, 102: 281-288.

6. Zeitouni AG, Yamamoto YL, Black M, Gjedde A Functional imaging of head and neck tumors using positron emission tomography. J. Otolaryngol. 1994, 23: 77-80.

7. Laubenbacher C, Saumweber D, Wagner Manslau C, Kau RJ, Herz M, Avril N, Ziegler S, Kruschke C, Arnold W, Schwaiger M. Comparison of fluorine 18 fluorodeoxyglucose PET, MRI and endoscopy for staging head and neck squamous cell carcinomas. J. Nucl. Med. 1995, 36: 1747-1757.

8. Greven KM, Williams DW 3rd, Keyes JW Jr, McGuirt WF, Watson NE Jr, Randall ME, Raben M, Geisinger KR, Cappellari JO. Positron-emission-tomography of patients with head and neck carcinoma before and after high dose irradiation. Cancer. 1994, 74: 1355-1359.

9. Austin JR, Wong FC, Kim EE Positron emission tomography in the detection of residual laryngeal carcinoma. Otolaryngol. Head Neck Surg. 1995, 113: 404-407.

10. Jabour BA, Choi Y, Hoh CK, Rege SD, Soong JC, Lufkin RB, HanafeeWN, Maddahi J, Chaiken L, Bailet J, et al. Extracranial head and neck: PET imaging with 2 [F18]fluoro-2-deoxy-D-glucose and MR imaging correlation. Radiology. 1993, 186: 27-35.

11. Rege S, Maass A, Chaiken L, Hoh CK, Choi Y, Lufkin R, Anzai Y, Juillard G, Maddahi J, Phelps ME. Use of positron emission tomography with fluorodeoxyglucose in patients with extracranial head and neck cancers. Cancer. 1994, 73: 3047-3058.

12. Rege S, Maass A, Chaiken L, Hoh CK, Choi Y, Lufkin R, Anzai Y, Juillard G, Maddahi J, Phelps ME. Use of positron emission tomography with fluorodeoxyglucose in patients with extracranial head and neck cancers. Cancer. 1994; 73: 3047-3058.

Radioactive Isotopes in
Clinical Medicine and Research XXIII
ed. by H. Bergmann, H. Köhn and H. Sinzinger

THE ROLE OF FDG-PET AND MIBI INVESTIGATIONS IN THE RESTAGING OF TREATED PATIENTS WITH MALIGNANT LYMPHOMAS

M. Papós, Z. Borbényi, L. Trón, A. Cserháti, E. Ambrus, I. Marton, Gy. Varga, L. Csernay, L. Pávics

Department of Nuclear Medicine, 2nd Department of Medicine, and Department of Radiology, Albert Szent-Györgyi Medical University, Szeged, Positron Emission Tomography Centre, University Medical School, Debrecen, Hungary

SUMMARY: In 14 patients (9 with Hodgkin disease (HD) and 5 with high-grade non-Hodgkin lymphoma (NHL)), 16 FDG-PET and MIBI investigations were carried out. The CT findings suggested a residual tumour mass in all of the patients. FDG-PET was found to most sensitive method for detection of residual tumor mass that MIBI investigation. However, our results lead us to conclude that a positive FDG-PET finding is of relatively low predictive value as regards the clinical relapse of HD and NHL. A positive result of MIBI investigation predicts the later activation of the lymphomas and the need for second-line therapy.

INTRODUCTION

In patients with Hodgkin disease (HD) or with high-grade non-Hodgkin malignant lymphoma (NHL), successful treatment may lead to a state free from an active tumour. For the detection of a residual tumour mass, chest X-ray investigations, computed tomography (CT) and magnetic resonance imaging (MRI) are routinely used. Nuclear medicine imaging techniques have made it possible to characterize the biological features of residual tissue masses. Fluoro-deoxyglucose positron emission tomography (FDG-PET) is a method that affords high accuracy in the evaluation of malignancy. FDG-PET is also effective in the staging of lymphomas (1,2,3,4). However, the predictive value of positive FDG-PET results as concerns recurrence of the disease seems doubtful (5). Besides FDG-PET, a few alternative methods such us 99mTc-MIBI seems also promising for the assessment of several types of tumours (6).

The aim of the present study was to compare the efficacies of MIBI and FDG-PET investigations in the evaluation of the residual active tumour tissue in treated lymphoma patients. The value of each method for the prediction of clinical recurrence was also analysed.

PATIENTS AND METHODS

Patients

16 FDG-PET and MIBI investigations (repeated investigations in two patients) were performed in 14 treated lymphoma patients (5 with NHL, 9 with HD, 7 males, 7 females, aged 19-68 years, mean: 35 years) in whom there was a suspicion of a residual mass after chemotherapy and/or irradiation or surgery. CT was applied for estimation of the involved regions or organs. B symptoms and an elevated lactate dehydrogenase level were regarded as signs of clinical activity.

After completion of the therapy, physical examination, clinical chemical tests, CT, FDG-PET and MIBI investigations were performed for restaging. . Four to 6 weeks after the FDG-PET and MIBI investigations, the physical examination and clinical biochemical tests were repeated and second-line therapy was provided as necessary. In cases without clinical activity signs or symptoms, a long-term clinical follow-up (24-60 weeks) was carried out to control the state of the disease.

CT

CT examinations were performed with Exel 2400 Elite equipment (Elscint, Israel). Following i.v. administration of contrast material, CT scans were performed from the thoracic inlet through the chest and recorded with lung, mediastinum and bone windows.

FDG-PET

After overnight fasting, 225-518 MBq of 18-FDG was administered to the patients. Sixty min after injection of 18-FDG, a whole body PET investigation concentrating on the suspected regions was performed with a PET device (GE 4096 plus, General Electric, UK). The slices were evaluated visually and interpreted by 3 well-trained specialists.

MIBI investigations

Images from the chest were acquired 5 and 90 minutes after administration of 720-804 MBq of 99mTc-MIBI. The MIBI investigations were carried out with a Siemens Icon Diacam SPECT device (Siemens, Germany). From the acquired data, transversal, sagittal and frontal slices were reconstructed. and additional planar images were also obtained. The pictures were interpreted visually by 3 well-trained specialists.

RESULTS

Restaging based on CT, FDG-PET and MIBI investigations

CT investigation revealed the morphological signs of a residual tumour mass in all patients in a total of 36 anatomical sites. FDG-PET demonstrated lesions with an increased glucose metabolism in 15 of the 16 cases, involving 38 lymphatic regions or organs. The CT and FDG-PET findings matched for 33 lesions. Five occult lesions were detected only by FDG-PET. Three CT-positive lesions did not exhibit an FDG uptake.

A pathological MIBI accumulation was detected in only 10 of the 16 cases, in regard to 14 regions or organs. The size of the MIBI-positive lesions was 2 cm or larger, while that of the involved lymph nodes missed by MIBI scintigraphy was in the range 1-4 cm (TABLE 1).

TABLE 1.

	Involved regions		
	CT	FDG-PET	MIBI investigations
cases	16	15	10
regions	36	38	14

Therapeutic consequences of FDG-PET and MIBI investigation results

Four to 6 weeks after the restaging, 9 of the 16 cases displayed clinical or biochemical activity signs of the disease. FDG-PET was positive in all of them. Eight of these patients had previously given positive MIBI investigation results. All these patients required second-line chemotherapy. Four of them proved to be therapy-responders on the basis of repeated CT investigation. No connection was detected between the MIBI-positivity and the later therapy response. Seven patients did not have B symptoms and exhibited a normal laboratory parameters, and second-line chemotherapy was therefore not applied. The positive predictive value of the FDG-PET and MIBI investigations as regards to the clinical relapse was 9/15 (60%) and 8/10 (80%), respectively. The negative predictive value of the MIBI investigation was 5/6 (83%) TABLE 2.).

TABLE 2.

	Clinial follow-up	
	active lymphoma	steady state
FDG+	9	6
FDG-	-	1
MIBI+	8	2
MIBI-	1	5

DISCUSSION

FDG-PET is frequently applied for lymphoma staging by Paul at al. (1) 99mTc-MIBI is also commonly utilized for the evaluation of different malignant diseases (6,7).
Our results suggested the value of FDG-PET in the detection of residual tumour tissue in lymphoma patients. The high sensitivity of this technique in our patient group was similar to that observed by Newman, Bares and Hoekstra (2,8,9).
MIBI investigation was found to be less sensitive method for the detection of residual lymphoma in agreement with others (6,10). Similarly to our findings, in a study of 17 HD patients Ziegels observed a relatively low sensitivity of MIBI investigations in the detection of residual lymphoma tissue (11). The low value of MIBI investigations for the detection of

residual tumour tissue in HD and NHL might be explained by the possible multidrug resistance of the tumour cells. In our study, however, there was no correlation between the MIBI-positivity and the response to the second-line therapy. Another possible explanation might be the difference between the spatial resolution of PET and SPECT. However, in our study a difference in resolution could not be responsible for the non-visualization of lymph nodes: the sizes of the MIBI-positive and MIBI-negative lymph nodes were in the same range.

The value of FDG-PET for prediction of the clinical recurrence of HD or NHL and the need for second-line therapy has rarely been investigated. The work of de Wit et al. revealed not only a high sensitivity, but also a relatively poor positive predictive value (57%) of FDG-PET investigations (5). Our results were similar; the positive predictive value of FDG-PET was 60%. The prognostic role of MIBI investigations in HD and NHL has not been studied previously. We found that the 99mTc-MIBI accumulation of the residual mass predicts the clinical recurrence of the disease, whereas the 18-FDG accumulation does not.

FDG-PET and MIBI investigations revealed different biological features of lymphomas. Further investigations, including *in vitro* studies, are needed to clarify the reasons for the different prognostic roles of the two methods.

CONCLUSIONS

Our results lead us to conclude that a positive FDG-PET finding is of relatively low predictive value as regards the clinical relapse of HD and NHL. A positive MIBI investigation result predicts the activation of a lymphoma and the need for second-line therapy.

REFERENCES

1. Paul R. Camparison of fluorine-18-2-fluorodeoxyglucose and gallium67 citrate imaging on detection for detection of lymphoma. J Nucl Med 1987; 28: 288-292.

2. Newman JC, Francis IR, Kiminski MS, Wahl RL. Imaging lymphoma with PET with 2-(F-18)-fluoro-2-deoxy-D-glucose: correlation with CT. Radiology 1994; 190: 111-116.

3. Okada J, Oonishi H, Yoshikawa K, et al. FDG-PET for predecting the prognosis of malignant lymphoma. Ann Nucl Med 1994; 8: 187-191.

4. Rigo P, Jerusalem G, Paulus P, Warland W, Fillet G. Positron emission tomography using fluorine-18deoxyglucose in response evaluation and follow-up of Hodgkin's disease and non-Hodgkin lymphoma. (abstract) Eur J Nucl Med 1995; 22: 786

5. de Wit M, Bauman D, Beyer W et al. Whole body positron emission tomography (PET) for diagnosis of residual mass in patients with lymphoma. Ann Oncol 1997; 8 (suppl 1): 57-60.

6. Aktolun C, Bayhan H, Kir MAD. Clinical experience with Tc-99m MIBI imaging in patients with malignant tumors. Preliminary results and comparison with Tl-201. Clin Nucl Med 1992; 17: 171-176.

7. Baillet G, Albuquerque L, Chen Q, Poisson M, Delattre JY. Evaluation of single-photon emission tomography imaging of supratentorial brain gliomas with technetium-99m sestamibi. Eur J Nucl Med 1994; 21: 1061-1066.

8. Bares R, Altehoefer C, Cremerius U et al. FDG-PET for metabolic classification of residual lymphoma masses after chemotherapy. (abstract) J Nucl Med 1994; 35: 131

9. Hoekstra OS, Ossenkoppele GJ, Gulding R et al. Early treatment response in malignant lymphoma, as determined by planar Fluorine-18-Fluorodeoxyglucose scintigraphy. J Nucl Med 1993; 34: 1706-1710.

10. Shirakawa T, Mori Y, Moriya E, Dohi M, Kawakami K, AkibaT, Nagata T. Uptake of Tc-99m hexakis 2-methoxy isobutyl isonitrile in lung or mediastinal lesions by SPECT. Nippon Igaku Hoshasen Gakkai Zasshi 1995; 55: 587-92.

11. Ziegels P, Nocaudie M, HugloD, Deveaux M, Detourmignies L, Wattel E, Marchandise X. Comparison of technetium-99m methoxyisobutylisonitrile and gallium-67 citrate scanning in the assessment of lymphomas. Eur J Nucl Med 1995; 22: 126-31.

Radioactive Isotopes in
Clinical Medicine and Research XXIII
ed. by H. Bergmann, H. Köhn and H. Sinzinger

ASSESSMENT OF PULMONARY NODULES AND COLORECTAL CANCER RECURRENCES BY FDG SCAN ON AN «ORDINARY» COINCIDENCE GAMMA CAMERA (CDET)

D. Grahek[1], F. Montravers[1], N. Ghazzar[1], S.Ait Ben Ali[1], N. Younsi[1], K. Kerrou[1], M. Wartski[2], E. Zerbib[2], J. Lumbroso[3], J.N. Talbot[1]

Services de médecine nucléaire (1) Hôpital Tenon, Paris ; (2) Centre Chirurgical Marie Lannelongue, Le Plessis Robinson ; (3) Institut Gustave Roussy, Villejuif. FRANCE.

SUMMARY

A FDG-CDET examination on a Picker gamma-camera equiped with coincidence detection and thick cristals was performed in 80 patients during the 2nd half of 1997. Sensitivity and specificity were both 100% for the detection of malignancy in primary lung tumours. Accuracy was 91% for the detection of hilar or mediastinal lymph nodes involvement vs 59% for CT ; lymphangitic carcinomatosis, metastases and concomittant tumours were also successfully detected and confirmed. FDG-CDET contributed to significant management changes in 30% of the patients referred for lung abnormalities. FDG-CDET was also usefull in "occult" recurrence of colorectal cancer with an accuracy of 78% vs 42% for CT in this difficult indication ; a longer follow-up is needed to be able to evaluate all the 25 patients whose management have been adequately modified in 60% of the cases. We conclude that the diagnostic performances of FDG-CDET derived from our current series cannot be distinguished from the corresponding results published with FDG-PET.

INTRODUCTION

For several years, [^{18}F]-fluorodeoxyglucose (FDG) has been recognized a proeminent imaging agent in oncology, using positron emission tomography (PET) scanners. These machines now provide whole body detection which is a clear advantage in oncology.

Two major indications of FDG-PET in oncology are the characterisation and the initial staging of pulmonary nodules or masses and the detection of recurrences of colorectal carcinoma.

However, PET scanners are expensive and not widely available (just one center with a whole body PET scanner in France, for example). Dual headed gamma cameras are much more widespread and disponible. Efforts have therefore been made to perform FDG imaging on ordinary gamma-cameras.

Attempts to fit ultra high energy collimators to dual head gamma cameras and obtain FDG images, regarding ^{18}F as a monoenergetic X-ray emittor of 511 keV, led to clinical performances significantly inferior to PET.

More recently, ordinary dual headed gamma-cameras were equiped with coincidence detection and thick cristals, to be able to detect FDG by means of the coincidence emission of the two 511 keV X photons, just as PET scanners do.

We have been granted such a CDET gamma-camera at the end of June 1997 and our aim was then to assess the clinical performances of FDG scintigraphy in two indications of great clinical importance where FDG-PET has proven useful : pulmonary nodules or masses and colorectal cancer recurrences. Since the unique PET center in the Paris area is relatively far from our department, we did not try a direct comparison in the same patients of the two modes of FDG detection. The direct confrontation of FDG-CDET scintigraphy to post surgical histology and follow-up data seemed more appropriate to assess the benefit that the clinicians could obtain from this new imaging technique.

PATIENTS, MATERIAL AND METHODS

Patients

In a prospective study, 80 patients had a FDG-CDET examination between July and December 1997, motivated by pulmonary nodule(s) or mass(es) in 53 cases or by suspicion of recurrence of a colorectal cancer in 27 cases. The examination was not performed in pregnant or lactating women and patients less than 18. In fact 3 patients met one of the other exclusion criteria which were infectious and/or inflammatory disease known to interfere (1 case of sarcoidosis), diabetes mellitus (1 case) advanced renal failure, surgical intervention or chemotherapy (1 case) or radiotherapy during the preceeding month. Eligible patients were then 52 for pulmonary nodules or masses or lung cancer recurrence and 25 for suspicion of colorectal cancer recurrence. A histological post surgical evidence was due to be obtained in all cases. However, the data were analysed while the results of post-surgical histology were not yet obtained in 29 cases, FDG examination being too recent in 9; the planed surgical intervention being canceled or postponed in 16 and no recent relevant information concerning 4 patients being forwarded to us.

Gamma-camera and FDG imaging methods

Since July 1997, we have used a Picker Prism 2000 dual head gamma camera equiped with coincidence detection and cristals 19 mm thick (instead of 9.5 mm in ordinary gamma-cameras). This gamma-camera is still able to perform high quality standard examinations of nuclear medicine, including those with isotopes emiting low energy photons (^{99m}Tc and ^{201}Tl). To detect ^{18}F, the colimators are removed and replaced by thin parallels bars which limitate the accepted incidence angle of the photons. Switching to coincidence detection mode is completly automated. An energy spectrum is displayed. We choosed to accept only those photons at 511 keV. However, it is also possible to accept photons of 350 keV, as proposed in order to obtain a more elevated counting rate. Each tomoscintigraphic acquisition involving a field of 35cm was performed using 30 steps of 6° lasting 70s when starting the acquisition (and then longer as ^{18}F decays). The duration of a tomoscintigraphic acquisition including patient positioning was typically 45min. The typical total counts per projection was 500 kcounts in thorax, 1500 kcounts in abdomen and 200 kcounts in brain. Slices are reconstructed by means of an iterative algorithm which minimizes artifacts in the vicinity of physiologically hyperactive organs such as urinary bladder, brain, heart...

Since the middle of september 1997, whole body imaging realised by rectilinear scanning has also become available as a «work in progress» feature. The acquisition lasts 30 min.

[^{18}F]-FDG was purchased from Hôpital Erasme, Université libre de Bruxelles, Belgique.

Imaging protocol

As this study was approved by an ethic comitee, patients gave their written informed consent. They were told to be fasting for at least 6 hours before the examination, with an abundant water intake. The IV injection of 150 to 200 MBq of FDG was done through an infusion line connected to saline. After injection, the patient stayed lying with a minimal musclar activity during 45 to 60 min ; he or she was then instructed to void his/her bladder and was subsequently positionned between the two heads of the gamma-camera for imaging.

Each patient had at first a tomoscintigraphic acquisition, centered on the thorax for pulmonary masses and on the abdomen for colorectal recurrences. Between July and mid-September, a second tomographic acquisition was then systematically performed and sometimes also a third one. As soon as whole body images could be obtained, a whole body scan was performed as the second acquisition and, depending on its result, the examination was either terminated or completed by another tomoscintigraphy, centered on abnormalities suspected on the whole body scan.

RESULTS

1) Pulmonary nodules or masses.

52 eligible patients had FDG-CDET in four different contexts :

1.1 Isolated pulmonary nodules.

16 patients were referred for an isolated nodule the diameter of which was less than 4 cm at CT, without histologic proof of malignancy (biopsy not done or negative). The nodules which were at FDG-CDET either not visible or with a counts ratio to contralateral parenchyma less than 3 were considered FDG negative.

Post surgical histology was obtained in 9 cases and therapeutic evidence in 1 case :

- 5 nodules were malignant, all FDG postive i.e. 5 true positive cases ; FDG-CDET was then also used in these patients for staging (see below 1.2) ;
- 4 were histologically proved to be benign and, in the last patient, a pulmonary abcess was subsquently completly cured by antibiotics ; all were FDG negative i.e. 5 true negative FDG-CDET examinations (Sp = 5/5 = 100%).

4 patients have not currently been operated : 1 was considered unoperable and only had a mediastinoscopy with biopsy on lymph nodes seen on CT but which were negative on FDG-CDET and which resulted to be benign ; 3 others patients had FDG-CDET less than one month ago. We have no recent news of the 2 last patients.

1.2 Staging of pulmonary masses

22 patients were referred for staging of a pulmonary mass, the malignancy of which was either demonstated by biopsy or very probable in view of the radiological and/or endoscopical aspect or shape of the tumour.

The tumour itself was proven by histology to be an adenocarcinoma or any other type of non-small cell lung cancer (NSCLC) in 19 cases, this evidence being obtained in a metastatic lymph node in 1 case or being lacking in 2 recent FDG examinations which are therefore excluded from the analysis. All tumours appeared FDG positive. The analysis of staging shall also include the 5 patients with a FDG positive isolated nodule who were operated ; altogether the sensitivity of FDG-CDET for detection of malignancy of primary NSCLC tumour was Se = 25/25 = 100%.

Homolateral lymph node involvement was histologically proven in 14 patients and was highly probable in 3 others with widespread pulmonary invasion confirmed by several imaging modalities and who were not operated. FDG-CDET was true positive in 14 of them (Se = 82%) ; the N1 lymph node invasion in the 3 false negative cases of FDG-CDET was not detected either by any other imaging modality or during surgical intervention : it was a post surgical microscopic discovery. Among the 8 patients with post surgical evidence of no homolateral lymph nodes involvement, FDG-CDET was evocative of a such invasion in 3 (Sp=63%) : one had a very extensive T4 tumour with a malignant thrombosis of vessels which was interpreted as a separate focus i.e. T3 N1 instead of T4 N0 without consequences on the patient management ; in the 2 other cases, histology revealed an inflammatory process around the tumour. The N1 stage, especially when confined to sattelite lymph nodes, was more difficult to differentiate from N0 than the N2 stage ; by using (as many authors in PET) the classification "hilar or mediastinal lymph nodes", the 3 FN and 1 FP of the N stage would then be correctly grouped (accuracy by reference to histology = (14+6)/22=91%).

Foci in the contralateral hemithorax were seen in 5 cases on FDG-CDET, which can correspond to N3 malignant lymph nodes or thoracic contralateral metastatic lesions. It was confirmed by other imaging techniques in 2 patients who were not operated but was neither brought in evidence nor ruled out in 3 patients who were operated on a single lung, the last examination being recent. Lymphangitic carcinomatosis, which gives a typical aspect of diffuse uptake on FDG scan, was proven in 1 patient and highly suspected in 2 others on concordant images with several modalities, all were FDG positive.

Extrathoracic metastases were suspected on FDG-CDET in 6 patients. In one case, a bone focus on the pelvic bone corresponded to an abnormal focus at bone scan and at a subsequent MRI ; the patient was considered uneligible for surgery. In another case, widespread metastases were noted at CT and a bilateral adrenal invasion was histologically demonstrated ; all these sites were FDG positive and FDG also revealed a large hyperactive mass on the right side of the right kidney and prevertebral lymph nodes. In none of the 4 other cases, concerning adrenal and/or bone metastases suspected on FDG-CDET, a histologic evidence could be obtained until now.
In one case, a very clear FDG focus was discovered in the caecum on the whole body scan ; the subsequent abdominal CT being unconclusive, colonoscopy was performed which confirmed the existence of a caecal tumour which was removed endoscopically and proved to be a villous tumour without evidence of malignancy on the examined specimens : FDG successfully brought in evidence an unsuspected tumour.

1 patient with a proven NSCLC was studied apart from the 22 others since he was referred prior to surgery only for confirmation of brain and adrenal metastases suspected on CT and MRI which were confirmed as FDG positive foci but no histologic proof was then obtained.

In summary, in the search for hilar or mediastinal lymph node involvement, the agreement rate with histology was 20/22 (91%) for FDG versus 13/22 (59%) for CT. All 5 metastastic cases confirmed histologically or highly probable on conventional imaging were FDG positive. One caecal concomittent tumor was discovered at FDG-CDET.

1.3 Search for recurrence of pulmonary cancer

7 patients previously operated for NSCLC were referred for suspicion of recurrence with, among other suspected sites, one or several pulmonary nodule(s) or isolated liver lesions in one case. Histologic evidence was just obtained in two cases. In one, the recurrence site suspected on

CT appeared much more extensive on FDG-CDET and was confirmed at post surgical histology. In the other, the small pulmonary nodule on CT was FDG negative (and remains apparently steady 3 months later) but a solitary focus of the knee, which was visible at bone scan, clearly took up FDG and was shown to be a recurrence on biopsy. Concerning the 5 other patients, FDG was in accordance with conventionnal imaging in 3, adding one other focus in one case, and discordant in 2, including one negative examination ; however histology is not avaliable until now and follow-up time still too short.

1.4 Search for secondary pulmonary masses

5 patients with known cancer and 1 with multiple metastatic lesions but unknown primary cancer were referred because of pulmonary nodule(s). The pulmonary nodule(s) were FDG positive in 4 cases, the secondary malignancy being confirmed in 1 case by post surgical histology and being probable in 2 cases due to agreement between imaging modalities ; the last case (a difficult one since the pulmonary FDG positive nodule was steady for several years and the patient had tuberculosis in the past) is not yet settled. In one patient referred after ablation of a skin nodule which proved to be melanoma, FDG was negative both around the excised primary lesion and at pulmonary nodules seen on CT ; a local reintervention with histology and the subsequent discovery of tuberculosis explaining the pulmonary lesions showed that both sites were true negative. In the last patient, FDG showed no uptake on the suspected pulmonary nodules shown on CT but detected an abdominal focus which is until now unexplored.

In summary, one can currently consider 3 TP and 1TN on 4 evaluated patients in this indication.

1.5 Modification of the patient management

Among 51 eligible patients referred for pulmonary nodule(s) or masse(s), we have until now been informed that FDG-CDET was contributive to the cancelation of the planed surgery and its replacement by proposed chemotherapy in 6 cases or abstention in 1 case without detectable relapse. On the other hand, FDG-CDET objectivated a lung cancer recurrence which led to surgery in one case and showed an unsuspected caecal tumor which was endoscopically removed in another case. The therapeutic adaptation rate was then 18% ; furthermore, suspicion of N3, metastatic or recurrent foci on FDG-CDET led to an adaptation and a special attention in the follow-up of 6 other patients (12%). Thus the overall rate of modification of patient management is currently 30% in this pathology, with no detrimental consequence reported.

2) Colorectal cancer recurrences.

26 FDG-CEDT have been performed in 25 eligible patients, in two different contexts : occult disease and search for other secondary locations when one recurrence site was demonstrated with conventional imaging techniques.

2.1. Occult disease.

Those 21 patients were refered with biological (CEA levels raising) or clinical (pain) symptoms evocative of recurrence but with negative (15 cases) or equivocal (6 cases) conventional imaging and endoscopy. CDET showed FDG positive foci in 14 of them constisting of a single focus in 9 cases and multiple foci in 5. FDG-CDET was therefore negative in 7 cases.

Post surgical histology was obtained in 7 cases. FDG-CDET was true positive in 5 patients and apparently false positive in 1 patient: in this patient, an initial FDG-CDET showed two abdominal foci ; only one was removed during a surgical reintervention and no evidence of malignancy was detected at histology ; the second focus appeared unchanged at a post-operative FDG-CDET examination and CEA levels are steady. In the last patient presenting with local pain but normal CEA levels, FDG-CDET was negative ; a surgical reintervention was finaly performed and no malignant lesion was objectivated : FDG-CDET is considered true negative. Surgery has been postponed waiting for other evidences in 2 FDG positive patients, or have not yet been performed in 3.

Radiotherapy was undertaken on the foci discovered on FDG-CDET, without histological proof, in 3 patients. It was associated to chemotherapy in one patient whom FDG-CDET demonstrated a presacral focus, with a remarquable success : CEA levels decreased from more than 20 ng/mL to normal levels ; after radiochemotherapy, the nodule was finally surgically removed but no malignant lesion could be demonstated in the necrotic remains. In the 2 other patients, radiotherapy is currently underway.

Concerning negative FDG-CDET, we have already mentionned one true negative case ; in contrast, another patient has probably to be considered false negative since he died several weeks after FDG with a cholestase probably related to the progression of his previous liver metastatic lesion, but without fresh histologic evidence. None of the 5 other patients has until now evidence of the disease : a purely symptomatic treatment was undertaken in one patient complaining from abdominal pain with normal CEA levels but a transient raise of CA 19.9, without any evidence of relapse after a 4 month follow-up ; 3 patients with elevated CEA levels and 1 with a small hepatic image at US and normal CEA levels are currently untreated for respectively 5, 2, 1.5 and 1 month with no carcinologic event.

2.2 Confirmation and/or extension of recurrence

In those 4 patients, conventional imaging and/or endoscopy detected or was highly suspicious of a relapse and FDG-CDET was indicated to confirm this finding and to detect possible other recurrent or metastatic lesions.

Each case has to be detailed. The first patient, whose local recurrence was seen at endoscopy and confirmed at biopsy, had a single focus at the same site at FDG-CEDT which was confirmed by the post surgical histology: true positive. The second patient was highly suspicious of perineal relapse on CT ; at FDG-CDET, this focus was confirmed and another bar-like focus was seen in the middle part of the abdomen ; the next day, US of the abdomen was equaly suspicious of peritoneal carcinomatosis which was confirmed later during a surgical exploration : FDG was true positive for peritoneal dissemination and true positive for the highly probable local relapse. Chemotherapy was then started. In the third patient, CT was evocative of a single relapse in a juxta renal lymph node ; FDG showed a single focus higher in the upper abdomen and radiotherapy was started on this focus ; malignant inguinal lymph node invasion became obvious during radiotherapy. By that time, FDG-CDET whole body scanning was not implemented and the inguinal region had not been imaged prior to radiotherapy. In the fourth patient, a local retrovesical relapse has been found on abdominal CT ; this finding was confirmed by FDG-CDET which also brought in evidence pulmonary invasion on whole body scan, as did later thoracic CT : chemotherapy was then indicated.

2.3 Modification of the patient management.

Among 25 patients referred for colorectal recurrence, we have been informed in 12 cases (48%) of a modification of the patient management as a consequence of FDG-CDET, either by objectivating a target for surgery or radiotherapy or by refraining from intervention on equivocal foci shown by other imaging techniques which were not confirmed at FDG-CDET. This modification can be until now considered beneficial in all patient but two (40%) (one false positive in the site which was operated and one recurrence in another site during radiotherapy). Furthermore, by confirming foci seen on other imaging examinations or the absence of focus, FDG-CDET helped decision making in 5 other patients (20%).

DISCUSSION

Our first results concerning FDG-CDET detection of lung cancer presenting as a solitary nodule (Se=Sp=100%) are in accordance with those of FDG-PET which demonstrated an average sensitivity of 96% (1) and a high specificity when granulomatous diseases are excluded e.g. 2 FP on 17 benign nodules reported by Hustinx et al. (1). One patient referred for suspicion of coolorectal cancer recurrence also suffered from histologically proven sarcoidosis and was then excluded from the protocol ; the thoracic lesions of sarcoidosis were visible at FDG-CDET. Use of FDG-CDET in characterisation of pulmonary nodules could, as for FDG-PET, lead to significant savings in addition to reducing the complications during management e.g. 26% of pneumothorax as a consequence of tranthoracic fine needle aspiration reported by Devan et al. (2).

For preoperative staging of NSCLC, one has first to consider the detection of hilar or mediastinal lymph node involvement. FDG-CDET results of the present study are within the range of published FDG-PET values i.e. Se= 82-100, Sp=73-100% (1) ; FDG-CDET Se and Sp are still of the order when taking into account the N1 sattelite lymph nodes the diagnosis of which is more difficult (and which were responsible for the 3 FN of our series). For example, Valk et al. (3) reported with PET Se=4/7=57% for N1 versus Se=20/24=83% for N2. In our series, accuracy of FDG-CDET (20/22=91% in the operated patients) compete very favourably with that of CT (13/22=59%), as FDG-PET does : in the study by Wahl et al (4) including 19 NSCLC, the accuracy was 81% for FDG-PET versus 52% for CT ; in the work of Valk (3), it was 88% (73/83) for FDG-PET versus 65% (54/83) for CT ; in the series of the team of Rigo (1) it was 82% (41/50) for FDG-PET versus 66% (33/50) for CT. The very interesting accuracy of FDG-CDET to demonstrate more widespread lymph node metastasis giving lymphangitic carcinomatosis was noted by the referring clinicians ; FDG-CDET suspicion of N3 involvement in 3 cases remains to be histologically evaluated as were the 2 equivalent cases in the study of Valk et al (3).

All the confirmed metastases of NSCLC were seen on FDG-CEDET, the frequency of this discovery (6/25) being comparable to that of PET studies i.e. 19/61 (1) or 11/99 (3). Several authors reported high diagnostic accuracy of FDG-PET in the detection of NSCLC recurrence e.g. in 39 patients Se=100%, Sp=62% (5) , in 24 patients Se=94%, Sp=94% (1). In our series, FDG-CDET proved to be able to detect (and at least in one case to rule out) such recurrences, as well as to image unsuspected commitant tumours or lung metastases of other cancers.

FDG-PET contributes to significant management changes in lung tumour patients as first assessed by Lewis et al. (6) in 14/34 (41%) cases ; our current rate with FDG-CDET being 30%.

In the detection of recurrence of colorectal cancer, an histological evidence has been until now much rarer (9/25 patients) to assess FDG-CDET ; a longer follow-up time will be necessary to better evaluate FDG-CDET in this indication since only 3 non-operated patients can currently be evaluated with confidence on other imaging modalities and follow-up. However, very interesting results have been obtained in the “occult recurrence” group, the accuracy of

FDG-CDET being 7/9=78% while it is almost 0% by definition of this group for other imaging techniques including endoscopy with biopsy. Globally, the evaluation of FDG-CDET accuracy is 10/12=83%, somewhat less than the typical value for FDG-PET i.e. over 90% (7) but better than the typical value for CT i.e. 65% in 76 patients (8). However, one should take into account that all these PET series have included much less "occult recurrence" patients than ours (21/25=84%). The recurrence foci of this patients are more difficult to detect : the accuracy for CT in our series was just 5/12 =42%. As a consequence of the demand of the clinicians in the difficult cases they referred us, FDG-CDET influenced very frequently the patient management with a rate of 60% of justified modifications due to FDG-CDET, higher than that reported by Schiepers (8) i.e. 14/35=40% for FDG-PET.

In conclusion, FDG-CDET, performed on a Picker gamma-camera with cristals of 19 mm, tomoscintigraphy plus whole body scanning and image reconstruction by an iterative algorithm, gave, in pulmonary nodules or masses and in suspicion of colorectal cancer recurrence, relevant indications on the nature of the abnormalities seen with other imaging techniques and revealed their extension, local or metastatic, more accurately than does CT. In opposition with preliminary results, published until now as abstracts, comparing PET with CDET performed without all these features, no difference was observed between the clinical efficacy of FDG-CDET and the reported values for FDG-PET in the present indications, in terms of accuracy and of modification of patients management. However, dedicated PET machines will undoubtably be required in those centers specialised in oncology due to the previsible increase of the number of patients following the demonstration of utility of FDG examination in a large number of oncologic indications.

REFERENCES

1. Hustinx R, Paulus P, Rigo P, Yeung HW., Macxapinlac HA, Larson SM. In : Clinical PET in oncology. Lung tumors. GE Medical Systems Editor; 1996 : 16-31.
2. Dewan NA, Reeb SD, Gupta NC et al. PET-FDG imaging and transthoracic needle lung aspiration biopsy in evaluation of pulmonary lesions. A comparative risk-benefit analysis. Chest 1995; 108: 441-446.
3. Valk PE, Pounds TR, Hopkins DM et al. Staging non-small cell lung cancer by whole body positron emission tomographic imaging. Ann Thorac. Surg. 1995; 60 : 1573-82.
4. Wahl RL, Quint LE, Greenough RL et al. Staging of mediastinal non-small cell lung cancer with FDG PET, CT and fusion images : preliminary prospective evaluation. Radiology 1994; 191 : 371-377.
5. Inoue T, Kim EE, Komki R et al. Detecting recurrent or residual lung cancer with FDG-PET. J Nucl Med 1995; 36: 788-793
6. Lewis P, Griffin S, Marsden P et al. Whole body 18F-fluorodeoxyglucose positron emission tomography in preoperative evaluation of lung cancer. Lancet 1994; 344 : 1265-1266.
7. Hustinx R, Paulus P, Rigo P, Yeung HW., Macxapinlac HA, Larson SM. In : Clinical PET in oncology. Tumors of the gastro-intestinal tract. GE Medical Systems Editor; 1996 : 32-45.
8. Schiepers C, Penninckx F, De Vadder N et al. Contribution of PET in the diagnosis of recurrent colorectal cancer. Eur J Surg Oncol 1995; 21 : 517-522.

This work was supported by a clinical research grant «PHRC», coordinator : Pr J.L. Moretti.

Acknowledgements : The authors want to greatfully acknowledge
- Dr S. Goldman and M. P. Damhaut, cyclotron de l'Hôpital Erasme, Bruxelles, for the supply of [^{18}F]-FDG,
- and the referring clinicians : Dr André, Dr Baldeyrou, Dr Balosso, Pr Barbier, Dr Bard, Dr Bellaïche, Dr Benazra, Dr Bernier, Pr Cadranel, Pr Delfraissy, Dr Ducreux, Dr François, Dr Gharbi, Dr Gil Delgado, Dr Houry, Pr Housset, Pr Izrael, Dr Jauffret, Dr Lasser, Dr Lotz, Dr Magdeleinat, Dr Maltère, Pr Maylin, Pr Misset, Dr Monchâtre, Dr Milleron, Dr Regnard, Pr Rougier, Dr Rosencher, Dr Salmeron, Pr Sézeur, Dr Tashjian, Pr Tiret, Dr Tigaud, Dr Weissman.

Radioactive Isotopes in
Clinical Medicine and Research XXIII
ed. by H. Bergmann, H. Köhn and H. Sinzinger

CLINICAL UTILITY OF ^{18}FDG-PET WITH MOLECULAR COINCIDENCE DETECTION (MCD) AND A MODIFIED SPECT-CAMERA

H. Erler, E. Donnemiller, C. Bacher-Stier, M.Oberladstätter, G. Riccabona, R. Moncayo
Department of Nuclear Medicine, University of Innsbruck, A-6020 Innsbruck, Austria

INTRODUCTION

In clinical nuclear medicine there has been an increased demand for positron emission tomography (PET) studies in the last years. Clinical use has been defined and refined constantly [1]. While dedicated ring camera systems are optimal, but still expensive, alternatives have emerged with the development of hybrid camera systems that have the capability of detecting 511 KeV energy [2]. With ^{18}FDG becoming available through cyclotron centers, end users can rely upon delivery of the radiopharmaceutical in order to carry out the investigations.

The aim of this report is to describe our initial 1-year experience working with an ADAC-Vertex-camera equiped with 511 keV collimators and molecular coincidence detection (MCD). Most of the investigations were carried out using the newly described molecular coincidence detection (MCD), specially when dealing with oncological patients, while for cardiological studies 511 keV collimators were used [3]. We describe routine working protocols, imaging technique, and results obtained so far.

MATERIALS AND METHODS:

Camera system: All studies were done with a two-head digital gamma camera (Vertex EPIC, ADAC Laboratories, California, USA) equiped with 511 keV collimators in order to image ^{18}FDG. In addition the molecular coincidence detection (MCD) method developed by ADAC laboratories, which allows imaging of positron emitting isotopes by electronic coincidence [3], was also used. The operating characteristics for the system are: detector: non-Anger digital with 1 ADC per PM; field of view: 38 x 51 cm; cristall thickness: 5/8″; photo multiplier tubes: 55; analyzers: 3; lead shielding: 511 keV; resolution: ≤ 4,2 mm (^{201}Tl).

Patients: Between October 1996 and October 1997 a total of 157 studies in 153 patients were done. Ninety studies were carried out using MCD, while 67 were performed only with 511 keV collimators during the initial months of camera operation. Oncological and neurological studies are done routinely with MCD, cardiological ones without MCD. The majority of patients were refered to our department because of malignancy or suspected malignancy (n=101). In 26 cases the nature of detected lesions was not known. Oncological staging was done in 58 cases, and follow-up studies after therapy in 17 cases. Cardiological studies were done in 31 cases in order to evaluate myocardial viability. Neurological patients presented with either epilepsy (n=6) or with degenerative brain disorders (n=3). In addition heart and brain studies were conducted in 16 patients presenting systemic lupus erythematosus [4].

Evaluation parameters: The results of the PET scans were compared with conventional diagnostic methods. These included: surgical reports and histology, conventional x-ray, CT, MRI, EEG, bone scans, ^{131}I-scans, tumor markers, coronary angiography (CAG), myocardial perfusion-SPECT, as well as the effects of PCTA/bypass surgery. The comparison allowed us to classify the results as true positive, true negative, false positve, and false negative.

Handling of ^{18}FDG: ^{18}FDG was produced at the Radiopharmaceutical Unit of the Department of Nuclear Medicine, Klinikum Rechts der Isar, Technische Universität München. After transport (approximately 2 hours) to Innsbruck, the tracer was diluted to a handling volume of 5 ml and the total amount of radioactivity was recorded. The tracer was stored in a specially shielded container (COMTEC-Laborgeraete GmbH, Vienna) from which individual patient doses were prepared by aspiration into a shielded syringe. Before dose application an indwelling catheter was placed into a fore-arm vein of the patient. The effective dose to the patient was approximately 10 mSv for a given activity of 370 MBq ^{18}FDG.

Routine study protocols: Based on standard PET procedures [5] we designed individual protocols for all studies (Table 1). Blood sugar levels up to 140 mg/dl were considered the upper level of acceptable glycemia for the studies. In cases of diabetic patients, the corresponding upper level was set at 170 mg/dl. Patients with higher glycemic levels received fast acting insulin i.v. (1E / 30 mg/dl glycemia above 140 or 170 mg/dl, respectively) before ^{18}FDG application.

Table 1. **^{18}FDG Study Protocols for Clinical Routine Studies**

	Oncology	Cardiology	Cardiology in Diabetics	Neurology
Fasting before study	4-6 hours	4-6 hours	usual breakfast and medication	4-6 hours
Start clinical control before FDG application	30 minutes	2 hours	2 hours	1 hour
Preparation: place indwelling i.v. cannula	check glycemia	check glycemia meal [1]	check glycemia meal [1]	check glycemia cover eyes 15 minutes before FDG application
If glycemia >140 mg/dl	fast acting insulin [2]	fast acting insulin [2]	fast acting insulin [3]	fast acting insulin [2]
Furosemide 20 mg i.v.	yes	yes	yes	no
Acipimox 250 mg p.o.	no	yes	yes	no
Further medication or preparation	500 ml Ringer lactate infusion void bladder before imaging	500 ml Ringer lactate infusion void bladder before imaging	500 ml Ringer lactate infusion void bladder before imaging	relaxation for 20 minutes in a quiet, dim room
^{18}FDG Dose	approximately 148 MBq	370 MBq	370 MBq	-50 kg: 147 MBq -60 kg: 185 MBq -70 kg: 207 MBq -80 kg: 222 MBq -90 kg: 260 MBq
Time until imaging	60 min	60 min	60 min	30 min
Duration of imaging process	60 to 90 min (2 or 3 scans)	about 30 min	about 30 min	about 45 min

1: 70 g carbohydrates, 41 g protein, 21 g fat (= 639 cal), e.g. rye bread, cheese, ham, lemonade
2: 1E pro 30 mg/dl glycemia above 140 mg/dl
3: 1E pro 30 mg/dl glycemia above 170 mg/dl

RESULTS

Camera characteristics: Previous to the clinical studies, tests were performed to find the range of count rates which can be used safely in a clinical environment without the risk of producing artefacts due to too high count rates. Singles count rates in the range of 1 to 1,5 Mc/s per detector head were associated with the onset of artefacts. This figure corresponds to app. 50% of the specified maximum count rate for the camera. For safety reasons, i.e. to avoid diagnostic images with artefacts, the usable singles count rates per detector were limited to $\leq$ 1,3 Mc/s (see also M. Oberladstätter, this volume).

Oncological studies: The overall results are shown in Table 2. Five cases having an inflammatory or infectious process, e.g. tuberculosis, pulmonitis, gluteal abscess, questionable thyreoiditis and colitis, and showing a faint to mild ^{18}FDG uptake were misclassified as positive before the final diagnosis was known. The smallest malignant lung lesion showing a positive FDG image was seen in a 40-year old female patient with a solitary nodule of 8 mm diameter.

Table 2. Results of Oncological Studies [1]:

Scan Result	Clin. Positive	Clin.Negative
Positive	69	5
Negative	1 [2]	23

1: Sensitivity: 98,6%. Specificity: 82,1%. Positive predictive value: 93,2%. Negative predictive value: 95,8%.
2: low grade CNS lymphoma

Cardiological studies: Patients with coronary heart disease were studied either after previous ^{201}Tl scans (n = 22) or coronary angiography (CAG) (n = 6) or both (n = 12). Ten cases showed no ^{18}FDG uptake in areas having an irreversible ^{201}Tl defects, while 9 patients had ^{18}FDG uptake in these segments (hibernating myocardium). In 12 cases defects in ^{18}FDG uptake showed the same localization as seen in CAG. Since the same camera system is routinely used also for thallium perfusion studies, comparisons between both studies were easily done.

Neurological studies: Only few patients with a neurological syndrome were investigated. In 8 cases the positive findings correlated well with the clinical picture, including 6 cases of epilepsy. The pathology in the remaining case is uncertain at present.

DISCUSSION

The development of hybrid camera systems for PET studies, together with the availability of ^{18}FDG, has improved the coverage of clinical demand. While hybrid cameras still do not bring the high resolution which can be achieved with dedicated ring detection systems, the relatively low hardware cost of the former makes the method more accessible. In addition, the SPET capability of hybrid cameras leads to a reduction of the FDG dose, reducing consequently the cost of the studies.

In our 1-year experience we have been able to carry out PET studies on a regular basis using a hybrid camera system. Concerning spatial resolution and correlation with the size of lesions seen with other diagnostic methods, we were able to observe a positive FDG uptake in cases for lesions of 8 mm diameter, as described in CT. This is of importance since the great majoritiy of cases included oncological patients. In these cases sensitivity and specificity were 98,6%, and 82,1%, respectively. These figures are similar to those obtained with ring detector systems [6]. On the other hand indeterminate results arising from conventional imaging methods such as CT or MRI could be corrected or discarded depending on the PET results. Cardiac studies showed also a good correlation with thallium perfusion or CAG results.

Potential pitfalls in PET imaging constitute inflammatory processes [6] which look like a possible malignant process, therefore, false positive results can arise relatively frequently. Full PET systems can classify such cases better by carrying out quantitative uptake determinations. This feature, however, is currently missing in hybrid camera systems, even though it is expected to be resolved soon. In general, however, these problems are also known for ring cameras, showing that quantification may not be able to assess malignancy [6].

In conclusion, PET studies are feasible using hybrid camera systems that are able to detect 511 keV energy. The performance data regarding specificity and sensitivity are similar to those reported for ring cameras. Cardiac studies profit through data acquisition using the same hardware.

REFERENCES

1. Konsensus Onko-PET. Deutsche Gesellschaft für Nuklearmedizin e.V. Nuklearmedizin 1997; 45-46.

2. Drane WE, Abbott FD, Nicole MW, Mastin ST, Kuperus JH. Technology for FDG SPECT with a relatively inexpensive gamma camera. Work in progress. Radiology 1994; 191:461-465.

3. ADAC Laboratories. Molecular coincidence detection operator's manual.1997 Rev. 1.7.1:1-1-2-2.

4. Moncayo R, Kowald E, Schauer N, Pachinger O, Schmuth M, Fritsch P, et al. Detection of myocardial involvement in systemic lupus erythematosus (SLE) by means of 18FDG investigations. 1998 in preparation.

5. Rigo P, Paulus P, Kaschten BJ, Hustinx R, Bury T, Jerusalem G, et al. Oncological applications of positron emission tomography with fluorine-18 fluorodeoxyglucose. Eur J Nucl Med 1996; 23:1641-1674.

6. Bury T, Dowlati A, Paulus P, Corhay JL, Benoit T, Kayembe JM, et al. Evaluation of the solitary pulmonary nodule by positron emission tomography imaging. Eur Respir J 1996; 9:410-414.

Radioactive Isotopes in
Clinical Medicine and Research XXIII
ed. by H. Bergmann, H. Köhn and H. Sinzinger

DEOXYGLUCOSE UPTAKE BY APOPTOSING AND PROLIFERATING COLONIC TUMOUR CELLS

T.A.D. Smith, S.M. Ronen, J.C. Titley and V.R. McCready

Departments of Nuclear Medicine, NMR and Cell and Experimental Pathology, Royal Marsden NHS Trust and Institute of Cancer Research, Sutton, Surrey SM2 5PT UK

SUMMARY: The relationship between proliferation and glucose consumption was examined in two colonic tumour lines SW480 and SW620 by seeding cells from the two lines into each of 20 tissue culture flasks and determining the uptake of 2-deoxy-D-(1-^{3}H)glucose (^{3}H-DG) and S-phase fraction (Spf) at various time points after passaging. Strong correlations between Spf and ^{3}H-DG uptake were noted for both the SW480 ($r=0.73$ $p<0.01$) and the SW620 ($r=0.87$, $p<0.001$) cell line. The effect of treatment of SW620 cells with doxorubicin, which induces apoptosis, on ^{3}H-DG uptake by attached cells was also examined. By 24 hours uptake per viable cell had dropped to less than 50% of control.

INTRODUCTION

Tumours exhibit enhanced rates of glycolysis in the presence of glucose and glycolysis has been considered a more important source of ATP in tumours than oxidative phosphorylation (1). The glucose analogue, 2-Deoxy-D-glucose (DG) which after phosphorylation to the 6-phosphate derivative undergoes only minor further metabolism, accumulates in high levels in malignant tissue. A number of studies involving serial quantitative FDG-PET scanning of several different tumour types including lymphoma (2), glioma (3) and breast cancers (4) suggest that therapeutic responsiveness may be detected using this technique. Responding tumours showing decreased uptake of FDG after therapy, in some cases before a clinical response was observed, compared with pretreatment scans (2). The clinical role of PET-FDG in therapeutic response will depend on which feature of malignancy is most related to its uptake. Some in-vivo studies (5,6) have observed strong correlations between DG uptake and proliferative indices, although other workers (7,8) have failed to observe such an association. Response to therapy is often accompanied by decreased proliferative fraction and apoptosis. Presently we have examined the relationship between proliferation (S-phase frction (Spf)) and ^{3}H-DG uptake by two colonic tumour lines. Treatment of one of the lines (SW620) with doxorubicin (Dox) results in apoptosis. Using this system ^{3}H-DG uptake by cells destined to apoptose has been investigated.

MATERIALS AND METHODS

Cells: SW480 and SW620 cell lines were grown in Dulbecco's MEM containing 4.5 mM glucose (Gibco, UK) with 10% foetal bovine serum (Sigma Chemical Co, UK) and penicillin /streptomycin. Trypsinized cells (about 3 x 10^5) were then seeded into twenty 25 cm^2 tissue culture flasks (Nunc, UK) in 3ml of complete medium and maintained at 37°C in 5%Co_2:95% air. Two days after seeding and for upto 12 days the incorporation of ^{3}H-DG was determined in triplicate flasks of cells. This produced populations of cells with increasing cell density which also resulted in a range of proliferative fractions.

Doxorubicin treatment: Media in twelve flasks of confluent cells was replaced with doxorubicin (100μg/ml) containing media. ^{3}H-DG uptake was determined in triplicate flasks and controls 4, 8, 15 and 24 hours after treatment.

Determination of ^{3}H-DG incorporation:Medium was replaced in flasks 1 hr prior to determination of ^{3}H-DG incorporation. ^{3}H-DG (185 Kbq) was added to each flask which were then incubated for 30 min at 37°C. The medium was then poured off and the flasks washed 5 times with PBS (10 ml per wash). After trypsinizing, cells were dissagreggated by aspirating the suspension up and down a 1 ml pipette tip. Two 0.5 ml aliquots were added to scintillation vials containing 5ml of Ultima Gold (Packard) scintillant and ^{3}H-DG uptake determined in a beta-counter. A further 0.5 ml sample of cell suspension was centrifuged at 400g for 10 min and after removing supernatant the cells were resuspended in 200 μl of PBS. After addition of 0.7 ml of ice cold ethanol the fixed cells were stored at 4°C for determination of Spf using flow cytometry. Viable cell numbers were determined on 100 μl aliquots of the cell suspension.

Determination of apoptosis: Presence of a sub G1 peak was determined using flow cytometry

RESULTS

Figure 1 shows the uptake of ^{3}H-DG per 10^3 cells versus Spf. The correlation coefficients indicate significant correlations between proliferative fraction and ^{3}H-DG uptake by SW480 ($r=0.72$, $n=15$, $p<0.01$) and SW620 ($r=0.87$, $n=18$, $p<0.001$) cells.

Fig 1: Spf vs ^{3}H-DG uptake by SW480 (A) and SW620 cells

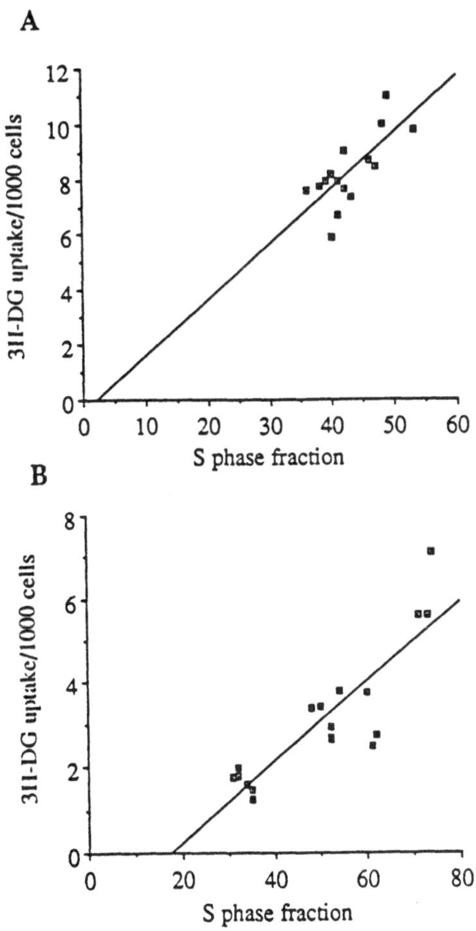

Figure 2 shows the number of attached cells and the uptake of ^{3}H-DG with time after treatment with Dox as a percentage of control. During the first 16 hours there is no change in the number of attached cells. However after 24 hours the number of attached cells had decreased to 66% of untreated. The uptake of ^{3}H-DG was lower by treated cells after only 4 hours and continued to decrease with time after treatment. In each case viability of attached cells was ≥98%. Cells which were attached even 24 hours, after exposure to Dox, did not appear to be apoptotic. However after 4 hours exposure to Dox 22% of detached cells were apoptotic which increased to 100% after 24 hours suggesting that cells which became detached were destined to apoptose.

Fig 2: Adherent cell number and ^{3}H-DG uptake by SW620 cells treated with Dox

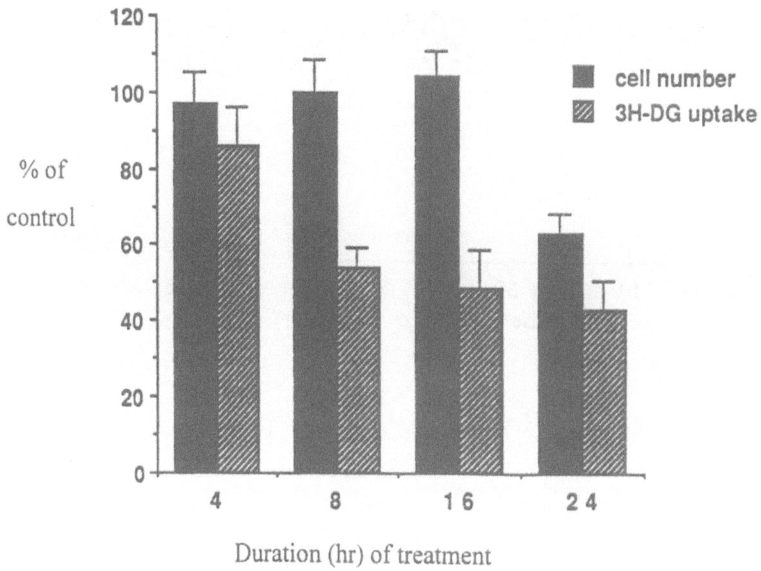

DISCUSSION

In the present study we have shown that the uptake of ^{3}H-DG by SW480 and SW620 colonic tumour cells correlates with Spf. The incorporation of DG into cells is dependent on its transport across the cell membrane and susequent phosphorylation by hexokinase (HK). Facilitative glucose transport is achieved by the protein products of a family of glucose transporter genes termed Glut1-5. Previous studies (9,10) have correlated hexokinase and Glut1 expression with proliferation. In a study of human breast tumours Younes et al found that Glut1 protein level correlated with the proliferative indicator, Ki67. Glut1 content and HK activity of rapidly growing clones of cultured C6 glioma cells (10) were found to be higher than in slower growing clones. Thus the association between proliferation and ^{3}H-DG uptake by SW480 and SW620 cells observed in the present study, may be a consequence of upregulation of Glut 1 and/or HK expression in the populations of cells with high proliferative fraction.

We have also shown that cells induced to apoptose take up less DG than untreated cells. Therapeutic agents including cisplatin (11) and radiotherapy (12) have been demonstrated to induce apoptosis. Previous works strongly suggests that tumour response to therapy is accompanied by decreased FDG uptake (2-4). The results of the present study suggest that decreased FDG uptake by responding tumours at least in some cases reflects the presence of apoptosising cells.

REFERENCES

1. Wienhouse S, The Warburg hypothesis fifty years later (guest editorial). Z Krebsforsch. 1976; 87:115-126

2. Hoekstra OS, Ossenkoppele GJ, Golding R. Early treatment response in malignant lymphoma, as determined by planar fluorine-18-fluorodeoxyglucose scintigraphy. J Nucl. Med 1993; 34:1706-1710

3. Mineura K, Yashuda T, Kowada M, et al. Positron emission tomograpic evaluation of radiochemotherapeutic effect of regional cerebral hemocirculation and metabolism in patients with gliomas. J Neuro Oncol 1987; 5:277-285

4. Wahl RL, Zasadny KR, Hutchins GD, Weber M, Cody R. Metabolic monitoring of breast cancer chemohormonotherapy using positron emission tomography (PET): initial evaluation. J Clin Oncol 1993; 11:2101-2111

5. Watanabe A, Tanaka R, Takeda N, Washiyama K. DNA synthesis, blood flow, and glucose utilization in experimental rat tumors. J Neurosurg. 1989; 70:86-91

6. Minn H, Joensuu H, Ahonen A, Klemi P. Fluorodeoxyglucose imaging:a method to assess the proliferative activity of human cancer in vivo. Cancer 1988; 61:1776-1781

7. Haberkorn U, Ziegler SI, Oberdorfer F. et al. FDG uptake, tumor proliferation and expression of glycolysis associated genes in animal tumor models. Nucl Med Biol 1994; 21:827-834

8. Brown RS, Leung JY, Fisher SJ, Frey KA, Ethier SP and Wahl RL. Intratumoral distribution of tritiated fluorodeoxyglucose in breast carcinoma: I, are inflammatory cells important? J Nucl Med 1995; 36:1854-1861

9. Younes M, Brown RW, Mody DR, Fernandez L and Laucirica R. Glut1 expression in human breast carcinoma: correlation with known prognostic markers. Anticancer Res. 1995; 15:2895-8

10. Nagamatsu S, Nakamichi Y, Inoue N, Inoue M, Nishino H and Sawa H. Rat C6 glioma cell growth is related to glucose transport and metabolism. Biochem. J. 1996; 319: 477-82

11. Eastman A. Activation of Programmed Cell Death by Anticancer agents: Cisplatin as a Model System. Cancer Cells 1990; 2:275-280

12. Blank KR, Rudoltz MS, Kao GD, Muschel RJ, Gillies McKenna W. The molecular regulation of apoptosis and implications for radiation oncology

CARDIOLOGY

Radioactive Isotopes in
Clinical Medicine and Research XXIII
ed. by H. Bergmann, H. Köhn and H. Sinzinger

RELATION BETWEEN VIABILITY, IMPROVEMENT OF LVEF AND HEART FAILURE SYMPTOMS AFTER REVASCULARIZATION.

J.J. Bax*, F.C. Visser**, G.W. Sloof**,
A. van Lingen**, P.M. Fioretti#,
J.H. Cornel## and C.A. Visser**.

From:

*: University Hospital Leiden, The Netherlands
**: Free University Hospital Amsterdam, The Netherlands
#: Istituto di Cardiologia, Udine, Italy
##: Medical Center Alkmaar, The Netherlands.

SUMMARY: In 32 patients undergoing revascularization, viability assessment by FDG SPECT was related to improvement in LVEF and heart failure (HF) symptoms (graded according to the NYHA criteria). In 18 patients with substantial viability, the LVEF improved from 27±8% to 34±9% ($P<0.05$) and the NYHA functional status improved from 2.9±0.3 to 1.5±0.7 ($P<0.01$). In 14 patients without viability, the LVEF (31±8% vs 31±8%, ns) and the NYHA status (2.6±0.5 vs 2.4±0.7, ns) remained unchanged. Hence, FDG SPECT can predict improvement in LVEF and HF symptoms after revascularization.

INTRODUCTION

Revascularization may lead to improved left ventricular (LV) function in patients with coronary artery disease if viable myocardium is present (1,2). Reversibility of *regional* dyssynergy after revascularization can be predicted with PET or SPECT in combination with F18-fluorodeoxyglucose (FDG) (3,4). From the clinical point of view, improvement of *global* LV function (ejection fraction, EF) may be more important, particularly in terms of prognosis. Also the quality of life, in terms of improvement of heart failure (HF) symptoms after revascularization, is important (5). In the current study, we have addressed the issues and determined whether viability testing by FDG SPECT before revascularization, can predict improvement of 1) LVEF and 2) HF symptoms after the revascularization.

MATERIALS AND METHODS

Patients. Thirty-two patients with depressed LV function secondary to chronic ischemic heart disease, scheduled for revascularization, were included (28 men, mean age 59±8 years). All patients had a previous myocardial infarction. They had a mean number of stenosed vessels of 2.7±0.6 and a mean LVEF of 28±6%.

SPECT studies. Each patient underwent early resting Tl-201 SPECT to evaluate regional perfusion, followed by FDG SPECT during hyperinsulinemic glucose clamp. The SPECT studies were performed with a dual head rotating gamma camera system (ADAC Laboratories, Milpitas, CA, USA), equipped with 511 keV collimators for the FDG study. Corresponding series of Tl-201 and FDG images (long- and short-axis) were displayed on a videoscreen. Circumferential profiles were obtained and displayed in a polar map. The polar maps were divided in 13 segments: 1 apical, 6 distal and 6 basal segments (anterior, anterolateral, inferolateral, inferior, inferoseptal and anteroseptal). The segmental activities were calculated and compared with normal reference values (6). Segments with a Tl-201 activity <2SD below the normal reference value were considered abnormal. Criteria for viability on SPECT were: 1) if the perfusion was normal, or 2) if the FDG uptake was relatively increased (6) in a perfusion defect (flow-metabolism mismatch). Segments with a perfusion defect and concordantly decreased FDG uptake (flow-metabolism match) were considered necrotic (6).

Regional LV function before/after revascularization. Regional wall motion was evaluated with 2D echo before and 3 months after revascularization. The left ventricle was divided into 13 segments, matching the SPECT segments. Each segment was assigned a wall motion score (WMS), ranging from 0: normal to 3: dyskinetic. Recovery was defined as improvement in WMS ≥ 1 grade after revascularization.

Global LV function before/after revascularization. Global LV function (LVEF) was assessed by radionuclide ventriculography/echocardiography before and 3 months after revascularization. The same technique was always used before and after revascularization. An improvement of of LVEF $\geq 5\%$ was considered significant (7).

Heart failure symptoms before and after revascularization. Clinical assessment of signs of heart failure was assessed by grading the functional status using the New York Heart Association (NYHA) criteria, before and 3 months after revascularization.

Statistical analysis. Results are expressed as mean$\pm$1 SD. Data were compared using the Student's t-test for (un-) paired data. A P-value < 0.05 was significant.

RESULTS

Adequate revascularization was obtained in 215 dysfunctional segments; 70 improved in function after the revascularization, 139 remained unchanged and 6 deteriorated. Fifteen dysfunctional segments had normal perfusion on Tl-201 SPECT, while 200 segments had a perfusion defect; 78 perfusion defects showed increased FDG uptake (mismatch pattern) and 122 had concordantly decreased FDG uptake (match pattern). Thus, according to the "viability criteria" on SPECT imaging, 93 segments were viable.

Sixteen (50%) patients demonstrated improvement of LVEF ($\geq 5\%$) after the revascularization. No significant differences between the 2 groups were noted, except for the number of viable segments on SPECT (Table 1).

In the patients (n=18) with ≥ 3 viable segments on SPECT, the LVEF improved significantly from $27\pm8\%$ to $34\pm9\%$ ($P<0.05$). In contrast, in the patients (n=14) with 2 or less viable segments on SPECT, the LVEF remained unchanged ($31\pm8\%$ versus $31\pm8\%$, ns). In the patients with ≥ 3 viable segments on SPECT, the mean NYHA status improved from 2.9 ± 0.3 to 1.5 ± 0.7 ($P<0.01$). In the remaining patients the NYHA functional status remained unchanged (2.6 ± 0.5 vs 2.4 ± 0.7, ns). Considering 3 or more viable segments on SPECT predictive for improvement of heart failure symptoms, SPECT had a positive predictive value of 87% and a negative predictive value of 70%.

Table 1. Patient characteristics (group I=with improvement of LVEF, group II=without improvement of LVEF).

	Group I (n=16)	Group II (n=16)	P-value
Age (yrs)	63±8	60±11	ns
Sex (M/F)	1/15	3/13	ns
Q wave MI	12	9	ns
HF (NYHA)	2.8±0.4	2.7±0.4	ns
VD	2.8±0.6	2.7±0.6	ns
LVEF	30±9%	28±7%	ns
Nr of viable segments on SPECT	4.8±2.1	1.6±1.5	<0.05
Nr of nonviable segments on SPECT	3.3±2.8	3.6±1.7	ns

DISCUSSION

From the present data it can be concluded that patients with substantial viability (in this study defined as ≥3 viable segments on SPECT) improve in LVEF and HF symptoms after revascularization. In contrast, the patients without viability do not improve in LVEF or HF symptoms. Patients with severely depressed LV function were included in this study; in these patients the improvement of LVEF renders the greatest benefit in terms of prognosis (8). Moreover, it appeared from the current data that an improvement of LVEF ≥5% is clinically important (an issue frequently discussed), since these patients do als o improve their functional status (graded according to the NYHA criteria).

Although it should be recognized that this classification is subjective, it is the most commonly used classification for the quality of life for patients with HF symptoms.

Over the past 5 years, FDG SPECT has developed as an accurate technique to assess viable myocardium. Prediction of improvement of *regional* LV function was demonstrated previously (4); the current data it appears that the technique is also capable to identify the patients who are likely to improve in *global* LV function and HF symptoms.

REFERENCES

1. Dilsizian V, Bonow RO. Current diagnostic techniques of assessing myocardial viability in patients with hibernating and stunned myocardium. *Circulation* 1993;87:1-20.

2. Vanoverschelde JLJ, Wijns W, Borgers M, Heyndrickx G, Depre C, Flameng W, Melin JA. Chronic myocardial hibernation in humans. From bedside to bench. *Circulation* 1997;95:1961-1971.

3. Tillisch J, Brunken R, Marshall R et al. Reversibility of cardiac wall motion abnormalities predicted by positron tomography. *N Engl J Med* 1986;314:884-888.

4. Bax JJ, Cornel JH, Visser FC et al. Prediction of recovery of myocardial dysfunction after revascularization. Comparison of fluorine-18 fluorodeoxyglucose/thallium-201 SPECT, thallium-201 stress-reinjection SPECT and dobutamine echocardiography. *J Am Coll Cardiol* 1996;28:558-565.

5. Bonow RO. Identification of viable myocardium. *Circulation* 1996;94:2674-2680.

6. Bax JJ, Visser FC, Blanksma PK et al. Comparison of myocardial uptake of F18-fluorodeoxyglucose imaged with positron emission tomography and single photon emission computed tomography. *J Nucl Med* 1996;37:1631-1636.

7. Vom Dahl J, Eitzman DT, Al-Aouar ZR et al. Relation of regional function, perfusion and metabolism in patients with advanced coronary artery disease undergoing surgical revascularization. *Circulation* 1994;90:2356-2366.

8. The Multicenter Postinfarction Research Group. Risk stratification and survival after myocardial infarction. *N Eng J Med* 1983;309:331-336.

Radioactive Isotopes in
Clinical Medicine and Research XXIII
ed. by H. Bergmann, H. Köhn and H. Sinzinger

ATTENUATION CORRECTED Tl-201 SPECT USING A Gd-153 MOVING LINE SOURCE: CLINICAL VALUE AND THE IMPACT OF ATTENUATION CORRECTION ON THE EXTENT AND SEVERITY OF PERFUSION ABNORMALITIES

Hans Jürgen Gallowitsch[1], Josef Sykora[2], Oliver Unterweger[1], Peter Mikosch[1], Ewald Kresnik[1], Georg Grimm[2], Peter Lind[1]

[1]Department of Nuclear Medicine and Special Endocrinology, [2]Department of Cardiology, Landeskrankenhaus Klagenfurt, Austria

SUMMARY: The aim of the study was to test the clinical value and the impact of attenuation-corrected Tl-201 SPECT (AC), using a moving Gd-153 line source, on the extent and severity of perfusion abnormalities in a clinical setup of patients planned to undergo coronary angiography because of clinically suspected coronary artery disease. 107 patients, planned to undergo coronary angiography, were included in our study. In each patient, AC and NC (non-corrected)- Tl-201 SPECT was performed. AC and NC were evaluated visually as well as by a 31-segment-semiquantitative analysis and correlated with angiographic results. Patients were assigned to two different groups: group A with angina and no previous cardiac infarction or intervention (Specificity NC 68.7 %, AC 83.9 %) and group B with known CAD because of previous myocardial infarction or intervention (Specificity NC 91.3 %, AC 100 %). The extent and the severity of perfusion abnormalities were significantly influenced using AC by demonstrating significantly less abnormal and less severe abnormal segments in the segmental analysis compared to NC, especially for the vascular territory of the LAD and RCA.

INTRODUCTION

Myocardial perfusion scintigraphy with Tl-201 is a widespread method to gain information about impaired perfusion either in clinically suspected or known coronary artery disease (CAD). While the method exhibits sufficient sensitivity, it lacks in specificity because of attenuation artefacts in the anterior or posterior wall caused by the eccentric cardiac position in the thorax. With nonhomogenous, patient specific attenuation correction, using transmission computerised tomography (TCT), several authors reported a improved homogeneity of myocardial tracer distribution in patients with low risk of CAD and a significant increase in specificity, especially in the posterior, posterolateral and posteroseptal wall (1-5).

Apart from evaluating the specificity and sensitivity of attenuation-corrected Tl-201 SPECT with a moving line source, we also wanted to examine whether AC has an impact on the extent and severity of perfusion abnormalities and to compare the results with angiographic data.

MATERIALS AND METHODS:

PATIENTS: 107 consecutive patients (69 males, 38 females; mean age 63.8 ± 9.5, range 33-77 yr.), planned to undergo coronary angiography because of suspected CAD were included in our study. Only patients with left bundle branch block (LBBB) were excluded.

The patients were assigned to two different groups: Group A (n = 49) with chest pain and no history of cardiac infarction or intervention and group B (n = 58) with known CAD, 42 of them had previous myocardial infarction, 30 of them had a previous cardiac intervention (22 PTCA and 8 CABG), 17 both intervention and infarction.

In all patients, simultaneous attenuation - corrected (AC) and non - corrected (NC) Tl-201 stress / redistribution SPECT were performed. Coronary angiography was carried out consecutively in each patient within a time interval of 1-14 days.

ATTENUATION CORRECTED/NON CORRECTED Tl-201 SPECT: Tl-201 SPECT stress imaging was started approximately 5 min after injection of 111 MBq Tl-201 given at the peak workload after symptom - limited maximal treadmill exercise according to the Bruce-protocol (68 pts) or pharmacological stimulation with Dipyridamol (39 pts). Redistribution images were acquired approximately 180 min after Tl-201 injection. The acquisition was performed in a step-and-shoot mode over 180 degrees (6 ° angle steps, 35 sec/step). Emission and transmission data were acquired simultaneously using a biplane high-resolution gamma camera (Apex SP-X Cardia-L, Elscint®) with a moving Gd-153 line source (Transact®, Elscint, Haifa) using three different energy windows and a low - energy - all -purpose (LEAP) parallel - hole collimator.(6,7).

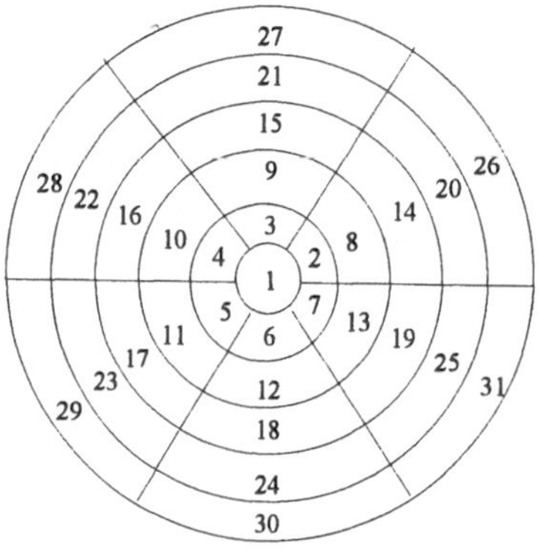

Figure 1

INTERPRETATION: NC and AC slice reports were qualitatively interpreted by two independent interpreters for positivity (+ , -) and reversibility on the redistribution images.

Additionally, a semiquantitative analysis was performed using polar maps for NC- and AC stress and redistribution short axis and vertical long axis (apex) slices and circumferential count profiles (Fig.1). Mean count rates / pixel were evaluated for 31 segments, normalised on the maximum and the percentage of maximal count rate was calculated for each segment (mean Cts/ pixel / max. in %) (Fig.1). Segmental perfusion abnormalities were classified as mild to moderate perfusion defect (50-75% of maximal counts - $PD_{50\text{-}75}$), severe segmental perfusion defect (25-50% - $PD_{25\text{-}50}$) and complete segmental perfusion defect (0-25% - $PD_{<25}$). The extent of ischemia was determined by the number of affected segments in comparison to the total number of segments (segments/31 *100). The data of visual and semiquantitative analysis were compared with the digitally evaluated angiographic data using a degree of 70 % stenosis as a cut-off level of significance. Data were expressed as mean ± SD. The Student's t-test for paired samples ($p<0.05$) was used to determine the differences in intrasegmental relative count density rates between NC and AC studies and between the mean number of segments with impaired perfusion, $PD_{50\text{-}75}$, $PD_{25\text{-}50}$ and $PD_{<25}$. Mc Nemar's test was used to determine the differences in paired data samples. Fig.1. Segmental polar-map analysis

RESULTS:

VISUAL ANALYSIS: The results for the visual *Overall analysis, the subgroup analysis of group A and B, male and female patients and bicycle vs. dipyridamole examination are shown in table 1.*

		true +	true	false +	false -	sensitivity	specificity
Total	NC	42	43	11	11	79.2	79.6
n = 107	AC	50	49	5	3	94.3	90.7
Group A	NC	16	22	10	1	88.9	68.7
n = 49	AC	17	26	5	1	94.4	83.9
Group B	NC	26	21	2	9	74.3	91.3
n = 58	AC	33	23	0	2	94.3	100
male	NC	31	25	8	5	86.1	75.8
n=69	AC	34	30	3	2	94.4	90.9
female	NC	11	18	3	6	64.7	85.7
n=38	AC	16	19	2	1	94.1	90.5
bicycle	NC	30	22	10	6	83.3	68.8
n=68	AC	35	28	4	1	97.2	87.5
dipyridamole	NC	12	21	1	5	70.6	95.4
n=39	AC	15	21	1	2	88.2	95.4

Tab. 1 Visual analysis NC = non corrected, AC = attenuation corrected

SEGMENTAL ANALYSIS: *Differences in count rate densities.* 3317 segments were evaluated by semiquantitative analysis for both NC and AC studies. NC demonstrated significantly lower relative count densities than AC in the posterior (segment 6,12,18,24,30), posterolateral (segment 7,13,19,25,31), posteroseptal (segment 5,11,17,23,29), anteroseptal (segment 4,10,16,22,28) and basal anterior wall (segment 27) and higher densities in the anterolateral (segment 8,14,20) and apex near anterior segments (segment 3, 9) ($p<0.05$). No significant differences were seen in segments 1,2, 15, 21,26 (Fig. 2).

Overall analysis of pathological segments. Semiquantitative analysis detected a total of 1494 segments (45 % of all evaluated segments) with impaired perfusion (<75 %/Max) with NC and 1171 segments with AC (35.3 %)($p<0.05$). NC showed significantly more segments with impaired perfusion (<75%/max) than AC in the posterolateral (13,19, 25, 31), posterior (12, 18,24,30); and septal wall (10, 11, 16, 17, 22, 23, 28, 29) and the basal anterior segment (27) (p=<0.05). In the anterolateral (2,8,14,20,26) and anterior wall (3,9,15,21), there were no significant differences in number of segments with impaired perfusion <75 % despite lower count rate densities with AC in several segments. This could also be demonstrated for the apex (segment 1). The results for the extent and severity of segmental hypoperfusion of the *Overall analysis* and the *Subgroup analysis for group A and B* are shown in table 2.

total	NC	mean segments	AC	mean segments	p
TOTAL	1494	13.9 ± 6.85	1171	10.9 ± 6.6	0.000
PD_{50-75}	1190	11.1 ± 4.9	1001	9.35 ± 4.8	0.001
PD_{25-50}	283	2.6 ± 4.2	150	1.4 ± 3.1	0.000
$PD_{<25}$	20	0.2 ± 0.7	20	0.19 ± 0.7	n.s.
Group A					
TOTAL	593	12.1 ± 7.3	474	9.7 ± 6.6	0.001
PD_{50-75}	490	10 ± 5.1	432	8.8 ± 5.3	n.s.
PD_{25-50}	96	2 ± 4.3	36	0.7 ± 2.0	0.001
$PD_{<25}$	5	0.1 ± 0.4	6	0.1 ± 0.5	n.s.
Group B					
TOTAL	901	15.5 ± 6.0	697	12.0 ± 6.5	0.000
PD_{50-75}	700	12.1 ± 4.7	569	9.8 ± 4.3	0.002
PD_{25-50}	185	3.2 ± 4.2	114	2.0 ± 3.8	0.000
$PD_{<25}$	5	0.3 ± 0.9	14	0.2 ± 0.8	n.s.

Tab.2 Segmental analysis NC = non corrected, AC = attenuation corrected, PD_{50-75} = mild to moderate segmental perfusion defect (50 - 75 %/ max), PD_{25-50} = severe segmental perfusion defect (25 - 50 % /max), $PD_{<25}$ = complete segmental perfusion defect (< 25 %/max)

SUBGROUP ANALYSIS FOR VASCULAR TERRITORIES: *LAD.* Only segments 1, 3, 4, 9, 10, 15, 16, 21, 22, 22, 27, 28 were included in this analysis: A total number of segments with impared perfusion <75 % were found in 505 segments with NC and 325 with AC. PD_{50-75} were found in 401 (NC) and 271 (AC) segments, respectively, PD_{25-50} in 90 (NC) and 41 (AC) segments and $PD_{<25}$ in 14 (NC) and 13 (AC) segments. The mean number of affected segments in the vascular territory of the LAD was 4.7 ± 3.9 (NC) and 3.0 ± 3.3 (AC) segments ($p<0.05$). The relation between PD_{50-75} and PD_{25-50} was 4.4 (NC) and 6.6 (AC), respectively.

LCX. Segments 2, 8, 14, 20, 26 were included in this analysis. Segments 7, 13, 19, 25, 31 were only included in case of a dominant left coronary artery: 385 (NC) and 387 (AC) segments with impaired perfusion < 75 %/max were totally seen. PD_{50-75} were found in 305 (NC) and 331 (AC) segments, respectively, and PD_{25-50} in 80 (NC) and 56 (AC) segments. No $PD_{<25}$ were seen with both methods. The mean number of affected segments in this vascular territory was 3.6 ± 2.5 (NC) and 3.6 ± 2.5 (AC) (n.s). The relation between PD_{50-75} and PD_{25-50} was 3.8 in case of NC and 5.9 in case of AC.

RCA. Segments 5, 6, 11, 12, 17, 18, 23, 24, 29, 29, 30 were included in this subanalysis. Segments 7, 13, 19, 25, 31 were only included in case of a dominant right coronary artery: A total of 604 (NC) and 459 (AC) segments with impaired perfusion could be found. PD_{50-75} were found in 484 (NC) and 399 (AC) segments, PD_{25-50} in 113 (NC) and 53 (AC) and $PD_{<25}$ in 7 (NC) and 7 (AC) segments. The mean number of affected segments was 5.6 ± 2.5 in case of NC and 4.3 ± 2.5 in case of AC ($p<0.05$). The relation between PD_{50-75} and PD_{25-50} was 4.3 in case of NC and 7.5 in case of AC.

DISCUSSION:

As previously reported with Tc-99m Sestamibi and an Am-241 line source, Tc-99m tetrofosmin and a Gd-153 or Tl-201 and a Tc-99m line source, we observed a significant increase in sensitivity and specificity using TCT also in our study with Tl-201 SPECT using a moving Gd-153 line source (3-5).

Comparing male and female patients, attenuation correction seems to influence specificity more in male than female patients with an increase in specificity of 15.1 % in male vs. 4.8 % in female patients, whereby the differences in specificity are more pronounced in group A patients.

Comparing the data after ergometric and pharmacological stress we found no significant increase in specificity in the smaller group stressed by dipyridamole whereas in case of bicycle workload an increase in specificity of 18.7 % could be observed. Concerning sensitivity, both methods showed comparable increases by using AC with 17.6 % (dipyridamole) and 13.9 % (bicycle), respectively.

In our study using a moving Gd-153 line source, and an 31-segment analysis, the total number of affected segments and the number of PD_{50-75} and PD_{25-50} was significantly higher with NC compared to AC. Additionally to the previously reported effect on the posterior wall, we observed a significant decrease in the extent of ischemia in the posteroseptal, posterolateral and anteroseptal segments while the extent of anterolateral and apex near anterior wall defects appeared to be unchanged with AC. The decrease in count density in the anterolateral and apex-near anterior wall had no impact on the extent of ischemia in this region.

Additionally to the extent of perfusion abnormalities, also the scintigraphic aspect of the severity of ischemia seems to be influenced by attenuation correction (1,5). Whereas the relation between the segments with 50-75% (PD_{50-75}) and 25-75 % (PD_{25-50}) of maximal perfusion was 4.2 in case of NC, it significantly increased to 6.7 in case of AC when including both groups. This points out that the severity of perfusion abnormalities is usually overestimated in the posterior and septal wall without attenuation correction. Concerning vascular territories, both the extent and severity of perfusion abnormalities seemed to be influenced significantly by AC for the LAD and RCA. For the left circumflex artery (LCX), significance could only be demonstrated for the posterolateral segments but not for the whole vascular territory.

REFERENCES:

1. Ficaro EP, Fessler JA, Ackermann RJ; Rogers WL, Corbett JR, Schwaiger M. Simultaneous transmission-emission thallium-201 cardiac SPECT: effect of attenuation correction on myocardial tracer distribution. J Nucl Med 1995; 36 (6): 921-31
2. Prvulovich EM, Lonn AHR, Bomanji JB, Jarritt PH, Ell PJ. Effect of attenuation correction on myocardial thallium - 201 distribution in patients with a low likelihood of coronary artery disease. Eur J Nucl Med 1997; 24: 266-75
3. Ficaro EP, Fessler JA, Shreve $PD_{<25}$ et al. Simultaneous transmission/emission myocardial perfusion tomography. Diagnostic accuracy of attenuation-corrected Tc-99m Sestamibi SPECT. Circulation 1996;93:463-473
4. Kluge R, Seese A, Sattler B, Knapp WH. Non-uniform attenuation correction for myocardial SPECT using two Gd-153 line sources. Nuklearmedizin 1996; 35(6): 201-11
5. Knesewitsch P, Walser R, Kantlehner R, Munzing W, Hahn K. Tl-201 myocardial SPECT. First experiences with a simultaneous transmission-emission acquisition protocol for patient-specific attenuated correction. Nuklearmedizin 1996; 35 (3): 78-85
6. Tan P, Bailey D, Meikle S et al. A scanning line source for simultaneous emission and transmission measurements in SPECT. J Nucl Med 1993; 34:1752-1760
7. TRANSACT® Operation Manual. 1996. Elscint LTD, Technical Writing Department, Haifa, Israel

Radioactive Isotopes in
Clinical Medicine and Research XXIII
ed. by H. Bergmann, H. Köhn and H. Sinzinger

CORRELATION OF EBCT AND TL-201-SPECT SCINTIGRAPHY IN PATIENTS WITH CORONARY HEART DISEASE

Aigner R.M., Kern R., Rienmüller R., Fueger G.F. and Nicoletti R.
Karl-Franzens-University of Graz, Dept. of Radiology, Graz, Austria

SUMMARY

The aim of the study was to compare the findings of EBCT with those of Tl-201-scintigraphy. 12 patients with CAD were investigated. The 14 fixed Tl-defects were associated with coronary artery stenosis of more than 50% in 5 cases, with atherosclerotic plaques in 2 cases. The 7 non-persisting defects were associated with coronary artery stenosis of more than 50% in 3 cases, with irregularities of the arterial wall in 3 cases, and with atherosclerotic plaques in 2 cases. Contractility and athrophy as seen on EBCT did not correlate with typical findings on scintigraphy. The preliminary data show that EBCT and Tl-scintigraphy do not replace but complement each other.

INTRODUCTION

The objective diagnosis of coronary heart disease (CAD) is based on coronary catheterization and angiography. Regional myocardial perfusion, however, is considered one of the most important functional diagnostic parameters of the heart. Its direct measurement (e.g.by Xe-133 wash-out) requires invasive catheterization and permits little regional differentiation beyond the left and right coronary arteries. Various indirect diagnostic modalities are used to determine the effects of coronary blood flow and myocardial perfusion. These are myocardial stress/rest scintigraphy (SPECT and PET), stress echocardiography and, as a newer technique, electron-beam-computed-tomography (EBCT, ultrafast computed tomography). The aim of this study was to compare the findings of EBCT with those of myocardial scintigraphy with 201-thallium-chloride (Tl-201).

MATERIALS AND METHODS

Twelve consecutive patients, 6 female, 6 male, aged between 46 and 74 years were investigated, eleven had proven coronary heart disease, one was suspected, but turned out normal. The study protocol consisted of clinical investigation, laboratory values, spiroergometry, echocardiography, Tl-201-SPECT stress/rest scintigraphy, EBCT and coronary angiography. EBCT: For acquisition, electron beam computed tomography equipment was used (CT-Evolution, Siemens, Erlangen, Germany, Imatron Inc, San Francisco, CA). A preview scan of the chest was obtained in order to localize the area of the sinus valsalvae of the aorta for further planning of the examination. Native scan for coronary calcification was obtained using the single slice mode (SSM) with 1.5 mm slice thickness, 100 ms exposure time at 130 kV and 630 mA, and ECG gating at 80% of the R-R-interval in suspended inspiration. In this mode, 40 adjacent slices were performed (40 seconds duration at a heart rate of 60/min). The measurement of contrast medium transit time was done after the native scan. The left ventricular myocardial perfusion was assessed using the short axis view. This position was obtained by moving the table 25 degrees to the patient's right and 15 degrees caudally. To determine the position of the left ventricle, a localization scan was obtained in multi-slice mode using all 4 target-rings, thus obtaining 8 tomographic levels over 68 mm (each tomographic level having a slice thickness of 7 mm, with an interslice gap of 4 mm between each two adjacent tomographic levels). In the short axis position, using the multi slice flow mode with 3 target-rings and after administration of 50 ml of contrast medium intravenously with a flow of 3 ml/second six tomographic levels were imaged. Each tomographic level was obtained 13 times at 80% of the R-R-interval at each 2 or 3 heart beat (ECG-gated). The left ventricular myocardial contrast enhancement was measured by drawing manually the outline of the left ventricular myocardium using time-density-software of the Imatron^{R} workstation.Using the slope method on EBCT it was possible to access the distal coronary perfusion in ml/100g/min. The results are expressed as the maximum slope of enhancement of the myocardium divided by the difference of the precontrast and peak CT-value in the left ventricle. The global myocardial perfusion was calculated as a mean of all evaluated tomographic levels. Myocardial scintigraphy (Tl-201): After an overnight fast, all patients underwent symptom-limited bicycle exercise testing according to a standardized multistage protocol with continuous monitoring of heart rate and rhythm, blood pressure and symptoms. Exercise was begun at 25 W and increased each 2 min in 25 W increments. 111 MBq (3 mCi) of Tl-201 were injected at peak exercise, the patients were encouraged to exercise for one further minute to maintain stress while the tracer was taken up by the myocardium. Within 5-10 min of Tl-201 injection, ECG triggered acquisition of tomographic images was started using a rotating triple-head scintillation camera (Picker^{R}, Prism 3000), equipped with a general purpose collimator and connected to a dedicated computer system (Odyssee). Patients were ambulatory and continued fasting during the interval between stress and rest images. For interpreting the left ventricular myocardium was divided in the usual standardized segments: septum, anterior wall, apex, inferior wall and posterolateral wall.

RESULTS

Scintigraphy: A total of 14 segments with localized, fixed thallium defects was seen in 8 patients, a total of 7 segments with non-persisting defects was seen in 5 patients, a total of 7 segments with reverse redistribution was seen in 6 patients. The regional distribution of these segments is given in table 1. Myocardial scintigraphy was normal in 1 patient.

Table 1: A = anterior wall, P = posterolateral wall, I = inferior wall, F = free wall, S = septal Wall, X = apex wall, N = non-persisting defect, F = fixed defect, R = reverse redistribution, H = focal hypertrophy, S = stenosis, I = irregularities

Comparison of scintigraphy and EBCT

Id.Code	Sex	Age	scintigraphy	EBCT
AUE	F	66	AF, XF	$LAD_{s>50}$, RCA_{I}, LCX_{I} thrombus apex
BEN	M	57	ASF, IN, SR	$LAD_{s>50}$, $LCX_{s>50}$
BEK	M	67	XF, SN	$LAD_{s>50}$, $LCX_{s>50}$
BOE	M	46	SR	$LAD_{s>50}$
BUC	F	74	XF, ASN, PH	$LAD_{s>50}$, $RCA_{s<50}$ dilation
DIS	M	61	IF, PF, SR	plaques
FRE	M	41	SN, ASR, PR	LAD_{I}
GRA	F	70	AF, IN, PR	LAD_{I}, -plaques dilation
MEI	F	47	SF, ASF, IF, PH	LCA-plaques
HUS	M	54	AF, ASF, IF	plaques
HOD	F	47	PH	-
OBE	F	47	IN, SN, XR, APR	LAD_{I}, LCX_{I}, RCA_{I}

EBCT: Stenosis of more than 50% of the LAD was seen in 5 patients; this finding was associated with further findings as follows: (a) stenosis of more than 50% of the LCX in 2 patients, (b) stenosis of less than 50% of the RCA and dilatation of the left ventricle in 1 patient, irregularities of the RCA and the LCX and (d) a thrombotic plaque in the apex in 1 patient. Atherosclerotic plaques of the LAD in 1 patient, and of the RCA in 1 patient. Irregularities of the LAD, the LCX and of the RCA were observed in 1 patient. EBCT was normal in 1 patient, the same who had the normal thallium study. Localized reduced wall thickness was observed in 4 patients. Reduced ability in localized wall thickness changing during end systole and end diastole was observed in 5 patients.

Comparison of scintigraphy and EBCT (see table 1): The 14 persisting thallium defects were associated with coronary artery stenosis of more than 50% in 5 patients (LAD stenosis in 5 patients, and additionally the LCX in 2 patients). In 2 further patients the fixed defects were combined with atherosclerotic plaques of the LAD. The 7 non-persisting defects were associated with coronary stenosis of more than 50% in 3 patients. In 3 further patients the non-persisting defects were combined with irregularities of the arterial wall, and in 2 patients with atherosclerotic plaques. Impairment of contractility and atrophy, as seen on EBCT, did not correlate with any characteristic findings on scintigraphy.

Figure 1: Thrombus at the apex of the left ventricle. Id. Code Aue, female, 65 years

a: Thallium scintigraphy - fixed defect at the anterior wall and the apex

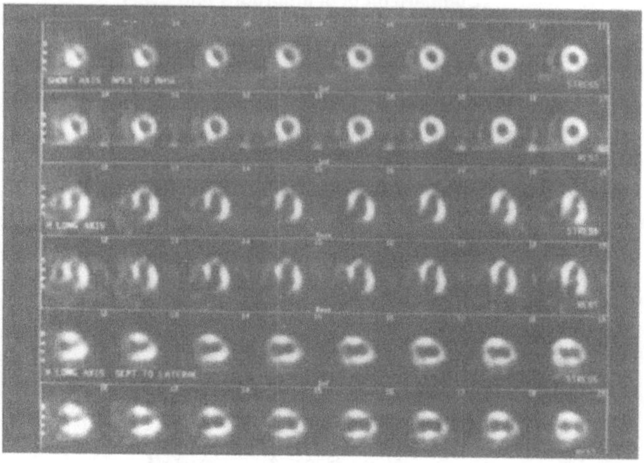

b: On EBCT study localized thinness of the anteroseptal, apical and posterolateral segment of the left ventricular myocardium

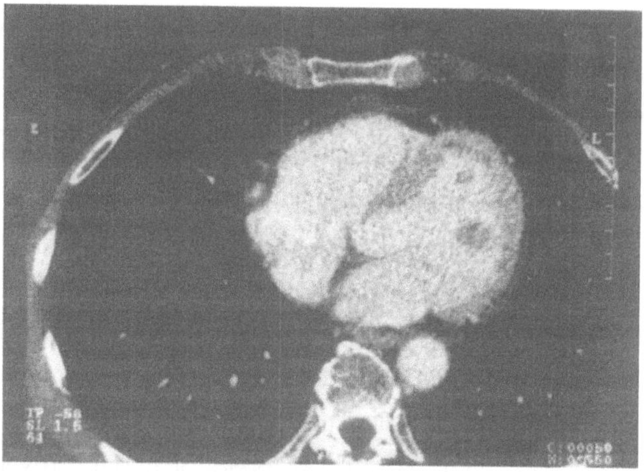

DISCUSSION

Myocardial competence resides in muscular strength and endurance. Myocardial atrophy and fibrotic degeneration weaken systole and stroke volume. The effects of coronary stenosis or occlusion on myocardial competence are judged clinically and by pharmacologic or bicycle ergometry. The objective diagnosis of coronary heart disease relies most strongly on vascular integrity as seen by angiography, and secondly on identification of vascular calcifications. Anatomical thickness, not necessarily integrity, of the myocardium is best seen by electron-beam-computed-tomography (EBCT), but not by angiography (1). Regional myocardial quality (muscular, fibrotic, membranous) and viability is demonstrated best by thallium-scintigraphy. Regional perfusion may be measured reliably by Xenon-133, but requires catheterization, and is therefore undesirable. Correlating the results of EBCT and thallium scintigraphy we investigated whether EBCT can predict the results of thallium scintigraphy. Tl-201 stress/rest scintigraphy (planar or SPECT, triggered or untriggered) is a widely used diagnostic modality for assessing myocardial perfusion and viability. It is non-invasive and cost effective, and is therefore regarded as a useful gate keeper study prior to coronary angiography. The uptake of thallium into the myocardium is determined by regional blood flow, concentration of the tracer in the plasma, and of cell membrane integrity. Using both early and delayed thallium images, („Tl-redistribution") the differentiation between non-persisting (ischemic) and persisting (fixed) defects („infarcted myocardium") is possible. But the definite diagnosis of viable or necrotic myocardium (as well as the etiology of the pathological findigns) still remains uncertain, even with late delayed images (8-72 hours post injection), or in combination with diverse forms of quantification. Thallium scintigraphy allows to stratify patients with CAD in recognizing the myocardial consequences of the disease (2,3,4). EBCT has limited availability. It yields tomographic images of the heart, of focal coronary artery calcifications, precise measurements of wall thickness and changes in wall thickness between diastole and systole. It has been proposed to use non-invasive EBCT as a sole method to diagnose CAD, especially (if available) to replace scintigraphy and angiography. So far, EBCT and thallium scintigraphy were compared only in a small number studies whereby most of the investigations were performed with the ultrafast CT scanner designed by Boyd and associates (5). Typical findings of EBCT in CAD are coronary artery stenosis, its percentage of luminal constriction (more or less than 50%), calcifications, irregularities of the wall or tortuosity of the coronary arteries and their branches. In our study group we found no predictable association of the EBCT findings with the findings of Tl-scintigraphy. (6,7,8,9,10). Stenosis of more than 50% of the LAD on EBCT was associated with normal Tl-findings, with non-persisting Tl-defects, or persisting Tl-defects or reverse redistribution within this area of distribution. One further important oberservation was that localized thinness of the myocardium on the EBCT studies was not always associated with defects, neither fixed, nor non-persisting. Therefore EBCT and Tl-scintigraphy evidently can not replace each other but may complement each other. The two imaging techniques are based on different tissue qualities. It was not possible to correlate objectively the results of EBCT and Tl-studies. Tl-scintigraphy provides a simple, non-invasive and economical method for the functional evaluation. Its information can readily be combined with the anatomic parameters as demonstrated by EBCT. Additional studies are necessary to determine if a normal thallium study should be followed by EBCT, and if a negative EBCT investigation should be followed by thallium scintigraphy. One further question is, where both diagnostic modalities are available, what method of investigation should be the primary screening method. Although EBCT is technically advanced, the investigations are expensive, it is not widely available and it requires application or potentially harmful iodinated contrast media. Nowadays the evaluation of myocardial perfusion at rest and after physical exercise or after pharmacologic provocation continous to represent the state of the art in imaging the assessment of ischemic heart disease; whenever difficulties exist in the evaluation of the difference between the stress and rest states, particularly in the quantification of the perfusion reserve upon stimulation.

RESULTS

1. Judkins MP. Selective coronary arteriography: a percutaneous transfermoral technique. Radiology 1967; 815-824
2. Dilsizian V, Rocco TP, Freeman NM et al. Enhanced detection of ischemic but viable myocardium by reinjection of thallium after stress-redistribution imaging. N Engl J Med 1990; 323:141-146
3. Altehoefer C, von Dahl J, Büll U, Uebis R, Kleinhans E, Hanrath P. Comparison of thallium-201 single-photon emission tomography after rest injection and fluoro-deoxyglucose positron emission tomography for assessment of myocardial viability in patients with chronic coronary artery disease. Eur J Nucl Med 1994; 21:37-45
4. Pohost GM, Henzlova MJ. The value of thallium-201 imaging. N Engl J Med 1990; July19,190-192
5. Boyd DB. Computerized transmission tomography of the heart using scanning electron beams. In Higgins C.H.(ed): Computed tomography of the heart and the great vessels, Futura Publishing, New York, 1983,45
6. Rienmüller R, Baumgartner C, Kern R, Harb S, Aigner RM, Fueger G, Weihs W. Quantitative Bestimmung der linksventrikulären Myokardperfusion mittels EBCT. Herz 1997; 22:63-71
7. Agatson AS, Janowitz WR, Hildner FJ, Zusmer NR, Viamonte M, Detrano R. Quantification of coronary artery calcium using ultrafast computed tomography. J Amer Coll Cardiol 1990; 15:827-832
8. Canty J. Measurement of myocardial perfusion by fast computed tomography. Amer J Cardiol 1993; 309-316
9. Georgiou D, Wolfkiel C, Brundage BH. Ultrafast computed tomography for the physiological evaluation of myocardial perfusion. Amer J Cardiol 1994; 151-158
10. Wolfkeil CJ, Brundage BH. Measurement of myocardial blood flow by UFCT: towards clinical applicability. Int J Cardiol 1991; 89-100

Radioactive Isotopes in
Clinical Medicine and Research XXIII
ed. by H. Bergmann, H. Köhn and H. Sinzinger

INFLUENCE OF RIGHT VENTRICULAR STIMULATION SITE ON LEFT VENTRICULAR FUNCTION IN ATRIAL SYNCHRONOUS PACING

C. Alexander[1], B. Schwaab[2], G. Fröhlig[2], D. Hellwig[1], J.B. Bader[1],
H. Schieffer[2], C.-M. Kirsch[1]

Department of Nuclear Medicine[1] and Cardiology[2], Saarland University Medical Center;
D-66421 Homburg; Germany

SUMMARY: In 14 patients with 3rd degree AV block, one pacing lead was implanted in the right ventricular apex, the septal electrode was attached to that site exhibiting the smallest QRS complex. During atrial synchronous ventricular pacing, AV delay was optimized individually for each stimulation site. Phase distribution of left ventricular contraction and systolic function were randomly determined for each pacing site by radionuclide ventriculography. Decreased QRS duration was correlated with less dyssynergy of contraction and with an increase in systolic function. In atrial syncronous pacing, this can be obtained if the pacing site is optimized by surface ECG guidance and the AV delay is adapted individually.

INTRODUCTION

It is well known that ectopic artificial stimulation of the heart results in asynchronous, prolonged contraction with lower dP/dt and a reduced pressure maximum (1, 2). In animal studies alternate pacing sites yielded inconsistent results. Pacing the right ventricular outflow tract, the right ventricular septum or the bundle of His increased systemic arterial blood pressure, peak left ventricular pressure, dP/dt and cardiac output, it normalized the biventricular activation and contraction patterns and it illustrated normal cellular morphology as compared with right ventricular apical, inflow tract or epicardial free wall pacing. However, other investigators did not find any significant differences with regard to left ventricular function or blood pressure between these stimulation sites in animals. In man literature reports a significant increase in left ventricular function by right ventricular septal or outflow tract pacing as compared with apical single chamber pacing. Other work deny such a favorable outcome.

In this study, we defined alternate pacing functionally looking for that particular right ventricular stimulation site that provides for the shortest surface QRS duration possible. The AV interval was also optimized individually and separately for septal and apical stimulation because an adequate AV delay is essential for left ventricular function during atrial synchronous pacing. The aim of this prospective study was: 1. To test whether right ventricular implantation using this technique is feasible by means of commercially available pacing leads. 2. To investigate the correlation between surface QRS duration and left ventricular function if this implantation technique is used and the AV delay is optimized.

MATERIALS AND METHODS

Fourteen consecutive patients , 6 men, 8 female, mean age 71 ± 8 years (range 63-87 years) were included. All were in sinus rhythm and were paced with a DDD system for third degree AV block.

Implantation: All atrial leads were attached to the right atrial lateral wall. During replacement of an exhausted pulse generator, patients had the ventricular lead implanted in the right ventricular apex and received the temporary pacing lead in septal position. During a new implantation, the temporary pacing lead was implanted conventionally in apical position before the permanent electrode was attached to the septum.

QRS duration: During operation, surface ECG was recorded. In order to determine the spatial conduction of the electrocardiogram the orthogonal leads of Frank were used. QRS duration was measured from the earliest to the latest deflection of the QRS complex in any of the Frank leads. The difference in QRS duration between septal and apical stimulation (d xyz) was calculated.

Instrumentation: Communication between the permanently implanted pacing system and the temporary ventricular pacing lead was maintained by means of an external DDD pacemaker. The internal pacemaker was programmed to AAT in order to be triggered by intrinsic P waves. The external device was programmed in the DDD mode with the pacing rate well below the intrinsic atrial rate. Atrial sensitivity of the external device was programmed to insure the proper detection of atrially triggered spikes of the internal pacemaker by means of skin electrodes, thus providing for atrial synchronous ventricular pacing.

Optimization of AV delay: The optimum AV delay during atrial synchronous ventricular pacing was determined by maximizing left ventricular stroke volume equivalents using impedance cardiography or using pulsed Doppler echocardiography of the transmitral blood flow. Optimization was performed in every patient and for each stimulation site.

Radionuclide ventriculography: Red blood cell labelling was performed in vivo with 800 MBq Tc-99m. For scintigraphy a small-field-of-view gamma camera (APEX 210M, Elscint, Haifa, Israel) was used. An ECG-triggered, gated scintigraphy of the left ventricle was performed from the left anterior oblique (45°) view. Sixty-four frames per cardiac cycle were acquired in phase mode and a 32x32 pixel matrix. Total counts acquired was 6 million. Measurements were taken randomly 15 minutes after programming.

For evaluation, a master left ventricular region of interest (ROI) was created after standardized background subtraction. This Master ROI was held constant for the processing of all intraindividual studies acquired. It was used to define the working area for an atomatic edge detection creating the ROI on each frame. After generation of the time activity curve, global ejection fraction (EF) and absolute ejected counts (EC) were calculated. Data were corrected for physical decay. Amplitude and phase images were generated by Fourier analysis and a phase distribution histogram was documented. The area unter the curve (AUC) of the left ventricular peak in phase distribution histogram was calculated as were the relative differences between septal and apical right ventricular stimulation for all parameters (d AUC, d EF, d EC). All scintigraphic measurements were evaluated by the same physician who was blinded for the actual pacing modes.

Statistics: Linear regression analysis was performed for d xyz and d AUC, d EF, and d EC, respectively. In 8 patients randomly chosen, acquisition was performed twice for each pacing mode. The ratio between standard deviation and mean value was taken as the coefficient of variation. Paired data were compared by the nonparametric Wilcoxon test. A p value < 0.05 was considered significant.

RESULTS

By the technique described, QRS duration was shorter in 9 out of 14 patients (64 %) with septal pacing as compared with apical pacing. In one patient there was no difference and in 4 patients (29%), QRS duration was longer despite a septal implantation site. Average QRS duration did not differ significantly between septal and apical pacing.

Optimization of the AV delay was performed by impedance cardiography in 5 patients, by mitral valve doppler echocardiography in 9. In 8 out of 14 patients (57 %) the optimized AV delay was shorter with septal pacing, in one patient there was no difference and in 5 patients (36 %) it was shorter with apical pacing. The mean optimized AV delay did not differ significantly between septal and apical pacing. Left ventricular systolic function was not severely depressed in the patients as indicated by their ejection fraction ranging between 38 % and 74 %. The coefficient of variation of the repeated measurements obtained by radionuclide ventriculography was 0.06 ± 0.08, 0.07 ± 0.05 and 0.05 ± 0.03 for the AUC, EF and EC, respectively.

There was a significant, linear, positive correlation between the difference in QRS duration obtained by apical and septal pacing and the change in phase distribution histograms of left ventricular contraction, evaluated as the area under the curve (d AUC, $r = 0.66$, $p= 0.010$) with 7 patients being outside the 95 % confidence limit (Fig 1). The difference in QRS duration was linearily and negatively related to the difference in left ventricular systolic function measured as ejection fraction (d EF, $r=0.71$, $p=0.004$, Fig 2) and absolute ejected counts (d EC, $r=0.74$, $p=0.002$, Fig 3) with 6 and 4 patients, respectively, being outside the 95 % confidence limit.

DISCUSSION

This study shows that right ventricular lead implantation guided by surface QRS duration is feasible by means of commercially available electrode. Using this technique, the reduction of QRS duration obtained by alternate pacing sites is linearily related with less dyssynergy of left ventricular contraction and with improvement of the systolic function. This study does not prove in general right ventricular septal pacing to be superior over apical pacing but emphazises the need for further clinical trials on this topic. However, the stimulation site under study must be clearly defined, whereby a functional definition such as surface QRS duration should be established instead of a sole topographic definition of alternate pacing. In patients with sinus rhythm and AV synchronous pacing, the AV delay should be optimized individually and separately for each stimulation site. It might be that these methodological considerations are responsible for the fact that recent studies failed to confirm any consistent benefit of DDD pacing in severe heart failure using one single alternate pacing site and that at least biventricular or even multisite pacing was needed to achieve this.

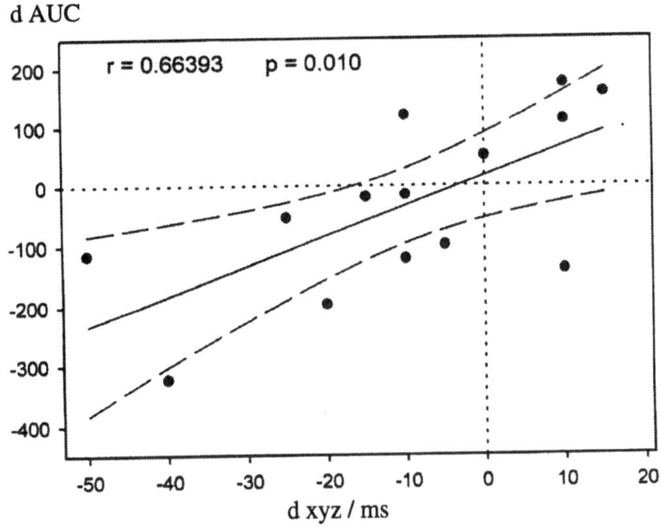

Fig 1.

The difference in QRS duration obtained with septal and apical pacing (d xyz (ms)) plotted against the difference in the area under the curve of the phase distribution histogram as obtained with septal and apical pacing (d AUC; n=14). Full line = regression line; dashed line = 95 % confidence limit; r = coefficient of regression; p = level of significance.

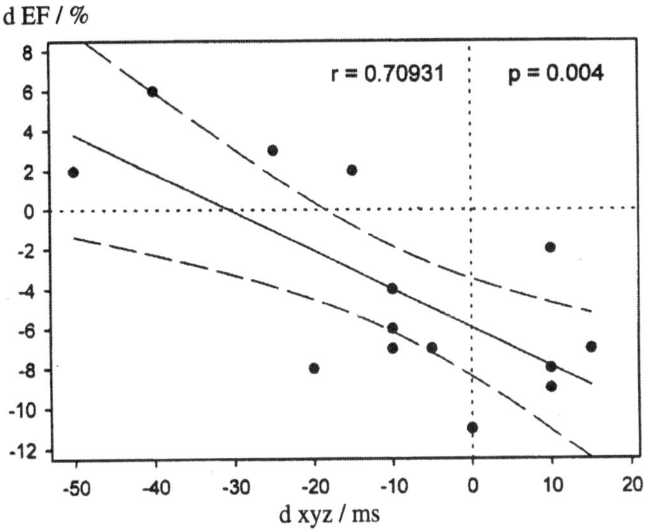

Fig 2.

The difference in QRS duration (d xyz) plotted against the relative difference in the ejection fraction as obtained with septal and apical pacing (d EF (%); n=14).

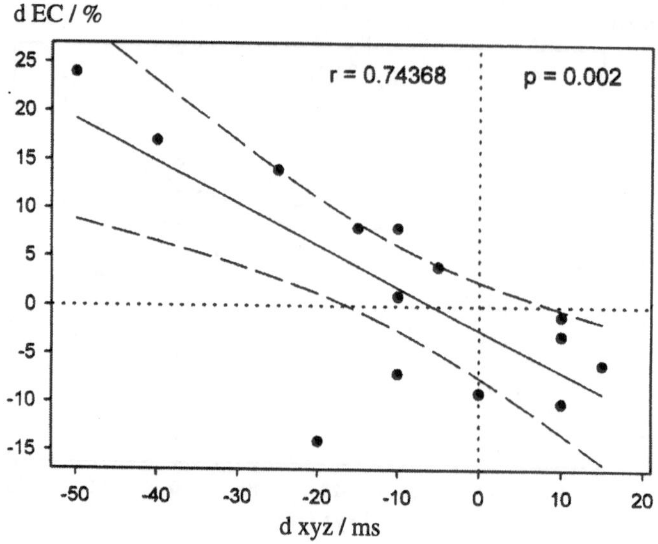

Fig 3.

The difference in QRS duration (d xyz) plotted against the difference in the systolic ejected counts as obtained with septal and apical pacing (d EC (%); n=14).

REFERENCES

1. Koch E. Der Kontraktionsablauf an der Kammer des Froschherzens und die Form der entsprechenden Suspensionkurve, mit besonderen Ausführungen über das Alles-oder-Nichts-Gesetz, die Extrasystole und den Herzalternans. Pflügers Arch Physiol 1920; 181: 106-129.

2. Wiggers CJ. The muscular reactions of the mammalian ventricles to artificial surface stimuli. Am J Physiol 1925; 763: 346-378.

VARIA

Radioactive Isotopes in
Clinical Medicine and Research XXIII
ed. by H. Bergmann, H. Köhn and H. Sinzinger

^{153}SM- EDTMP FOR PAIN RELIEF IN MALIGNANT AND BENIGN BONE AND JOINT DISEASES

Kendler D., Donnemiller E., Riccabona G., Mur E.,
Depts. of Nuclear Medicine and Internal Medicine, University of Innsbruck, Austria

INTRODUCTION

Management of bone pain in patients with disseminated skeletal metastases and also in patients with widespread benign inflammatory joint diseases unresponsive to all conventional treatment is a significant clinical problem.

Many years ago Phosphorus-32 has been used as systemic radioisotope therapy for the treatment of bone pain but its use is limited because of frequent bone marrow depression. More recently strontium-89 has been used for the management of bone pain. A very good clinical response with acceptable haematological toxicity have been observed (1,6).

Since several years however two new bone-seeking radiopharmaceuticals were introduced for this purpose: ^{186}Re- HEDP and ^{153}Sm- EDTMP (2,3,4,5). Both are emmiting besides therapeutically effective ß- radiation also low energy γ- radiation useful for imaging after therapy. As their metabolism is very similar to ^{99m}Tc-phosphonates used for bone scanning it seems feasible to use parameters of bone scans (regional uptake, whole body retention, biological half life and tumor volume estimates) for adequate dosimetry. ^{153}Samarium- EDTMP can be ordered according to need and is therefore less costly for each patient.

So far recommended „dosage" was 18,5 - 55,5 MBq kg body weight. We tried to analyze important factors (number of lesions (BSI), tumor volume, regional uptake) for individual dosimetry in relation to therapeutic results in patients with bone metastases and inflammatory joint diseases.

MATERIAL AND METHODS

So far 13 patients with bone metastases (7 prostate Ca, 3 breast Ca, 1 ovarian Ca, 1 renal cell Ca and 1 SQC Ca) and 5 patients with benign joint disaeases (2 with psoriatic arthropathy and 3 with rheumatoid arthritis) unresponsive to conventional treatment (10 males, 8 females; mean age: 62 years) were treated. 3 of our patients died soon after therapy but not due to treatment with ^{153}Sm EDTMP. Only 14 cases could therefore be evaluated in follow-up studies of more than 4 weeks (1 patient had the therapy only 3 weeks ago).

Pain and mobility scores were obtained from all patients. 11 of our patients needed morphine or similar alcaloids 3 or more times/ day and 8 of them were bedridden or with severely restricted mobility. All patients received a pain diary for individual assessment of therapy effects (pain intensity and analgesic medication was recorded).

All patients were investigated by whole body bone scan 2-3 hours after the injection of 555 MBq ^{99m}Tc DPD, 2 patients had SPECT of the trunk. ^{99m}Tc HIG scans (bloodpool phase, 6 and 24 hours after 555 MBq ^{99m}Tc HIG) were performed in patients with inflammatory diseases only. In both kinds of scanning thyroid uptake was blocked with 400 mg NaClO4. 24 hours after treatment with ^{153}Sm EDTMP whole body planar scintigraphic images in all patients were obtained.

The studies were aquired with a dual head camera Elscint Helix equipped with LEAP-collimators. For reporting the data were processed on an APEX- SPX and Hermes workstation.

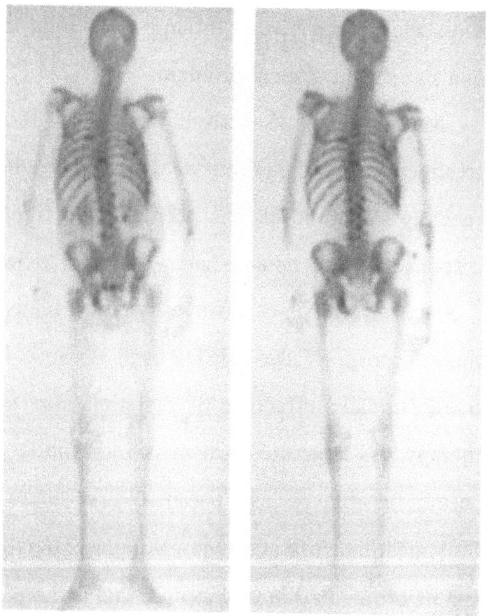

Figure 1. ^{99m}Tc DPD whole body bone scan and whole body planar scan 24 hours after treatment with ^{153}Sm EDTMP in patient with disseminated skeletal metastases

Bone scan indices were calculated from whole body bone scans (6). Count ratios tumor/ normal bone were calculated from conjugated views of bone scans comparing count rates in lesions and reference ROIs. Moreover whole body ^{99m}Tc-DPD retention was measured indirectly by collecting 24 hours-urine-samples and compared with ^{153}Sm- EDTMP- retention after therapy.

Estimation of volume of bone metastasis was tried by comparing lesion size with sources of defined volumes on planar scans (by 3 independent observers) and by SPECT using a Jasczak-phantom filled with activity concentrations „lesion" to background 3:1 and with „lesion" volumes 2- 125 ml aquired with aquisition matrix 64 x 64 and 128 x 128. For semiquantitative analysis the projection data were transferred to a NUD Hermes workstation (processing software by Nuclear Diagnostics). Data were reconstructed by back projection using a Wiener filter. For volume estimation the program MultiModality from NUD was used. In patients we used the same approach, drawing regions of interest manually around areas of abnormal uptake and counting pixels to obtain an estimate of tumor volume. Because of the well-known problems with volume estimation particularly in small lesions we recommend this procedure for volume estimation only for large and irregularly formed areas while in small lesions it can produce considerable errors.

We then applied still standardized therapy doses of 28 (n = 3), 37 (n = 9) and 55 (n = 6) MBq/ kg body weight. The mean activity applied was 2896 MBq (1480 - 4958 MBq).

All patients were followed according to a defined protocol with pain diary, haematological samples weekly, clinical exam every 3- 4 weeks by nuclear physicians (in patients with benign joint diseases by rheumatologists), if needed by X- ray and 3, 6 and 12 months following treatment also by scintigraphic procedures (bone scans and bone combined with HIG scans in patients with benign diseases).

RESULTS

Bone scan indices were calculated in all 13 patients with malignant bone lesions. They showed big differences (14 - 112). In patients with benign diseases we found particularly high bone scan indices (in all patients above 90) because of the high number of very small lesions in small finger and toe joints.

Count ratios tumor/ normal bone in bone scans in 10 patients with bone metastases varied also (1,2 - 14; mean 1,95).

Counts ratios lesion/ normal bone in HIG scans in 5 patients with rheumatoid arthritis or psoriatic arthropathy were more homogeneus (1,2 - 6,1; mean 2,2).

24 hours whole body retention values of 99mTc DPD (mean 72%) and 153Sm EDTMP (mean 68%) were similar (mean difference < 10%).

Estimated tumor volume in all 13 patients with malignant lesions showed a mean of 120 ml (range 48 - 264 ml).

Using the previous data from bone scans and whole body retention as parameters for dose estimation as well as MIRD formulas (Figure 2.) assuming a homogeneus uptake of the radiopharmaceutical in the lesion we arrived at a mean dose estimate of 64 Gy (range 9 - 124 Gy) in our cases.

Dose (Gy) = A x t x S

A = max. activity in lesion
t = residence time
= eff. half- life/ ln2
S = 4,21 x 10^{-3} mGy/ MBq /s

Figure 2. MIRD formula for dosimetry

In all 14 patients observed longer then 4 weeks so far there was only 1 non- responder, who developed pathological fractures in his ribs. In all patients with benign diseases we observed positive treatment effects (2 patients with improvement of >2 grades and 3 patients with improvement of 1-2 grades on the pain scale). Duration of pain relief lasted at least 6 weeks, the longest seen effect is at present 11 months in a patient treated for psoriatic arthropathy (Table 1)

outcome n/ total	improved ++ 7/14	improved + 6/14	no change 1/14	worse -
duration of effects n	< 2 months 4	> 2 months 2	> 4 months 5	> 8 months 3
additional therapies n	radiation 2	chemotherapy 3	hormone therapy 2	immun suppr. therapy 0

Table 1. Clinical results after treatment with ^{153}Sm EDTMP

Haematological toxicity was defined by signes of bone marrow depresion. In 11 of 16 cases we observed thrombopenia which was transient and never severe. In patients with bone marrow pathology before therapy with ^{153}Sm EDTMP because of previous treatment (chemotherapy, radiation therapy) or by severe bone marrow metastases we observed also leukopenia in 3 cases and anemia in 6 cases (2 of them needed treatment).

Moreover we registered the effect of ^{153}Sm therapy on tumor markers and other parameters recorded during follow-up. We observed a decrease of alcaline phosphatase in all cases with bone metastases and a decrease of inflammation parameters (ESR, CRP) in patients with inflammatory joint diseases.

DISCUSSION

So far several ß-emitting radionuclides are being tested clinically. A number of reports showed that ^{153}Sm EDTMP can be used successfully to control pain from bone metastases (3, 4) and from benign inflammatory joint diseases (7, 8).

In our study we found that a single administration of ^{153}Sm EDTMP was more effective in palliation pain (90% responders) than ^{89}Sr (68% responders) in patients with bone metastases. Moreover we observed no correlation of therapy effect or side effects with bone scan index (number of lesions) and no corelation of treatment effect with whole body retention/ kg body weight.

On the contrary we found a good correlation of therapy effect with ^{153}Sm activity retained in ml tumor volume. Using the data from bone scans, effective half time und 24 hrs whole body retention of ^{153}Sm EDTMP as well as MIRD formulas for dose estimates in the lesions we could assume that 37 MBq ^{153}Sm EDTMP gives approximately a dose of 20 Gy to a tumor of 10 ml with homogenous uptake of the radiopharmaceutical in the lesion. In our cases dose estimates ranged from 9 - 124 Gy. Obviously the uptake is not homogeneous, but will occur mainly in the border zone of tumor and bone lesion, so that there the radiation dose will be higher. At present there are still problems, however to assess regional ^{153}Sm and ^{99m}Tc DPD uptake as well as lesion volume especially by SPECT. Moreover this dosimetric approach is impossible in patients presenting „superscans“ due to diffuse bone infiltration by tumor. We hope that these problems can be overcome in the near future so that usually a satisfactory dosimetry can be obtained which could improve therapy results even more.

Finally we are satisfied with the positive treatment results also in patients with rheumatoid arthritis and psoriatic arthropathy and we hope that this kind of treatment can improve the life quality of these patients significantly.

REFERENCES

1. Robinson-RG.,et al.: Radionuclide therapy of intractable bone pain: emphasis on strontium-89; Semin-Nucl- Med. 1992 Jan; 22(1): 28-32

2. Clarke -SE.: Radionuclide therapy in oncology; Cancer-Treat-Rev. 1994 jan; 20(1): 51-71

3. Turner JH, Martindale AA, Sorby P, et al. Samarium-153 EDTMP therapy of disseminated skeletal metastasis. Eur J Nucl Med. 1989; 15:784-95.

4. Turner JH, Claringbold PG. A phase II study of treatment of painful multifocal skeletal metastases with single and repeated dose samarium-153 ethylenediaminetetramethylene phosphonate. Eur J Cancer. 1991; 27:1084-6.

5. Ahonen A, Hiltunen J, Härkönen R, Jakobsen M, Jurvelin J, Joensuu H, Kumpulainen E, Kulmaml J, Nikula T. Pharmakokinetics of Samarium-153-EDTMP in Connection with a Treatment of Patients with Bone Metastases. Eur J Nucl Med 1992; 18:623

6. Blake GM et al., 89Sr therapy: Strontium kinetics in disseminated carcinoma of the prostate. Eur J Nucl Med 1986; 12:447-454

7. Alberts AS, Brighton SW, Kempff P, et al. Samarium-153-EDTMP for palliation of ankylosing spondylitis, Paget's disease and rheumatoid arthritis. J Nucl Med. 1995; 36:1417-1420

8. Marinho NVS, Nobre MRC, Coelho IJ, et al. Samarium-153-EDTMP for pain palliation in patients with rheumatoid arthritis. Eur J Nucl Med 1997; 24:963

Radioactive Isotopes in
Clinical Medicine and Research XXIII
ed. by H. Bergmann, H. Köhn and H. Sinzinger

TC-99M-TETROFOSMIN SPECT SCINTIGRAPHY IN THE POST-OPERATIVE FOLLOW-UP OF MICROVASCULAR ANASTOMOSED FLAPS IN FACIAL RECONSTRUCTION

Aigner R.M., Fueger G.F., Ruda C.*
Karl-Franzens-University of Graz, Dept. of Radiology, *Dept. of Maxillo-Facial-Surgery, Graz, Austria

SUMMARY

The early post-operative evaluation of perfusion and viability of microvascular anastomosed flaps is most important. We analyzed Tc-99m-tetrofosmin scintigraphy for that purpose in 15 patients during their immediate post-operative period. Early, localized muscular necrosis was seen on the SPECT studies in 5/15 cases, on the planar images in 4/15 cases. Absence of perfusion was seen in 2 cases. We consider Tc-99m-tetrofosmin scintigraphy as a sensitive diagnostic tool for the early detection of inadequate implantation and viability of the microvascular anastomosed flaps. It was more sensitive and accurate than the early clinical investigation.

INTRODUCTION

Using microvascular anastomosed flaps in maxillofacial surgery is important for reconstruction of bone and muscular defects caused by tumour resection. The early evaluation of perfusion and viability of the microvascular anastomosed flaps is most important in the immediate post-operative period. This prospective study analyzes the diagnostic value of Technetium-99m-tetrofosmin for that purpose.

MATERIALS AND METHODS

In fifteen patients mandibular reconstruction had been performed with autologous vascular pedicled grafts (microvascular flaps), after more or less partial resection of the mandible for malignancy. These patients, 5 female, 10 male, aged between 31 and 66 years were investigated at our nuclear medicine department 4-5 days post-operatively. As a tracer Tc-99m-tetrofosmin was used in a dose of 555 MBq (15 mCi) intravenously. Scintigraphy was done firstly on a dual-headed Elscint gamma camera (Helix^{R}) and consisted of radionuclide angiography (16 frames à 4 seconds) and static planar images in four projections at 10 minutes post injection. Immediately afterwards the SPECT images were done; a Picker-triple headed camera (Prism 3000) was used for that purpose.

RESULTS

An uncomplicated healing process was observed in 10/15 patients. A complicated healing process was demonstrated in 5/15 patients: (1) Absence of perfusion associated with localized absent tracer uptake on the static images was visualized in one patient. These findigs were interpreted as early, localized muscular necrosis. (2) Localized inhomogenous decreased tracer uptake was seen in 4/154 patients, which could be better analyzed on the SPECT studies than on the static planar images. Associated hypoperfusion was seen in one of these patients. These findings were interpreted as inadequate healing process, as incipient early necrosis of the soft tissue component, respectively.

Figure a and b: Complete early necrosis of the soft tissue component in the right buccal region
Pat. Id. MAY, male, 37 years

a: anterior view

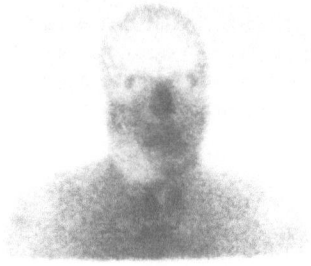

b: posterior view

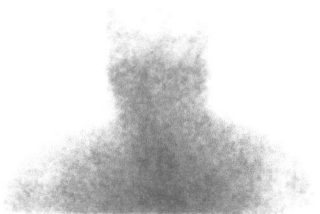

DISCUSSION

The successful incorporation of microvascular anastomosed flaps depends on a biologically complex process. One of these parameters are sufficient blood supply, i.e. adequate localized perfusion, vitality of the muscular cells and of the osteoblasts (1). Clinical and radiological diagnostic modalities, even magnetic resonance imaging can not provide an early assessment of graft outcome. Perfusion is one of the diagnostic tools of bone scintigraphy. Complications in cortical and cancellous bone graft incorporation or viability can be recognized by bone scintigraphy with Technetium-99m-labelled-(di)phosphonates (2,3,4,5). Therefore, therapeutic intervention is possible before the osseous portion of the microvascular anastomosed flaps become non-viabel, necrotic or infected. But the objective follow-up of the soft tissue component still remains uncertain. There is a lack for the early and sensitive recognition of complications of the muscular component of the graft. We hypothesized that the widely accepted myocardial perfusion imaging tracer Tc-99m-tetrofosmin(1,2-bis(bis(2-ethoxy-ethyl)-phosphino)-ethane) could possibly offer advantages for that purpose (6,7,8). The uptake mechanism of tetrofosmin is explained on the basis of (increased) perfusion, mitochondrial membrane activity, mitochondiral count, and cell metabolism. As shown in the result section tetrofosmin scintigraphy is a sensitive diagnostic tool for the early detection of (in)adequate healing of the microvascular anastomosed flaps. It is even more sensitive and accurate than the early clinical investigation. Using radionuclide-angiography the (in)adequate localized perfusion can be visualized. Adequate perfusion is the basic parameter for the observation of vitality of the muscular cells. On the other hand the SPECT technique is more sensitive for the early and sensitivie recognition of the healing process than static planar imaging. The SPECT technique provides better recognition and localization of focal muscular complications of the healing process. Therefore, better and earlier therapeutic intervention can be done. The earlier prompt and effective therapy can be instituted, the better late and severe complications can be avoided.

REFERENCES

1. Neukam FW, Scheller H, Günay H. Experimentelle und klinische Untersuchungen zur Auflagerungsosteoplastik in Kombination mit enossalen Implantaten. Z Zahnärztl Implantol 1989; 5:235-241
2. Stevenson JS, Bright RW, Dunson GL et al. Technetium-99m phosphate bone imaging: a method for assessing bone graft healing. Radiol 1974; 11:391-349
3. Dee P, Lambruschi PG, Hiebert JM. The use of Tc-99m MDP bone scanning in the study of vascularized bone implants. J Nucl Med 1981; 22:522-525
4. Matin P. Bone scintigraphy in the diagnosis and management of traumatic injury. Semin Nucl Med 1983; 13:104-122
5. Lee HK, Markowitz J. 99m-Technetium diphophonate bone scanning of the mandibular bone graft. Oral Surg 1980; 49:471-473

6. Jones S, Hendel RC. Technetium-99m-tetrofosmin: a new radiopharmaceutical for myocardial perfusion imaging. J Nucl Med 1993; 34:222-227

7. Aigner RM, Ruda C, Fueger GF, Kärcher H. Combined Tc-99m-MDP and Tc-99m-tetrofosmin scintigraphy in the follow-up of microvascular anastomosed flaps. Eur J Nucl Med 1997; 24:974

Radioactive Isotopes in
Clinical Medicine and Research XXIII
ed. by H. Bergmann, H. Köhn and H. Sinzinger

LONG-TERM FOLLOW-UP STUDY OF GASTRIC EMPTYING AND *HELICOBACTER PYLORI* ERADICATION AMONG PATIENTS WITH FUNCTIONAL DYSPEPSIA

Koskenpato J(1), Korppi-Tommola T(2), Kairemo K(3), Färkkilä M(1)
Dept. of Gastroenterology (1); Clin. of Radiology (2); Dept. of Clinical Chemistry(3), Helsinki University Central Hospital, Haartmaninkatu 4, Helsinki, Finland

SUMMARY

Studies on the influence of *Helicobacter pylori* gastritis on gastric motility have produced inconclusive results. We examined the effect of *Helicobacter pylori* eradication therapy on gastric emptying in patients with functional dyspepsia. A standardized scintigraphic double-tracer examination was used. There was no difference in gastric emptying among *H.pylori* eradicated and *H.pylori* positive patients after one year follow-up. However, the reproducibility of the scintigraphic study was good.

INTRODUCTION

Functional dyspepsia is a clinical syndrome defined as upper abdominal symptoms without cause that can be identified by conventional diagnostic evaluation (1). *Helicobacter pylori* is associated with chronic gastritis, peptic ulcer disease and gastric malignancies (2) but the studies on the influence of *H.pylori* on gastric motility and on the symptoms of functional dyspepsia (3-6) have provided inconclusive results. Healing of the gastritis after *H.pylori* eradication takes months or even longer (7). At present, scintigraphy is the most reliable method for measuring gastric emptying, and it remains the gold standard (8). A standardized double-tracer scintigraphy (9) with one year follow-up time was employed to investigate the effect of *H.pylori* eradication therapy on gastric emptying in functional dyspepsia.

MATERIALS AND METHODS

Twenty-nine *H.pylori* positive patients (6 men and 23 women) with functional dyspepsia participated in the study after giving their informed constent. Each subject underwent a normal physical examination. None of the study subjects had evidence of any systemic disease known to affect gastrointestinal motility. Every patient was evaluated by gastroscopy and ultrasonography of the upper abdomen before the study.

After an overnight fast lasting at least 12 hr, the patients were given 5 min to eat a warm 200 g standard test meal within 5 min. (lactose-free meat cabbage casserole; Ruoka-Saarioninen Oy, Sahalahti, Finland) labeled with In-111 (9.25 MBq). The energy content of the meal was 220 kcal. After consuming the meal, the patients drank 150ml Tc-99m labeled (75 MBq) water just prior to the study. The gamma imaging system of a Picker „Prism 2000XP" dual-headed gamma camera connected with an „Odyssey VP" image processing computer was used. Tc-99m (140keV; 20% window) and IN-111 (247keV; 20%window) activity distributions of the abdominal area were recorded simultaneously by using medium energy collimators. After a 5-min eating period, the patient was placed into a supine imaging position. The dynamic double iosotope study having a 30-sec acquisition time included images of the gastric area in anterior and posterior projections for a total of 90 minutes. Four different, simultaneous image files were recorded during each study. The size of the acquisition matrix was 128x128 pixels.

The regions of interest (ROIs) were drawn, including the areas of the intire stomach, proximal (corpus) and distal (antrum) parts of the stomach and the distal part of the oesophagus. The oesophagal ROI was drawn in order to detect any reflux that occurred during the study. The background area was drawn outside, near the medial side of the stomach. The time-activity curves were calculated as geometric means of the total counts of the anterior and posterior ROIs. The mirrored ROIs were used for postero-anterior images to produce geometric mean values. The background subtraction was made using the information of the background curve generated by the In-111 and Tc-99m Compton scatter. Correction of Tc-99m decay was performed. The 50% post-lag retention time (T50) for solid substances and the gastric emptying half-time (T1/2) for liquid substance were determined separately from the dynamic curves. The lagtime in solid emptying was determined at the turning point of the descending part of the time activity curve of the entire stomach. At the turning point, the second derivative equals zero.

After the scintigraphic examination fourteen patients received *H.pylori* eradication therapy with amoxycillin, metronizadole and omeprazole, and the eradication was successful among 13 patients. The medication was double-blinded and placebo controlled. After a one year follow-up period the scintigraphic study was repeated and the postlag 50% retention time for solids, the gastric emptying half-time for liquids and the solid lag duration were determined. Data were evaluated using paired *t*-tests and simple linear regression analysis (BMDP new system 1.1).

RESULTS

In the whole study population the solid T1/2 was 108±79.8 min in the beginning of the study and 96±53.2 min one year later (p=ns). The liquid T1/2 was 33.4±9.7 min in the beginning and 33.1±9.0 one year later (p=ns). The solid lagtime duration values were 3.6±3.5 min and 4.4±3.0 min (p=ns). There were no statistically significant differences between the *H.pylori* eradicated patients and *H.pylori* positive patients.

Table 1: Gastric emptying parameters of *H.pylori* positive and negative patients at the end of one year follow-up. (ns = statistically nonsignificant)

	T50 / solids (min)	T1/2 liquids (min)	solid lagtime (min)
H.pylori +	89.1 ± 45.7 (ns)	33.0 ± 8.8 (ns)	4.7 ± 2.9 (ns)
H.pylori -	104.3 ± 61.0 (ns)	33.2 ± 9.6 (ns)	4.1 ± 3.1 (ns)

The correlations between the first and the second scintigraphy study results of each individual subject in the whole study population were statistically significant in solid postlag 50% retention time (p = 0.20, PearsonR = 0.43) (Fig.1) and in liquid gastric emptying half-time (p = 0.018, PearsonR= 0.43) (Fig.2).

Figure 1: Postlag 50% retention time in solids. Values of the whole population at the beginning and after one year follow-up (p = 0.20, PearsonR = 0.43)

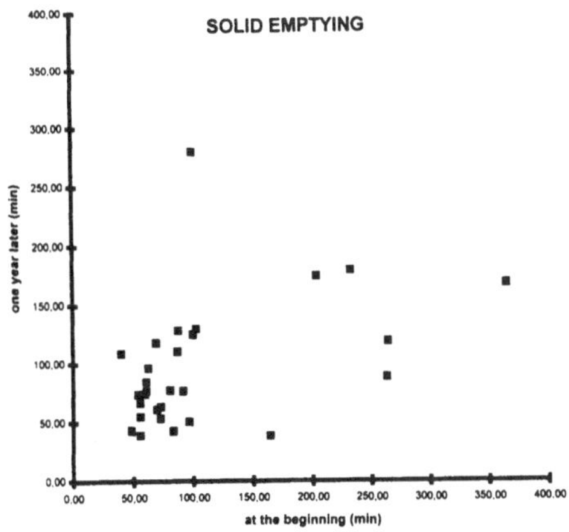

Figure 2: Emptying half-times in liquids. Values of the whole population at the beginning and after one year follow-up (p = 0.018, PearsonR = 0.43)

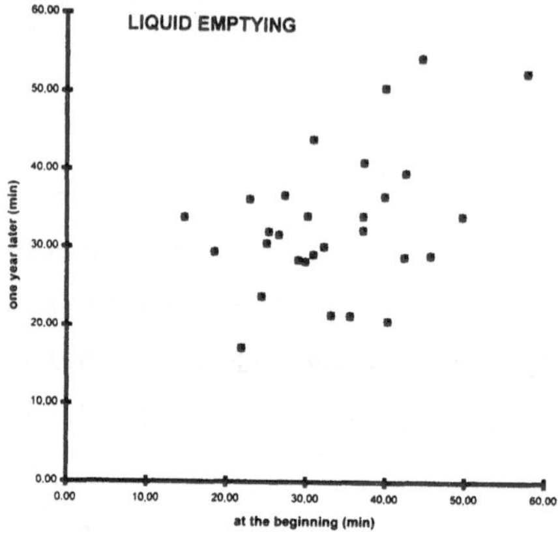

DISCUSSION

Our study shows that *Helicobacter pylori* eradication therapy does not alter the gastric emptying in patients with functional dyspepsia. It seems, however, that the repetitiveness of a standardized double-tracer scintigraphic study of gastric emptying of solids and liquids is good in one year follow-up period.

ACKNOWLEDGEMENTS

This study was supported by a grant from the Yrjö Jahnsson Foundation.

REFERENCES

1. Talley NJ, Colin-Jones D, Koch KL, Nyren O, Stanghellini V. Functional Dyspepsia: A Classification with Guidelines for Diagnosis and Management. Gastroenterology Intl 1991; 4:145-157
2. Current European concepts in the management of Helicobacter pylori infection. The Maastricht Consensus Report. Gut 1997; 41:8-13
3. Caballero-Plasencia AM, Muros-Navarro MC, Martin-Ruiz JL, Valenzuela-Barranco M, de los Reyes-Garcia MC, Casado-Caballero FJ et al. Dyspeptic symptoms and gastric emptying of solids in patients with functional dyspepsia. Role of Helicobacter pylori infection. Scand J Gastroenterol 1995; 30:745-751.
4. Scott AM, Kellow JE, Shuter B, Cowan H, Corbett AM, Riley JW et al. Intragastric distribution and gastric emptying of solids and liquids in functional dyspepsia. Dig Dis Sci 1993; 38:2247-2254
5. Tucci A, Corinaldesi R, Stanghellini V, Tosetti C, Di Febo G, Paparo GF et al. Helicobacter pylori infection and gastric function in patients with chronic idiopathic dyspepsia. Gastroenterology 1992; 103:768-774

6. Chang CS, Chen GH, Kao CH, Wang SJ, Peng SN, Huang CK. The effect of Helicobacter pylori infection on gastric emptying of digestible and indegestible solids in patients with nonulcer dyspepsia. Am J Gastroenterol 1996; 91:474-479
7. Valle J, Seppälä K, Sipponen P, Kosunen T. Disappearance of gastric after eradication of Helicobacter pylori: a morphometric study. Scand J Gastroenterol 1991; 26:1057-1065
8. Fried M. Methods to study gastric emptying. Moderator's comments. Dig Dis Sci 1994; 39:114-115
9. Kairemo KJA, Koskenpato J, Korppi-Tommola ET, Färkkilä M. A double-tracer method for studying intragastric distribution and gastric emptying of solids and liquids in fuctional dyspepsia: Nucl Med Comm, in press

Radioactive Isotopes in
Clinical Medicine and Research XXIII
ed. by H. Bergmann, H. Köhn and H. Sinzinger

The value of renal scintigraphy under controlled diuresis in children with hydronephrosis

Steiner D., Bauer R., Steiss J.O., Rascher W., Miller J., Weidner W.
Clinic for Nuclear Medicine, Children's Hospital, Clinic for Urology,
Justus-Liebig Universitaet Giessen, Germany

Summary

Dynamic renal scintigraphy (DRS) during controlled diuresis is the method of choice to diagnose the functional relevance of urinary tract obstruction in children with sonographically demonstrated hydronephrosis. However, there are no commonly accepted scintigraphic criteria of indication for surgical intervention. According to our findings, we propose three stages of washout (WO) of tracer following diuresis: In stage I, WO > 50%, neither further diagnosis nor intervention is necessary, in stage II, 50% ≥ WO ≥ 10%, repeat DRS is advised within 2-3 months. Only in stage III, WO< 10%, surgery should be done immediately. This regime reduces (unnecessary) surgical interventions to 50% without bearing the risk of remaining renal damage.

Introduction

Congenital anomalies of the urinary tract are common, showing a frequency of 1:650 to 1:1000. Usually, they are detected early during pre- or postnatal screening procedures (1,8,10). Stenosis of the proximal ureter is the most common anomaly, causing dilation of the renal pelvis and thus hydronephrosis (6). These findings are easily detected by ultrasound. Further diagostic and therapeutic procedures have certainly changed during the last years. At that times mictions-cysto-urography, i.e. intravenous urography, and renal scintigraphy were performed. Thereafter, surgery was performed depending only upon the degree of hydronephrosis. Thus, stenoses of the ureter were surgically cured which might have caused only partial obstruction without being urodynamically fully effective.

At present, DRS using MAG-3 is the most important investigation to answer the question if the known stenosis is urodynamically effectiveneeding surgical intervention or not. Whereas the value of DRS is commonly accepted, there is no agreement concerning the relation between scintigraphic findings and indication for surgical intervention. According to Koff (5) and Ransley (9), surgery may be postponed in children in whom the affected kidney shows normal function, having divided clearance of at least 40% of the global clearance. These authors recommend surgical intervention, if repeated controls show worsening of divided clearance. Thus, these groups take into account only the tubular function, neglecting the washout of the tracer. Other groups critizise these procedure; there is no guarantee, that reduced tubular function of hydronephrotic altered kidney will completely recover after surgery. In contrary, other investigators relay mostly upon the washout kinetics of the tracer prior to decide on surgical intervention. There are many recommendations to classify stenoses of the urinary tract as relevant, if less than 50% of the remaining tracer is excreted after application of Furosemide. According to our experience, also this opinion should be discussed.

Patients and methods

During the last 40 months 86 children (33 girls and 53 boys) were investigated by DRS using Tc99m-MAG-3. All these children were younger than 2 years, age range was between 1 and 24 months, median was 5 months. In 65 children uretero-pelvic obstruction, in the other 21 children uretero-cystic obstruction was suspected.

Immediately after birth, glomerular filtration rate (GFR) is low but increases markedly during the next four weeks. Thus, in newborns scintigraphy was performed not earlier than after the fourth week of life. In all the children hydronephrosis with dilation of the renal pelvis of more than 12 mm was diagnosed by ultrasound. Four hours prior to scintigraphy, children were hydrated by infunding a solution of glucose and electrolytes (Ionosteril PED III). Within 4 hours a total volume of 30-40 ml / kg b.w. was given. If necessary, the children were sedated by orally administered Chloralhydrate (0.56 - 1.0 mg / kg b.w.).

DRS was performed with 8 MBq/kg b.w. Tc99m-MAG-3, administering at least 20 MBq. Scintigrams were recorded in posterior view using a Siemens Diacam™. Recording protocol was 20 scintigrams at a rate 2 sec/frame, 20 at 10 sec/frame and 40 scintigrams at a rate 60 sec/frame. Zoom was between 2.0 and 3.0. In patients in whom a stenosis of the outflow tract was suspected during the first 15 minutes of investigation, Furosemide was administered intravenously 20 minutes after start of the investigation at a dose of 0.5 - 1.0 mg/kg b.w. to achieve forced diuresis. At the end of the investigation, divided clearance was evaluated. In addition, the wash-out (WO) of the tracer was estimated by comparing the activity 30 minutes after application of Furosemide, A_{30}, with the maximum activity, A_{max}:

$$WO = 100 * A_{30} / A_{max} .$$

Results

The results of renal scintigraphy are demonstrated in table 1. In 54 out of the 86 children, WO was above 50%, in 16 children, WO was above 12% but below 50%, 2 children had a borderline value of WO ≈ 10%, whereas 14 children had no increase of tracer washout after Furosemide, WO being less than 8%. All the children with WO > 8% had normal divided clearance, the diseased kidney with suspected obstruction of the urinary tract showed a clearance of at least 40%. In none of these children infection of the urinary tract could be diagnosed, neither by clinical nor by serological findings. Therefore, none of these children had primary surgery, instead, sonography of the kidneys and the urinary tract was repeated in regular intervals.

14 of the 16 children with WO between 12% and 50% had repeat DRS 2-4 months after the first investigation. 13 children showed a marked improvement of WO as it is shown in fig. 1. Only one child had deterioration of renal washout. The other two children with primary WO between 12% and 50% had marked improvement of sonographical findings; therefore, scintigraphy was not repeated. In addition, also the two children with WO ≈ 10% showed marked improvement at control scintigraphy (fig. 1).

The 14 children with no increase of tracer washout after Furosemide (WO < 8%) had surgery soon after scintigraphy. In 13 of the 14 children tracer washout increased to 50% or more, in the remaining 1 child WO increased to ≈ 30%. 8 of these 14 children had normal divided clearance above 40%, the other 6 children had diveded clearances between 30 and 40%.

wash-out WO	*n*	*(%)*	*n*	*(%)*
WO > 50%	54	63		
50% > WO > 12%	16	19	16	50
12% > WO > 8%	2	2	2	6
8% > WO	14	16	14	44
total	86	100	32	100

Table 1: Wash-out (WO) after forced diuresis

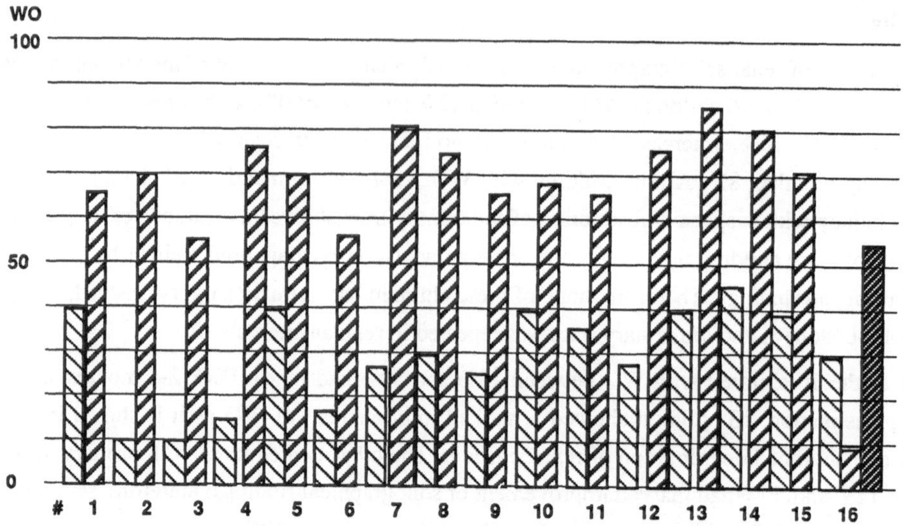

Figure 1: Wash-out (WO) of tracer during first DRS and control 2-4 months later

Discussion

Early diagnosis and therapy of functionally relevant urinary-tract obstructions is very important to avoid chronic renal damage. However, there is no agreement in the appropriate diagnostic modalities to discriminate relevant and non-relevant obstructions. Sonography is suited to demonstrate the anatomical situation. It can be repeatedly applied without radiation burden. However, the relevance of obstructions of the urinary tract cannot be assessed. Intravenous urography is used to clarify the anatomical situation, but again, this method is not suited to give the indication for surgery of known stenoses of the urinary outflow tract.

DRS using Tc99m-MAG-3 is the only non-invasive modality to assess the functional relevance of urinary tract obstructions, provided it is performed during standardized forced diuresis (4, 12). Compared to i.v. urography, radiation burden of the bone marrow is less than 20%, with respect to the gonads the advantage in reduction of radiation burden is even higher (2).

Renal function improves rapidly during the first weeks after birth. Whereas glomerular filtration rate (GFR) is as low as 5-10 ml/min/1.73 m^2, it increases to 40-50 ml/min/1.73 m^2 at the end of the fourth week (3). Therefore, DRS should be applied not earlier than 4 weeks after birth. To achieve reproducible results, babies and small infants have to be intravenously hydrated (4, 12). Otherwise, the kidneys cannot increase urinary flow following forced diuresis.

stage	*wash-out WO*	*procedure*
I	WO > 50%	no further treatment
II	50% ≥ WO ≥ 10%	follow-up by DRS within 2-3 months
III	10% > WO	surgery

Table 2: Functional grading of impaired wash-out and implication on further procedures

Recent publications stress the opinion that diuresis-induced wash-out of tracer (WO) of less than 50% is indicative for surgical intervention (7, 11). These results are in contradiction to our findings. According to our results, we define three stages of impaired wash-out as defined in table 2. If the children with morphological stenosis are free from clinical signs of urinary tract infection and have normal divided clearance (≥40%) of the diseased kidney, we recommend the following procedure:

1) Stage I: WO > 50%, neither further diagnosis nor surgery is necessary.
2) Stage II: 50% ≥ WO ≥ 10%, surgery can be postponed. Follow-up has to be performed within 2-3 months.
3) Stage III: WO < 10%, surgery has to be done soon after DRS.

In our patient's population, we had 32 children with WO < 50% at initial scintigraphy. Only 14 had low WO and surgery immediately after DRS. The other 18 children had a follow-up study. Even two children with WO as low as 10% improved and had normal WO kinetics 2 months later. Only one child with initial WO of 30% deteriorated to WO = 9% at follow-up. Now it had surgery; WO normalized to 55%, divided clearance was 45%.

Discriminating three different stages of wash-out WO after forced diuresis, frequency of surgery can be reduced to 50% or less as compared to subdivide only into two classes. In "borderline" WO of stage II, no remaining renal damage is to be expected if follow-up DRS is performed within 2-3 months. On the other hand, if indication for surgery is based only upon the result of divided clearance, the frequency of follow-up studies is higher and the risk of remaining renal damage might be increased.

References:

1 Ashley D.J.B., Mostofi F.K.: Renal agenesis and dysgenesis. J. Urol. 1960; 83:211-230.
2 Buttermann G.: Radioaktivität und Strahlung. Verlag RS Schulz, Percha 1987.
3 Guignard J.P.: The neonatal stressed kidney. In: Gruskin A.B.: Pediatric Nephrology
4 Howman-Giles R., Uren R., Roy L.P., Filmer R.B.: Volume expansion diuretic renal scan in urinary tract obstruction. J. Nucl. Med. 1987; 28: 824-828.
5 Koff S., Campbell K.D.: The nonoperative management of unilateral neonatal hydronephrosis: natural history of poorly functioning kidneys. J. Urol. 1994; 152: 593-595.
6 Lettgen B., Brudererk C., Meyer-Schwickerath M., Kröpfl D., Bonzel K.E.: Angeborene Dilatationen und Stenosen des Harntrakts. Monatsschr. Kinderheilkunde 1996; 144: 918-923.
7 Liepe K., Kropp J., Böhme B., Manseck A., Rupprecht E., Wirth M., Franke W.G.: Die Nierensequenzszintigraphie unter Furosemidbelastung bei Neugeborenen mit kongenitaler Hydronephrose. Nuklearmedizin AB 1997; 36: A19.
8 Najmaldin A.S., Burge D.M., Atwell J.D.: Outcome of antenatally diagnosed pelviuretric junction hydronephrosis. Br. J. Urol. 1991; 67: 96-99.
9 Ransley P.G., Dhillon H.K., Gordon I., Duffy P.G., Dillon M.J., Barratt T.M.: The postnatal management of hydronephrosis diagnosed by prenatal ultrasound. J. Urol. part 2 1990; 144: 584-587.
10 Rascher W., Bonzel K.E., Guth-Tougelidis B., Kröpfl D., Meyer-Schwickerath M., Reiners C.: Angeborene Fehlbildungen des Harntrakts. Monatsschr. Kinderheilkunde 1992; 140: 78-83.
11 Reisinger I., Kettner B., Kirchmair F., GellermannJ.: Verlaufsuntersuchungen obstruktiver Nephropathien mittels der Diureseszintigraphie. Nuklearmedizin AB 1997; 36: A18
12 Sukhai R.N., Kooy P.P.M., Wolff E.D., Scholtmeijer R.J., van Heijden H.J.: Evaluation of obstructive uropathy in children. 99m-Tc-DTPA-renography studies under conditions of maximal diuresis. Br. J. Urol. 1985; 57: 124-129.

Radioactive Isotopes in
Clinical Medicine and Research XXIII
ed. by H. Bergmann, H. Köhn and H. Sinzinger

ASSESSMENT OF BRAIN PERFUSION BY ECD-Tc99m SPET IN RETT SYNDROME

L. Burroni, D. Volterrani, Y. Hayek*, P. Bertelli, A. Vella, M. Zappella* and A. Vattimo

Departments of Nuclear Medicine and *Infantile Neuropsychiatry, University of Siena, Policlinico "Le Scotte", 53100 Siena, Italy

SUMMARY

Rett syndrome (RS) is a progressive neurological pediatric disorder which affects only girls. The aim of our study is to determinate if brain perfusion abnormalities might be able to explain the clinical manifestations and progression of the disease. Quantitative global and regional brain blood flow was evaluated in 25 RS girls and compared with a reference group of 9 children. SPET revealed a considerable global reduction in cerebral perfusion in the group of RS girls and a great statistical difference was recorded when compared with the control group. The reduction of cerebral perfusion reflects the functional disturbances in the brains of RS girls, which might be associated with precocious brain atrophy, even when morphologic imaging (MRI) appears normal.

INTRODUCTION

Rett Syndrome (RS) was first described in 1966 by Andreas Rett [1], but was neglected for some time. The prevalence is currently estimated at about 1:10000-15000 in girls [2]. RS is an early-onset progressive neurological disorder of childhood, seen exclusively in females. Early development is apparently normal. The initial clinical manifestations are deceleration of head growth with consequent microcephaly, impaired communicability, loss of manual skill and speech, stereotypies, gross motor dysfunction and mental deterioration leading to dementia. Other supporting symptoms include intermittent hyperventilation, periodic apnoea during full wakefulness, epilepsy (in up to 80% of patients), bruxism and scoliosis observed in early adolescence [3]. The disease has four clinical stages based on the extent of mental deterioration according to the staging system proposed by Hagberg and Witt-Engerström [4]. Etiology and pathogenesis are still unknown. Genetic factors presumably play a fundamental role; it has also been hypothesized that some autoimmune phenomena may be involved. Neuropathological studies have revealed reduced brain size, reduced size of certain neurones with a decrease in the number of dendrites, cortical and sub-cortical atrophy [5]. In absence of any biological or genetic markers, the diagnosis is essentially based on clinical grounds. A classical form and some variants have been recognized [6]. EEG and traditional neuroradiology often fail to be informative [7]. In recent years, an approach based on tomographic methods for studying cerebral blood flow (rCBF) with Xenon-133 [8], metabolism with PET [9] and anatomical variations with MRI [10] has been introduced. SPET for studying rCBF is now largely used for the examination of patients with various brain diseases and dysfunctions. Recently new tracers (Tc99m-ECD and Tc99m-HMPAO) have been introduced for cerebral blood flow imaging with SPET. The aim of our study was to establish a relationship between regional cerebral blood flow assessed with Tc99m-ECD and the clinical manifestation and progression of the disease, comparing the results with those obtained in a control group of normal children.

MATERIALS AND METHODS

25 young females (aged 3 to 19 years) displaying the classical form of RS [3], recruited from the Department of Infantile Neuropsychiatry, were examined. 16 of them were found to be in clinical stage III and 9 were in clinical stage IV. All girls underwent careful, detailed clinical examination, an EEG investigation and brain MRI. Since normal children cannot be examined for ethical reasons, nine non-Rett patients, referred after one attack of pyretic seizure, were recruited as controls on the basis of their regular neurologic development and normal brain MRI. None of them had any history or signs of neurologic or systemic diseases. Brain SPET was performed on all the children using Tc99m-ECD (10 MBq Kg^{-1}) administered i.v. in a quiet environment. In all RS patients the acquisition was performed under monitored sedation administered following injection of the tracer. 96 frames (40 seconds per frame in a 128x128 pixel matrix) were acquired over a circular orbit with a dual head rotating camera fitted with LEHR collimators. Raw data were reconstructed as one pixel thick slices using a Butterworth filter (order: 10; cut-off: 0.45 Nyquist) in the transaxial fronto-occipital line and in the coronal and sagittal planes. No attenuation correction was performed. Transaxial slices were selected in correspondence with 3 different planes (15.5 mm. thick) passing through the cerebellum (cerebellar level), the basal ganglia and thalamus (mid-thalamic level) and the centrum semiovale (supra-ventricular level). Regions of interest (ROIs) were drawn manually in the cerebellum and, for each side, in the frontal, temporo-parietal, parietal, occipital cortex and in the caudate nucleus and in the thalamus at the described levels. Mean counts per pixel were calculated for each ROI and these measures were used to obtain two indexes: the perfusion index (PI), calculated as the ratio between each ROI and the cerebellum, and the asymmetry index (AI) using the following formula: $AI=(r-l)/[(r+l)/2]x100$ (r = right; l = left). The Mann-Whitney U test for unpaired data was used for comparing the relative regional perfusion and asymmetry in RS girls with the corresponding values of controls. The

reference group was compared separately with the stage III subjects and the stage IV subjects using the Kruskal-Wallis statistical test. $P<0.05$ was considered statistically significant in both tests.

RESULTS

Magnetic resonance imaging revealed no evident abnormalities in 19 patients, mild or moderate cerebral atrophy in five others and ventricular asymmetry in two; one displayed both atrophy and ventricular asymmetry. Of these six pathological patients, five were in stage IV and one was in stage III. No focal lesions were revealed using MRI. Qualitative SPET revealed a hypoperfusion in the left temporo-parietal region in only one stage IV RS girl: none of the others presented focal blood flow alterations. All the children of the reference group revealed a normal cerebral perfusion without regional abnormalities. In comparison with the reference group, quantitative SPET revealed a considerable reduction in cerebral perfusion in all the regions evaluated (Fig. 1).

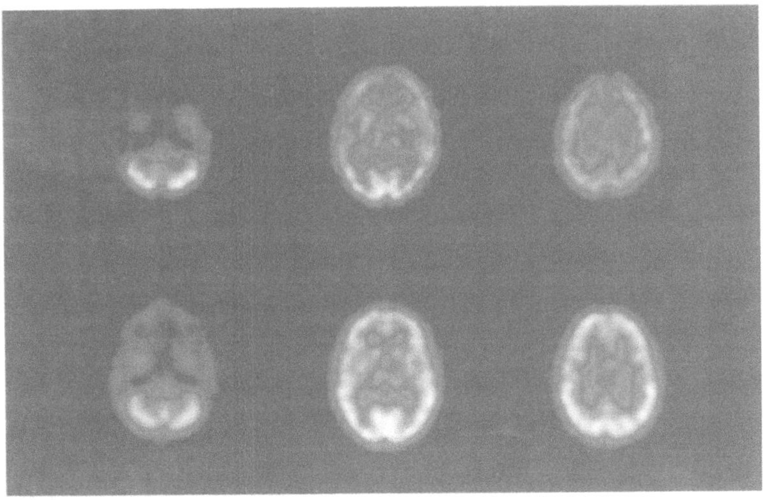

Fig. 1: Three different planes in two age-matched children: a diffuse cortical blood flow reduction is evident in the girl with RS (top) in comparison with a normal children (bottom).

A great statistical difference was found in all the ROIs and in both hemispheres, although more evident in the frontal and temporo-parietal regions and less evident in the thalami (Fig. 2). The difference is more evident when comparing the reference group with stage IV girls than when comparing it with stage III girls (Fig. 3). No significant asymmetry of regional perfusion was found in the RS patients or in the reference group.

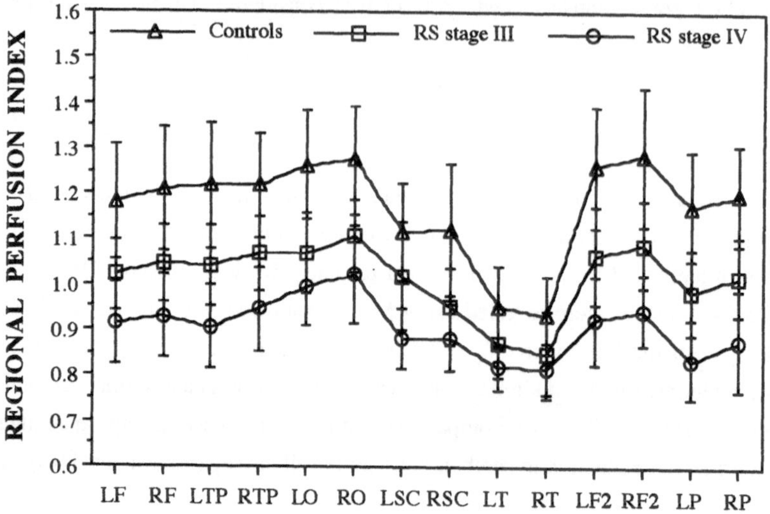

Fig. 2: Means and standard deviations of perfusion index measured in the ROIs drawn on cortical and subcortical structures (Mid-thalamic level: LF and RF = Left and Right Frontal area; LTP and RTP = Left and Right Temporo-Parietal area; LO and RO = Left and Right Occipital area; LSC and RSC = Left and Right Striatum; LT and RT = Left and Right Thalamus. Supra-ventricular level: LF2 and RF2 = Left and Right Frontal area; LP and RP = Left and Right Parietal area).

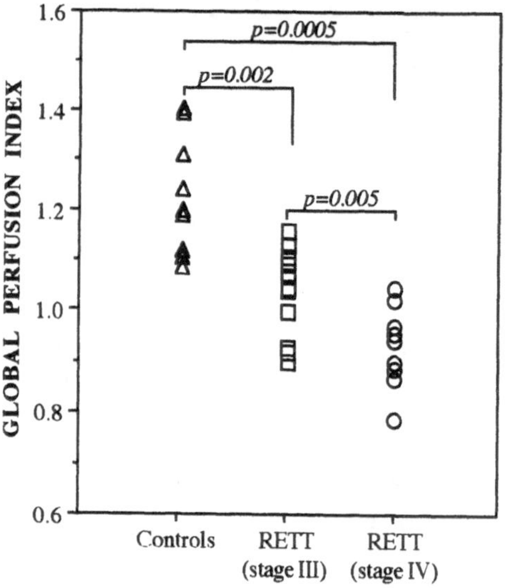

Fig. 3: Relationship beetwen the global perfusion index in controls and stage III and stage IV RS patients

DISCUSSION

Our study revealed a reduced cerebral blood flow in both hemispheres, especially in the frontal and fronto-parietal regions bilaterally, in the group of RS patients. A great reduction of perfusion occurs at the cortical level and the thalami seem to be less effected, as other papers have confirmed [10]. It is believed that the arrest of brain development underlies a complex symptomatology in Rett syndrome. The observation of the more extensive brain perfusion abnormalities found in stage IV Rett patients more frequently than in their stage III counterparts also supports this hypothesis. The age difference discerned between stage III and stage IV RS patients is furthermore due to the fact that although the illness advances with time, its course is irregular. Therefore brain blood flow reduction is probably a sign of the clinical progression of the disease. We also witnessed reduced cerebral blood flow in patients with normal brain MRI; this feature indicates that SPET analysis may reveal a functional alteration such as reduced blood supply, before morphological or structural damage is appreciable, since morphological imaging has demonstrated structural lesions more frequently in stage IV patients than in stage III patients. It is debatable whether the cerebral perfusion impairment is also the cause of direct involvement of cerebral arteries and arterioles. In this regard a similarity exists between SPET findings in RS and in the connective tissue (systemic lupus erythematosus) [11] and endocrine system (diabetes) [12] diseases, in which vascular lesions are responsible for brain damage. No significant right-to-left asymmetry was found to recur in all ROIs of the cortex; this data confirms that RS is a diffuse and non-focal or non-side neurological disorder. This study has found Tc99m-ECD SPET to be sensitive in revealing focal or diffuse brain blood flow abnormalities closely related to EEG alterations, even when MRI patterns are normal. Since RS children are non-cooperative patients, head movement is a potential drawback, which may be prevented with mild sedation.

REFERENCES

1. Rett A: Über ein eigenartiges hirnatrophisches syndrom bei hyperammonämie im kindesalter. Wien Med Wochenschr 1966; 116: 723-726.

2. Hagberg B: Rett syndrome: swedish approach to analysis of prevalence and cause. Brain Dev 1985; 7: 277-279.

3. The Rett syndrome diagnostic criteria work group: Diagnostic criteria for Rett syndrome. Ann Neurol 1988; 23: 425-428.

4. Hagberg B, Witt-Engerström I: Rett syndrome: a suggested staging system for describing the impairment profile with increasing age towards adolescence. Am J Med Gen 1986; 24 (suppl.): 47-59.

5. Armstrong D: The neuropathology of Rett syndrome. Brain Dev 1992; 14: 89-94.

6. Hagberg B, Skjeldal OH: Rett variants: a suggested model for inclusion criteria. Pediatr Neurol 1990; 47: 982-986.

7. Elian M, Rudolf N de M: EEG and respiration in Rett syndrome. Acta Neurol Scand 1991; 83: 123-128.

8. Nielsen JB, Friberg L, Lou H, Lassen NA, Sam ILK: Immature pattern of brain activity in Rett syndrome. Arch Neurol 1990; 47: 982-986.

9. Yoshikawa H, Fucki N, Suzuki H, Sakuragawa N, Ilio M: Cerebral blood flow and oxygen metabolism in the Rett syndrome. Brain Dev 1992; 14 (suppl.): S69-S74.

10. Reiss AL, Faruque F, Naidu S, Abrams M, Beaty T, Bryan RN, Moser H: Neuroanatomy of Rett syndrome: a volumetric imaging study. Ann Neurol 1993; 34: 227-234.

11. Colamussi P, Giganti M, Cittanti C, Dovigo L, Trotta F, Tola MR, Tamarozzi R, Lucignani G, Piffanelli A: Brain single-photon emission tomography with 99mTc-HMPAO in neuropsychiatric systemic lupus erythematosus: relations with EEG and MRI findings and clinical manifestations. Eur J Nucl Med 1995; 22: 17-24.

12. Keymeulen B, de Metz K, Cluydts R, Bossuyt A, Somers G: Technetium-99m hexamethylpropylene amine oxime single-photon emission tomography of regional cerebral blood flow in insulin-dependent diabetes. Eur J Nucl Med 1996; 23: 163-168.

Radioactive Isotopes in
Clinical Medicine and Research XXIII
ed. by H. Bergmann, H. Köhn and H. Sinzinger

DETECTION OF INFLAMMATORY BOWEL DISEASES IN CHILDREN WITH 99m Tc ANTIGRANULOCYTE Mab (BW 250/183) SCINTIGRAPHY

Aprile C, De Giacomo C, Valdambrini V, Cannizzaro G, Saponaro R.

Fondazione «S.Maugeri»,IRCCS- Nuclear Med Serv.;
S.Matteo University Hosp.,IRCCS – Pediatric Clinic , Pavia, Italy

SUMMARY

Twelve children with IBD (5 Crohn's disease and 7 Ulcerative colitis) were studied with the 99mTc labelled antigranulocyte Mab BW 250/183 (early and late planar scans, early SPET). The SPET study offered higher sensitivity than both early and late planar studies. Endoscopic and scintigraphic results were concordant in 17/25 and 17 /28 segments respectively in the Crohn and ulcerative colitis group of pts. On an individual pt. basis all Crohn pts were true +ve, while in the ulcerative colitis group 3 were true+ve, 1 false-ve and 1 false +ve.

INTRODUCTION

Leukocyte scintigraphy is a well established technique for the diagnosis of inflammatory bowel diseases (IBD)(1-3). The in vitro technique, however, requiring a large amount of blood, may be impracticable in children. Our aim was to evaluate the accuracy of the antigranulocyte Mab BW250/183 in children with Crohn'disease (CD) and ulcerative colitis (UC)(4-8) .

MATERIALS & METHODS

Twelve children (5 males and 7 females; median age 13 yrs and 2 mo., range 4-18 yrs), 5 with florid CD and 7 with UC (4 active, 3 inactive) underwent scintigraphic detection after iv. administration of the antigranulocyte Mab BW 250/183 (Behring-CIS bio Int.), whole IgG

0.3-0.5 mg, labelled with 300-600 MBq of 99mTc. Planar scans of the abdomino-pelvic area were taken 4-6 hrs (early scan) and 20 hrs (late scan) p.i. in the anterior, posterior and caudal view when needed. The SPET study was performed immediately after the early scan with reconstruction of transverse, sagittal and coronal slices.

To evaluate the extent of the disease the abdomen was divided into five segments: 1-small-bowel, 2-caecum and ascending, 3-transverse, 4-descending colon and 5-rectosigmoid region, and a simple visual grading scale was used: 0-no activity, 1-moderate, 2-prominent uptake both in the planar and the SPET studies, since the comparison with the bone-marrow could be misleading.

At the time of the study 2 children were on prednisone therapy, 6 were on ASA, 2 on ASA & prednisone and two did not take any medicament. A five-point inflammatory score was used as the sum of pathological parameters (ESR, CRP, platelets, α1-antitrypsin, α1-glycoprotein). Within three weeks from the scan all children underwent colonoscopy with multiple bioptic specimens. Activity and severity of the disease were evaluated by means of the pediatric Crohn's disease activity index (PCDAI) and the ulcerative colitis activity index (9,10).

RESULTS

All pts in the CD group had florid disease, and colonoscopy & histology detected disease activity in 21/25 bowel segments; in the UC group in 5/28 segments only there was active disease, in 4 cases involving the rectosigmoid region.

Sensitivity, specificity and accuracy of the scintigraphic imaging on a per segment basis are reported in tab.1, the colonoscopy and histology being the reference value. In the UC group, only 4 segments were considered, the small bowel being unaffected in all cases. The number of segments visualized was higher in the late scans and more significant with SPET; in no case, however, a segment proved positive by the late scan was missed by SPET, nor the positivity observed in early planar scans turned to negativity in the late scans. Thus, there was concordance in 17/25 and 17/28 segments respectively in the CD and UC group.

If the same results are expressed on a per patient basis and, therefore, if we consider positive a result when at least a single segment is visualized, then all CD pts were true positive, while in the UC group 3 pts were true positive, 2 true negative and 1 pt was false negative and false positive.

No significant correlation was found between the sum of the scan score results and the inflammatory index, even if all CD pts had a positive scan with positive inflammatory score (one 3, three 4 and one 5 points); no clear relationship was found between UC activity index and scan score, while there was a straight relationship between PCDAI and cumulative SPET score (Fig.1).

	CD (n.5 pts;25 segm.)			UC (n.7 pts.; 28 segm)		
	Early	*Late*	*SPET*	*Early*	*Late*	*SPET*
Sens	.33	.52	.62	0	.40	.60
Spec	1	1	1	.95	.82	.60
Acc	.44	.60	.68	.60	.75	.60

Tab. 1. Sensitivity, specificity and accuracy of the BW 250/183 scan in children with Crohn's disease (CD) and ulcerative colitis (UC), on a per segment basis

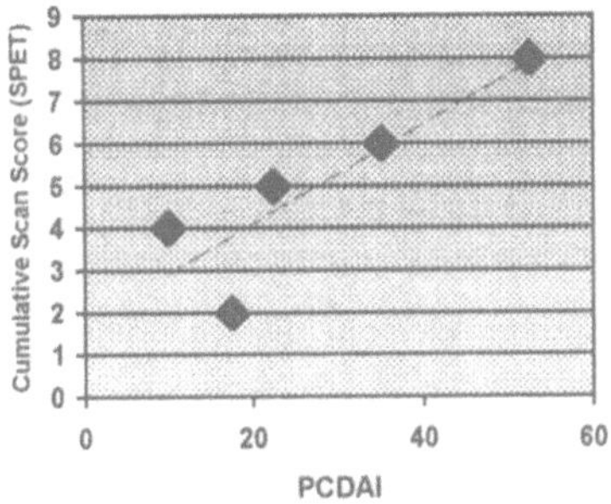

Fig.1 Relationship between Pediatric Crohn's Disease Activity Index (PCDAI) and the cumulative scan score (SPET study) in 5 children with active disease.

DISCUSSION

The more evident pattern in our results is the discrepancy of accuracy between CD and UC, the results in the CD group being more favourable from the clinical point of view. As previously reported by others (11), a better sensitivity is obtainable in late scans , and this fact has been related to a more complicated biokinetics of the Mab labelled granulocytes in comparison with that occurring after in vitro labelling (4), while in the European Multicenter trial there was no evidence of additional information in the late scan. On the other side the SPET scan, as previously reported by Kroiss and us (12,13), allowed to obtain a further increase of sensitivity, even if with some reduction of specificity. This behaviour could not be related to biokinetics, but rather to the fact that a better contrast is obtainable in SPET studies, thus allowing the detection of early accumulation. In fact, a major limit of the antigranulocyte scan is the marked bone–marrow uptake, that in the particular case of IBD can mask visceral abdomino-pelvic accumulation (6). Therefore, SPET scan may be proposed as the unique approach to study IBD with this tracer, thus reducing the imaging time.

An effect of steroid treatment in addition cannot be excluded, even if there is no agreement in the literature that steroids can decrease the accuracy of the leukocyte scintigraphy (14).

In the same way, the number of false positive segments tends to increase in late scans and is more pronounced with SPET. There is not complete agreement about this aspect. In fact, some claim the absence of non-specific bowel uptake even in the late scan (4,5), while others (15,16) noted late low-intensity uptake located mainly in the ileocaecal region and ascending colon. In our experience (pts. without IBD in whom the abdomen was included in the SPET view) , there is no significant non-specific uptake in the early SPET study as well as in the late planar scan. In this IBD pts group false +ve were recognized by SPET only in three UC pts (2 inactive and 1 active case): 4 caecum/ascending, 3 transverse and 2 descending, therefore without a significant trend of location, but in the active case contiguous to an involved segment. Therefore it is not possible to exclude that this uptake might represent some degree of inflammation missed by the endoscopy.

Another element that can reduce the test accuracy is the difficulty to relate exactly the segment localization of an endoscopically and histologically observed inflammation with the scintigraphic location, thus contributing to a reduced concordance between endoscopy and scan results (14). When accuracy assesment is based on individual patients, however, the results obtained in the CD group are satisfactory, allowing to reach diagnosis in all patients. From the clinical point of view this aspect is most important, because in CD pts initial symptoms are frequently non specific and lead to a diagnostic delay of several years; in addition, the lesions are discontinous thus rendering the endoscopic assessement more difficult (1).

When comparing the antigranulocyte approach with the HMPAO labelled leukocytes (7,8,17), the accuracy of the results seems to be higher employing the in vitro approach. Our results, however, seem to demonstrate that the use of the Mab in association with early SPET scan offers acceptable diagnostic accuracy in children in whom the in vitro technique may be unquestionably more difficult and sometimes impracticable due to the large amount of blood required.

REFERENCES

1. Kipper SL. Radiolabeled leukocyte imaging of the abdomen. In: Nuclear Medicine Annual 1995. Freeman LM,ed. New York: Raven Press,1995:81-128.
2. Charron M,Orenstein SR,Bhargava S. Detection of inflammatory bowel disease in pediatric patients with technetium-99m-HMPAO-labeled leukocytes. J Nucl Med 1994;35:451-455
3. Shah DB,Cosgrove M,Rees JI,Jenkins HR. The technetium white cell scan as an initial imaging investigation for evaluating suspected childhood inflammatory bowel disease. J Pediatr Gastroenterol Nutr 1997;25:524-528.
4. Joseph K,Hoffken H,Bosslet K,Schorlemmer HU. In vivo labelling of granulocytes with 99mTc anti-NCA monoclonal antibodies for imaging inflammation. Eur J Nucl Med 1988;14:367-373.
5. Mahida YR,Perkins AC,Frier M,Wasie ML,Hawkey CJ. Monoclonal antigranulocyte antibody imaging in inflammatory bowel disease:a preliminary report. Nucl Med Commun 1992;13:330-335.
6. Steinstrasser A, Oberhausen E. Granulocyte labelling kit BW 250/183.Results of the European Multicenter Trial. Nucl- Med 1996;35:1-11
7. Segarra I,Roca M,Baliellas C et al. Granulocyte-specific monoclonal antibody technetium-99m-BW 250/183 and indium-111 oxine-labelled leucocyte scintigraphy in inflammatory bowel disease. Eur J Nucl Med 1991;18:715-719
8. Almers S,Granerus G,Franzen L,Strom M. technetium-99m scintigraphy: more accurate assesment of ulcerative colitis with exametazime-labelled leucocytes than with antigranulocyte antibodies. Eur J Nucl Med 1996;23:247-255
9. Hyams JS,Ferry GD,Mandel FS et al. Development and validation of a pediatric Crohn's disease activity index. J Pediatr Gastroenterol Nutr 1991;12:439-447
10. Rachmilewitz D. Coated mesalazine (5-aminosalycilic acid) versus sulphasalazine in the treatment of active ulcerative colitis: a randomized trial. B M J 1989:298:82-86.
11. Becker WS,Saptogino A,Wolf FG. The single late 99mTc granulocyte antibody scan in inflammatory diseases:a preliminary report. Nucl Med Commun 1992;13:186-192.
12. Kroiss A,Weiss W,Auinger C et al. Immunoscintigraphy (IS) with I-123 and Tc-99m labeled granulocytes antibody (Ab) in patient with inflammatory bowel diseases. Prog Clin Biol Res 1990;31:319-325
13. Aprile C, Saponaro R,Cannizzaro G. Leserbriefe. Nucl-Med 1996;35: (65)
14. Almer S,Franzen L,Peters AM et al. Do technetium-99m hexamethylpropylene amino oxime-labeled leukocytes truly reflect the mucosal inflammation in patients with ulcerative colitis?. Scand J Gastroenterol 1992;27:1031-1038.
15. Ivancevic V,Munz DL. Non specific bowel activity in 99mTc-labelled monoclonal anti-granulocyte antibody imaging.Nuc Med Commun 1992;13:899-900
16. Ivancevic V, Schworer H,Sandrock D et al. Falsely negative 99mTc-Antigranulocyte immunoscintigraphy and positive 99mTc-HMPAO-labelled leukocyte scan in active Crohn's disease. Nucl- Med 1995;34:248-251.
17. Papos M,Nagy F,Narai Gy et al. Immunoscintigraphy (IS) with antigranulocyte monoclonal antibody and HMPAO-labeled white blood cell scintigraphy (WBS) in inflammatory bowel disease (IBD).Eur J Nucl Med 1993;20:938 (abst).

PHYSICS, RADIATION PROTECTION

Radioactive Isotopes in
Clinical Medicine and Research XXIII
ed. by H. Bergmann, H. Köhn and H. Sinzinger

ATTENUATION CORRECTION IN PET USING CS-137 SINGLES TRANSMISSION AND ITERATIVE RECONSTRUCTION.

Gerd Muehllehner[1], Eugene Gualtieri[1], Joel S. Karp[2] and Robin J. Smith[2]

UGM Medical Systems[1] and University of Pennsylvania[2], Philadelphia, PA, USA

SUMMARY: Attenuation correction in PET using a coincidence method typically leads to 10-20 minute acquisition time per axial bed position in order to obtain adequate counts. This makes it impractical for whole body tumor surveys requiring 7-12 axial positions in a typical dedicated PET scanner. In order to reduce the acquisition time we employ a Cs-137 point source in singles mode (gamma ray energy 662 keV).

Performing a transmission scan in 75 seconds in singles mode allows us to collect adequate count density to obtain good quality transmission images. By using an iterative reconstruction for both the transmission and the emission scans, streak artifacts usually associated with attenuation corrected images can be avoided.

Contrary to results reported by others, we find that attenuation corrected images not only allow accurate quantitation, but significantly enhance the visual interpretation of PET scans.

INTRODUCTION

Post injection coincidence transmission has been implemented in PET cameras both with septa (1,2) and those operating without septa (3). Typical transmission scan durations are 10-15 minutes per axial position (2) although a system without septa uses a much lower activity source. Thus quantitative whole body imaging of the whole human torso may consist of 60 minutes of emission imaging followed by 60 minutes of transmission scanning to acquire sufficient counts for low noise attenuation correction. The use of a singles transmission source for PET has recently been investigated (4,5) to use the high singles gamma ray flux for short duration, high count density scans. This paper reports on the practical implementation of post-injection singles transmission in PET. To do this a ^{137}Cs point source emitting 662 keV gamma rays is used. These singles transmission scans have two major advantages over coincidence transmission: (1) singles countrates are typically 10-20 times coincidence countrates, since only single gamma rays are detected in the crystals opposite the transmission source, and (2) since the transmission source produces 662 keV gamma rays and emission activity produces 511 keV gamma rays, a different transmission energy window can be used to suppress emission contamination due to the good energy resolution of NaI(Tl).

Several practical problems have to be addressed with post-injection singles transmission. Since 662 keV gamma rays are being used for transmission scanning, measured attenuation coefficients will be 10% lower than for the 511 keV gamma rays of emission data. Also, the scatter and emission background are potential problems, even with a higher energy window, since it is not possible to apply a collinearity gate as is done in coincidence transmission. The magnitude and significance of these effects have been studied as well as several methods to correct them (6).

Combining the use of singles transmission scanning with fast iterative reconstruction using the OSEM (Ordered Subset, Estimation Maximization) reconstruction (7,8) results in attenuation corrected emission scans which avoid many of the problems, such as streak artifacts and increased noise, usually associated with attenuation correction in PET.

METHOD

The camera used for all of these studies is the volume imaging PENN PET 240H camera (marketed by GE under the name Quest). This consists of 6 large NaI(Tl) detectors (50 x 20 x 2.5 cm) in a hexagonal arrangement. The camera has an active 12.8 cm axial and 51.2 cm diameter transaxial FOV (9,10).

Singles transmission scans are performed by rotating a 6 mCi ^{137}Cs point source (30 y half-life) at a radius of 37 cm and at the center of the axial FOV. The source is shielded from the near detector by a 1 cm block of lead, to reduce light buildup in the near crystal, and rotates around the patient at about 1 revolution/minute. The energy window for the transmission scan is set as high as possible (625-800 keV) to suppress contamination of the scan by 511 keV emission gamma rays. Lines of response are constructed from the detected gamma ray position and the known source position, and the axial slice location is determined from the weighted average of these two positions. The bed position is displaced 5.6 cm between transmission scans to maintain uniform axial sensitivity. Following photopeak energy gating, singles transmission countrates are typically 180 kcps compared to coincidence transmission countrates of 35 kcps in the PENN PET 240H scanner. A single rotation of the point source results in approx. 1.5 Mcts/slice.

Accelerated maximum likelihood (OS-EM) reconstruction (7,8), with 2 or 4 iterations and 8 ordered subsets, of both the transmission and emission data improves image quality and avoids filtered back projection reconstruction artifacts from lower count density data. This reconstruction method is used for all clinical studies.

To use singles transmission scans performed post-injection for quantitative attenuation correction in PET one needs to correct the measured transmission data for emission spillover, scatter, and the lower attenuation coefficients for 662 keV versus 511 keV gamma rays. In order to subtract the emission contamination in the singles transmission scan, a short emission contamination (EC) scan is performed. This is a transmission scan with all appropriate settings but without a transmission source, and measures the emission contamination directly. Since the emission contamination of a singles transmission scan has a relatively uniform spatial distribution (6) a short EC scan (8 seconds/axial position) may be performed and smoothed for subtraction. The transmission scan minus the EC scan is then scaled in order to correct for the different attenuation coefficients for 662 versus 511 keV gamma rays and for the residual scatter in the singles transmission scan. The corrected transmission image is then forward projected for attenuation correction of the emission data.

RESULTS

Figure 1 demonstrates the benefit of iteratively reconstructing both the emission data and the transmission data using transverse section data from a cardiac FDG scan. Without attenuation correction the data collected from different angles are inconsistent, since usually the attenuation in the anterior-posterior direction is significantly less than in the left-right direction. Both the filtered backprojection as well as the iteratively reconstructed images (Left top row and left bottom row respectively) show non-uniform uptake in the myocardial wall and lack of demarcation between the lung, which typically has very low glucose metabolism, and the surrounding tissue.

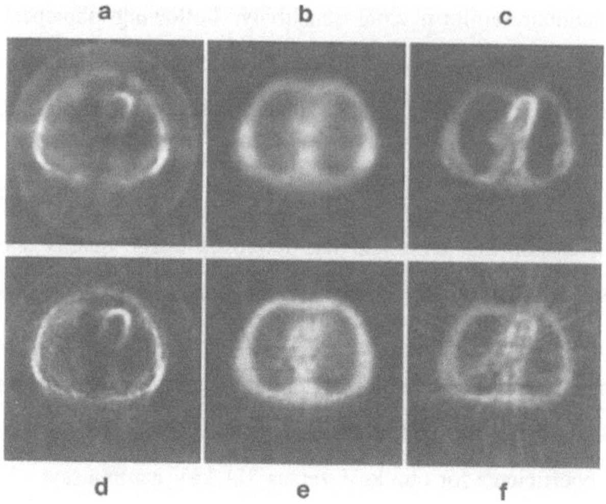

Fig. 1: a) Iteratively reconstructed emission image without attenuation correction

b) Iteratively reconstructed transmission image

c) Iteratively reconstructed emission image with attenuation correction

d) Filtered backprojection emission image without attenuation correction

e) Filtered backprojection transmission image

f) Filtered backprojection emission image with attenuation correction

While the transmission image itself appears actually to be better defined in the filtered backprojection reconstruction (e) compared to the iteratively reconstructed image (b), the sharply reduced statistical noise in the iteratively reconstructed transmission scan allows the final emission scan to be reconstructed with improved image quality. The iteratively reconstructed image with attenuation correction (c) shows uniform uptake in the cardiac wall and clear delineation between the tissue and lung without the streak artifacts normally seen in filtered backprojection images, specially after attenuation correction (f).

Figure 2 compares coronal images in a cancer patient using iterative reconstruction and the Cs-137 singles transmission scan (top row) with the non-attenuation corrected emission image reconstructed with a filtered backprojection algorithm. The images in the bottom row show several artifacts due to overlying breast tissue (horizontal bands) and areas of low intensity located laterally next to several tumors, particularly larger ones with high FDG uptake. The clear delineation of the lung regions with attenuation correction aids in describing the location of the tumors. It should be noted that even small areas of increased uptake are already visible in the images without attenuation correction; however, the confidence in identifying and localizing abnormalities is clearly improved with attenuation correction and iterative reconstruction.

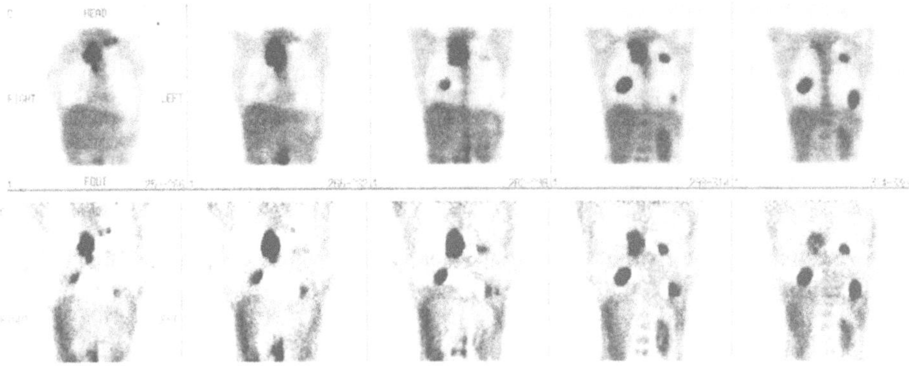

Fig. 2: The same patient data are reconstructed with singles attenuation correction and iterative reconstruction (top row) and compared to non-attenuation corrected images obtained with a filtered backprojection algorithm (bottom row).

CONCLUSION AND DISCUSSION

Singles transmission scans performed post-injection have been implemented in a septaless PET scanner using a point source of Cs-137. These provide low noise attenuation correction using one minute/axial position scans. In order to achieve high quality, quantitatively accurate results both scatter and emission contamination must be minimized and the remaining contamination must be subtracted. Both scatter and emission contamination can be reduced by applying tight energy gates to the transmission data and by optimizing the effective energy resolution at all countrates to discriminate between 511 and 662 keV gamma-rays. The application of narrow energy gates results in emission contamination of less than 25% and a scatter fraction of less than 15% due to the good energy resolution of NaI(Tl) of approximately 12% under clinical conditions.

Combining fast, singles transmission scanning with iterative reconstruction improves image quality by eliminating attenuation artifacts as well as streaks in the images.

REFERENCES

1. Daube-Witherspoon ME, Carson RE and Green MV: Post-Injection Transmission Attenuation Measurements for PET. IEEE Trans Nucl Sci 1988; 35: 757-761.

2. Thompson CJ, Ranger NT et al: Simultaneous Transmission and Emission Scans in Positron Emission Tomography. IEEE Trans Nucl Sci 1989; 36: 1011-1016.

3. Smith RJ, Karp JS and Muehllehner G: Post Injection Transmission Scanning in a Volume Imaging PET Camera. IEEE Trans Nucl Sci 1994; 41: 1526-1531.

4. Karp JS. Muehllehner G, Qu H and Yan X-H: Singles Transmission in Volume Imaging PET with a ^{137}Cs source. Phys Med Biol 1995; 40: 929-944.

5. de Kemp RA and Nahmias C: Attenuation Correction in PET using Single Photon Transmission Measurements. Med Phys. 1994; 21: 771-778.

6. Smith, R. J, Karp, J. S, Muehllehner, G, Gualtieri, E and Benard, F: Singles Transmission Scans Performed Post-Injection for Quantitative Whole Body PET Imaging. IEEE Trans Nucl Sci 1997; 44(3), 1329-1335.

7. Hudson HM and Larkin RS: Accelerated Image Reconstruction Using Ordered Subsets of Projection Data. IEEE Trans Med Imag 1994; 13: 601-609.

8. Meikle SR, Hutton BF et al: Accelerated EM reconstruction in total body PET: potential for improving tumor detectability. Phys Med Biol 1994; 39: 1689-1704.

9. Karp JS, Muehllehner G, Mankoff DA et al: Continuous slice PENN-PET: a positron tomograph with volume imaging capability. Journal of Nuclear Medicine 1990; 31: 617-627.

10. Karp JS, Kinahan PE, Muehllehner G: Effect of increased axial field of view on the performance of a volume PET scanner. IEEE Trans Med Imag 1993; 12: 299-306.

Radioactive Isotopes in
Clinical Medicine and Research XXIII
ed. by H. Bergmann, H. Köhn and H. Sinzinger

OPTIMIZATION OF ACQUISITION PROTOCOLS BASED ON 18F-FDG PHANTOM STUDIES USING A DUAL HEAD SPECT CAMERA IN COINCIDENCE MODE

Zaknun John, Oberladstätter Michael, Wenger Martin

University Clinic of Nuclear Medicine, University Hospital. A-6020 Innsbruck, AUSTRIA

Summary : using different phantoms with variation of energy window parameters and reconstruction algorithms, various variables related to the performance of a dual head PET camera were better characterized. As a result acquisition protocols using stringent energy window settings for brain imaging with 18F-FDG with improved image quality along with fine tuning of patient injected dose for optimal acquisition were defined. Furthermore the characterization of camera performance with regard to the detection of small hot and cold lesions, scattering problems and other pitfalls contributed to a better interpretation of clinical data.

Materials and Methods

Applying different energy windows width (10-30%) in a Photopeack-to-photopeack acquisition mode (PP) with or without Compton-photopeak (PC) set to 30 % width. The following phantoms were investigated.

1. A Jaszczak-phantom of 19.5x19cm (diameter x height, volume 5.6l) with different inserts; a. 3 cylinders with a diameter of 5 cm each filled either with water or consisting of Teflon to simulate bony structures. Target to background ratios (T/B) ranged from 0-8. b. "Hot" spheres phantom, consisted of 6 hot balls with their centers aligned along a circle 6cm deep (relative to the edge). Diameter of the spheres were 10,13, 17, 22, 28 and 37mm. The T/B-ratio as measured by Gamma counter was 4:1. Total phantom activity by start was 41MBq of 18FDG. c. The Plexiglas cold rods phantom insert (Data Spectrum standard 6250) consisted of 6 triangular regions. The diameters of the cold rods within each region were 9.5, 11.1, 12.7, 15.9, 19 and 25.5 mm. This insert was embedded in a 21.5 x 19 cm (diameter x height, volume 7.1l) cylinder. Total activity by start was 18.2MBq 18FDG. Studies of the 2D-Hofman brain phantom in air using coincidence mode detection were acquired with an activity concentration of 37kBq/ml. The quality of the reconstructed images applying filtered back projection (FBP) were compared to a planar image using 99mTc with a high resolution collimator while the phantom disk laying immediately on top of the collimator.

All cylinder studies except these with the Hofman phantom were acquired using a 23.3 cm radius of rotation. In the Hofman phantom the radius was 20.7cm. The ratios of activity in different compartments was calculated by counting aliquots in a gamma well counter. These ratios were compared to ratios derived from ROIs. The range of activity concentration in different compartments at start was 2-55kBq/ml. In all experiments total activity of the phantoms at start did not exceed 62MBq. The shifting of the PP position from its original location was monitored on the pulse-height analyzer (PHA) screen at immediately before and at the end of different patient studies.

Results

Estimation of target to background activity concentration 5 cm cylinders:

Table 1 summarizes the effect of variation of photopeak width and compton window on estimating T/B activity ratio and magnitude of contrast enhancement.

The nearest estimation of the hot/background activity-ratio was achieved by applying a narrow PP window and inhibition of photopeak-compton option (true 3.6 vs. 3.51 measured, 97.5%). Operating with only a 30% PP gave also very good results (~95% precision).

The ratio derived from cold/background activity (cylinder filled with water) indicates the magnitude of activity spill-over. This ratio increases by 26% for PP of 30% compared to 15% PP. However a significant increase of almost 90% is found when PC is activated. This suggests that the main increase is due to scattered events. Improving activity estimation or image contrast is associated with significant loss of events. This loss could be compensated by increasing acquisition time, however not always by increasing patient dose due to system saturation. Similar results as shown in table 1 were achieved for T/B ratios of 2.3 and 4.5. A significant underestimation of T/B ratio recovery (55-70%) was calculated for a target value of 8. More over one of the cylinder inserts, made of Teflon (5 cm φ), could not be visualized as a cold circle mainly due to significant scattering !. Clinically this phenomenon was observed in patients unable to empty the bladder resulting in a "hot" sacrum due to scatter. This phenomenon may cause difficulties to interpret findings in patients referred due to rectum carcinoma.

The images in figure 1 show two contiguous transaxial slices at the central level of the 6 spheres phantom. The pair of slices in the first raw was acquired using 15% PP and PC off, those in the second raw with 30% PP and PC on. The smallest sphere with 10 mm diameter was seen in none of the combinations 15%, 20% 30% with PC off nor with 30% PP and PC on. The next sphere with a 13 mm diameter could only be visualized applying 15% PP and PC off.

Enhancing image Contrast :

As suggested by the experiments involving 5cm cylinders, image contrast can be improved by inhibiting PC-acquisition. Furthermore this observation was supported by the fact that variation of PP width did not effect image quality of the 2D Hofman brain phantom *in air*. For further investigation a phantom study using cold rods (smaller structures) was done. Representative slices of the phantom applying 15% PP with PP of vs. 30% PP and PC on are shown in figure 2. The 9.5 , 11.1 and 12.7 mm rods are better identified with 15% PP. Due to lower total study counts (for equal effective acquisition time in both studies) images with 15% PP appear somewhat noisy due to significant loss of counts.

Discussion

The presented data support the notion that scatter correction can be implemented at the photon energy level when operating a NaI(Tl) crystal system which has in comparison to the BGO crystals a significantly higher energy resolution. Accuracy of activity concentration estimation in studies using photopeak/photopeak (PP)- and photopeak/Compton (PC)-coincidences is better with narrow photopeak windows. A further improvement is achieved when PC-coincidences are inhibited (PC-off). This effect is more pronounced with phantoms of larger volumes.

Photopeak shift: Observing the behavior of the PHA, we registered during clinical patient studies a down-shift in the PHA spectrum of 10 and up to 14 keV. This phenomenon may lead to significant reduction in count rates due to a gradual shift of the preset energy window to seemingly higher energy regions of the spectrum. The magnitude of the drift is related to the change over time in the intensity of photon flux. This phenomenon may be relevant for longer studies as for whole body scans where changes in the photon flux intensity may occur when moving from chest to pelvis acquisition or vise versa. By laying the patient on the acquisition table thus exposing the system to the expected photon flux (same radius of acquisition) the initial drift of energy spectrum stabilizes within ~5-7 min.

Conclusion

The accuracy of activity concentration estimation in studies using photopeak/photopeak (PP)- and photopeak/Compton (PC)-coincidences is better with narrow photopeak energy window. A further improvement is achieved when PC-coincidences are inhibited (PC-off). This effect is more pronounced with phantoms of larger volumes. Regarding detection of small hot lesions system performance improved only when applying a narrow energy window (15% PP) and inhibition of PC. The visualization of 13 mm hot spheres in water at a target to background ratio of 4:1 is then possible. Smaller cold structures also are better visualized with 15% PP window and PC-off. This indicates that mainly scattered events are responsible for loss in contrast when studying large and bulky phantoms. For clinical studies one must however take into account the significant loss in count statistics which may otherwise increase image noise. Special attention must be applied to the possibility of a drift of energy spectrum which is more pronounced if a study with high singles count rates is immediately started before allowing the system to stabilize. Based on this data, 18-FDG brain studies for epilepsy are currently acquired using an 20% window over the PP and inhibition of the PC. To compensate for the resulting loss of events, acquisition is started at singles-count-rates of $1,3x10^6$ just below the threshold for pearl-string artifacts. This is reached by adjusting individual patient injected dose calculated in a weight-dependent fashion according to the formula; Activity [mCi] = 0.05xBW[Kg] + 1.2. For different camera versions, slight correction of K (0.9-1.5) may be needed. Readjusting the window position over the PP is mandatory prior to each acquisition start.

1 . . . . ADAC VERTEX plus EPIC/MCD

Table 1 : 2 cylinders of 5 cm in diameter placed in a Jaszczak cylinder were filled with water. The T/B ratios were zero and 3.6. Total phantom activity at start was 30MBq. Acquisition and reconstruction parameters were: matrix 128x128, zoom factor 1.57. FBP reconstruction after ribinning applying Wiener filter 0.75, average slices 5, attenuation coefficient 0.095/cm and non-uniform scatter correction. Rectangular regions were drawn over the hot and cold cylinders and 2 ROIs for background estimation placed close to and distant from the hot cylinder.

Start time min	Azimuth sec	Coinc./s $x10^3$	Avg. singles $x10^6$	Total events $x10^6$	PP %	PC	T/B hot	T/B cold	Avg.T/B (% recov.)	Cold/B
0	50	13.9	0.82	35.2	30	On	3.29	2.9	3.08 (85)	0.42
38	56	6.3	0.67	17.8	30	Off	3.72	3.14	3.41 (94.7)	0.29
78	63	6.0	0.56	10.7	15	Off	3.99	3.13	3.51 (97.5)	0.23

Fig 1. : Images in the first and second raw are contiguous 2.8 mm transaxial slices at the central level of the 6 spheres phantom described in methods. Data in the first raw were acquired with a 15% photopeak-photopeak energy window and inhibition of photopeak-Compton option, while data in the second raw were acquired with 30% PP and PC on. Average slices was set to 3 otherwise data reconstruction was a described in table 1. At a T/B ratio of 4:1 stringent energy window settings lead to a significant improvement in detecting hot lesions (13 mm sphere) .

Fig. 2 :The cold rods phantom is described in methods. Total phantom activity at start was 18.38 MBq 18FDG (3 kBq /ml). The effective acquisition time was comparable for both studies, starting with 45 sec/azimuth. Acquisition radius 23.2, zoom 1.57 , matrix 128x128. Reconstruction: using FBP with butterworth filter, cutoff 0.68, order 5, attenuation coefficient 0.095/cm and non uniform scatter compensation. Total events were 25.8 $x10^6$ for the study with 15% photopeak and inhibition of the photopeak-Compton option (left) vs. 75.8$x10^6$ applying 30% PP and PC-on (right). Note that the contrast enhancement achieved by applying a narrow photopeak is accompanied by increased image noise.

FnBadg2.doc

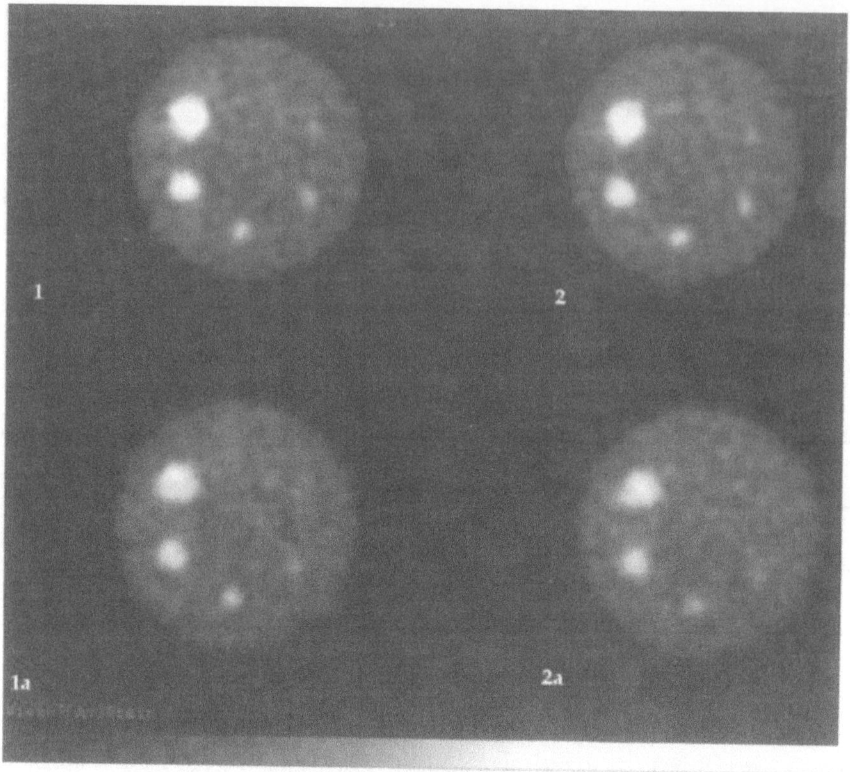
1
2
1a
2a

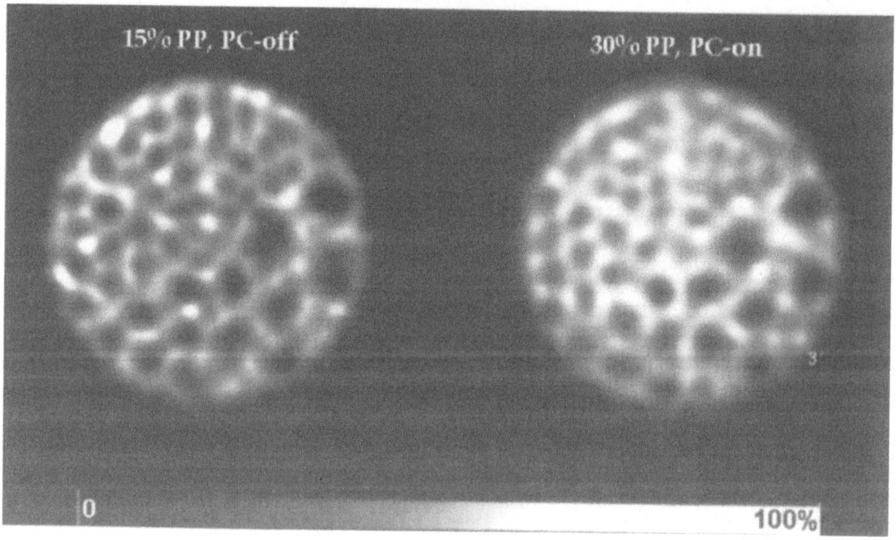
15% PP, PC-off
30% PP, PC-on
3
0
100%

Radioactive Isotopes in
Clinical Medicine and Research XXIII
ed. by H. Bergmann, H. Köhn and H. Sinzinger

RADIATION PROTECTION IN I-131-LIPIODOL THERAPY IN LIVER NEOPLASMS

Risse JH, Grünwald F, Ponath C and Biersack HJ.

Nuclear Medicine Dep., University of Bonn,
Sigmund-Freud-Str. 25, D - 53105 Bonn

SUMMARY: Radiation doses (RD) to fingers, eyes, and whole body of the medical staff during 17 angiographic applications of I-131-Lipiodol in 11 patients with liver malignancies were assessed. An automatic injector reduced the high finger dose of 20 mSv / application to 5 mSv but yielded contamination problems. A new developed special container reduced the finger RD to < 10 μSv. Additional radiation protection equipment resulted in a significant dose reduction to the eyes from 90 μSv to < 5 μSv and to the whole body from 120 μSv to 20 μSv.

INTRODUCTION

One of the most common malignant tumors worldwide is primary liver cancer (1). Surgical resection may lead to long-term survival, but the resectability rate in HCC may be as low as 1 % (2). Non-surgical regional therapy like transarterial chemoembolisation (TACE) or percutaneous ethanol injection (PEI) have shown some effect but have several limitations (3, 4). Intraarterial (i.a.) iodine-131-Lipiodol has been shown to be effective in HCC (5). In contrast to TACE, I-131-Lipiodol therapy is also suitable in portal vein thrombosis (6). Since many HCC patients initially present with portal vein thrombosis and multinodular disease, the treatment with I-131-Lipiodol may primarily be the only regional therapy option. Nevertheless, no experience with intraarterial I-131-Lipiodol has been reported from Germany or Middle Europe yet.

Besides introducing the therapy in Germany we wanted to assess the radiation doses to the medical staff during and after angiography-guided i.a. application of I-131-Lipiodol; because of the first measurement results showing high values particularly for the fingers, we started to develop a special radiation protection equipment.

MATERIALS AND METHODS

11 patients with liver malignancies were treated by 17 selective intraarterial (i.a.) administrations of I-131-labeled Lipiodol (Lipiocis[R]) during hepatic angiography via the femoral artery.

The mean administered I-131 dose was 45.4 ± 5.6 mCi (1680 ± 207 MBq) with a range from 30 - 52 mCi (1110 - 1924 MBq). For radiation protection reasons the patients had an 8 days hospital stay each time.

Preparation and application of Lipiocis[R] were initially performed as usual: A wolfram shielded syringe containing the nuclide is transported to the angiography room in a syringe carrier (3 mm pb shield). At the angiography site, the syringe is manually connected to the angiography catheter and injection is performed in 3 minutes. The catheter is cleaned by a new saline filled syringe. After catheter withdrawal, the femoral artery is compressed until coagulation at the puncture site is sufficient, taking 8 - 20 minutes. The final dressing takes another 5 minutes.

This procedure was performed in the first two patients (same day). Because of the high radiation load to the medical staff combined with contamination problems it was changed.

An automatic injector (Perfusor[R] M1, B. Braun) with an infusion rate of 2 ml in 3 minutes was used for the next three applications. The procedure is the same as described above except that the nuclide filled syringe is not injected manually. But other problems occured.

Finally, a new device was developed which should enable the medical staff to transport and to inject the radionuclide without high radiation loads or contamination problems. This construction represents a lead shielded container with an unhinged lead lid and 2 narrow outlet canals in the upper wall surface of the main container. The outlet canals are angled so that no radiation from inside the container can leave. A saline filled tube in the container with the tube ends laying in the outlet canals is filled with the radionuclide; another saline filled tube is connected to the contaminated end of the first tube and this connection site is also put into the container. Thus the container provides complete radiation protection from the radionuclide inside, allowing transport and injection of the nuclide inside without further manual handling of a „hot" syringe. Furthermore, the injection may be performed from a great distance using a long tube between the applying physician and the container tubes. Hence, there is virtually no radiation load to the staff during the application when the radioactivity leaves the container. The patent is pending.

Additionally, we use further equipment to protect the staff from the radiation coming from the patient´s liver after the injection. A mobile lead wall (50 mm pb) is positioned between patient and physician. After withdrawal of the catheter we put a lead cover (1 mm pb) on the patient´s abdomen, leading to a radiation reduction of about 30 %. During the femoral artery compression the physician sits behind the lead wall trying to hide his eyes whenever possible.

Radiation doses (RD) to the fingers, eyes, and whole body during injection and postangiography patient care were determined. For fingers and eyes RD were calculated from measurements of the integrals of the surface dose rate. The whole body RD was taken from measurements of the surface dose in µSv at the level of the upper thorax.

RESULTS

The finger dose during the injection of I-131-lipiodol as described in the initial procedure was calculated from a 2 ml syringe with 60 mCi (2,22 GBq) I-131, wolfram shielded, mean distance of the radionuclide to the fingers 10 mm, injection time 3 minutes, and yielded 19.5 mSv per application. The whole body dose including postangiographic patient care, i.e. femoral artery compression, dressing etc. with a total exposure time of 25 minutes, distance to patient´s liver 50 cm, and 30 % dose reduction in the patient was calculated to be 60 µSv per application.

In contrast, the whole body measurements during the first two applications yielded 108 and 119 µSv, respectively. From these values, total eye RD was estimated to be about 130 µSv (90 µSv during injection and 40 µSv thereafter) because the eyes were always exposed whereas the surface measurement did not get the radiation exposure when sitting behind the mobile lead wall. Additionally, the manual handling of the nuclide filled syringe (52 and 50 mCi (1850 and 1924 MBq), respectively) including syringe exchange took more than 3 minutes in total. During syringe exchange there was in one case some contamination of the underlying coverings which had to be removed completely. After the procedures, the hands of the involved staff were severely contaminated despite wearing sterile gloves. The total finger radiation dose was estimated to be about 25 mSv for each of these first applications.

The automatic injector was used to reduce at least the finger RD. The syringe handling time with the injector was ½ to 1 minute, giving a finger dose of about 5 mSv per application, i.e. a reduction of 75 %. On the other hand, the injector yielded handling problems: only 10 ml syringes fit herein, and it is difficult to handle 2 ml of an oily and viscous substance in such a big syringe. Additionally, a three-way stopcock does not fit to the syringe inside the injector. Finally, the syringe exchange is more complicated. These handling problems resulted in contamination of the injector in all three application procedures.

The last 12 application procedures were performed with the new developed transport and application container allowing transport and injection of the nuclide without further manual handling, thus resulting in virtually no more radiation to the fingers (< 10 μSv) and eyes (< 5 μSv). The injection is performed from a great distance to the patient (3-4 m), thus avoiding radiation exposure when the radionuclide leaves the container. The lack of manual handling resulted in the elimination of contamination possibilities.

During the postangiographic patient care the total eye RD could be reduced to 13 μSv by having the eyes behind the mobile lead wall as much as possible; the abdominal lead cover reduced the radiation to the eyes when looking at the puncture site. Thus eye RD during femoral artery compression was about 3 μSv; making the dressing yields about 10 μSv. The radiation load to the fingers is unavoidably 120 μSv because the fingers are not protected by this equipment.

The whole body measurements in the last 12 applications showed mean values of 20 μSv with a range of 14 - 26 μSv per application, compared to 108 and 119 μSv in the first two procedures.

DISCUSSION

I-131-Lipiodol therapy for HCC has been investigated for safety and effectiveness in previous studies (5-11). But, to our knowledge, there is no published measurement of the radiation load to the medical staff, particularly to the applying physician. In this study, we found a high radiation load particularly to the fingers (as high as 25 mSv), but also to the eyes and whole body when performing the procedure under usual conditions. The i.a. I-131-Lipiodol therapy had not been introduced in Germany or Middle Europe before. Several reasons may be responsible for this lack of use of a liver cancer therapy option. Besides others, there are rigid radiation protection laws in these countries and the injection procedure itself carries a risk for the medical staff as shown by our investigation. The oily substance seems to penetrate the sterile gloves. In our experience, the resulting hand contamination is difficult to remove.

We tried to ameliorate the situation by using an automatic injector. It was chosen after we had made laboratory experiments with several types of injectors. But in the real angiography situation the injector yielded other problems with syringe handling and contamination so that we were forced to change the procedure again.

The development of the new transport and application container solved the problems generated by the manual syringe handling. First, the manual syringe handling outside the „hot" preparation room in the nuclear medicine department is completely eliminated. The radioactivity does not leave the container until it is applied to the patient. Second, the hot syringe is shielded by a real thick lead container. Third, the device allows application from a long distance, thereby reducing the radiation load to the applying physician when the radioactivity leaves the container; and last but not least it reduces the risk of contamination. Together with the mobile lead wall and the abdominal lead cover we achieved a significant reduction of the radiation load to the medical staff. The new developed container will work for all liquid radionuclides including those with high viscosity and high activity.

In many instances people without nuclear medicine knowledge have fear of open radionuclide handling, even the medical staff who does not belong to a nuclear medicine department. As members of this department we are faced to such radiation fears daily; this was also true for the recently introduced i.a. I-131-lipiodol therapy. With the presented equipment we could already reduce, besides the radiation doses, the fears of the medical staff of other departments at our university hospital, and we believe that in general the compliance for such procedures should improve.

REFERENCES

1. London W. Primary hepatocellular carcinoma - etiology, pathogenesis and prevention. Hum Pathol 1981; 12: 1085-1097.

2. Maraj R, Kew MC, Hyslop RJ. Resectability rate of hepatocellular carcinoma in rural southern Africans. Br J Surg 1988; 75: 335-338.

3. Groupe d`étude et de traitement du carcinome hepatocellulaire. A comparison of Lipiodol chemoembolisation and conservative treatment for unresectable hepatocellular carcinoma. N Engl J Med 1995; 332: 1256-1261.

4. Livraghi T, Bolondi L, Lazzaroni S et al. Percutaneous ethanol injection in the treatment of hepatocellular carcinoma in cirrhosis: a study on 207 patients. Cancer 1992; 69: 925-929.

5. Bretagne JF, Raoul JL, Bourguet P et al. Hepatic artery injection of I-131-labeled Lipiodol. Part 2: Preliminary results of therapeutic use in patients with hepatocellular carcinoma and liver metastases. Radiology 1988; 168: 547-550.

6. Raoul JL, Guyader D, Bretagne JF et al. Randomized controlled trial for hepatocellular carcinoma with portal vein thrombosis: intra-arterial iodine-131-iodized oil versus medical support. J Nucl Med 1994; 35: 1782-1787.

7. Leung WT, Lau WY, Ho S et al. Selective internal radiation therapy with intra-arterial Iodine-131-Lipiodol in inoperable hepatocellular carcinoma. J Nucl Med 1994; 35: 1313-1318.

8. Novell R, Hilson A and Hobbs K. Ablation of recurrent primary liver cancer using ^{131}I-lipiodol. Postgrad Med J 1991; 67: 393-395.

9. Kobayashi H, Hidaka H, Kajiya Y et al. Treatment of hepatocellular carcinoma by transarterial injection of anticancer agents in iodized oil suspension or of radioactive iodized oil solution. Acta Radiol [Diagn] 1986; 27: 139-147.

10. Yoo HS, Lee JT, Kim KW et al. Nodular hepatocellular carcinoma. Treatment with subsegmental intraarterial injection of iodine-131-labeled oil. Cancer 1991; 68: 1878-1884.

11. Raoul JL, Bourguet P, Bretagne JF et al. Hepatic artery injection of I-131-labeled Lipiodol. Part 1: Biodistribution study results in patients with hepatocellular carcinoma and liver metastases. Radiology 1988; 168: 541-545.

Radioactive Isotopes in
Clinical Medicine and Research XXIII
ed. by H. Bergmann, H. Köhn and H. Sinzinger

RADIATION EXPOSURE DERIVING FROM PATIENTS TREATED WITH ^{165}Dy-FERRIC HYDROXIDE

Havlik E.[1,3], Karanikas G.[2], Pirich Ch.[2], Preitfellner J.[2], Schaffarich P.[1], Sinzinger H.[2]

[1] Department of Biomedical Engineering and Physics, University of Vienna, Austria
[2] Department of Nuclear Medicine, University of Vienna, Austria
[3] The Ludwig Boltzmann Institute of Nuclear Medicine, Austria

SUMMARY: In radiation synovectomy 1-10 GBq Dysprosium-165 ferric hydroxide is injected into the joints. To estimate the radiation exposure of persons in the neighbourhood of the patients measurements of the dose rates were performed in 5cm, 0.5m, 1m and 2m distance of the surface of the treated joints (knees) until 200 min after the application.
The highest doses were estimated for the fingers of the technologist (212 μSv) and for the physician (550 μSv). In order to reduce the doses we constructed special shieldings for the syrings. The whole body doses were 79 μSv for the technologist and 24 μSv for the physician. After the discharge to a ward or at home other persons in 1m distance from the patients can receive 72 μSv, which is 4.8% of the permissible dose.

INTRODUCTION

Radiation synovectomy is an alternative treatment of chronic synovitis. Dysprosium-165 ferric hydroxide (DFH) macroaggregates proved to be clinically effective (1). In connection with this treatment it is asked to what extent radiation protection precautions might be necessary. The aim of the recent study was to get quantitative information about the dose rates and the maximum achievable doses near the treated patients and to estimate the radiation exposure of the staff and of other persons.

^{165}Dy is an element belonging to the group of lanthanoids. In Table 1 physical data of the radionuclide are summarized. The mean penetration distance of the beta radiation is in the desired range, and the 95 keV-gamma rays are suitable for scintigraphy and for leakage control.

Table 1: *Physical data of dysprosium-165 (2), (3)*

Physical half-life: 2.33 h
Decay product: holmium-165 (stable)
Main beta transitions: 0.3 MeV (1.7%), 1.2 MeV (15%), 1.3 MeV (83%)
Mean beta energy: 0.44 MeV
Max. range in soft tissue: 5.7 mm, mean range in soft tissue: 1.0 mm
Main gamma transitions: 95 keV (4.0%), 361 keV (0.8%)
total: ≈0.08 gammas per disintegration
Gamma dose rate constant Γ: $2.8 \cdot 10^{-6}$ Gy·m²·GBq^{-1}·h^{-1}

PATIENTS AND METHOD

Some skill is necessary to inject the radioactive solution in the right site where it will not protrude from the capsule. One hour and 3 h after application of 1 to 10 GBq ^{165}Dy the joints - mainly the knees - were investigated and scintigraphies were performed.
In order to reduce the finger doses to technologists and physicians during preparation and application of the activity we constructed special shieldings for the syrings, combining 5.5mm perplex and 2mm lead. This shielding is absorbing completely the beta-rays and reducing 77% of the dose rate due to the gammas and bremsstrahlung on the surface.

Leakage control was performed either by blood sample measurements or by using a whole-body counter with activity profile device. The spatial resolution enables the detection of small amounts of activity outside the treated joint, like in lymph nodes or in the urinary bladder (4). Because of the short half-life of ^{165}Dy the patients were discharged from the nuclear medical department after 5 to 6 hours. The same time period is recommended for at-ease positioning of the treated joint.

Sixteen patients were included in the study. The dose rates were measured in a room with low background radiation, using a calibrated portable radiation detector (Berthold LB 133®). The measurements were performed at distances of 5cm, 0.5m, 1m and 2m from surface of the treated knees at 10 minutes, 40 min, 100 min and 200 min after the injection.

RESULTS

In Table 2 the initial values of the dose rates and the theoretically maximum doses in the neighbourhood of the patients - in four distances - are listed.

Table 2: *Initial dose rates and maximum achievable doses near patients treated with ^{165}Dy-DFH (mean±SEM, n=16)*

Distance (m)	$\dot{D}$ (μSv/h)	D_{max} (μSv)
0.05	3170 ±2950	12 990
0.5	119 ± 19	474
1	72 ± 18	271
2	10 ± 1,6	36,3

By integrating the time courses of the dose rates and fitting exponential functions the time courses of the doses, the maximum radiation doses as well as the doses for any time period near the patients - necessary for the following dose estimates - were calculated. Because of the practically lack of distribution of radioactivity the effective and physical half-lives are identical.

DISCUSSION

The presumptions made for the estimations of finger doses and whole-body doses are shown graphically in Figs. 1 and 2.

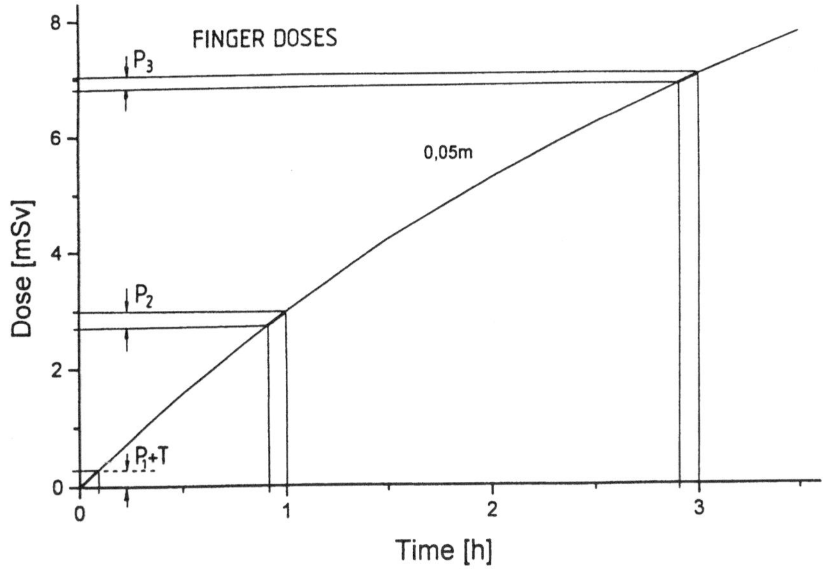

Fig. 1: *Finger doses, derived from the time course of the dose in 0.05m distance from the treated joint*

Finger doses: The physician and the assisting technologist are manipulating for 4 min during the time of application in an average distance of 5cm (indicated by P_1 respectively T in Fig.1). The physician then is investigating the treated knee before each scintigraphy - 1h and 3h after the injection - for another 5 min each (P_2 and P_3 in Fig.2). The results are: a dose of 550 μSv for the physician, which is 0.073% of the permissible dose of 750 mSv per year, and 212 μSv for the technologist respectively less than 0.03% of the permissible annual dose.

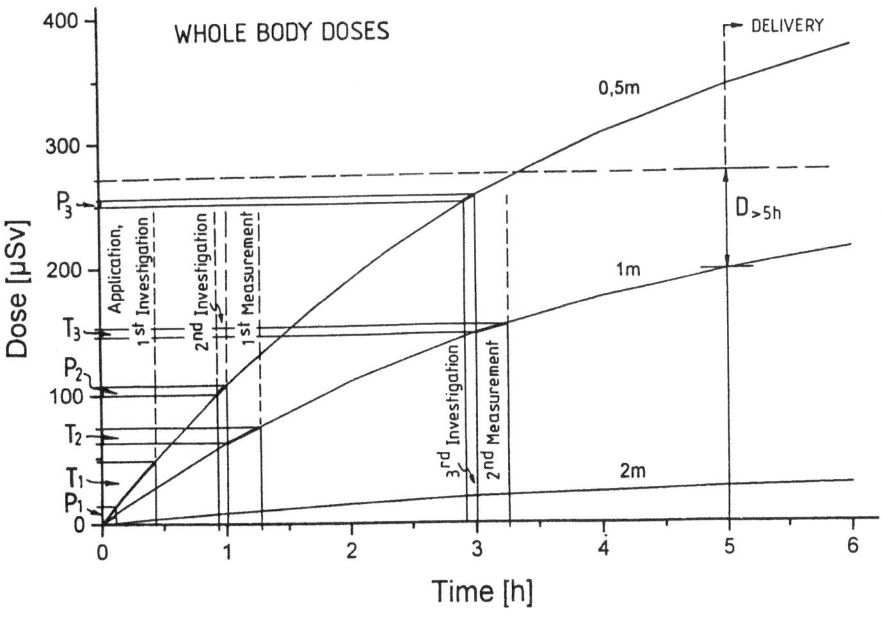

Fig. 2: *Whole-body doses, derived from the time courses of the doses in 0.5m and 1m from the treated joint*

Whole-body doses: The physician receives his dose three times for 6 min each in 0.5m distance from the joint (indicated by P_1, P_2 and P_3 in Fig.3). The technologist is taking care for the patient for the first 24 min in an average distance of 0.5m and then performing two measurements (14 min each) in 1m distance (T_1, T_2 and T_3 in Fig.3). The whole-body doses then are 24 μSv for the physician and 79 μSv for the technologist, corresponding to less than 0.05% and less than 0.16% of the permissible annual whole-body dose for radiation workers, respectively.

Table 3: *Doses due to radiation exposure near patients treated with ^{165}Dy-DFH (in brackets: percent of permissible annual doses)*

Group of persons	Finger doses	Whole-body doses
Physicians	550 μSv (0.073%)	4 μSv (0.048%)
Technologists	212 μSv (0.028%)	79 μSv (0.158%)
Other persons (after discharge of the patient)	-	72 μSv (4.8 %)

Doses to non-radiation workers: The patients are isolated from other patients or accompanying persons in a special resting room after the injection of ^{165}Dy-DFH, between the measurements, and before their delivery from the nuclear medicine department. They are in closer contact with other persons, at home or in a ward, at the earliest 5 h after the application. In 1m distance from the treated joint other persons may receive 72 μSv. That means 4.8% of the permissible annual dose for members of the general public, which in Austria - as well as in many other countries - is 1.5 mSv per year.

CONCLUSION

Our results demonstrate, that even under restrictive presumptions the radiation exposure of persons near patients after the administration of ^{165}Dy are far below the limit to members of the staff as well as to non-radiation workers set by radiation protection regulations. Attendances, family members, nurses and other patients and people in the neighbourhood of "radiating" patients can meet such situations about 20 times a year without receiving the maximum permissible dose. If, in accordance to a recommendation of the European Commission (5) the limit is decreased to 1 mSv per year, this figure of course will become accordingly lower.

REFERENCES

1. Hnatowich DJ, Kramer RI, Sledge CB, Noble J, Shortkoff S: Dysprosium-165 ferric hydroxide macroaggregates for radiation synovectomy. J Nucl Med 1977; 19: 303-308
2. Lederer CM, Shirley VS (eds.): Table of isotopes. Wiley & Sons, 7th ed. 1978
3. ICRP Publication 38: Radionuclide transformations. Pergamon Press 1983
4. Pirich C, Prüfert U, Havlik E, Schwarmeis E, Flores J, Kvaternik H, Angelberger P, Aiginger H, Wanivenhaus A, Sinzinger H: Monitoring of the biodistribution and biokinetics of dysprosium-165 ferric hydroxide with a shadow-shield whole-body counter. Eur J Nucl Med 1997; 24: 398-402
5. Basic Safety Standard 96/EURATOM

Radioactive Isotopes in
Clinical Medicine and Research XXIII
ed. by H. Bergmann, H. Köhn and H. Sinzinger

RECONSTRUCTION OF SPECT DATA USING AN ARTIFICIAL NEURAL NETWORK

Peter Knoll[1,2,3], Siroos Mirzaei[1], Martin Neumann[3], Karl Koriska[2], Horst Köhn[1]
Dept. of Nuclear Medicine,
[1] Wilhelminenspital, [2] Kaiserin Elisabeth Spital,
[3] Institute of Experimental Physics, University of Vienna,
Vienna, Austria

Summary:

At present, algorithms used in nuclear medicine to reconstruct single photon emission computerized tomography (SPECT) data are usually based on one of two principles: filtered back projection and iterative methods. In this paper a different algorithm, applying an artificial neural network (multilayer perceptron) and error backpropagation as training method are used to reconstruct transaxial slices from SPECT data. The algorithm was implemented on an Elscint XPERT workstation (i486,50 MHz) used as routine digital image processing tool in our departments. Reconstruction time for a 64x64 matrix is approximately 10 seconds per transaxial slice. The algorithm has been validated by a mathematical model and tested on heart and Jaszczak phantoms. The very first results show in comparison with filtered back projection an improvement in image quality.

Introduction:

Generally, a scintigram represents the two-dimensional projection of a three dimensional activity distribution. Most of the information on the three dimensional activity distribution gets lost if only planar acquisition is performed. In order to utilize this information rotating, Anger gamma cameras have been developed. SPECT (Single Photon Emission Computerized Tomography) is widly used in nuclear medicine to obtain tomographic information about the regional activity concentration in the organ of interest. During standard acquisition the head of the gamma camera rotates around the patient. The images obtained in that way represent the projection of the activity concentration within the examined object. Using filtered back projection (FBP), which is the current standard reconstruction technique in nuclear medicine, the resulting reconstructed slices are usually blurred by the presence of noise. The very poor collimator efficiency and the relatively low injected activity, dictated by the radiation burden to the patient, limit the count rates achieved by the gamma camera. The FBP algorithm can produce serious artifacts in the reconstructed imgage slice. These artifical structures can be controlled to some extent by the choice of the filter function, but they cannot be totally eliminated [1]. The limitations of filtered back projection are well known to clinicans, but this method nevertheless remains the standard method in nuclear medicine to reconstruct SPECT data because of fast reconstruction time. In order to extract the maximum amount of information from our data, we need to be able to describe the aquisition process as accurate as possible. Instead of backprojecting the projection data to reconstruct the object, we propose a method to learn this image function. The ability to learn is not unique to the biological world. Neural computing is one of the most rapidly expanding areas of current research. The standard workhorse of artificial neural networks (ANN) is the family of multilayer feedforward network. This network architecture consists of a set of neurons which are logically arranged in two or more layers. There is an input and an output layer, each containing at least one neuron and sandwiched between them there are usually one or more hidden layers. The widespread applicability of feedforward networks is due to the following fact that, three layer feedforward networks are universal approximators, which means, that this kind of network can be used to approximate any „reasonable" function [2]. In nuclear medicine some applications, such as to analyze SPECT brain [3] or renal dynamical data [4] have been presented recently.

Methods:

The head of the gamma camera, rotating around the patient, aquires the projection data. A multilayer feedforward network (Fig. 1) is used in the present model to approximate the imaging function we want to describe.

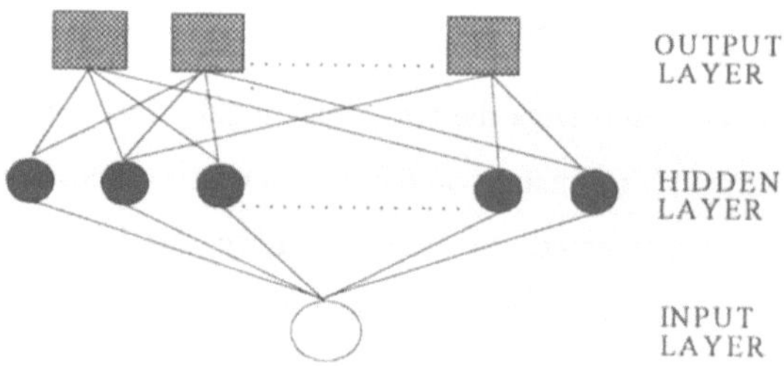

Fig. 1: Schematic representation of the multilayer feedforward network used for reconstruction.

In the following i,j represents the x,y coordinates of the object slice to be reconstructed and k the angular position of the gamma camera. The input layer is used as a dummy and set at the beginning at 1. For a given matrix n_x x n_y, the number of output nodes is calculated by multiplying n_x with the number of angular positions of the gamma camera n_θ wheras the number of hidden nodes results from n_x times n_y.

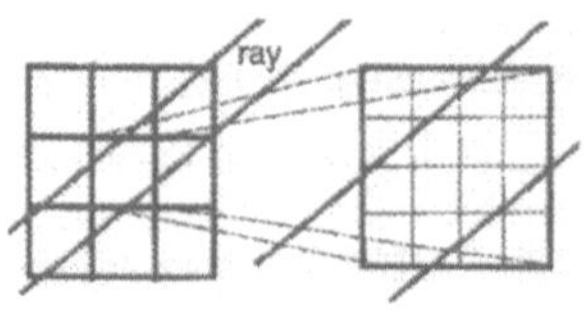

Fig. 2: schematic presentation of the voxel volume correction [6]

The values of the output layer are the registered counts of the gamma camera. The weights of the second layer represents the fraction of the voxel volume given by the intersection of voxel i,j and angular position k of the gamma camera (Fig. 2). The value of this volume correction v_{ijk}^{corr} is between 1 and 0 and represents the fraction of the voxel volume, which contributes to the raysums. This purely geometrical correction is calculated for each voxel at the beginning [6] and is not changed during the network learning process. All weights in the first layer w_{1ij} are initially set randomly at the beginning and are adjusted during the training process using the error back propagation method [7]. Error back propagation was the first practical method for training a multilayer feedforward network. Using this method, the output layer errors are successively fed backwards through the network. Because the weights of the second layer are known a priori, only the weights of the first layer have to be changed and therefore only this part of the error back projection algorithm [7] needs to be performed. In the model, used in the present paper the value of the input layer is equal to 1 and therefore the hidden layer h_{ij} is simply

$$h_{ij} = w^1{}_{ij} \qquad (1)$$

To calculate the output of the net the following condition is used:

$$\text{if Voxel} \quad V_{ij} \in ray \Rightarrow S = S + v_{ijk}^{corr} h_{ij}$$

$$\text{else} \quad S = S$$

where S is the value of the raysum. As transfer function the hyperbolic tangent was chosen [5]. The output of the net a_{ijk} is therefore

$$a_{ijk} = \tanh(S)$$

and the difference between the target z_{ijk} (normalized pixel value measured on the gammacamera) and S is given by

$$\varepsilon_{ijk} = z_{ijk} - S \qquad (2)$$

The weights of the first layer are iterativly readjusted by backpropagating the local error ε_{ijk}

$$w^{1^{n+1}}{}_{ij} = w^{1^n}{}_{ij} + \alpha\varepsilon_{ijk} h_{ij}\left(1-\tanh\left(a_{ijk}\right)\right) + \beta\left(w^{1^n}{}_{ij} - w^{1^{n-1}}{}_{ij}\right) \qquad (3)$$

until the root mean square global error is a minimum. The output of the net, a_{ijk} is the result of the value of the hidden layer times the weights of the second layer by a non linear transfer function. The variable *nx and ny*, used in (4) represent the matrix size, θ the number of acquisition angles. The parameters α, β generally should be a number between 0 and 1. In the present algorithm α is set to 0.9 at the beginning, β to 0.5 and then successivly decreased during the learning process. The procedure results in the transaxial slice of the aquired object, which is stored in the hidden layer. Using the presented network where the input remains constant, the output is changed for different acquisitions, means that the function we are looking for will differ from slice to slice. Therefore, training of the network has to be repeated for every transaxial image slice. Reconstruction time applying the presented algorithm takes only about 10 seconds per transaxial slice using a 50 MHz i486 processor and the Elscint XPERT software.

Results and discussion:

To validate the reconstruction algorithm a Jaszczak phantom as well as patient data sets were investigated.

Jaszczak phantom:

The Jaszczak phantom, filled with 370 MBq 99m Tc pertechnetat, was imaged using an Elscint Helix HR gamma camera. The aquisition parameters were 360° SPECT, 6°/step, 30 sec./frame . The collimator used was a MEGP (*middle energy general purpose*) collimator. A rotation radius of 250 mm was chosen to simulate routine conditions of patient imaging. The results of FBP and ANN are shown in Fig. 3a,b. The advantage of the present algorithm over to the filtered backprojection is clearly shown in the attenuation corrected (Chang method, attenuation coefficient= 0.125/cm) transaxial slices of the Jaszczak phantom.

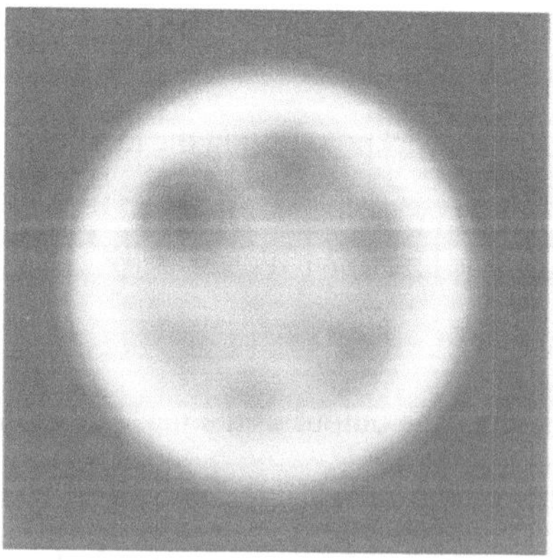

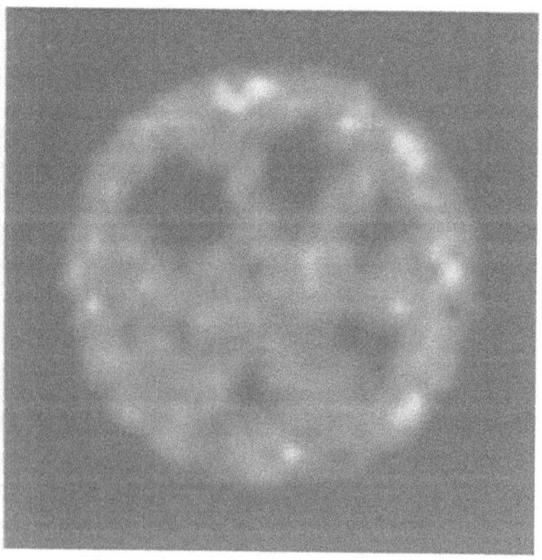

Fig.3: Reconstructed Jaszczak phantom: a) FBP, b) ANN

In Fig. 3a, showing the FBP slices (reconstruction filter Metz, power=3, FWHM=10mm) only 4 spheres, while slices, reconstructed by ANN show 5 spheres are clearly visible (Fig. 3b).

Patient study:

The patient SPECT study reconstructed by the ANN was a 99m Tc MDP SPECT. The matrix used for this studies was 64x64. After application of 374 MBq 99m Tc MDP 360 ° SPECT aquisition was performed using an Elscint Helix dual head gamma camera. The SPECT study was performed to localize better the lesions in the spine, found on the planar image. Aquisistion parameters were 360°, 6°/step, 35 sec./frame and a *LEHR (low energy high resolution)* collimator was used. The image after FBP (reconstruction filter=Metz) and ANN reconstruction, respectively, are shown in Figs. 4a,b.

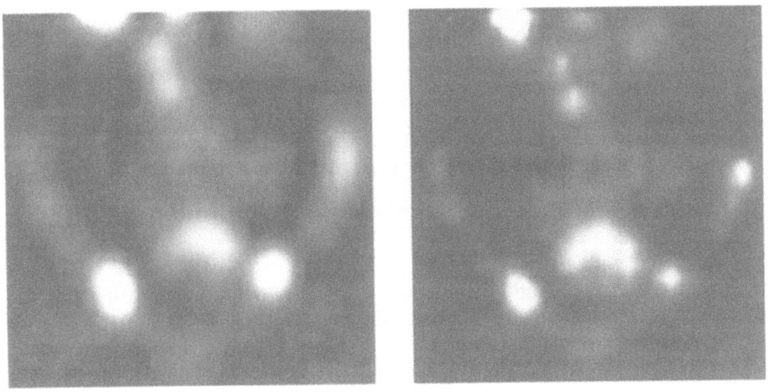

Fig. 4: 99m Tc MDP Bonescintigraphy: a) FBP coronal slice, b) ANN coronal slice

The coronal slices, reconstructed by FBP (Fig. 4a) shows 2 not clearly defined lesions in the lumbar spine. Also an exact localization of the hot lesions is not possible. In contrast, the ANN images (Fig. 4b) shows 2 clearly seperated lesions and their exact localization in the 3. and 4. lumbar vertebra.

Conclusion:

The very preliminary results of our study indicate that the quality of reconstruction by an artifical neural network and error backpropagation as training method is superior to that by FBP. Both, the reconstructed phantom and the presented patient studies demonstrate the advantage of ANN over the standard reconstruction method. The blurring effect of noise is significally less in the ANN slices than in the FBP images. This leads to clearer defined structures resulting in a better assessment of the size of the lesions. Although we used a computer with a processor (i486) that is not „state of the art", the reconstruction time is still acceptable even for clinical routine. The easy of handling, the totally automatic processing of the algorithm and the reproducibility of the results are other advantages of the present method. The use of different learning algorithms, like *fast delta rule based algorithm* or *fast eleanne* 7[8], will help to improve the speed of convergence and therefore shorten the reconstruction time. A faster processor will substantially improve application of this algorithm too. This also provide the possibility to implement physical properties (e.g. resolution) of the gamma camera into the algorithm and further improving the image quality after reconstruction.

Acknowledgement:

P. Knoll and S. Mirzaei would like to thank Dr. Riedl, MedPro and Ing. F. Schedlmayer, BSM for supporting this work. P. Knoll would like to thank E. Nir, ElGems for providing the necessary software tools.

References:

[1] H. Luig, W. Eschner, M. Bähre, E. Voth, G. Nolte: Eine iterative Strategie zur Bestimmung der Quellverteilung bei der Einzelphotonentomographie mit einer rotierenden Gammakamera.
Nucl.-Med 1988;27:140-146

[2] K. Hornik, M. Stinchcombe, H. White: Multilayer feedforward networks are universal Approximators.
Neural networks 2 (1989): 359-366

[3] D. Hamilton, D. O'Mahony, J. Coffey, J. Murphy: Comparison of artificial neural network and discrement analysis for the classification of mild alzheimer's disease using SPECT data.
Eur. J. Nucl.Med 24,8,1997

[4] J. Rudzka, K. Rudzki, S. Nowak: Application of artificial neural network in analysis of renal dynamic studies.
Eur. J. Nucl. Med. 24,8,1997

[5] Kalman, B. L., Kwasny, S. C.: Why tanh? Choosing a sigmoidial function.
International conference on neural networks, Baltimore, M.D.

[6] Knoll P., Mirzaei S., Koriska K., Köhn H.: Modifizierter iterativer Rekonstruktionsalgorithmus für SPECT Daten
Nukl. Med. 1997;36

[7] Kinnebrock W.: Neuronale Netze: Grundlagen, Anwendungen, Beispiele
Oldenburg Verlag, München 1992

[8] Karayiannis N, Venetsanopolus A: Fast learning algorithm for neural networks
Artificial neural networks, Elsevier Science Publishers B.V. (north Holland), 1991,1141-1144

WORLD WIDE WEB; WWW DEMO

Radioactive Isotopes in
Clinical Medicine and Research XXIII
ed. by H. Bergmann, H. Köhn and H. Sinzinger

THE USE OF INTERNET AS A MODE OF DELIVERY FOR NUCLEAR MEDICINE POSTGRADUATE EDUCATION

R. Anayat[1], J. Hendriks[2], A. Shah[1], A. Smith[1], B. Allen[3].

[1]. Discipline of Medical Radiation Science, University of Newcastle, Australia.
[2]. IESD, University of Newcastle, Australia.
[3]. Department of Nuclear Medicine, Waikato Hospital, New Zealand.

SUMMARY: The recent advances in computer hardware/software and the Internet have opened new channels of communication: e-mail, bulletin boards, voice mail, the World Wide Web(WWW), Internet chat/phone & Internet video conferencing/clips. The University of Newcastle is the first University to offer a postgraduate distance education (DE) award course using both traditional mode and via the internet. The students are continuously monitored for their performance and interaction. We have found that the Internet is a secure, reliable and adaptable method for course delivery which allows more interaction than traditional modes of DE.

INTRODUCTION

"We must not begin with what the new technology offers. Examining instead what students need, we are led to a quite different analysis of how new technology can help."

[Laurillard D, 1996 (1)]

There is a need for providing postgraduate education to full time workers within the field of Nuclear Medicine who do not wish to or are unable to take study leave in order to upgrade their qualifications. However, the Internet brings to DE new ways to deliver information and interact with students. In developing postgraduate Nuclear Medicine education for Internet delivery we have tried to take advantage of the ability to reach new students by-passing existing channels; the WWW's multimedia capability and the ability to distribute information (2).

DISTANCE EDUCATION: BACKGROUND

The concept of Distance Education (DE) has been around for many years. Australia has been a pioneer in this field, because of the isolation of some students who live on cattle stations and farms hundreds of kilometers away from the nearest school (3). An integral part of distance education was to ensure student participation via voice interaction between them and their teachers.

Tertiary level DE was once looked upon as the poor cousin of on-campus education. The course material consisted mostly of stacks of printed material delivered to the student via 'snail-mail'. The student had to read through the material and either complete a set of assignments or sit for an exam at the end of the year. The more advanced courses offered audio-tapes and more recently video-tapes. There was limited interaction between the students and the subject coordinator or between the students themselves, which is an important part of education at any level.

DE has now become an integral part of education, it has even been integrated within the regular on-campus education with video link-ups and virtual classrooms. The worldwide growth in DE has been stimulated by many factors, the most important being a massive growth in number and diversity of student populations and a shift in focus from teacher-centred to learner-centred teaching (3).

THE NEW TECHNOLOGY: INTERNET, INTRANET & EXTRANET

Electronic mail (e-mail) is the simplest starting point which allows the exchange of messages on-line with other connected parties, and also includes the ability to send data files such as Word documents and even audio/video files. Advantages over fax, phone and mail include lower costs, greater flexibility and increased efficiency.

An Intranet is a method of storing and manipulating information within the organisation using web protocols. It is easy and cheap to set up. This method is used to deliver information to our on-campus students. It is possible to deliver text, graphics, audio and video clips.

A public Web site is accessible to all Internet users, whereas a closed site, known as an Extranet, is accessible only to nominated people. To limit access, software is needed to organise log in access, the level of access and record management. Only students who are enrolled can have access to the material and each student is able to communicate with the subject coordinator and other students enrolled within that subject.

TopClass™ (WBTSYSTEMS: www.wbtsystems.com) was considered to be the superior software amongst many other options on the market. The other products evaluated were LearningSpace™ (www.lotus.com) and Authorware 4™ (www.macromedia.com). TopClass™, LearningSpace™ and Authorware 4™ allow cross-platform development, while the other solutions are Windows-only on the development side.

TopClass™ is a learning environment which distributes course materials for viewing on any PC compatible or Macintosh computer. It also provides communications functions to enable instructors and students to stay in touch. TopClass™ runs over TCP/IP networks such as the Internet, or a corporate or campus LAN (local area network) using World Wide Web protocols. TopClass™ allows great flexibility in data and student management (5).

TopClass™ stores all information on users and courses on a central server. Students, instructors and administrators can access that server from anywhere on the network using a standard Web browser such as Netscape® Navigator™ or Microsoft® Internet Explorer™. Once a student has officially enrolled in the course, an account is set up within TopClass™.

Students can be given access to all or a part of the online material. Accounts can be set up for individual subject coordinators and classes can be created as needed. Each class has its own bulletin board for interaction between students. The students can send e-mail to their subject coordinators and to each other. There are options for a personal profile, including pictures of lecturers and students (5).

The system was tested for reliability and security. A New Zealand student and a remote Australian student were chosen as the subjects of this trial. There were initial teething problems with server access and speed. These were rectified quickly. No instructions were given to the students regarding the use of the software, however, the students found the TopClass™ environment to be user friendly and intuitive.

We have been able to integrate graphics within the system and have also successfully tested audio and video clips in RealAudio™ (www.real.com) format. The use of audio and video clips requires the student to download RealAudio™ software which is freely available on the internet (freeware).

There are links to relevant online journals and sites within the texts, which makes the program more interactive. There are also many image libraries online which are accessible to students by providing a regularly updated links page.

STUDENT ASSESSMENT & EVALUATION

Student assessment is progressive, consisting mostly of minor projects, assignments and short and long answer questions. The only subject which requires a supervised examination, as an accreditation requirement, is Nuclear Medicine Science. A local senior Nuclear Medicine Technologist, Physicist or Physician is nominated to supervise the student during the examination.

We had 11 students in our first year, 8 of which had direct access to e-mail, including 3 with direct access to the WWW. Students with e-mail access receive their modules as attached documents. The student discussion and feed-back is also via e-mail. Students with no Internet access receive their modules via snail-mail.

The difference in performance between students with Internet access and those without is being monitored. Students are also surveyed to identify any possible gaps in the delivery of information to those without Internet access. Students without Internet access may be provided with CD-ROM containing the material available on the web pages.

CONCLUSION

With further development in mind, voice and video conferencing are being tested for reliability and speed. Freeware allows both voice and video conferencing at no cost (except Internet connection costs). The only constraint will be the disparity between the different time zones. We are planning to provide video clips of lectures and laboratory demonstrations for our on-campus and DE students. CD-ROM version of the lecture materials will be made available with optional links to the Internet site.

We have found that the Internet is a secure, reliable and adaptable method for course delivery which allows more interaction than traditional modes of DE course delivery.

ACKNOWLEDGEMENTS:

This project would not have been possible without the generous contribution of Information and Education Services Division at the University of Newcastle.

REFERENCES:

1. Laurillard D. The Changing University. ITFORUM Paper #13. Online Instructional Technology Forum ITFORUM@uga.cc.uga.edu Posted: 30 April, 1996.

2. Cuming D. Internet Considerations for any Small Business. Global Web Directory Australia. December 1997: Issue 2: www.globalwebdir.com.au

3. Smith K. Diversity Down Under in Distance Education. Darling Downs Institute Press 1984.

4. The University of Newcastle, Australia. Flexible Learning: Improving Student Access and Learning, 1997.

5. TopClass™ online instructions: www.wbtsystem.com

Radioactive Isotopes in
Clinical Medicine and Research XXIII
ed. by H. Bergmann, H. Köhn and H. Sinzinger

TWO YEARS EXPERIENCE WITH AN EXCLUSIVELY INTERNET-BASED VIRTUAL LECTURE FOR MEDICAL STUDENTS AND POSTGRADUATES

H.Kritz, H.Sinzinger
Rehabilitation Center „Engelsbad“, Baden, Austria and Department of Nuclear Medicine, University of Vienna, Austria

SUMMARY Since a littel while ago Internet had only an additive function in the education of students. Internet has now become easy and cheap, so that a complete lecture about atherosclerosis, which can be consumed exclusively about the Internet, has been created (http://www.univie.ac.at/nuklearmedizin/). New applications in the World Wide Web (WWW) and the use of interactive elements like Java applets, are useful features for teaching medical students and graduated doctors. The course of a complete term, available about the WWW, is structured. This system allows the student to evaluate his condition of knowledge. At the end of each chapter the acquired knowledge is evaluated with a questionnaire and dependent on the quality of the given answers, the student is authorized to go forward to the next chapter. Because of reference sites no additional educational aids are necessary. About e-mail and Internet Relay Chat the student is in contact with his teacher and the course is finished with a certificate (e-mail) about participation and success. First experiences (e.g. still now 80 users with increasing tendency) and problems (e.g. velocity of image transfer about our virtual lecture since the summer term 1996) will be discussed. The issue „atherosclerosis“ seems to be an useful model for structured courses with additional success control.

INTRODUCTION

Advances in telecommunication technologies in the last decade have fostered the development of computer networks that allow to access fast amounts of information and services (1). Of the many computer networks that have been developed, the most prominent is the Interent. Orginally intended to be a way to share computing resources among academic and research institutions in the United States, the Internet has gradually evolved into a worldwide network of computers that proves various services reflecting the eclectic nature of component networks. The recent upsurge in interest in the Internet is due to several mutually reinforcing factors: increased ease and availability of access to the Internet, lower access charges, faster communications, and more organizations offering commercial and noncommercial services over the Internet.

Of particular interest to the medical community is the large and increasing number of technical, scientific and biomedical resources that can be accessed through the Internet. Most large medical centers have publicly accessible information, and some large organizations have extensive databases and services that can be used by medical researchers, clinicians, educators and students. The increasing availability and use of computer networks and the Internet are producing a changing climate in health care as well as in education (2). Moves away from traditional face-to-face teaching with a campus institution to widely distributed interactive multimedia learning will affect the roles of students and teachers (3).

METHODS

Hard- and Software

Starting our lecture in 1996 as hardware in the first time a Siemens Nixdorf PT 103 (Pentium 120, 64MB RAM, 2 GB hard disk), a H P Scanner 4P and a US Robotics 28800 Voice modem and a software Windows 95 and the Office Package were used. Later on a HP (Pentium 266, 128 MB RAM, 4 GBH hard disk), Windows NT 4.0 and an ISDN Creatix Omni.net had been installed. As web-editors first Word Assistant, HTML edit, and Homesite for Windows 95 were used and since summer 1997 Microsoft Front Page 1.1 later on Microsoft Front Page 97/98, MS Office 97, Paint Shop Pro 4 and the Real Publisher were available. As Browser first Netscape Version 3.0, since October 1997 the Netscape Communicator or Explorer 4.0 were installed.

Structure of the term

We used two models of structure for our lecture. The first model was a structured lecture divided in traditional chapters. With a questionnaire the acquired knowledge at the end of each chapter was evaluated. Dependent on the quality of given answers the student was authorized to go forward to the next chapter. In our lecture no additional education aids like printed material was necessary to follow the lecture. To get in contact with the students online, discussions with the teacher and other participants via Chat, IRC or i-Chat, were offered. Offline discussions were done via e-mail. Each student got a certificate about his participation and success per e-mail. To evaluate the acceptance of the lecture statistics about the response and logfiles were used.

The second model was a lecture with actual and variable topics (i.e. endothelial dysfunction, PGE_1-therapy in peripheral vascular disease, homocysteine). Working groups were built to develop the content of the lecture using the online resources of the WWW. A further tool was an intesive discussion between students/students and students/teacher. The reviewed and discussed content of the chats was online published as a lecture by the teacher. In this second model no evaluation forms were used and at the end of the lecture each participant got a certificate.

RESULTS

Our number of participants increased from 7 students at the beginning up to more than 80 students per term. The geographical distribution showed a leading part of students from overseas (60 persons), followed by 40 participants from Europe and only 3 to 4 from Austria. The distribution students to postgraduates was 1:3 . A comparison between the two models of lecture and the number of participants which only tried out the term and the one which finished the program showed that in the structured lecture 80% tried out and 20% finished the program, while in contrast in the working groups model 60% tried out and 40% finished the term.

DISCUSSION

The first experiences with a virtual lecture were mainly positive and the issue „atherosclerosis“ was a useful model to develop an Internet based lecture model. New forms of structuring the contents were possible and no additional educational aids were necessary. There is cost-effectiveness for both, the teacher and the student. The virtual way of teaching and learning might represent a solution for the explosion of costs at the Universities and the rapidly increasing international interest (Virtual University) is a new challenge for the teaching staff. The online resources are not only used for training, but also for continuing education and reference. Text and compressed images are sufficient to transport the content of the lectures.

With the new developed browsers and media players since December 1997 new structures can be evaluated (web casting projects). There was a great interest from the federal communities and world-wide (USA, Asia and Australia). The discussion via chat had a good response and the participants of our term showed a relatively high standard of knowledge. As help for beginners the structure of our lectures is available as a template on CD. There is also online help per e-mail. As help for experts there is a real publisher-web casting project (video), frontpage bots for the login procedure, evaluation sheets, a discussion forum and chats.
Our negative experiences were that the transfer of detailed images (x-ray, audio and videofiles) is too slow for non-ISDN lines. The rapid development of new advantages of the software (frontpage extension, Java) are incompatible with „old“ servers. Also European university servers are often slower than private providers. A problem is also the quick technical progress even during the period of one lecture, like there are new versions of browsers, new web-editors, animated graphics and Java-applets. Evaluation of knowledge via a multiple-choice form was found not to be a useful tool. Chats within a group seem to be important for the participants but this can be eventually better solved with web-phone conferences. Java-applets and CGI-scripts are too complicated for non-experienced teachers, but new browsers and editors allow a qick and competent preparation of data (tables, frames, script wizard, discussion rounds and templates).

CONCLUSION

As a result of the increasing use of computer networks and the Internet, educational institutions may see their role change (4). Campus universities where students travel to study may become more like the open university in remote provision of education, validation and kitemarking of courses (5). It should be remembered that in medical training and many other practice-based disciplines, hands-on experience cannot be replaced, but the way in which it is provided and the underlying knowledge gained are likely to change. Finally, if new technologies are to be effectively used to enhance clinical teaching, clinical teachers must provide leadership not only for their learners but also for their institutions, guiding both, students and colleagues, in making the best use of new technologies. They must show their institutions how investing in new technologies will be helpful, and they must assist in the actual implementations of new systems. Administrators will need to be reminded that clinical teaching should not stand still, and that the efforts to enhance it will require the investment of resources, including the presence and time of faculty. Colleagues will need help in acquiring and organizing new information resources and information-gathering and -assessment techniques. Finally, learners will need to see that emerging information technologies can make an immediate contribution to their daily endeavors. Clinical small-group teaching is demanding. The many constraints posed by clinical settings require discipline and focus on the part of the instructor if learners are to get the most benefit from each encounter. Information technologies now available can make immediate and significant contributions to clinical teaching if instructors are open to the possibilities they offer and prepared to take advantage of them. The rewards will make the effort worthwhile.

REFERENCES

1. Glowniak JV. Medical resources on the Internet. Ann Intern Med 123: 123-131, 1995
2. Sandroni S. Enhancing clinical teaching with information technologies: what can we do right now? Acad Med 72: 770-774, 1997
3. Ward R. Implications of computer networking and the Internet for nurse education. Nurse Educ Today 17: 178-183, 1997
4. Skiba DJ. Nursing education to celebrate learning. N HC Perspect Community 18: 124-129, 148, 1997
5. Frost M. An analysis of the scope and value of problem-based learning in the education of health care professionals. J Adv Nurs 24: 1047-1053, 1996

Radioactive Isotopes in
Clinical Medicine and Research XXIII
ed. by H. Bergmann, H. Köhn and H. Sinzinger

TELE NUCLEAR MEDICINE ON THE WORLD WIDE WEB

L. Svensson and B. Sarby

Department of Hospital Physics, Huddinge University Hospital, Sweden.

SUMMARY: Two-way interactive communication with full diagnostic capabilities is achieved using work stations.`Gamma camera patient studies at remote hospitals can be fully analysed and quality controlled. By means of modern PC technology and the possibilities offered by the WWW a cost effective diagnostic tool can be accomplished using standard hard- and software. Referring doctors can get access to images and curves as well as to reports from a database using a standard PC and WWW browser. Diagnostic work can easily be performed at home with these techniques.

INTRODUCTION

Since 1991 we have utilised a network at Huddinge Hospital, where digital images from patient studies are transferred between the gamma cameras, MRT- and CT-units. During the first years this network was used mainly for moving images between these units. Patient data were analysed using multi modality techniques, chiefly brain examinations.

The network has then been extended to referring clinics as e.g. the Geriatric Clinic and the Department of Clinical Physiology in our hospital. During the last years other hospitals within the Stockholm County Council as well as other referring Medical Centres have been connected. The gamma cameras at two of these hospitals, Sophiahemmet and S:t Görans Sjukhus are today directly accessible for continuos support, mathematical image analysis and quality control using Hermes Systems (Nuclear Diagnostics, Sweden).

The appearance of images displayed on a modern PC has today a good quality both in colour and black/white. Thus, a natural process has been to move on to modern PC technology and the possibilities offered by the World Wide Web for access and exchange of patient images, other examination data and medical reports.

MATERIALS AND METHODS

An interactive Web Site has been developed in co-operation with Nuclear Diagnostics, Sweden, where patient reports and images can be accessed by authorised physicians (Figure 1). The software, hwww, written in Pearl, is fully integrated into the Hermes System.

After a patient examination has been completed and analysed the most relevant images are documented using the standard hard copy utility. However, instead of sending a hard copy through the printer system, the image is stored together with the answer from the reporting doctor in the hwww database. The doctor signs the report and makes it accessible for the referring physician. In this way the referring physician can only read patient documents made accessible for him when logging on to the Web Site.

If the analysis of the patient study is done by some other member of the staff, the documents are made accessible for the reporting doctor and stored. Later these documents can be accessed through the Web, the report can be entered and the referring physician authorised.

The reporting doctor is available for completing questions and exchange of experience using the WWW e-mail utility.

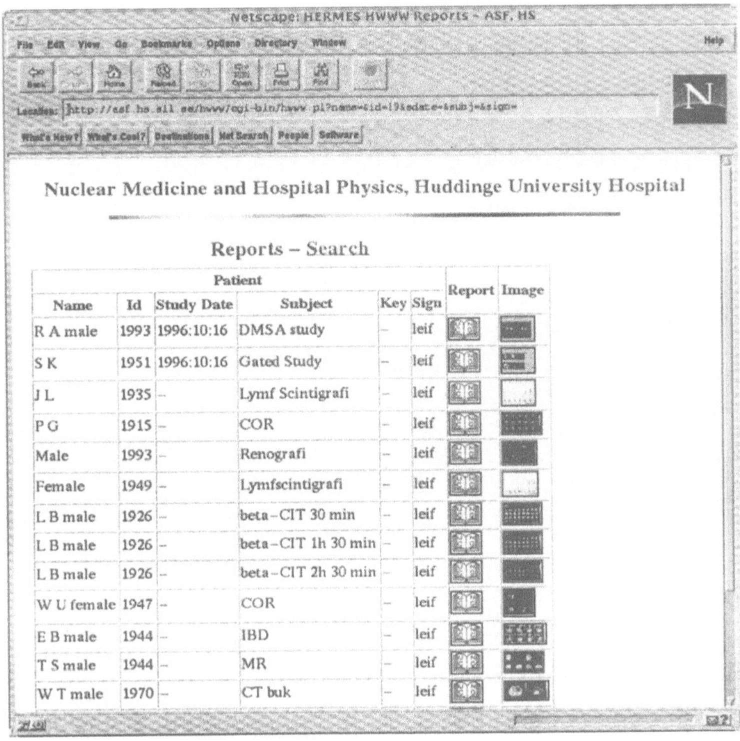

Figure 1. WWW page showing some studies used for demonstration purposes. These report pages can be reached by authorised physicians from the Web Site at the Department of Hospital Physics and Nuclear Medicine, Huddinge University Hospital.

RESULTS AND DISCUSSION

Among the most frequent diagnostic applications are: Brain studies due to symptoms of dementia referred from the Geriatric Clinic (Figure 2), heart studies for the Cardiac Unit and kidney studies for the Paediatric Clinic and the Transplantation Unit. During the last months some hundred documents have been entered into the hwww database each month.

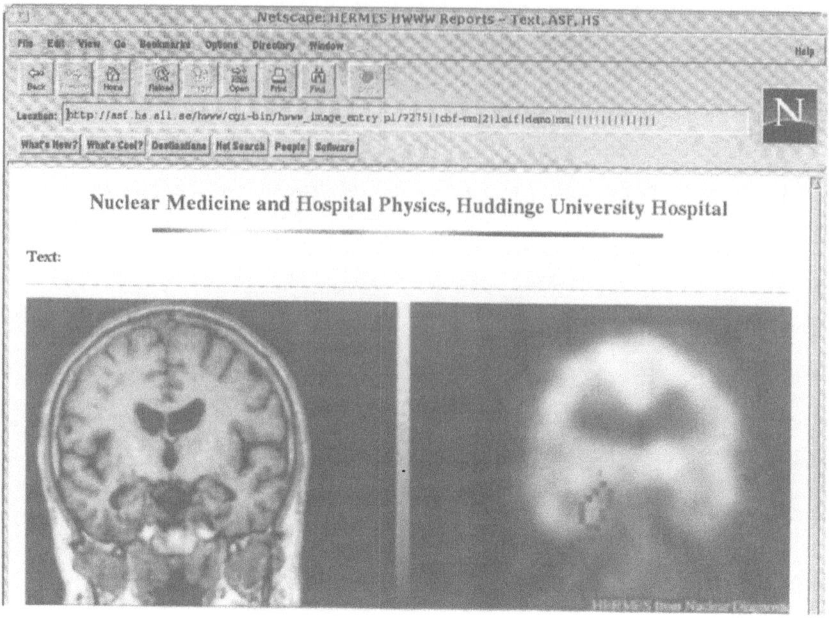

Figure 2. Aligned tomographic sections of the brain from a patient examined with MRT (left) and SPECT (right). The MRT image gives the anatomical definition while the SPECT image represents the blood flow distribution. A decrease in blood flow in a specific anatomic region, outlined in the MRT image, can then be concluded from the gamma camera examination.

According to our experiences tele nuclear medicine on the World Wide Web leads to an expanding interest in nuclear medicine methods from referring units. They can now take a more active part in a mutual diagnostic work and get a better knowledge about the methods. Furthermore, a better availability for second opinion has been achieved. Larger common databases for diagnostic references are available for the daily routine as well as for education and scientific work. Standardisation of methods among different hospitals are facilitated.

To ensure the patient integrity the following measures are taken:

1. User identification by password.
2. Only known and registered systems (IP address) have access to the hwww database.
3. Cryptation using the browser built-in functions.

CONCLUSION

Cost effective solutions have been achieved using standard hardware and software on two levels:

1. Referring doctors can get fast access to images and curves as well as reports from the database in our department using a standard PC and WWW browser.
2. Two-way interactive communication with full diagnostic capabilities is achieved using a Hermes System (Nuclear Diagnostics, Sweden).
3. Patient studies on gamma a camera at remote hospitals can be fully analysed and quality controlled.
4. Doctors can be on duty at home for analysing and reporting patient examinations.
5. A better co-operation and exchange of knowledge with referring units.
6. Archives for education and research can easily be put together.

Radioactive Isotopes in
Clinical Medicine and Research XXIII
ed. by H. Bergmann, H. Köhn and H. Sinzinger

A JAVA-ENHANCED NUCLEAR MEDICINE TEACHING FILE

Jerold W. Wallis*, Michelle M. Miller*, and N. Xan Phung**

*Mallinckrodt Institute of Radiology,Washington Univ. School of Medicine, St. Louis, MO USA,

**Faculty of Medicine, Univ. of Sydney, Australia

SUMMARY: The WWW-based MIR nuclear medicine teaching file started in 1994, and is one of the most complete on-line teaching collections in the field, with over 160 cases viewable either as unknowns (without diagnoses) or with the diagnosis and discussion. Creation of teaching file cases was facilitated by means of an HTML forms-based system coupled with automated CGI-scripts. A Java-based image viewer has been developed to enhance teaching file image interpretation, which permits zooming, color table manipulation, cine & tiled viewing modes, and image filtering.

Introduction

Collections of sample patient images, sometimes referred to as "teaching files", play an important role in radiology education. The clinical case collection is typically built up over many years, as studies of particular interest or learning value are encountered in clinical practice. Although a large part of radiology education is via supervised interpretation of routine patient exams, training time in each branch of radiology is limited and residents may not encounter a sufficiently wide spectrum of disease in their time on a specific clinical service. Teaching files are therefore used to supplement resident education by providing exposure to both typical and unusual radiologic manifestations of a variety of disease processes.

Digital teaching files have several advantages over film-based teaching files [1, 2]. A network-based teaching file can be viewed from many locations both locally and worldwide, images are rarely misplaced or lost, searching capability can allow rapid access to specific cases, and it is possible to include cine and image manipulation capability.

The Mallinckrodt Institute of Radiology Division of Nuclear Medicine (MIR-NM) teaching file [2] was start in 1994. The World-Wide-Web (WWW) was chosen as the vehicle for electronic transmission, since it allows rapid transfer of images and text, computer platform independence, multiple simultaneous users while sparing computer resources, and its hypertext markup language (HTML) allowed relatively easy formatting and case development. This paper discusses the design choices and development of the MIR-NM digital teaching file, which is located at <http://gamma.wustl.edu/home.html>.

Teaching file design

Ease of importing nuclear medicine images (scintigrams) into web format is essential for the development of teaching file cases. We currently view clinical images on UNIX workstations, and can select portions of the viewing screen to save as an X-windows screen dump. Using locally-developed software, these saved images are then automatically converted to GIF format (using the freely available NetPBM package),and sent to our web server by electronic file transfer (FTP). These images are then stored in a holding area for addition to teaching file case pages.

Several image file format options [3] are available for use on the web. GIF (Graphics interchange format) images allow several-fold compression of 8-bit image data, without any loss of image detail ("lossless" compression). It employs the Lempel-Ziv-Welch (LZW) compression algorithm developed by Unisys. The smaller file size allows easier storage and more rapid network transmission of image data. The GIF format was the first and perhaps most widespread image format used on the World-Wide-Web. It is particularly effective for simple images such as line-drawings, but also offer reasonable levels of compression for image data.

JPEG compression (developed by the Joint Photographics Expert Group) allows even greater compression by removing high image frequencies that are unlikely to be appreciated visually, and thus very slightly alters the image. This "lossy" compression employs the discrete cosine frequency transformation (DCT) as well as Huffman encoding, and allows the user to set an "image quality factor" on a 1-100 scale; a higher value results in better image quality but larger file size. Both 8-bit grayscale and 24-bit color images can be compressed as JPEG images. The degree of file compression of a bone scintigraphy study is shown in Table 1 [4].

Table 1. Effect of image compression on file size

Image	File size
Uncropped 16-bit grayscale image	1000 kb
Cropped 16-bit image (246 x 818 pixels)	402 kb
Cropped 8-bit image (used as basis for images below)	201 kb
GIF compression	85 kb
JPEG compression (Q=88)	29 kb
JPEG compression (Q=50)	11 kb
JPEG compression (Q=15)	5 kb

The MIR-NM teaching file primarily uses GIF images, however a shift to JPEG images is being considered. Experimentation has shown that a JPEG compression setting of 88 is adequate for teaching purposes [4], and achieves about a 3-fold greater compression than use of the GIF format.

An example of a case page can be seen in Figure 1. We elected to store the primary nuclear medicine image as an in-line image (i.e., the image appears in the same computer window as the text of the case). Ancillary images are available as links from the main case page. A case may be either with the diagnosis and discussion shown (as a "known" case), or without the diagnosis (as an "unknown"). Viewing of cases as unknowns allows a resident to more closely model the clinical environment—after forming an option about the displayed images, he may click on the "show diagnosis" link to get feedback on his assessment of the case.

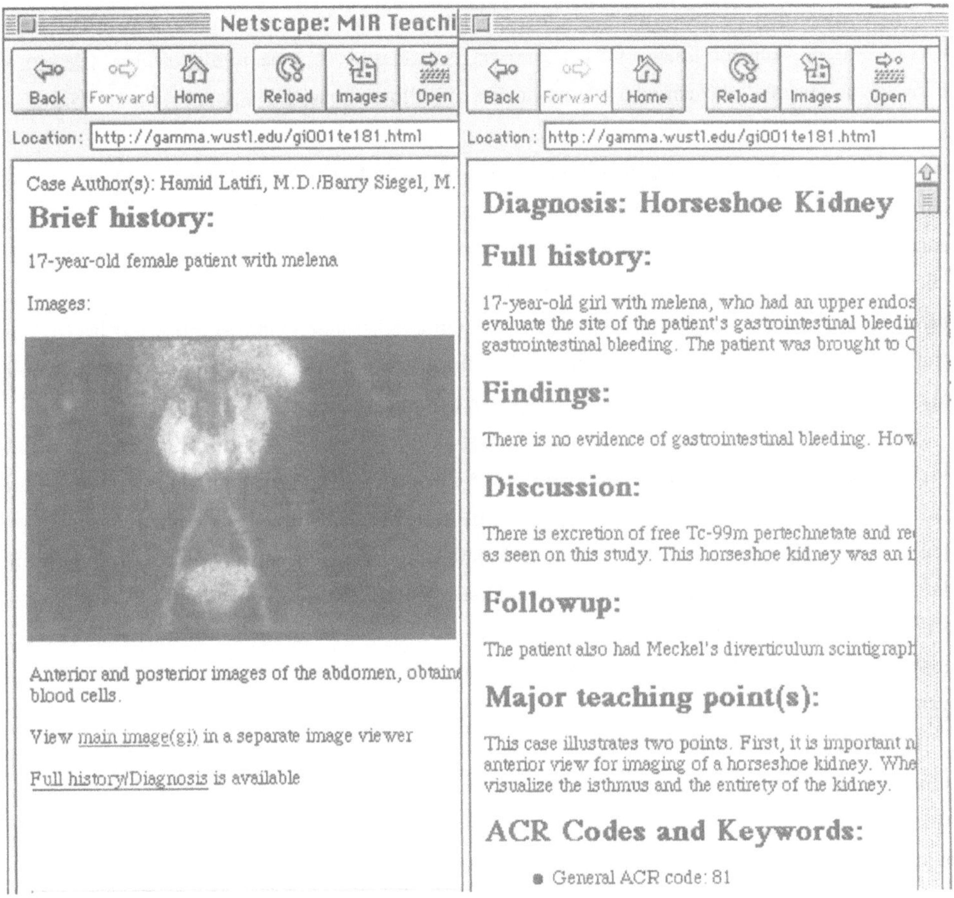

Figure 1. Example of a digital teaching file case. Initial viewing, without diagnosis, would reveal only the information on the left above. If the diagnosis were requested, additional information would appear below (shown at right in this figure).

Initial prototyping of the MIR-NM teaching file was done by creating hand-crafted HTML documents in a text editor. While this allowed maximum flexibility in exploring presentation formats, it rapidly became clear that use of some type of authoring software would be desirable. A "standard" teaching file description was created, including places to designate the brief history, full history, findings, discussion, teaching points, figure captions, and follow-up. These were then incorporated into an HTML form, allowing case information to be entered on-line in a WWW browser from any Internet-connected computer.

A computer program was then developed to reside on the web server to receive and process the submitted data. (This type of program is sometimes referred to as a CGI application.) When executed, it follows a template to create the "known" and "unknown" case pages described above. It also generates case numbers, renames image files to reflect the case number and image type, inserts links to the selected images into the case pages, and adds the case to the teaching file index. A copy of the completed form is also kept on-line, to allow access for any subsequent editing of the case.

An alternate design format would have been to save all the information in a database, and assemble the components dynamically upon request for a case page. This would make it easy to change the design of a standard case page in the future, and have the changes instantly reflected in all the existing teaching cases. We elected instead to create and store pre-assembled case pages, to minimize web server overhead. Changing our standard format would require editing of our "template" page, and then clicking "edit" and "submit" for each case, however this still would likely be less work than developing and managing a dynamic database.

Cases are indexed using the American College of Radiology (ACR) indexing scheme, which classifies studies based on anatomic and pathologic categories. The broad anatomic categories are {skull, face/neck, spine, heart, lung, gastrointestinal system, genitourinary system, vascular/lymphatic, and breast}. The broad pathologic categories are {normal/congenital, inflammation/infection, neoplasm, trauma, metabolic/endocrine, other systemic disorder, organ specific disorder, miscellaneous, and artifact}. Finer subdivisions in each of these categories are available in the on-line ACR classification, down to specific diagnoses. Search capability includes searching by diagnosis, by case difficulty, and by broad or exact ACR classification.

In order to prevent partially completed cases from being viewed over the Internet, the teaching file has two levels of access. Other institutions may view only cases which have been completed by the residents and approved by the nuclear medicine attending. Local users are also able to access incomplete cases for editing and review.

There has been dramatic growth in usage of the teaching file, approximately doubling every 9 months since 1994. The teaching file currently consists of over 160 cases, and approximately 12,000 cases are accessed each month from sites worldwide. Local usage accounts for less than 10% of total access.

Although there are many advantages to a digital teaching file, there are some limitations as well. It is more difficult to create a digital teaching file case than one for local usage only, resulting in some resistance in adding new cases. Unless one has an (expensive) digital projector system, it remains easier to show cases in conferences using slides or film than using a digital computer.

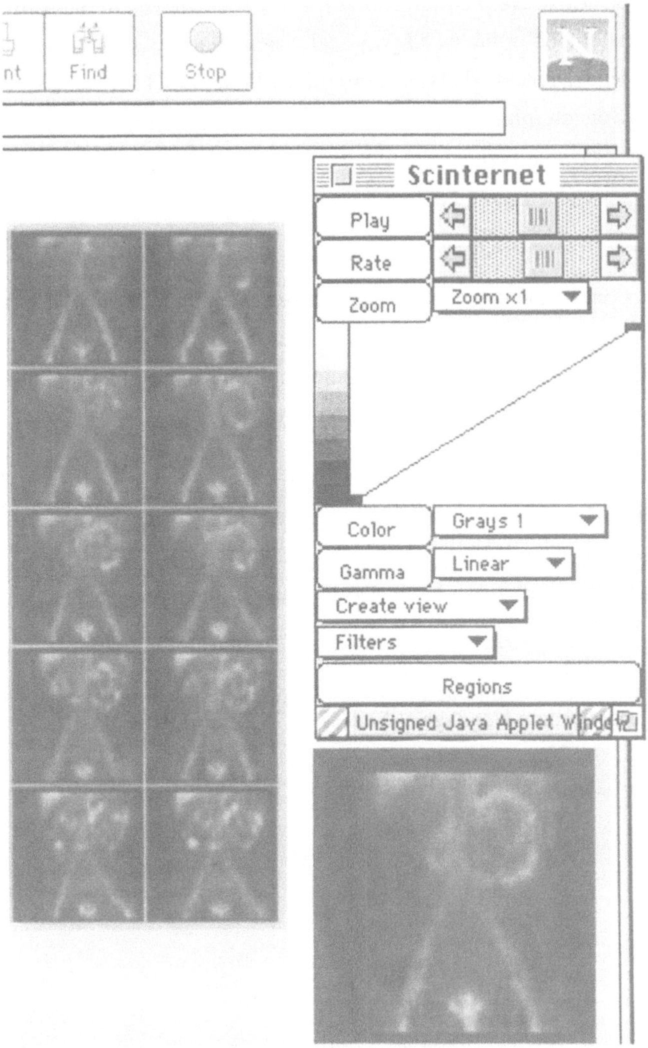

Figure 2. Portion of the display of our Java image viewing applet. The image controls are shown at the upper right. If the "Play" button is pressed, the cine window (bottom right) will show the study as a movie. Cine speed may be controlled by the slider. Pop-up buttons (currently marked "Grays1" and "Linear" control the overall color lookup table, and selective upper and lower level adjustments may be made by dragging the boxes at the end of the diagonal line. Other controls are available as well. In addition to the movie display, the study is also shown as individual frames, partly visible at the left of this figure.

Java

The Java computer language, developed by Sun Microsystems, is designed in a way so as to permit programs to be downloaded to your computer as part of a World-Wide-Web viewing session. These Java programs are designed to be computer platform independent, so that they can run under any operating system. To achieve this, modern WWW browsers have built-in a Java interpreter (or just-in-time-compiler), which receives and executes the Java program.

We have developed a Java program [4] that allows viewing and manipulation of nuclear medicine images, shown in Figure 2. This Java program allows images to be viewed in tile format or in cine display, supports image zoom, color table and gray scale manipulation, image filtering, and orthogonal slicing of tomographic data sets. This Java program will be used for teaching file cases which require cine displays for interpretation. Development and debugging was slightly hindered by the slightly differing non-standard implementations of Java interpreters on the different computer platforms.

Conclusion

The MIR-NM teaching file is one of the largest nuclear medicine teaching tools available on the Internet. Addition of new cases and viewing of existing cases is aided by use of the forms and CGI capabilities of the World-Wide-Web, and nuclear medicine specific image manipulation capabilities have been developed using the Java programming language.

References

1. Parker J, Wallis J, Halama J, Brown C, Cradduck T, Graham M, Wu E, Wagenaar D, Mammome G, Greenes R , Holman B. Collaboration using Internet for the development of case-based teaching files. *J Nucl Med* 1996; 37: 178-184.
2. Wallis J, Miller M, Miller T , Vreeland T. An Internet-based nuclear medicine teaching file. *J Nucl Med* 1995; 36: 1520-1527.
3. Murray J , VanRyper W. *Encyclopedia of Graphics File Formats.* Sebastopol, CA: O'Reilly and Associates, Inc.; 1994.
4. Phung N , Wallis J. An Internet-based, interactive nuclear medicine image display system implemented in the Java programming language. *J Nucl Med* 1997; 38: 210P.

Radioactive Isotopes in
Clinical Medicine and Research XXIII
ed. by H. Bergmann, H. Köhn and H. Sinzinger

EMERALD - EUROPEAN MEDICAL RADIATION LEARNING DEVELOPMENT - FOR VOCATIONAL TRAINING AND INTERACTIVE LEARNING ON WORLD WIDE WEB - NUCLEAR MEDICINE TRAINING MODULE

S.E.Strand[3], F.Milano[1], S.Tabakov[2], C. Roberts[2], I.L. Lamm[3], M Ljungberg[3], A. Benini[4], G. da Silva[5], B.A.Jonsson[3], L. Jonsson[3], C.A. Lewis[2], N.Teixeira[5], A. Compagnucci[1], L. Riccardi[1]

[1] University of Florence, Italy; [2] King's College London, UK; [3] University of Lund, Sweden; [4] International Centre for Theoretical Physics, Italy, [5] University of Lisbon, Portugal.

SUMMARY: EMERALD is an EC-funded Leonardo da Vinci pilot project in which three common transnational vocational training modules in Medical Radiation Physics are developed; Physics in Diagnostic Radiology, Nuclear Medicine and Radiotherapy. They will be delivered for training of graduate and postgraduate students. Each module, following a syllabus and a workbook for students, will last about four months. It incorporates material for interactive computer-based learning and distance learning on CD-ROMs, as well as a database of technical and physical images (i.e. equipment, phantom images, simulated images, artefacts, etc.). An extension of the EMERALD project considers the design of an electronic course and conversion to network-based material on interactive WWW-pages for on-line initial vocational training (IVT) and continuing vocational training (CVT) in "life long learning and training".

INTRODUCTION

The European Union has assigned a key role to vocational education and training because of the close correlation between economic and social progress and high quality vocational education and training policies. An effective vocational training system is based not only on the high level performance of the training institutions but also on the effectiveness of the training support services. Modern medicine requires well-trained medical physicists. However, sophisticated and expensive equipment actually used clinically, cannot be purchased solely for training needs, and in addition, only a very limited time is in general available on clinical equipment for training purposes. To come out of this situation, special Training Modules, based on interactive multimedia material and databases of medical images on CD-ROMs, are being developed by a consortium of European Universities and Hospitals involved in training in health care in the field of Medical Radiation Physics; the EMERALD project - European MEdical RAdiation Learning Development.

The adoption of this form of multimedia-based training will improve the quality of learning and will permit an easy transfer to the net for future distance "life long learning/training", available "when and where it is needed".

TRAINING MODULES

Three Training Modules are being developed in Physics of I) Diagnostic Radiology, II) Nuclear Medicine and III) Radiotherapy. Each module, addressed to graduate and post graduate students in Medical Physics, will correspond to a total of 80 days, i.e. four months of study. This will not enable the students to achieve full competence in each area, but completion of the Modules will be sufficient to give a sound foundation for further training.

The Modules incorporate material for distance learning including a CD database of medical images and interactive multimedia. According to the syllabi and curricula of the training scheme, the students will use the interactive multimedia materials to study the operation and safe use of the medical radiation equipment to achieve the necessary basic skills. After reaching a certain level of knowledge with distant learning, the students will practice the skills acquired on real equipment under guidance. Each completed part of the training in a Module will give the student certain credits, which will be further used for mutual recognition of the training within the EMERALD consortium to start with. It is expected that the EMERALD Training Structure, after presentation and dissemination, could be used by various National and International Institutions and Organisations providing Medical Radiation Physics training.

THE EMERALD TRAINING STRUCTURE

The EMERALD Training Structure will be based on the three Training Modules and organized by the EMERALD project coordinators with Local Training Coordinators (Trainers) and Supervisors. The Training Supervisor has to share the responsibility of the training with the Trainee in a well-structured way. Thus a contract in the format of a Pro-Forma Statement of Mutual Interest should be signed, before the training starts, by both Trainer and Trainee. It is recognised that the entrance requirement for a Trainee is to have reached a level of attainment in Physical Science equivalent to at least a BSc.

The EMERALD-project started 1996 and will last till 1998. In January 1998, drafts of the Teacher's Guide and Student Manuals / Task Workbooks are available, and the basic images of the image data base (IDB). The first Trainees (more experienced students) have been selected to test the Training Modules, starting in autumn 1997. During the first half of 1998 the IDB will be engraved on a CD and the full versions of the three Student Manuals and the Teacher's Guide printed. The Training Modules will be tested fully with Trainees at the different EMERALD sites. For the second half of 1998 the following activities will be initiated; 1) Hyperlink-connections for the Multimedia, 2) A European Conference for Medical Radiation Training (presentation of the EMERALD results) and 3) An international student exchange project.

The Teacher's Guide will include the guidelines for those responsible for the organization and supervision of training for the medical radiation physicist, and should be used together with the Student Manuals, available either as hard copy with accompanying CD-ROM or in a CD-ROM multimedia version.

The skills and competencies addressed in the Modules are based on the recommendations given by EFOMP (European Federation of Organisations for Medical Physics). According to the EFOMP structure of competency-based training and career development in medical physics, five levels of competence are defined (2). The medical physicist is recognised as competent to work in the clinic without direct supervision after having reached competency level 3, which includes requirements on both theoretical education and practical training. This is also the level of competence required to be accepted in a National register of Medical Physicists according to EFOMP recommendations (3). The EFOMP competency level 3 corresponds to the level of Corporate Membership of the IPEM (Institution of Physics and Engineering in Medicine) in the United Kingdom. In the EMERALD Training Modules, the competencies addressed are listed according to the IPEM structure, as Basic (B) and Corporate (C) competencies (4).

CONTINUOUS ASSESSMENT

If the structure of the training is to work effectively, the training has to be subjected to continuos assessment. To assist in this process firstly a weekly record of the work is required and secondly a meeting each two weeks between Trainee and Trainer/Supervisor, which should be addressed to discussion and recording of the competencies reached and tasks performed. These meetings should not only identify problems encountered but also promote the forward planning of the next task to be addressed.

The Trainee will most probably carry out parts of the training in a new department or even in a new country. Receiving feedback from both the Training Supervisor and the Trainees is important for those responsible for the whole EMERALD training scheme. At least 2-4 times during the work with the Training Module, a review with the Local Training Coordinator should take place. When submitting training course work to be assessed, the Trainee is presumed to undertake the responsibility that this is his or her own work. Instances of cheating in training course assessments are dealt with very severely. At the end of the training for each Module, the Trainee should finalise the Workbook and the portfolio, containing additional material, for final assessment and acceptance by the Supervisor.

MODULE; PHYSICS OF NUCLEAR MEDICINE

The Module Physics of Nuclear Medicine contains 15 Sub-modules. The idea is to cover all the aspects of a clinically working hospital physicist's daily duties and responsibilities. Included are maintenance and quality assurance of the different procedures in radiopharmacy, detection, imaging, image processing, evaluation and radiation protection. Both diagnostic and therapeutic applications are covered. In Table 1 is given a summary of the Student Manual / Task Workbook covering all the Sub-modules. For each Sub-module is also given the number of days, i.e. 8 hours working days, suggested that the student spends on that particular task.

Table 1. ***Task Workbook - Student Manual - Physics of Nuclear Medicine***

No.	Sub-module	Days
i	*Introduction. Basics in NM (visits). Using the training materials and multimedia.*	1
1	*General principles of radiation protection in NM (Introduction)*	2
2	*General principles of NM Quality Control organisation and equipment*	2
3	Basic properties of radiopharmaceuticals. Risk assessment in NM.	4
4	Pharmacokinetics and internal dosimetry.	5
5	Single detector systems and survey metres	4
6	General principles of scintillation camera systems	6
7	Single photon emission tomography (SPECT)	4
8	Positron emission tomography (PET)	2
9	Image evaluation and data analysis in NM	5
10	Preparation and QC of radiopharmaceutical	6
11	Quality assurance of equipments and softwares	8
12	Radionuclide therapy	6
13	Radiation protection of the NM staff	6
14	Radiation protection of the NM patient	5
15	National and EU legislation in radiation protection and radiopharmacy	9
ii	*Organising of the portfolio, training assessment, etc.*	5
	Total for 4 months: 16 weeks x 5 days = 80 days	***80***

INTERACTIVE DISTANCE TRAINING USING SIMULATIONS

In the EMERALD Training Modules, it is possible to supplement the clinical equipment not available for hands on training with images using interactive equations and simulations. An example of such a simulation program is the SIMIND-program. The SIMIND-program was originally developed by some of us (5) as a research tool for simulation of scintillation camera parameters, and it was recently presented as a chapter in a book on Monte Carlo methods in Nuclear Medicine (6).

The SIMIND program is under reprogramming as a Windows version, to be included in the Nuclear Medicine Training Module. Several windows with graphics routines have been implemented, showing in real time the buildup of the scintillation camera image and the energy pulse-height distribution while the simulation program is running (Fig 1). By using the 'point-and-click' technique, the user can easily select different imaging situations; from simple phantom studies to clinical situations, such as bone, heart and kidney

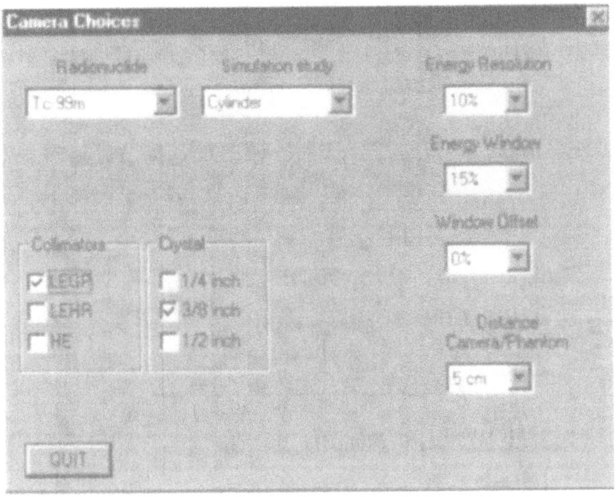

Figure 1: Window showing some of the parameters that can be selected for the simulation.

scintigraphy, using accurate anthropomorphic phantoms (Fig 2). Also, several camera parameters, such as collimator type, energy resolution, window setting and crystal thicknesses can be studied for most radionuclides.

Thus the student will, irrespectively of the availability of scintillation camera equipment, be able to perform calculations and evaluations based on these simulations.

The SIMIND simulation program will also facilitate the investigation of parameters not possible to measure or vary in the clinical situation. For example, the fraction of scatter contribution to the image and the connected quantification problem can be illustrated on the screen by using different colours for the primary and the scatter events in the image and in the energy pulse-height distribution. A future version of the program will also include a window where the photon tracks are drawn directly on the screen, thus giving the user a feeling for how the photon transport occurs in the patient.

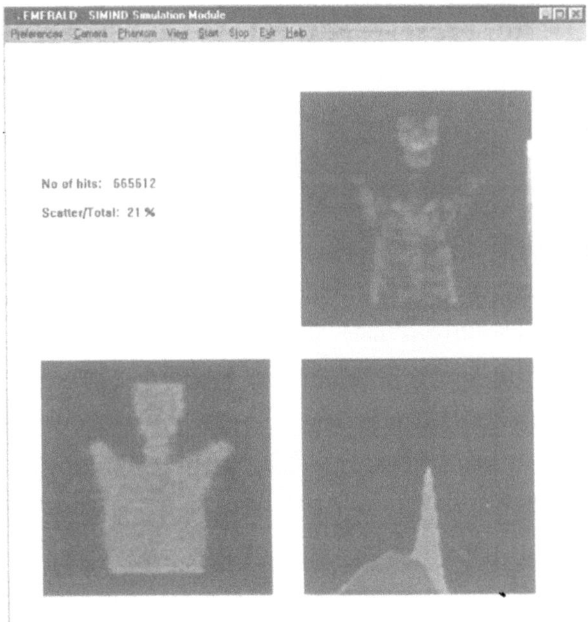

Figure 2: First version of the output window. Lower right image shows energy spectrum separated into primary and scatter events. Lower left image shows a 'persistence' like display. Upper right image shows the simulated image in grey- or colour scale and upper left shows parameters, calculated during the simulation.

MULTIMEDIA - COMPUTER BASED TRAINING

In the EMERALD project an interactive multimedia product for each Training Module will be designed, supplemented by an image database with images of equipment, measurement set-up, artefacts etc., as has been described earlier. The structure of the multimedia Training Module is presented in the flow chart below (Fig 3).

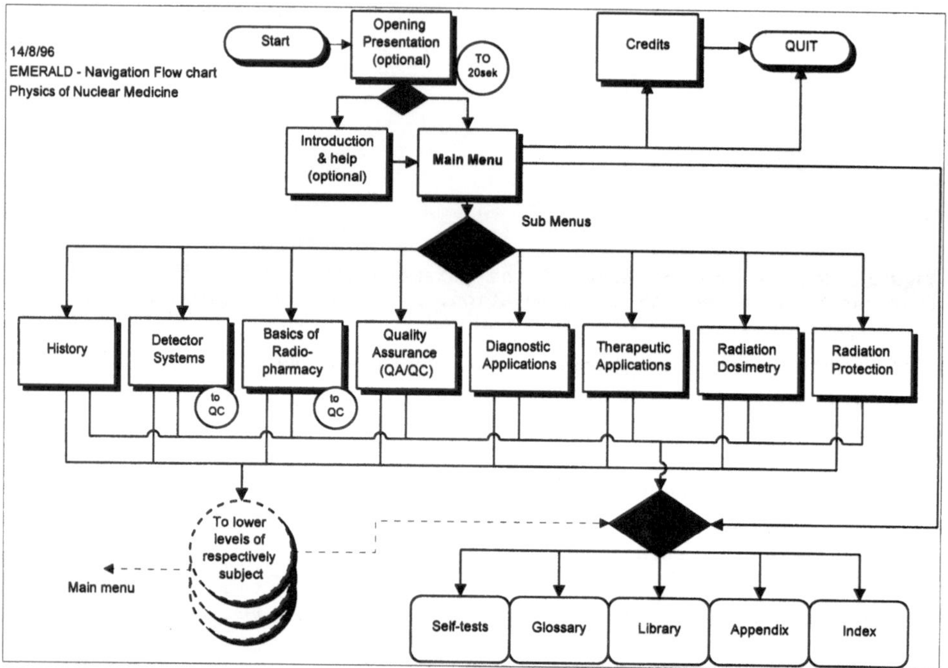

Figure 3. CD-ROM Navigation Flow Chart for the Module "Physics in Nuclear Medicine".

ACKNOWLEDGEMENTS

The work has been partly funded by the Leonardo da Vinci EC project 2620 (EMERALD) and by the participating universities and hospitals.

REFERENCES

1. The URL is **http://www.fysik.lu.se/~radiofys/emerald/**
2. Lamm I.L. Postgraduate Education in Medical radiation Physics - the EFOMP View. In: Medical Radiation Physics - a European perspective. Editors Roberts C., Tabakov S., Lewis C., London, 1995
3. EFOMP Policy Statement: Recommended Guidelines on National registration Schemes for Medical Physicists. Physica Medica 1995:XI(4); 157-159
4. Training Scheme Prospectus for Physical Scientists in health care. The Institute of Physical Science in Medicine, IPSM, 1994 (IPSM->IPEM)
5. Ljungberg M., Strand S. A Monte Carlo Program Simulating Scintillation Camera Imaging. Comput Meth Programs Biomed 1989;29:257-72.
6. Ljungberg M. The SIMIND Monte Carlo Program. In "Monte Carlo calculations in Nuclear Medicine - Applications in Diagnostic Imaging." 1998: in press

Radioactive Isotopes in
Clinical Medicine and Research XXIII
ed. by H. Bergmann, H. Köhn and H. Sinzinger

JAVA-BASED REMOTE VIEWING STATION FOR NUCLEAR MEDICINE IMAGES

Slomka PJ, Cheng D, Driedger AA.
Nuclear Medicine and Diagnostic Radiology. University of Western Ontario.
London Health Sciences Centre, 375 South Street, London, Ontario, N5A4G5

SUMMARY:

We propose Java-based remote viewing station (JaRViS) for reviewing of nuclear medicine images using Internet browser technology. The clinical imaging database can be searched via a browser interface and compressed patient images with the Java applet and color lookup tables are downloaded on the client computer from the departmental server. This paradigm does not require nuclear medicine software setup on remote viewing computers, simplifying support and deployment of such stations. Images can be interactively manipulated and displayed in a variety of layouts. Common image processing operations are supported. We conclude that it is feasible to setup a nuclear medicine reviewing station using Java and an inter- or intra-net browser.

INTRODUCTION

In nuclear medicine practice, the situation often arises where images have to be reviewed and reported from many locations outside the department. Typically, image hardcopy, is used for that purpose and although simple and portable, it takes valuable time and it does not offer electronic data search and image manipulation capabilities offered by Picture Archiving and Communications Systems (PACS) (1) or dedicated imaging workstations. Moreover, films cannot be shared simultaneously between multiple reviewers and often tend to get lost between imaging departments and referring centers. On the other hand, PACS systems cannot be easily deployed at numerous locations, because they are fairly expensive, and require dedicated hardware for image display, mainly to satisfy radiological requirements. Dedicated nuclear medicine workstations are usually too complex to use for the casual reviewer, and although they use the standard computer platform, they often require UNIX operating system or have some other advanced requirements (3). Even if the nuclear medicine workstation operated on a standard office PC, this machine would require considerable software setup and maintenance. In addition, licensing costs for nuclear medicine workstations can be prohibitive. Recently, a new software paradigm has been developed by Sun Microsystems (California, CA). Sun has introduced Java language (2), which, among other features, allows remote execution of applets (small programs) by the World Wide Web browsers. Such applets can be combined with the standard Hyper Text Markup Language (HTML) documents to provide interactive content to the web pages. Java applets are downloaded on-the fly from the server in an executable form called "bytecode". Current web browsers, running on ubiquitous office computers such as PC with Windows95/NT or Macintosh, support the execution of such bytecode. Conceivably, Java applets residing on the main imaging server could be used for on-line distribution of medical images and contain the code to perform interactive image analysis (4,5). Such an approach could enable the concept of the "department without walls", where the diagnostic images would be made available to the referring physicians involved in patient care, without equipping them with neither dedicated imaging workstations, nor installed software. In this paper, we describe our prototyping experience in utilizing Java for developing a remote nuclear medicine reviewing station (JARVIS) and discuss potential applications of such a system.

METHODS

JaRViS interfaces to the Interfile-based (6) clinical patient database on a HERMES Nuclear Diagnostics (Stockholm, Sweden) workstation. The patient search module on the client side is written in JavaScript and HTML. The search of the patient database on the server is implemented using the Perl 5.04 language (7). User name and password are provided using standard HTTP security mechanisms. Patient database can be searched by several keywords such as: patient name, study type, and acquisition dates.

Selected patient study is prepared for the downloading by compressing Interfile image data. Subsequently, the compressed nuclear medicine image series, together with the server color lookup tables (31 lookup tables each with 256 entries) and the Java applet bytecode for interactive image viewing and processing are downloaded to the browser. The applet described in this manuscript was written in Java 1.0. This applet includes common nuclear medicine operations such as image filtering, frame grouping, movie display, interactive color table manipulation, threshold manipulation, spatial and temporal filtering. An example of the JaRViS display page is shown in Figure 1.

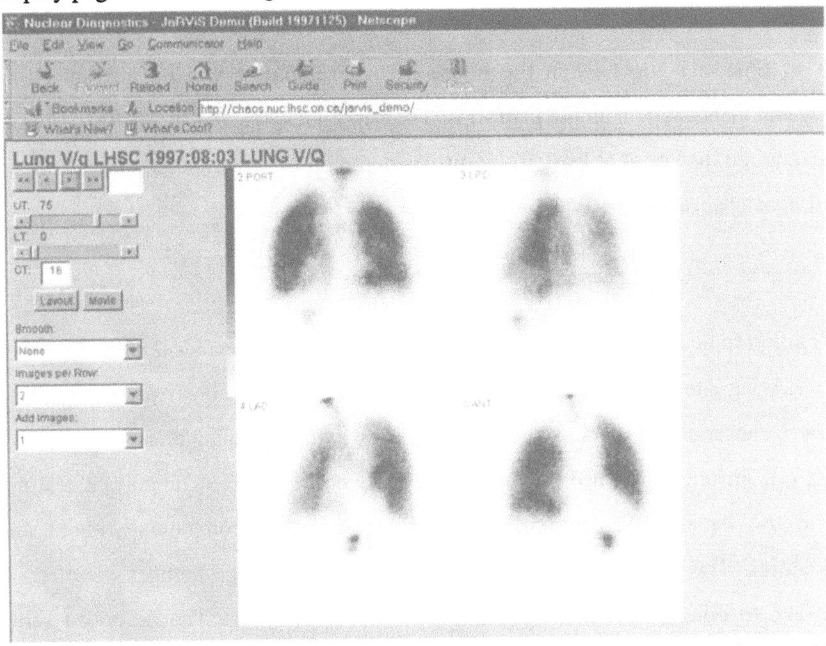

Figure 1. Static display page in Jarvis shown within Netscape Communicator (Mountain View, CA) browser

RESULTS

The average time to download 14 lung ventilation and perfusion images in 128x128 matrix (448 Kbytes raw data + header 8 Kbytes, 110 Kbytes bytes after compression), with Java bytecode (14 Kbytes) and color lookup tables (18 Kbytes) over 28.8 kbps modem is less than 2 minutes. The transfer time over the local area network is less than 1 sec. The time to spatially filter 14, 128x128 images on a Pentium 233 MMX running Netscape Communicator 4.04 with (Just-In-Time) JIT compiler is less than 1 second. Bilinear interpolation, threshold of lookup tables for visual presentation of images could be performed interactively in a 512x512 image window using the JIT compiler available in Netscape.

JaRViS application should be able to run on all computer platforms supporting Java Virtual Machine (2). We have tested JaRViS on the following platforms: Windows 95, Windows NT,

(Netscape, Internet Explorer) Solaris SPARC, Solaris x86, and Macintosh Apple (Netscape 4). We have experienced some small changes in the program behavior, such as different than specified font sizes, and some problems with window refresh on the Macintosh computer. Nevertheless, the program could be run on all these computers. We have found that such cross-platform testing consumes a lot of time and hopefully in the future Java development will be guaranteed to perform correctly and identically on all the platforms. The faithful display of at least 200 colors in the lookup table required the use of at least 16-bit display depth on these computers; this is due to the color allocation mechanism by the Web browsers.

DISCUSSION

The described solution to access nuclear medicine images has several advantages. No software is required on the viewing site, thus images can be made easily and cost-effectively available to referring physicians, cancer clinics within and outside of the hospital, providing a viable alternative to film media. In our limited experience this has already proven to be a very important feature. We were able to use the described system on a variety of remote computers without any installation procedures. This may prove of critical importance when large number of referring clinicians would like to reliably access the images from various locations. The described setup should ensure that everyone uses the same version of the software and that differences in configurations and type of remote computers are of no consequence. Several security issues including the spread of computer viruses are also well addressed in such a paradigm (2).

Such functionality overlaps with that offered by a fully-fledged Picture Archiving and Communications Systems (PACS) systems (1), in which medical images can be viewed on PACS stations across the institution. Currently, PACS systems require dedicated viewing hardware, software licenses for each display station, and maintenance support for each display station. A Java-based system like JaRViS, however, could potentially provide similar function using standard computers already present in many locations in a hospital setting, and therefore drastically reducing the cost of such solution and simplifying the training for the use of such system. Such a solution may be much more beneficial for nuclear medicine imaging. Indeed, a more controversial view could be that such system could be used for general radiology PACS purpose – perhaps with higher requirement on the display graphics board and monitors on the viewing side. A natural extension of such a system is the integration of viewing software with image reporting software, where patient reports could be stored in HTML format including captured images and animation. This function would be somewhat equivalent to the Screen Capture format (8), however more powerful since animations and text reports could be also included. The benefit of using the HTML format (perhaps encapsulating the DICOM definitions of medical terms) would be the simplification of the software needed to review such reports.

In addition to the use of such system as a component in the hospital PACS, an immediate practical application for JaRViS is home reporting of emergency procedures such as lung ventilation perfusion scans or dynamic studies. We found the speed of download over a standard modem sufficient for such use.

An often discussed issue is the performance of the code implemented in Java programming language (9), especially when it involves computationally intensive tasks, such as image processing tasks. In this project, we have found that the performance of Java code for bilinear interpolation, cine display and filtering, approaches that of standard imaging workstation if Just in Time (JIT) compiler is used. Therefore we do not perceive Java performance as an obstacle for this application, even if more sophisticated image algorithms are required.

REFERENCES:

1 Meyer-Ebrecht D. Picture archiving and communication systems (PACS) for medical application. Int J Biomed Comput, 35(2):91-124 1994

2. Arnold K, Gosling J. The Java programming language. Addison-Wesley, Reading, Mass. 1996.

3. Slomka PJ, Dey D. J Nucl Med 1996;37(9):25N-33N

4. Phung NX, Wallis JW. An Internet-based, interactive nuclear medicine image display system implemented in the Java Programming language. *J Nucl Med* 1997;38:210P

5. Wittry MD, Farris JS, Fletcher JW. Tiffnet: A Web-based PACS for nuclear Medicine *J Nucl Med* 1997;38:307P

6. Todd-Pokropek A, Cradduck TD, Deconinck F. A file format for the exchange of nuclear medicine data: a specification of INTERFILE version 3.3. *Nucl Med Commun* 1992;13:673-699.

7. Wall L, Christiansen T, Schwartz RL. Programming Perl. O'Reilly & Associates, Inc. Sebastopol, CA. 1996.

8. American College of Radiology, National Electrical Manufacturers Association. Digital imaging and communications in medicine (DICOM): conformance. Washington, DC: NEMA publication PS 3.2-1993, 1993.

9. Gosling J. The Feel of Java. *Computer*, 1997-June:53-57

POSTER SESSION I

Radioactive Isotopes in
Clinical Medicine and Research XXIII
ed. by H. Bergmann, H. Köhn and H. Sinzinger

PREOPERATIVE DETERMINATION OF STROKE RISK WITH ECD SPECT BEFORE THERAPEUTIC CAROTID ARTERY OCCLUSION

J.P. Wielepp[1,4], G. Schroth[2], R. Häusler[3], D. Lüscher[1], T. Mende[4], J.A. Kinser[1]

Department of Nuclear Medicine[1], Neuroradiology[2] and ENT[3], University of Berne, Switzerland; Department of Nuclear Medicine[4], Martin-Luther-University Halle, Germany

SUMMARY: The CBF evaluation with ECD SPECT allows a sensitive identification of clinically inapparent cerebral perfusion disturbances during the balloon occlusion test (BOT). A symmetric perfusion pattern or only slight defects with an asymmetry less than 9% and no neurological symptoms during the BOT means only a low risk for stroke after sacrifice of the ICA. However, a hemispheric or territorial perfusion defect with an asymmetry of greater than 9% or the occurence of neurological symptoms during the BOT is associated with a high risk for a stroke after permanent occlusion or resection of the ICA.

INTRODUCTION:

Inoperable aneurysms and malignant cervical tumors with involvement of the internal carotid artery (ICA) can make resection or permanent occlusion of the ICA mandatory. The main complication is a cerebral infarct due to embolus or ischemia as a result of inadequate collateral circulation (1). Complications, such as hemiparesis, hemiplegia, aphasia or even death, occur in 5-30% of patients after ligature of the ICA (2). Normally the circle of Willis provides the collateral circulation. However, this is intact in only 20%. That is the problem in the preoperative evaluation of the risk of brain damage resulting from inadequate collateral circulation. The balloon occlusion test (BOT), to simulate the planned intervention, plays a central role in the work-up of the resectability of the ICA. However, 5-20% of the patients with anatomically sufficient collateral circulation and without clinical changes during the BOT develop a brain infarct after permanent occlusion or resection of the ICA (1). Additional techniques for the preoperative prediction of adequacy of the collateral circulation are brain perfusion measurements with SPECT, transcranial doppler sonography, EEG and stump pressure measurements (1,3,4). The goal of our study is to examine the value of ECD SPECT for the determination of the infarkt risk before therapeutic sacrifice of the ICA.

METHODS:

During the preoperative work-up of the collateral circulation of the involved hemisphere, a BOT was carried out in 24 patients (4 giant aneurysms, 20 head-neck tumors, m:17, f:7; average age 52.8 ± 17.4 years), in 12 patients during induced hypotension. 10 minutes after begin of the occlusion 750 MBq ^{99m}Tc-ECD were injected iv and 60 minutes pi the aquisition was done on the 3-headed SPECT camera (Prism 3000). When necessary baseline SPECT was performed on the following day. For SPECT evaluation 3 representative transverse slices (slice thickness 7.5 mm) were chosen and ROI's were placed over the territories of the ACA, MCA, PCA, watershed zones and striatum. The semiquantitative evaluation was done by calculation of the asymmetry index (AI) and comparison to a control group (10 healthy volunteers, 52.5 ± 6.5 years).

RESULTS:

16 of 24 patients had an AI < 9% with only minimal solitary defects or a symmetric perfusion with an AI < 5% (Group A) and normal clinical and angiographic findings as well as outcome. In comparison to the control group, there was no significant difference in the AI ($p>0.05$ in all ROI's, w-test). 8 of 24 patients showed either hemispheric or territorial decreased perfusion (Group B) with an AI > 9% ($p<0.05$ in all ROI's, except the territory of the ACA and the cerebellum). 5 of Group B had an anatomically intact collateral circulation and no neurological symptoms during occlusion, and in 4 of them the decrease in perfusion occurred during induced hypotension. A definitive occlusion or resection of the ICA was done in 7 patients. (Table 1)

Table 1. SPECT findings in comparison to angiography, clinical symptoms and outcome

SPECT	BTO (n=24)		Clinic (n=24)		p.o.Outcome (n=7)	
	negative	positive	negative	positive	negative	positive
A (n=16)	16	0	16	0	5	0
B (n=8)	5	3	6	2	0	2

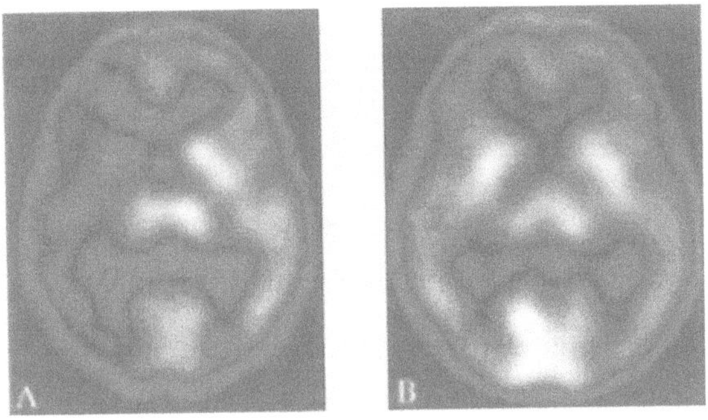

Figure 1. 53 years old female patient with an glomus tumor on the right side. The angiography shows a good collateral circulation over the right posterior communicating artery. Even after induced reduction of blood pressure she developed no neurological symptoms. The CBF SPECT shows an hemispheric hypoperfusion (A) with total normalization in the baseline SPECT performed on the following day (B).

DISCUSSION:

The temporary occlusion of the ICA with balloon mimics the vascular situation after permanent occlusion. Cerebral angiography during occlusion allows the anatomical demonstration of the collateral circulation in the areas of the carotis and basilar arteries. In contrast, SPECT gives information about the functional adequacy of the collateral circulation. Improved accuracy can be achieved by the simulation of stress situations which can occur intra- or postoperative and increase the risk of a delayed stroke due to poor blood flow reserves (5). For these reasons we carried out the BOT during induced hypotension which increased the predictive value of the procedure. In our study 88% (21/24) of the patients had an anatomically sufficient collateral circulation and 92% (22/24) tolerated the BOT without neurological symptoms. However, the SPECT showed in 33% (8/24) a clearly reduced perfusion as an indication of a functionally insufficient collateral circulation which was clinically and anatomically inapparent in 20% (5/24) of the patients at the time of the BOT, of these 4 (17%) after reduction of the blood pressure. All patients in whom an ICA resection or permanent occlusion was carried out and who had no neurological symptoms postoperatively had a symmetrical or only slightly asymmetrical perfusion. Thus, there is a high predictive value of a negativ CBF SPECT.

CONCLUSION:

SPECT allows a sensitive identification of clinically inapparent cerebral perfusion disturbances during BOT. The combination of BOT and SPECT enables a reliable estimation of the stroke risk before carotid sacrifice is carried out. An improvement in the test significance can be achieved by an reduction of the blood pressure during the test occlusion to estimate the cerebrovascular reserve capacity and by semiquantitative SPECT evaluation.

REFERENCES:

1. Erba SM, Horton JA, Latchaw RE, Yonas H, Sekhar L, Schramm V, Pentheny S. Balloon Test Occlusion of the Internal Carotid Artery with Stable Xenon/CT Cerebral Blood Flow Imaging. AJNR 1988; 9:533-538,
2. Miller J, JawadK, Jennet B. Safety of carotid ligation and ist role in the management of intracranial aneurysms. J Neurol Neurosurg Psychiatry 1977; 40:64-72
3. Leech PJ, Miller JD, Fitch W, Barker J. Cerebral blood flow, internal carotid pressure, and the EEG as a guide to the safety of carotid ligation. J Neurol Neurosurg Psychiatry 1974; 37:854-862
4. Keller E, Ries F, Urbach H, Gass S, Grünwald F, Solymosi L, Schild H. Endovaskulärer Ballonokklusionstest der A.carotis interna mit erweitertem hämodynamischen Monitoring zur Bestimmung der Durchblutungsreserve vor geplanten Kartisverschluss. Fortschr Röntgenstr1996; 4:324-330
5. De Vries EJ, Sekhar LN, Horton JA, Eibling DE, Janecka IP, Schramm VL, Yonas H. A new method to predict safe resection of the internal carotid artery. Laryngoscope 1990; 100:85-88

Radioactive Isotopes in
Clinical Medicine and Research XXIII
ed. by H. Bergmann, H. Köhn and H. Sinzinger

Asymmetry of the dopaminergic system in schizophrenic patients

U. Bauer[1], R. Bauer[2], M. Puille[2], G. Schüler[1], P. Rappelsberger[3], B. Gallhofer[1].
Center for Psychiatry [1], Clinic for Nuclear Medicine [2], Justus-Liebig-Universitaet Giessen, Institute for Neurophysiology [3], University of Vienna.

Summary

Alterations of the dopaminergic neurotransmitter system (DAS) in schizophrenia have been studied post mortem as well as in vivo with PET and SPECT techniques. We describe a new semiquantitative technique for assessment of DAS laterality by means of I-123-IBZM SPECT. We compared DAS laterality with functional neurophysiological parameters derived from qEEG recordings. Highly significant correlations between DAS asymmetry and EEG amplitude changes in response to sensory motor tasks were found. These results are in line with current concepts of the DAS.

Introduction

Dopaminergic dysregulation has been often discussed in schizophrenia because of psychosis-inducing effects of dopaminergic agonists and the antipsychotic potency of dopaminergic antagonists. The dopaminergic neurotransmitter system is asymmetrically distributed in the brain. Abnormal dopaminergic lateralization in schizophrenic patients compared to healthy subjects has been demonstrated in PET [1] and IBZM SPECT investigations of schizophrenic patients at least in subgroups [2]. During neuroleptic treatment reversal of dopaminergic lateralization has been described in some patients [3]. However, the changes obtained using usual ROI techniques (basal ganglia /frontal cortex) were small.

We introduce a new technique for the assessment of dopaminergic asymmetry. The derived index of lateralization is correlated with functional quantitative EEG parameters at rest and in response to sensory motor tasks.

Patients and Methods

23 patients with DSM-III-R diagnosis of schizophrenia were investigated. They were all right-handed. IBZM SPECT and functional qEEG were performed within three days. The patients were treated with atypical neuroleptics. No additional medication was allowed. Clinical symptoms were assessed with the Brief Psychiatric Rating Scale (BPRS).

180 MBq I-123-IBZM were intravenously injected for the IBZM SPECT study. Acquisition was started 80 min p.i., acquisition time was 40 min. 60 projections with angular steps of 6 degrees were recorded using the Siemens triple head Multispect equipped with medium energy collimators. Matrix size was 64 x 64.

Tomograms were interpolated to 256 x 256 matrices and reoriented to achieve orthogonal orientation. Squared ROI's of 10x10 pixels were selected in appropriate sagittal planes which covered the basal ganglia. The ROI's were copied to all sagittal slices, and the total counts within these ROI's were computed. The resulting line profil was interpolated to 100 data points. A schematical drawing of the evaluation is given in fig. 1. Weighted regression lines were computed as semiquantitative measure of lateral differences of IBZM activity. The index of laterality "L" was computed as the difference of the slope of basal and frontal lines as

$$L = \text{abs}(\, m(BG) - m(FC)\,)$$

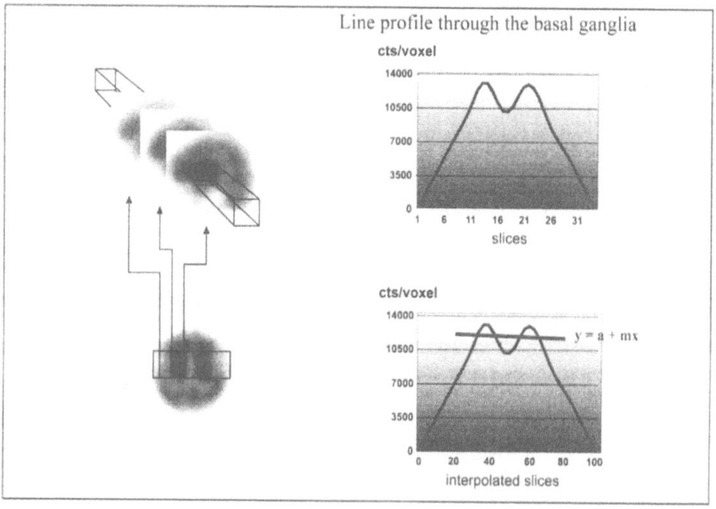

Fig. 1: Schematical drawing of IBZM SPECT evaluation

EEG was recorded at rest with eyes closed (EC) and eyes open (EO) in intervals of 30 sec and during three different sensory motor tasks (GT, AT, CT). Spectral amplitudes "FA" were calculated in the main frequency bands. Reactivities "R" at rest and in response to tasks were computed as the difference of spectral amplitudes :

$$R(task) = FA(task) - FA(EO) \text{ and } R(EO) = FA(EC) - FA(EO) .$$

Results

Schizophrenic patients had a wide range of laterality from nearly missing to pronounced interhemispheric differences. Whereas in healthy controls (n= 6) L was between 0.25 and 1.27, in schizophrenic patients L was in the range between 0.10 and 3.28 .

Patients with no laterality showed significant decrease of amplitudes in reaction to tasks in the alpha and beta bands, whereas patients with marked laterality had an increase. The correlations between the laterality L and different activational conditions are shown in Table 1.

Frequency band	delta	theta	alpha	beta
Condition				
FA (EO)	0.094	-0.123	-0.304	0.069
FA (EC)	0.120	-0.193	-0.369	0.183
R (EO)	-0.039	-0.223	-0.198	0.312
R (GT)	0.142	0.347	**0.725** [a]	**0.560** [b]
R (AT)	0.090	0.313	**0.669** [a]	**0.543** [b]
R (CT)	0.160	0.292	**0.670** [a]	**0.503** [b]
			[a] $p<0.001$	[b] $p<0.02$

Table 1: Correlation r between the index of laterality L and the spectral amplitudes as well as reactivity to tasks in the different frequency bands. Probability values are given.

Discussion:

Up to now dopaminergic asymmetries as demonstrated by means of IBZM SPECT had usually been evaluated by ROI technique. Obtained values were correlated with clinical data. However, no significant relationship could be found. In this paper two new aspects are introduced:

1) we assess dopaminergic asymmetry with activity histograms (line profiles) of voxels over both the basal ganglia and the frontal cortex and
2) we compare the calculated index of laterality with functional neurophysiological parameters derived from qEEG recordings.

A wide range of lateralization in patients was found which can indicate that subtle DA asymmetries can be evaluated by means of this method. The correlation with functional parameters is highly significant. The results are in line with recent concepts of the dopaminergic neurotransmitter system (DAS). Within striato-pallido-thalamo-cortical feedback loops DA has an important role in modulating the excitability of basal ganglia output [4]. Altered D2 receptor distribution becomes relevant when information is processed through the basal ganglia. In sensory motor tasks an involvement of the basal ganglia has been shown. EEG is an important tool to assess cerebral activation at rest and in response to sensory motor activation [5]. The results of the present study indicate such a correlation between lateralization effects in IBZM SPECT and stimulation-induced activation in the EEG. These findings suggest that dopaminergic lateralization plays an important role in EEG amplitude changes occuring in response to sensory motor tasks. IBZM SPECT and qEEG seem to be appropriate methods to assess this functional relationship.

References:
1. Farde L., Wiesel F., Stone-Elander S., and et.al. D2 dopamine receptors in neuroleptic-naive schizophrenic patients. *Arch Gen Psych* 1990; 47: 213-219.
2. Pilowsky L., S., Costa D., C., Ell P., J., Verhoeff N., P., Murray R., M., and Kerwin R., W. D2 Dopamine Receptor Binding in the Basal Ganglia of Antipsychotic-Free Schizophrenic Patients: An 123I-IBZM Single Photon Emission Computerised Tomography Study. *Br J Psychiatry* 1994; 164: 16-26.
3. Schröder J., Bubeck B., Silvestri S., Demisch S., and Sauer H. Gender differences in D2 dopamine receptor binding in drug-naive patients with schizophrenia: an (123)iodobenzamide single photon emission computed tomography study. *Psychiatry Res : Neuroimaging* 1997; 75; 115-123.
4. Smith A., D. and Bolam J., P. The neural network of the basal ganglia as revealed by the study of synaptic connections of identified neurones. *TINS* 1990; 13: 259-265.
5. Toro C., Cox C., Friehs G., Ojakangas C., Maxwell R., Gates J., R., Gumnit R., J., and Ebner T., J. 8-12 Hz rhythmic oscillations in human motor cortex during two-dimensional arm movements: evidence for representation of kinematic parameters. *Electroenceph clin Neurophysiol* 1994; 93; 390-403.

Radioactive Isotopes in
Clinical Medicine and Research XXIII
ed. by H. Bergmann, H. Köhn and H. Sinzinger

BLOOD FLOW CHANGES IN CEREBRAL AND CEREBELLUM CORTEX IN OBSESSIVE-COMPULSIVE DISORDER PATIENTS EVALUATED WITH ECD-Tc99m SPET

A. Vella, D. Volterrani, G. Pacciani*, P. Bertelli, L. Burroni, P. Castrogiovanni* and A. Vattimo

Departments of Nuclear Medicine and Psychiatry*, University of Siena, Policlinico "Le Scotte", 53100 Siena, Italy

SUMMARY

A semiquantitative analysis of brain perfusion was assessed with ^{99m}Tc-ECD SPET in 30 pts affected by Obsessive-Compulsive Disorder (OCD) and in 8 normal controls. In OCD drug-free pts a significant blood flow increase in both frontal, the right temporal, the left occipital cortex, the left thalamus and in the cerebellum was observed. Moreover, cerebellum perfusion was related with several brain regions only in drug-free pts. Treated patients did not show significant blood flow abnormalities. The presence of comorbidity in OCD patients was associated with a trend of hypoperfusion. The OCD duration showed a relationship only with lenticular nuclei perfusion.

Our findings suggest that OCD involves the limbic/paralimbic structures and the cerebellum.

INTRODUCTION

Several independent SPET studies of subjects with OCD have demonstrated an increased flow in the frontal lobes (1). PET studies have also demonstrated increased glucose metabolism in the frontal cortex of subjects with this disorder. Moreover, an involvement of the basal ganglia and thalamus bas been demonstrated, but not all studies have replicated the same findings (2). Recently, an involvement of the cerebellum in the output cognitive function has been reported in literature (3). Previous SPET and PET studies have not reported significant differences of cerebellum perfusion between OCD patients and normal controls. The aim of this study was to investigate differences of blood flow in the cerebral and cerebellum cortex, basal ganglia and thalamus in untreated and treated OCD patients matched with normal control subjects.

MATERIALS AND METHODS

Thirty patients (12 F, 18 M; mean age 35 yrs) with OCD and 8 control subjects (3 F, 5 M; mean age 25 yrs), free of past or existing neurological and psychiatric disease, were enrolled in the study.

Ten OCD patients were drug-free whereas 20 were psychopharmacologically treated.

Moreover, 10 out 30 OCD patients presented AXIS I (mood disorders) comorbidity. Subject behaviour was evaluted for severity of symptoms the day of the examination, prior to the SPET scans using the CGI test and the Yale-Brown obsessive compulsive scale (Y-BOCS).

Both patients and controls received 30 mCi iv of ^{99m}Tc-ECD in the supine position and in a room with a minimum of noise and low ambient light; SPET acquisition started 30 min. later using a dual-head rotating camera (ADAC-VERTEX) equipped with LEUHR collimators, on a 128 x 128 matrix, with a 1.46 zoom, and using 64 projections for 60 sec. over 360°. Raw data were reconstructed as 2 pixel thick (6.28 mm) slices using a Butterworth filter (cut off 0.45 Nyquist, order 10) in the transaxial fronto-occipital line. Attenuation correction was performed.

Four transaxial slices were selected in correspondence with the planes passing through the centrum semiovale (supraventricular level), the middle of the lateral ventricles (midventricular level), the basal ganglia and thalamus (midthalamic level) and the brain stem and cerebellum (cerebellar level). Squared ROIs of 16 pixels were drawn along the cortex, the head of the caudate nucleus, the putamen, the thalamus and the cerebellum.

Perfusion index (PI) for semiquantitative analysis was calculated as the ratio of the activity density for the ROI, divided by the activity density for the whole brain (averaging the activity density across the slices considered). The PI values of the OCD patients were compared with those of the controls using the Mann-Whitney U test. Futhermore, PI differences beetwen groups were assessed according to the severity of the OCD, the treatment, and the disease duration. A correlation analysis was also performed between cerebellum PI and each of the regional PI both in OCD patients and in normal controls.

RESULTS

SPET results demonstrated significant increase of the PI in drug-free OCD patients in comparison with normal controls in the following brain regions: right supraventricular prefrontal ($p=0.05$); left midventricular prefrontal ($p=0.03$), left occipital midventricular ($p=0.03$) and left occipital midthalamic ($p=0.01$), right orbito-frontal ($p=0.03$), right temporal ($p=0.01$), right thalamus ($p=0.02$) and cerebellum ($p=0.03$). Two cases of untreated OCD patient are reported in Fig.1.

Treated patients did not show significant differences in PI in comparison with the control group. However, when we considered treated patients only affected by a slight disorder, a trend of higher PI than in controls was observed. OCD patients with AXIS I comorbidity showed a trend of diffuse hypoperfusion in comparison with patients without comorbidity.

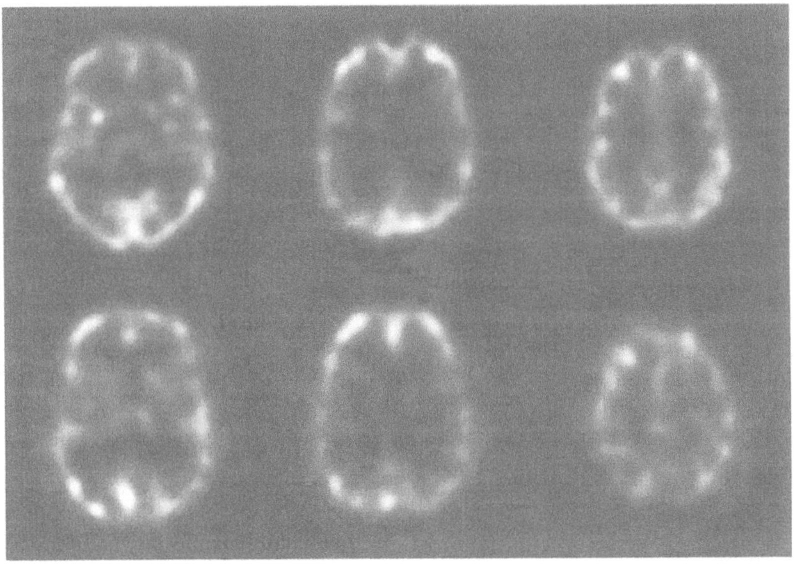

Fig. 1: (on top raw) hyperperfused areas in both frontal lobes and the right lenticular nucleus; (on bottom raw) hyperperfused areas in frontal lobes, right prefrontal and right temporo-occipital regions.

The intragroup correlation analysis, only in untreated OCD patients, demonstrated a direct correlation among the cerebellum and the right hemispheric cortex, right subcortical structures, left orbitofrontal and frontal-temporal cortex, and an inverse correlation with the left temporo-occipital. Moreover, according to disease duration, the only significant differences were found in the lenticular nucleus bilaterally: the highest value of PI related to both lenticular nuclei was that of the group in which the disease lasted for fifteen or more years.

DISCUSSION

Drug-free OCD patients showed a specific pattern of hyperfusions in cortical and subcortical structures, namely the bilateral prefontal cortex, right orbito-frontal, right temporal, left thalamus, left occipital and cerebellum. These results suggest that OCD symptoms are associated with a neurophysiologic dysfuction, involving limbic frontal-basal ganglia and the thalamus circuit (4). Recently the involvement of the cerebellum in output cognitive function has been reported in literature. Our data seem to confirm this hypothesis. In fact, we have found a strong statistically significant increase of cerebellum perfusion in OCD drug-free patients compared with normal controls. Furthermore, in the group of drug-free OCD patients we observed a correlation among cerebellum PI and the right hemispheric cortex, right subcortical structures, left orbitofrontal, frontal-temporal cortex and the left temporo-occipital. On the contrary, a limited number of correlations with different regions have been found in normal controls.

We have found no significant differences in all treated OCD patients when compared with normal controls. However, treated patients with a slight disorder showed a trend of diffused higher perfusion compared with controls. This finding could depend on the higher dosage of the drugs administered to OCD patients with a more severe disorder. In fact, several authors have previously described decreased brain blood flow or brain metabolic activity in patients psychopharmacologically treated (5).

Moreover, we have found that the presence of AXIS I comorbidity produces a trend of lower cerebral and cerebellum cortical perfusion in OCD patients when compared with those without comorbidity. In fact, the state of depression can be associated with the lower perfusion of the frontal and limbic cortex. In a PET study (6) it was reported that in OCD patients with depression, the glucose metabolic rates for the left dorsal anterolateral prefrontal cortex were significantly lower than values obtained for both normal controls and OCD subjects without depression.

A significant bilaterally increased perfusion of the lenticular nucleus was found only in patients that had been diseased for fifteen or more years. This finding suggests that pathophysiological changes of these subcortical structures could be related to the disease duration.

REFERENCES

1. Machlin S, Gordon JH, Pearlson GD, Hoehn-Saric R, Jeffery Petra and Camargo EE. Elevated medial-frontal cerebral blood flow in obsessive-compulsive patientes: a SPECT study. Am J Psychiatry 1991; 148: 1240-1242.

2. Perani D, Colombo C, Bressi S, Bonfanti A, Grassi F, Scarone S, Bellodi L, Smeraldi E and Fazio F.: 18FDG PET Study in Obsessive-Compulsive Disorder A clinical/metabolic correlation study after treatment. British Journal of Psychiatry 1995; 166:244-250.

3. Middleton F and Strick P: Anatomical evidence for Cerebellar and Basal Ganglia involment in Higher Cognitive Fuction. Science 1994;266:458-461

4. Modell J, Mountz J, Curtis G, Greden J. Neurophysiologic dysfuction in basal ganglia/limbic striatal and thalamocortical circuits as a pathogenetic mechanism of obsessive-compulsive disorder. J neuropsychiatry 1989; 1: 27 36.

5. Hoen-Saric R, Pearlson GD, Harris GJ., et al. Effects of fluoxetine on regional cerebral blood flow in obsessive-compulsive patients. American Journal of Psychiatry 1991; 148: 1243-1245.

6. Baxter LR, Phelps ME, Mazziotta JC et al: Local cerebral glucose metabolic rates in obsessive-compulsive disorder. a comparison with rates in unipolar depression and normal controls. Archives of General Psychiatry 1987; 44: 211-218.

Radioactive Isotopes in
Clinical Medicine and Research XXIII
ed. by H. Bergmann, H. Köhn and H. Sinzinger

^{99m}Tc-HMPAO SPECT IN BORDERLINE CONDITIONS RELATED TO THE AGING BRAIN

B. Palumbo, L. Cardinali, L. Parnetti, H. Sinzinger*, R. Palumbo
Nuclear Medicine, University of Perugia, Italy and *University of Vienna, Austria

Summary

We performed ^{99m}Tc-HMPAO SPECT in 25 patients with probable dementia of the Alzheimer type (AD), 25 with age-associated memory impairment (AAMI), and 25 healthy age-matched controls (C), repeating the examination at follow up (12-15 month later). 9 simmetrical bilateral ROIs were selected and analyzed semiquantitatively using cerebellum as reference region. The baseline analysis showed a significantly higher uptake ($p<0.001$) in AD, but not in AAMI and C, while the follow up analysis confirmed the trend for AD showing a significative uptake decrease for AAMI, more similar to AD group with respect to controls. In conclusion This approach, is valid to evaluate borderline conditions such as AAMI, nosological entity between normal and pathological aging brain, actually considered as an early monosymptomatic phase of Alzheimer.

INTRODUCTION

Cerebral ^{99m}Tc-HMPAO SPECT is useful to detect early perfusional modifications in aging brain (1). The border between normal and pathological aging brain is not well defined and, at the moment, only longitudinal observation shows the difference. Although Alzheimer's disease (AD) is the most common and the most known kind of dementia, not all the neurodegenerative diseases of elderly people are likely known. Age-associated memory impairment (AAMI), as defined by Crook's et al.'s criteria (2), is characterized just by a selective memory loss without other cognitive defects. This nosological entity is a borderline condition between normal and pathological aging brain and actually only follow-up study can reveal a progression in dementia or not. A lot of data are available about the scintigraphic pattern of AD , whilst scarce is the knowledge about AAMI. With the aim of further contributing to this knowledge, we performed ^{99m}Tc-HMPAO SPECT in subjects affected by AD, AAMI and in normal aged controls, repeating the exam after a period of one year without any pharmacological treatment.

MATERIALS AND METHODS

Among the subjects studied 25 suffered from Alzheimer's disease according to the NINCDS-ARDRA criteria (3) (11 males / 14 females, mean age 73.2 ± 1.4 years, mean disease duration 2-3 years), basal Mini Mental Examination (MMSE) (4) scores 18.9 ± 2.1, MMSE scores at follow-up (one year later) 16.7 ± 2.4 Global Deterioration Scales (GDS) (5) range : 3-5. Duration of disease varied from 2 to 3 years and no patient had an encephalic CT or MRI positive for focal lesions. 25 had age-associated memory impairment according to the Crook et al.'s criteria (2) (12 males and 13 females, mean age 71.9 ± 1.5, basal MMSE scores 26.8 ± 0.9, follow up MMSE scores 26.4 ±1 Benton Visual Ritention Test). 25 were normal healthy age-matched controls (12 males and 13 females, mean age 72.1 ± 1.3, basal MMSE scores 29.1 ± 1, follow up MMSE scores 28.8 ± 0.8). ^{99m}Tc-HMPAO SPECT was performed to each subject at baseline and at follow up after 1 year in absence of any nosological treatment.

SPECT scans were performed with a single-head γ-camera (Starcam, General Electric) coupled to a high resolution collimator. 20 mCi (740 MBq) of ^{99m}Tc-HMPAO SPECT (Ceretec, Amersham) were administered i.v. to the patients after 30 minutes of rest, lying in a bed with the eyes closed in absence of visive and auditory stimulations. 64 views of 30 seconds each over a 360° circular orbit were acquired on a 64 x 64 matrix with rilevator area parallel to the orbito-meatal line of the patients. Transaxial slices were produced using filtered back projection with a Butterworth filter and RAMP filter; the attenuation coefficient was 0.1 cm^{-1}.

18 simmetrical bilateral regions of interest (ROI) were selected, considering the cerebellar ROIs as reference regions and normalizing the count densities to these, to determine the regional cerebral blood flow (r CBFi). The different ROIs are reported in table 1.

The statistical analysis was carried out with univariate analysis and accepting as level of significance $p<0.05$.

RESULTS

Table 1 indicates the mean tracer uptake obtained in the ROIs examined at baseline and at follow-up, while table 2 reports the mean statistical significance of the differences in the ROIs considered in the different diagnostic categories. AD vs C showed, at baseline and follow-up, a significantly higher value ($p<0.001$) of the uptake differences, except for the right frontal posterior ROIs. AD group vs AAMI group showed at baseline and follow-up a statistical significance between the differences in the great part of the ROIs examined, not disclosing any significant trend in both right frontal posterior, temporo-parietal and left temporo-occipital. Interestingly at follow-up analysis the left frontal ROI (2 L/C) did not evidence any significance as compared with baseline data, while the right temporo-occipital (6 R/C) demonstrated a statistically significant value ($p<0.05$) with respect to the baseline. AAMI subjects vs controls showed at baseline a significant trend in bilateral frontal anterior, right temporo-occipital, bilateral perisylvian and temporal. On the other hand at follow-up in AAMI patients was observed a higher statistical significance ($p<0.001$) in comparison with controls in all the ROIs with exception of the left temporo-parietal and the reference regions. Therefore it is worth mentioning that the most sensitive and specific ROIs to evaluate cerebral perfusional pattern are the frontal-anterior (1), the perisylvian (7) and the temporal (8). No significant association was found between MMSE scores (at baseline and follow-up) and cortical tracer uptake in any group studied.

DISCUSSION

In conclusion the main results of this study are:

1) At baseline: a significant difference between AD and C was found by cerebral ^{99m}Tc HMPAO SPECT. Conversely AAMI patients disclosed a lower, although significant, tracer uptake, as regards to AD subjects, but not to controls.
2) At follow-up: the statistical significance was the same for AD vs C, showing a percentual value of 10% as cut off. On the other hand AAMI group evidenced a statistical significance only with respect to C group and not with AD.

Therefore our results confirm that ^{99m}Tc-HMPAO SPECT is a sensitive and an accuracy methodology to reveal early modifications of cerebral perfusion (1), allowing to evaluate differences between normal and pathological aging brain.

In particular, this is of great interest to study borderline conditions such as AAMI, nosological entity between normal and pathological aging brain, which in our data seems to be an early monosymptomatic phase of Alzheimer's disease, as it has been demonstrated by the great part of the international literature.

	AD (25)		AAMI (25)		C (25)	
	baseline	follow up	baseline	follow up	baseline	follow up
1 L/C	85±6.9	85±6.4	90.4±5.4	92±2.9	97.4±1.5	97±1.7
1 R/C	88±4.4	84.8±5	92.6±3.1	92.2±3.2	96.7±1.6	96.6±1.9
2 L/C	84.6±6	83.5±6	93±4.6	92±5	96.2±1.6	96.6±1.5
2 R/C	86±6.9	83.5±5.5	92.2±4.6	92.3±4	96.4±1.4	97±1
3 L/C	85.9±6	84±6.1	93.1±4	92.5±4	97.2±1.7	97.3±1.8
3 R/C	85.3±5	82.4±6.1	93.1±4.2	91.3±4.3	96.9±1.2	97.1±1.1
4 L/C	86.7±5	85±5.6	91.9±5	90.8±4.9	97.4±1.3	97.8±1.2
4 R/C	87.2±5	84.3±6.1	92.4±3.9	93.1±4	97.7±1.7	97.5±1.7
5 L/C	86.9±6	85.1±7.9	92.9±4	90.9±3	97.1±1	97.3±1.2
5 R/C	86.1±6	84.1±5	91.5±4.5	91.4±4.2	96.8±1.5	96.9±1.9
6 L/C	88±6.1	84.9±6.8	93.1±3.7	92.9±3.7	96.6±1.4	97±0.8
6 R/C	89.1±4	86.7±3.9	91.2±5	92.3±4.8	96.9±1	97.1±1.1
7 L/C	87±2.8	82.8±4.3	92.9±3	91.9±3.6	96.2±1.5	97.2±0.9
7 R/C	88±4.9	83.9±5	92.1±3.9	90.9±4	97.7±0.9	98.1±0.7
8 L/C	82±6.4	77.3±4.5	92.8±3.6	92.7±3.1	97.3±1.2	97.2±1.3
8 R/C	85.3±4	81.4±9	92.8±3	92.5±3.4	97.9±1.6	97.8±1.8
9 L/C	99.8±1	99.7±0.6	100±0.1	100±0.2	99.8±0.4	99.9±0.3
9 R/C	100±1	99.5±0.9	99.9±0.9	100±0.1	99.7±0.5	99.9±0.3

Table 1. Mean values of subjects' ROIs studied (baseline and follow up).

	AD vs C		*AD vs AAMI*		*AAMI vs C*	
	baseline	**follow up**	**baseline**	**follow up**	**baseline**	**follow up**
1 L/C	<0.001	<0.001	<0.05	<0.05	<0.01	<0.001
1 R/C	<0.001	<0.001	<0.05	<0.05	<0.05	<0.001
2 L/C	<0.001	<0.001	<0.001	ns	ns	<0.001
2 R/C	<0.001	<0.001	<0.01	<0.05	ns	<0.01
3 L/C	<0.001	<0.001	<0.01	<0.05	ns	<0.001
3 R/C	<0.001	<0.001	ns	ns	ns	<0.001
4 L/C	<0.01	<0.001	<0.05	<0.05	ns	<0.001
4 R/C	<0.001	<0.001	<0.01	0.01	ns	<0.01
5 L/C	<0.001	<0.001	ns	ns	ns	ns
5 R/C	<0.001	<0.001	ns	ns	ns	<0.001
6 L/C	<0.001	<0.001	ns	ns	ns	<0.005
6 R/C	<0.001	<0.001	ns	<0.05	<0.05	<0.001
7 L/C	<0.001	<0.001	<0.001	<0.001	<0.01	<0.001
7 R/C	<0.001	<0.001	<0.05	<0.01	<0.01	<0.001
8 L/C	<0.001	<0.001	<0.05	<0.05	<0.001	<0.001
8 R/C	<0.001	<0.001	<0.01	<0.01	<0.001	<0.001
9 L/C	ns	ns	ns	ns	ns	ns
9 R/C	ns	ns	ns	ns	ns	ns

Table 2. Statistical analysis results of subjects' studied (baseline and follow up).

REFERENCES

1. Read SL, Miller BL, Mene I et al. Spect in dementia : clinical and pathological correlation. JAGS 1995 ; 43 : 1243-1247.
2. Crook T, Bartus RT, Ferris SH et al. Age-associated memory impairment. Proposed diagnostic criteria and measures of clinical change-report of a National Institute of Mental Health work group. Dev Neuropsycol 1986 ; 24 : 261-276.
3. Mc Khann G, Drachman D, Folstein M et al. Clinical diagnosis of Alzheimer's disease : report of the NINCS-ADRDA work group under the auspices of Department of Health and Human Services Task Force on Alzheimer's disease. Neurology 1984, 34 : 939-944.
4. Folstein MF, Folstein SE, Mc Hugh PR. Mini Mental State : a practical method for grading the cognitive state of patients for the clinician. J Psychiatr res 1975 ; 12 : 189-198.
5. Reisberg G, Ferris SH, De Leon MJ et al. The global deterioration scale for assessment of primary degenerative dementia. Am J Psychiatry 1982 ; 139 : 1136-1139.
6. Benton AL, Eslinger PJ, Damasio AR. Normative observation on neuropsychological test performances in old age. J Clin Neuropsychol 1981 ; 3 : 33-39.

Radioactive Isotopes in
Clinical Medicine and Research XXIII
ed. by H. Bergmann, H. Köhn and H. Sinzinger

QUANTITATIVE BRAIN PERFUSION ANALYSIS IN HYPERTENSION DURING REST AND EXERCISE TECHNETIUM-99M-HMPAO SINGLE-PHOTON EMISSION COMPUTED TOMOGRAPHY

A. Klissarova[1], K. Nedelchev[2], D. Minchev[2], G. Tranulov[1] and E. Georgieva[1]

[1]Dept. of Nuclear Medicine, [2]Dept. of Neurology, Medical University of Varna, 55 M. Drinov Str., 9002 Varna, Bulgaria

SUMMARY: The study aims at assessing the regional cerebral blood flow (rCBF) in uncomplicated hypertension (HT). We investigated 21 patients in stage I and 11 patients in stage II of HT. Tc-99m-HMPAO SPECT was performed at rest and after exercise stress. The right to left ratio values, perfusion indices (PI), were calculated in 10 symmetric sectorial areas of 3 transversal slices. The PI at rest did not differ from the referent values, except for 4 patients in the II stage of HT. Abnormal PI after exercise stress were detected in stage I (n=17) and in stage II (n=10). The method provides an adequate assessment of CBF autoregulation.

INTRODUCTION

Hypertension influences profoundly the cerebral circulation by causing structural and functional hemodynamic changes in the resistant vessels. The structural remodeling of the smaller arteries and arterioles leads to vasodilatory reserve reduction and shifts the autoregulation of cerebral blood flow (CBF) toward higher levels on the blood-pressure axis. SPECT has recently been accepted as a method for investigating cerebral autoregulation because it allows a quantitative brain perfusion analysis (1,2). Previous investigations have been concerned mainly with two aspects: the vasomotor response to chemical stimuli (acetazolamid, hypercapnia) (2,3) and the variations in CBF induced by orthostatic hypotension and reactive hyperemia (4,5). The present study was designed to assess the regional cerebral blood flow (rCBF) in uncomplicated hypertension. We used exercise testing to induce changes in cerebral perfusion pressure, analysing the SPECT parameters that correlate best with CBF and that are most strongly influenced by blood flow resistance - the perfusion indices (PI), i.e., the right to left ratio of the activity rate.

MATERIALS AND METHODS

Subjects of the investigation were 32 patients (mean age 36.11±9.21 years) without clinical evidence of target organ damage. After excluding subjects with occlusive disease of the supraortic trunks revealed by extracranial Doppler sonography, the patients were allocated to two subgroups: group A, composed of 21 patients in the first stage of hypertension and group B, composed of 11 patients in the second stage of hypertension. Tc-99m-HMPAO SPECT was performed at rest and during bicycle ergometer exercise, two days later. Only an increase in mean arterial blood pressure (ABP) of more than 10% was considered to be a sufficient stimulus. A single-headed camera (Diacam, Siemens - Germany) with the following acquisition protocol parameters was used to estimate CBF : rotation angle - 360°; number of frames - 64; frame duration - 25 sec., matrix -64/64, zoom 1. A dose of 20 mCi (740 MBq) Tc-99m-HMPAO was administered intravenously. The perfusion indices (PI) for 10 symmetric sectorial areas in 3 OM-transversal slices and the interhemispheric index (PIi) were calculated by means of a brain quantification computer programme. A referent range within 0.95 - 1.05 was accepted. Limits of the normal range of PI were calculated from 2 SD below / above the mean.

The control group comprised 5 normotensive volunteers. Informed consent was obtained from patients and control subjects. The study was approved by the Ethics Committee of the University Hospital Varna.

RESULTS

The stepwise bicycle ergometer test was terminated after registering a sufficient increase in mean ABP and this was a well-tolerated procedure. The mean ABP increase achieved in satisfactory autoregulation runs was 25.8±5.3 mm Hg. There was no significant difference in magnitude changes of mean ABP between hyper-

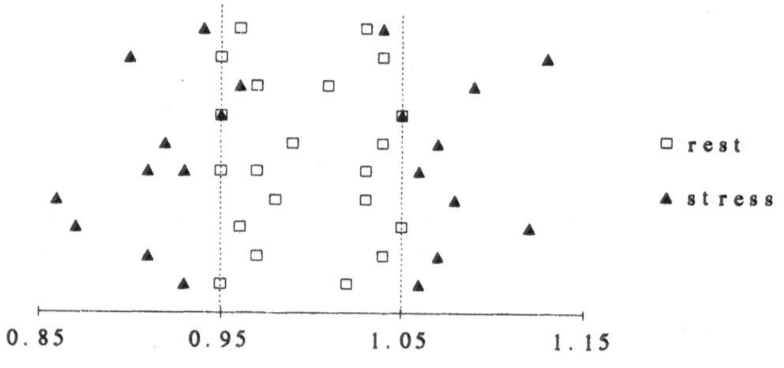

Fig. 1. Interhemispheric indices (PIi) at rest and during exercise (stress) in 21 patients with HT, stage 1. Dotted lines indicate limits of normal ranges.

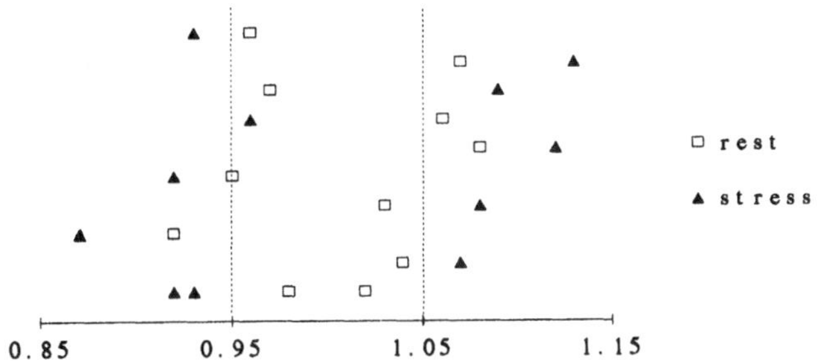

Fig. 2. Interhemispheric indices (PIi) at rest and during exercise (stress) in 11 patients with HT, stage 2. Normal range limits are shown by the dotted lines.

tensive patients and controls.

Resting PIi within the normal range were evaluated in group A. As shown in Fig. 1., abnormal interhemispheric indices were registered in 17 patients (80%) after exercise testing.

The data obtained in group B are summarized in Fig. 2. Interhemispheric indices (PIi) beyond normal range in 4 patients (36%) were detected at rest. After terminating the bicycle ergometer test abnormal PIi were demonstrated in 10 cases (90%).

The readings from the symmetric sectorial analysis of tracer's distribution are presented in Table 1. PI within the normal range were detected at rest in HT, stage 1. Resting PI with abnormal meanings were registered for temporal and parieto-temporal areas (3 cases and 2 cases, accordingly) in HT, stage 2. Under the conditions of physical challenge PI beyond normal range were obtained in most of the sectorial areas analyzed. Cases with abnormal PI were found mainly in parieto-occipital, temporal and temporo-occipital areas.

DISCUSSION

Our results demonstrated that in uncomplicated hypertension dynamic

Area	HT, stage 1 (n=21)		HT, stage 2 (n=11)	
	rest	stress	rest	stress
F	-	1	-	1
T	-	14	3	7
O	-	-	-	1
P	-	5	-	1
P-O	-	18	-	9
T-O	-	11	-	5
P-T	-	7	2	8

Table 1. Abnormal PI at rest and after exercise testing (n indicates the number of patients investigated; F, T, O, P, P-O, T-O and P-T indicate frontal, temporal, occipital, parietal, parieto-occipital, temporo-occipital and parito-temporal areas, accordingly).

autoregulation is impaired, as determined by the ability of the cerebral circulation to maintain an adequate CBF in response to a change of ABF. In a number of cases this technique identified impaired autoregulation in patients in whom resting activity rates were in the normal range. The disturbances were more expressed in stage II hypertension. This high sensitivity may make the technique useful in the clinical practice. The quantitative sectorial analysis of tracer's distribution supplies a more detailed information concerning the regional brain perfusion. The higher incidence of abnormal readings in areas irrigated from two different vascular beds may have a certain clinical importance. It may represent a marker of increased stroke risk, although this needs to be determined in prospective studies. Reduction of regional tracer uptake in temporal and parieto-temporal areas has been demonstrated in patients with vascular dementia (6).

SPECT studies with an acetazolamide challenge can detect the Stage II hemodynamic failure, as described by previous investigators (2,7). We designed this method of cerebral autoregulation testing to determine structural and functional hemodynamic changes in the resistant vessels. It is a well-tolerated procedure with no side effects in either the patient group or the control group.

Dynamic Tc-99m-HMPAO SPECT studies provide an adequate assessment of cerebrovascular autoregulation in uncomplicated hypertension.

REFERENCES

1. Knappertz V, Slevers C, Steinert H, Ulrich P, Kraemer G. Comparison of single photon emission computed tomography (SPECT), regional cerebral blood flow (rCBF) and transcranial Doppler (TCD) in assessing vascular reserve capacity in internal carotid artery occlusions (ICAO). Stroke 1994; 25:732.

2. Hirano T, Minematsu K, Hasegawa Y, Tanaka Y, Hayashida K, Yamaguchi T. Acetazolamide reactivity on ^{123}I-IMP Single-photon emission computed tomography in patients with major cerebral artery occlusive disease: correlation with Positron emission tomography parameters. J Cereb Blood Flow Metab 1994; 14:763-770.

3. Markus HS, Harrison MJG. Estimation of cerebrovascular reactivity using trans-cranial Doppler, including the use of breath-holding as the vasodilatory stimulus. Stroke 1992; 23:668-673.

4. Daffertshofer M, Diehl RR, Ziems GU, Hennerici M. Orthostatic changes of cerebral blood flow velocity in patients with autonomic dysfunction. J Neurol Sci 1991; 104:32-38.

5. Aaslid R, Newell DW, Stoos R, Sorteberg W, Lindegaard K-F. Assessment of cerebral autoregulation dynamics from simultaneous arterial and venous transcranial Doppler recordings in humans. Stroke 1991; 22:1148-1154.

6. Hadjiev D, Yancheva S, Ivanova L, Nikolova G, Raychev I. Early diagnosis of the vascular dementia. New Trends Clin Neuropharm 1988; 2: 305- 313.

7. Hellman RS, Tikofski RS. An overview on the contribution of regional cerebral blood flow studies in cerebrovascular disease: is there a role for single photon emission computed tomography? Semin Nucl Med 1990; 20: 303-324.

Radioactive Isotopes in
Clinical Medicine and Research XXIII
ed. by H. Bergmann, H. Köhn and H. Sinzinger

LONG-TERM SIDE EFFECTS AFTER HIGH DOSE RADIOIODINE THERAPY IN THYROID CARCINOMA PATIENTS

C. Alexander, B. Sax, J.B. Bader, D. Hellwig, C. Finke,
C.-M. Kirsch

Department of Nuclear Medicine, Saarland University Medical Center;
D-66421 Homburg; Germany

SUMMARY: The investigation is an evaluation of intermediate and long-term side effects in patients after high-dose radioiodine treatment due to differentiated thyroid carcinoma. The results demonstrate that severe long-term non-stochastic side effects are rare after high-dose radioiodine treatment of differentiated thyroid carcinoma. Moderate side effects are more common than mentioned in literature. Mostly they are the result of radiation damage to the salivary glands.

INTRODUCTION

In the last decades relevant information was accumulated concerning stochastic side effects of high-dose radioiodine therapy of thyroid carcinomas: The rates of miscarriage, prematurity, and major congenital anomaly is not significantly different from the general population. The post-therapeutic risk of other neoplasms is slightly increased for breast and bladder cancer, and the incidence of radiation leukaemogenesis is low. In summary, benefits do not appear to be outweighed by harmful effects.

Non-stochastic immediate side effects during hospitalization, such as radiation thyroiditis, nausea, vomiting, epigastralgia, and sialoadenitis, are common. Serious acute complications are extremely rare. However, little information is still available on non-stochastic intermediate and long-term side effects after discharge of patients (1-3).

The present investigation was a retrospective evaluation of intermediate and long-term complaints/side effects of patients after high-dose radioiodine treatment.

MATERIALS AND METHODS

In the course of follow-up of differentiated thyroid carcinoma from July 1996 to June 1997 170 patients were interviewed using a standardized questionnaire. Patients with additional percutaneous radiotherapy of head and neck were excluded. The period between the last radioiodine treatment and the interview was longer than one year.

The questionnaire included complaints which were reported regularly by follow-up patients, no matter if the cause was operation, radioiodine treatment, or unclear. They were divided into intermediate (from discharge up to 3 mo) and long-term (more than 3 mo after treatment) effects. For evaluation absolute and relative rates of side effects were counted for the total and for groups of different cumulative activities. Total activity administered ranged between 4.4 and 69.0 GBq. Five groups were formed: Cumulated activity was 0 to <5 GBq (0-<135 mCi) for group I (n=27), 5 to <10 GBq (135-<270 mCi) for group II (n=65), 10 to <18.5 GBq (270-<500 mCi) for group III (n=41), 18.5 - <37 GBq (0.5-<1 Ci) for group IV (n=22), and ≥37 GBq (≥1 Ci) for group V (n=15).

RESULTS

After radioiodine treatment 77.1 % of patients (131/170) reported intermediate or long-term complaints, of which 58.8 % (100/170) showed long-term side effects more than one year after the last I-131 application.

The intermediate complaints were documented as follows: Sialoadenitis occurred in 33.5 % of cases (57/170). In 80.7 % (46/57) the parotid gland (unilateral: 11; bilateral: 35) and in 47.4 % (27/57) the submandibular gland (unilateral: 6, bilateral: 21) was affected. The frequency of sialoadenitis showed a dose-dependence (p=0.003). Twenty-nine percent (49/170) suffered from a transient dose-dependent (p=0.003) loss of taste or smell. Another 29 % (49/170) of patients reported a transient episode of alopecia. Loss of taste/smell and alopecia mostly occurred one to several weeks after discharge and lasted for one to twelve weeks before normalization. In seven patients moderate alopecia persisted for more than one year, this side effect was not dependent on administered I-131 activity (p=0.802).

The following long-term complaints persisted during the intermediate period and were still present more than one year after the last radioiodine application: 42 % of patients (72/170) suffered from reduced salivary gland function which resulted in a dry mouth, increased production of viscous mucus, or morning expectoration. Complete xerostomia occurred in seven patients (4.1 %), in one female patient xerostomia resolved seven years after the last radioiodine treatment. A coincidence of dry mouth/xerostomia and post-therapeutic sialoadenitis occurred in 37 patients, a rate of 46.8 % (37/79). Thus, more than half the cases of reduced salivary gland function did not arise from clinically evident sialoadenitis. For dry mouth a dependence on cumulated activity was significant ($p=0.004$), but not for xerostomia ($p=0.352$).

In 39 cases chronic or recurrent conjunctivitis was reported (22.9 %), four patients underwent dacryocystorhinostomy. Twenty-two patients suffered from an increased frequency of influenza (12.9 %), but another 6 patients (3.5 %) reported a reduced occurrence of such infections. Both complaints were not dose-dependent ($p=0.011$ and $p=0.767$).

Haematological abnormalities were found in eight cases. These showed a moderate decrease of leukocytes in CBC. The values ranged between 3,200 and 4,200/μl (normal range: 4,300-10,000/μl). Thrombopenia, aplastic anaemia, and signs of leukaemia were not found.

The rate of the different intermediate and long-term side effects/complaints for groups of increasing cumulative activities is documented in figure 1. For sialoadenitis, loss of taste/smell, and dry mouth a dependence on accumulated activity is given.

DISCUSSION

The results demonstrate that severe long-term non-stochastic side effects are rare after high-dose radioiodine treatment of differentiated thyroid carcinoma. Moderate side effects are more common than mentioned in literature. Mostly they are the result of radiation damage to the salivary glands. The frequency of such complaints advocates a regular prevention of salivary gland damage and the development of more effective precautions. The description of transient alopecia and chronic conjunctivitis after treatment of thyroid carcinoma is novel and has not been described before. In our opinion it should be included in patient information before therapy to avoid unfounded worries after radioiodine treatment.

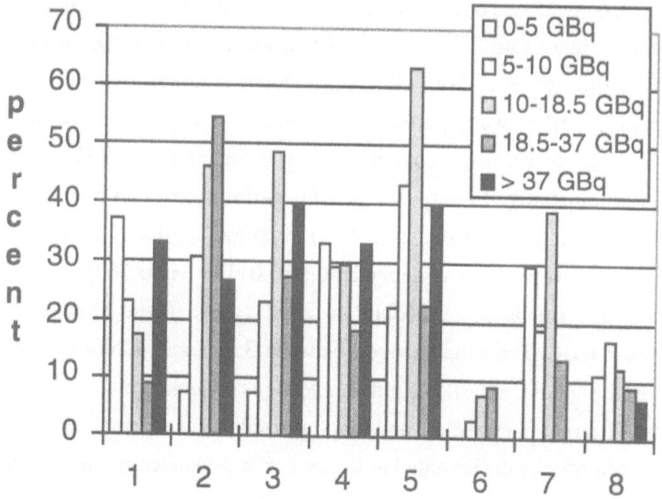

Fig 1. Side effects/complaints for groups of increasing cumulative activities: 1: no complaints, 2: sialoadenitis, 3: loss of taste/smell, 4: alopecia, 5: dry mouth, 6: xerostomia, 7: conjunctivitis, 8: increased frequency of influenza.

REFERENCES

1. Brown AP, Greening WP, McCready VR, Shaw HJ, Harmer CL. Radioiodine treatment of metastatic thyroid carcinoma: the Royal Marsden Hospital experience. Br J Radiol 1984; 57:323-327.

2. Edmonds CJ, Smith T. The long-term hazards of the treatment of thyroid cancer with radioiodine. Br J Radiol 1986; 59:45-51.

3. Van Nostrand D, Neutze J, Atkins F. Side effects of "rational dose" iodine-131 therapy for metastatic well-differentiated thyroid carcinoma. J Nucl Med 1986; 27:1519-1527.

Radioactive Isotopes in
Clinical Medicine and Research XXIII
ed. by H. Bergmann, H. Köhn and H. Sinzinger

INTRAARTERIAL I-131-MIBG TREATMENT - CLINICAL AND DOSIMETRIC RESULTS

Pinkert J.[1], Hliscs R.[1], Oehme L.[1], Hänig V.[2], Kühne A.[1], Neumann U.[2] and Franke W.-G.[1]

Dresden University of Technology, Depts. of Nuclear Medicine[1] and Radiology[2]
Fetscherstr. 74, Dresden, D-01307, Germany

SUMMARY: Treatment of APUDOMAs with I-131-MIBG is established by intravenous (i.v.) injection. In our present study we performed an intraarterial (i.a.) infusion of 2000-4000 MBq I-131-MIBG in 12 patients with inoperable progressive tumors through a superselective arterial catheter to enhance the tumor uptake. SPECT and whole body scans were performed for quantification of tumor uptake after i.v. tracer dose and i.a. therapy. The increase of tumor uptake was calculated as 187 % 24 h after i.a.-application vs. i.v.-injection. 5/5 symptomatic pts. showed a relief of pain and flush and 3/12 pts. a regression in tumor size. The radiation exposure after i.a. I-131 MIBG therapy remains in the range of published values for bone marrow.

INTRODUCTION

MIBG therapy via intravenous injection is well established for treatment of pheochromocytoma, neuroblastoma, or carcinoid tumors e.g. But the success of this kind of treatment is often limited due to low tumor uptake (1-3). Aim of the study was to evaluate the enhancement of tumor uptake, increase of tumor to nontumor ratios and the clinical value of intraarterially (i.a.) infused I-131-MIBG.

MATERIALS AND METHODS

20 i.a.-MIBG treatments (4 patients with repeated i.a.-treatments) were performed in 12 patients with inoperable progressive APUDOMAs (11 carcinoid tumors and 1 paraganglioma). All patients underwent clinical and lab examinations, contrast enhanced CT scans and angiographies prior to therapy. They gave their written consent for intraarterial treatment as a therapeutic trial. A tracer dose of 350 MBq I-131- MIBG was given intravenously one day before

the i.a. treatment for comparison with distribution pattern after i.a. I-131-MIBG application. Whole body scan and SPECT were done for measurement of tumor uptake and dosimetric calculations. The extent of the tissue supplied by the catheterized artery was determined by i.a. injection of Tc-99m-MAA.

The thyroid was blocked with a daily dose of 3x400 mg perchlorate for one week. 1000-4000 MBq I-131-MIBG in 30 ml were infused i.a. within 30 min according to the treatment protocol from SISSON (4) by means of a syringe infusion pump. The MIBG (specific activity >1.11 MBq/mg (1869 ±354) was purchased from Amersham Buchler (Braunschweig,Germany). During i.a. infusion the patient was connected to a monitor for control of heart rate, EKG, blood pressure and oxygen saturation. In 5 patients the infusion was monitored by planar sequence scintigraphy. SPECT and whole body scans using a dual head camera equipped with HEGP collimators were performed after 24 h, 48 h and 72 or 96 h. After iterative reconstruction and attenuation correction the tumor uptake was calculated from SPECT. Uptake in whole body, liver, lung, heart and bowel was determined from whole body scans in comparison with an external standard. Values for whole body, lung, liver, heart, bowel and bone marrow exposure and effective dose equivalent were calculated using the MIRDOSE 3.1 program and adult standard phantom. Lab examinations and physical examination were repeated for each patient before leaving the department (6-14 days p.i.). Follow-up was done by the referring physician and after 3-4 month in our department.

RESULTS

The tumor uptake 24 h after i.a. application increased by 187% (mean value) in comparison with intravenous injection in the areas supplied by the catheterized artery (42 lesions evaluated in the 12 patients). Individual values of enhancement of tumor uptake showed remarkable differences (see Fig.1). No significant enhancement was found in metastases not supplied by the catheterized artery. About 60 % of the uptake at 24 h was already reached 30 min after i.a. infusion. Time course measurements in tumor regions showed an increasing storage of MIBG with time compared to background only during i.a. infusion but not with i.v.-infusion. No side effects were noticed during intraarterial infusion and up to 24 h p.i. Except a decrease in blood count and increase of bilirubin (only one patient) no significant changes in lab examinations were found. A slight regression of tumor size was seen in 3/12 patients. Tumor related symptoms like pain and flush were reduced in 5/5 symptomatic patients.

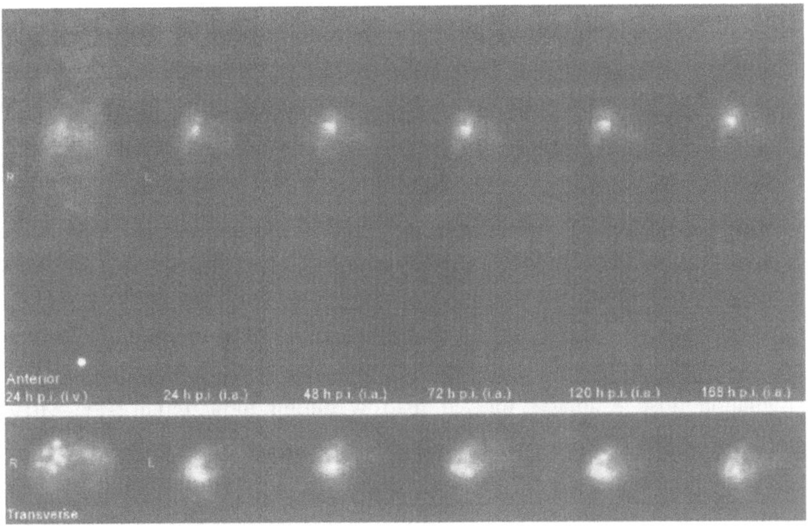

Fig. 1: 61 y., female, carcinoid, multiple liver metastases: whole body scans and SPECT slices after i.v. and i.a. infusion of I-131-MIBG (205 % increase of tumor uptake)

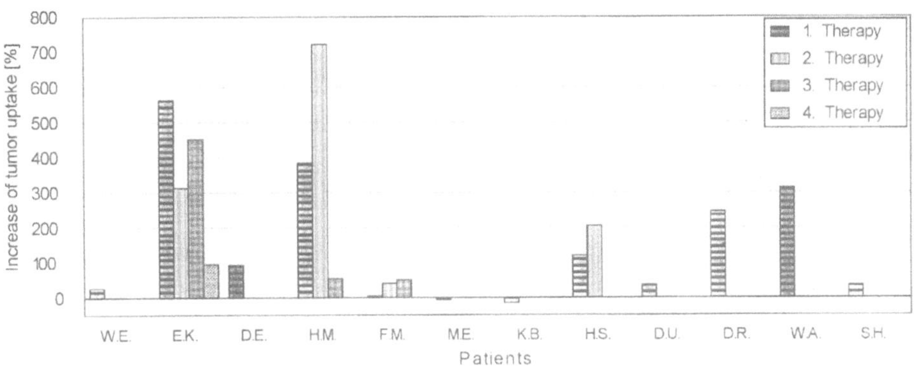

Fig. 2: Increase of tumor uptake after intraarterial application in comparison with intravenous injection of I-131-MIBG

The radiation exposure for whole body, heart, lung, liver, bowel and bone marrow exposure during i.a. MIBG therapy remains in the range of values published by other authors (0.09 mGy/MBq for bone marrow), but in case of multiple liver metastasis higher values up to 0.14 mGy/MBq were calculated (see Fig.3).

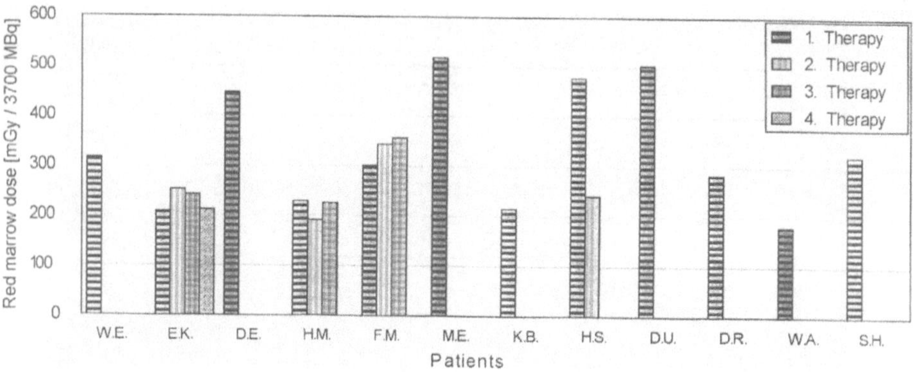

Fig. 3: Radiation dose estimates for red marrow during intraarterial I-131-MIBG therapy (normalized to 3700 MBq)

CONCLUSION

From our results we conclude that i.a. MIBG treatment is very promising in palliative therapy of APUDOMAs. Only minor side effects were observed.

Compared with high dose i.v. MIBG treatment the intraarterial treatment offers a clearly better target / background ratio with only small changes in blood count. To achieve the same tumor dose by i.v-application a greater activity of MIBG causing higher costs had to be applied. Our study will be continued to confirm initial results.

REFERENCES

1. Bestagno M, Pizzocaro C, Pagliaini R, et al. Results of [131I]Metaiodobenzylguanidine treatment of metastatic carcinoid tumors. J Nucl Biol Med 1991; 35: 277-279

2. Hoefnagel CA; Taal BG; Valdés Olmos RA. Role of [131I]Metaiodobenzylguanidine therapy in carcinoids. J Nucl Biol Med, 1991; 35: 346-348

3. Shapiro B. Summary, Conclusions and future directions of [131I]metaiodobenzylguanidine therapy in the treatment of neural crest tumors. J Nucl Biol Med 1991; 35: 357-363

4. Sisson JC, Frager MS, Val TW, et al. Radiopharmaceutical treatment of malignant pheochromocytoma. J Nucl Med 1984; 25: 197-206

Radioactive Isotopes in
Clinical Medicine and Research XXIII
ed. by H. Bergmann, H. Köhn and H. Sinzinger

DEVELOPMENT OF ^{166}Ho-Ho, Fe-HYDROXIDE (HFH) AND ^{166}Ho-HYDROXY-APATITE (HA) FOR RADIOEMBOLIZATION THERAPY OF LIVER MALIGNANCIES.

P. Angelberger, H. Kvaternik, J. Casta*

Abt. Radiopharmaka and *Abt. Forschungsreaktor, Austrian Resaerch Center Seibersdorf, A-2444 Austria

SUMMARY: The therapeutic radionuclide Ho-166 was produced in the Austrian Research Reactor Seibersdorf. Two potential radiopharmaceuticals, ^{166}Ho-Ho, Fe-Hydroxide (HFH) and ^{166}Ho-Hydroxyapatite (HA) designed for radioembolization therapy of liver malignancies were developed and investigated including biodistribution studies in rabbits. Both kinds of labeled particles were applied via the portal vein and showed a high retention of the Ho-166 in the liver after 4 days.

INTRODUCTION

Since hepatic tumor lesions receive most of their blood supply from the hepatic artery, the administration of beta-emitting particulate radiopharmaceuticals by this route is an attractive approach to deliver therapeutic irradiation differentially to tumors and metastases within the liver. Holmium-166 with a physical half-live of 26.9 h emits beta particles of max. energy 1.84 MeV resulting in a maximum soft-tissue-range of 8.4 mm. A low energy low abundance gamma emission of 81 keV (5.4 %) allows direct imaging with a gamma camera. Biodegradable Poly (L-Lactic Acid) microspheres containing neutron-activable ^{165}Ho were proposed (1) for this application, but we experienced significant instability (color, clumping, even disintegration) of such microspheres upon neutron irradiation associated with release of ^{166}Ho.

We therefore investigated the incorporation of ionic ^{166}Ho into preformed and presized particles. Based on our previous development of ^{165}Dy-Dy, Fe-Hydroxide for radiation synovectomy (2) we first used ferromagnetic Fe (II) Fe (III)-hydroxide particles as carrier for

^{166}Ho-hydroxide precipitation with NaOH. This allowed electromagnetic separation of ^{166}Ho-HFH under remote handling conditions. Since Hydroxyapatite was suggested as particulate carrier of ^{153}Sm for radiation synovectomy (3), we studied ^{166}Ho-labeling of HA-particles as an alternative radiopharmaceutical.

MATERIAL AND METHODS

0.5 mg Ho_2O_3 was dissolved in conc. HNO_3 and evaporated in a quartz ampoule at 240°C. The resulting $Ho(NO_3)_3$ was neutron irradiated in the 9 MW nuclear reactor of the Austrian Research Center Seibersdorf. The target was dissolved in 0.5 ml 0.1 M HCl and used for further preparation.

^{166}Ho-Ho, Fe-HYDROXIDE (HFH). 10^{-5} mol Ho-carrier was added to the ^{166}Ho-chloride solution and ^{166}Ho-HFH was precipitated by adding 2.5 ml 0.5 M NaOH containing 0.7 mg ferromagnetic "black" Fe(II)Fe(III)hydroxide particles. After heating for 5 min at 90°C the resuspended ^{166}Ho-HFH-particles were immobilized at the wall of the reaction vessel by applying an electromagnet and the solution was removed. The ^{166}Ho-HFH-particles were washed with 0.01 M NaOH/ 0.9% NaCl, resuspended in 0.01 M NaOH/ 0.9% NaCl and autoclaved (Fig.1) .

^{166}Ho-HYDROXYAPATITE (HA). ^{166}Ho-citrate was prepared by adding of 50 mM citric acid to the ^{166}Ho-chloride solution. After 30 min at room temperature the ^{166}Ho-citrate solution was transferred to a septum closed vial containing 40 mg HA-particles in the size range 15-40 µm obtained by ultrasonic sieving. The mixture was stirred and heated for 6 min at 95°C. Unincorporated ^{166}Ho-activity in the solution was removed via a 10 µm Nuclepore filter and the labeled ^{166}Ho-HA-particles were washed three times with water, suspended in saline and autoclaved.

RESULTS AND DISCUSSION

The irradiation of 0.5 mg (2.6 µmol) Ho_2O_3 in a neutron flux of 7×10^{13} n $cm^{-2}sec^{-1}$ for 2 hours produced ~ 400 MBq (~ 11 mCi) ^{166}Ho. The preparation of ^{166}Ho-HFH was performed with a radiochemical yield of 91 ± 3 % (n=8) and with a soluble fraction of 0.3 ± 0.1 % ^{166}Ho ("washout", determined by filtration through a 0.45 µm membrane) that did not increase through 24 hours. Serial Nuclepore membrane filtration revealed ~ 80 % of the particles to be in the size range 3 - 10 µm.

Fig.1: Remote handling apparatus for ^{166}Ho-HFH

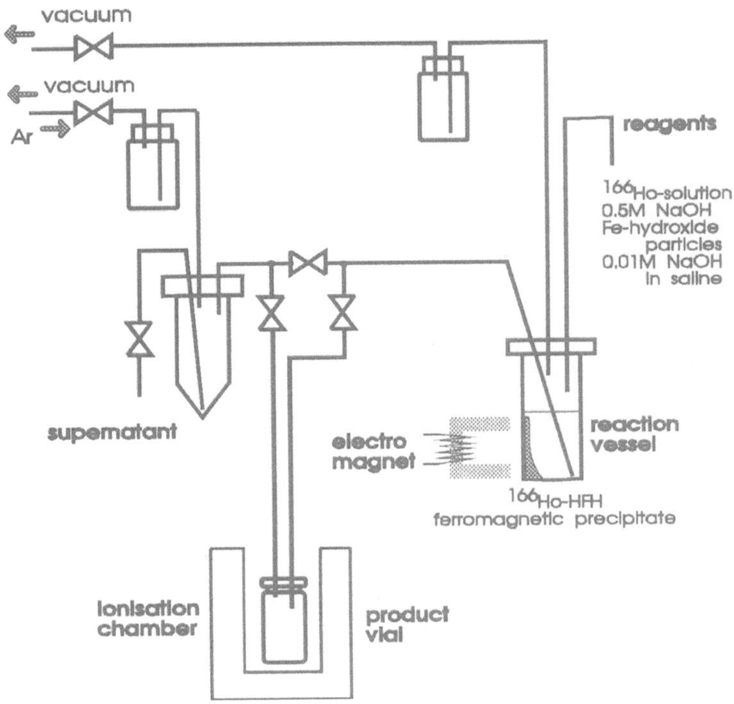

^{166}Ho-HA was obtained in 81 ± 5 % (n=5) radiochemical yield and with a soluble fraction of 0.4 ± 0.1 % ^{166}Ho ("washout") that was stable for 24 hours.

^{166}Ho-HFH and ^{166}Ho-HA were injected into the portal vein of NZW rabbits for deposition in the capillaries of the liver. The biodistribution is listed in Table 1.

Table 1: Biodistribution after injection into portal vein of NZW rabbits

	% dose/organ, 144 hours p.i.	
	^{166}Ho-HFH	^{166}Ho-HA
liver	91.7 ± 3.9	97.1 ± 1.6
blood (1)	< 0.01 ± 0.00	0.04 ± 0.04
kidneys	0.09 ± 0.02	0.09 ± 0.05
bladder	0.01 ± 0.01	< 0.01 ± 0.00
spleen	0.25 ± 0.04	0.10 ± 0.10
heart	0.01 ± 0.00	< 0.01 ± 0.01
lungs	0.07 ± 0.03	0.05 ± 0.01
gallbladder	0.09 ± 0.03	0.23 ± 0.13
stomach	0.74 ± 1.11	< 0.01 ± 0.00
intestine	0.14 ± 0.04	0.05 ± 0.06
urine + feces	1.35 ± 0.53	0.97 ± 0.25
bone (2)	4.80 ± 0.69	1.60 ± 0.97

(1) total blood = 6.5 % of body weight
(2) total bone = % ID one femur x 20

The biodistribution of ^{166}Ho-HFA showed high retention (< 91 %) in the liver but some activity in bone, stomach and urine. ^{166}Ho-HA displayed 97 % retention in the liver and appears to be a promising particulate radiopharmaceuticals for radio-embolization therapy of liver malignancies.

REFERENCES

1. Mumper R.J., Ryo U.Y., Jay M. Neutron-Activated Holmium-166-Poly(L-Lactic Acid) Microspheres: A Potential Agent for the Internal Radiation Therapy of Hepatitic Tumors. J. Nucl. Med. 1991; 32: 2139-2143

2. Kvaternik H., Angelberger P., Sinzinger H., et al. Dy165-Dysprosium-Eisen-Hydroxid: ein neues Radiopharmakon für die nuklearmedizinische Therapie. Radioaktive Isotope in Klinik und Forschung, F.K. Schattauer Verl., Stuttgart 1993; p. 274-278.

3. Chinol M., Vallabhajosula S., Goldsmith S.J., et al. Chemistry and Biological Behavor of Samarium-153 and Rhenium-186-Labeled Hydroxyapatite Particles: Potential Radiopharamceuticals for Radiation Synovectomy. J. Nucl. Med. 1993; 34: 1536-1542

Radioactive Isotopes in
Clinical Medicine and Research XXIII
ed. by H. Bergmann, H. Köhn and H. Sinzinger

POSSIBLE USE OF ^{11}C-LABELED 8-(3-CHLOROSTYRYL) CAFFEINE (CSC) MAPPING A_{2A} ADENOSINE RECEPTORS IN THE CNS AND MYOCARDIUM

Zs. Lengyel*, I. Boros*, T. Márián*, É. Sarkadi+, G. Horváth*, Z. Kovács+, M. Emri*, L. Trón*

*PET Centre of the University Medical School of Debrecen, Hungary, +Institute of Nuclear Research of the Hungarian Academy of Sciences, Debrecen, Hungary

SUMMARY: Here we report on the preparation of (E)-8-(3-chloro-styryl)-1,3-dimethyl-7-[^{11}C]methylxanthine ([^{11}C]-CSC) and present a preliminary evaluation of its potential as a tracer for mapping adenosine A_{2a} receptors by positron emission tomography (PET).

INTRODUCTION

The role of adenosine in modulating the function of the cardiovascular, endocrine, and nervous system has been known for several decades. The effect is mediated by two classes of receptors. The A_1-adenosine receptors exhibit higher affinity for adenosine and inhibit adenylate cyclase, the other class consists of lower affinity A_2-adenosine receptors which stimulate adenylate cyclase. Recently the adenosine/P_1 purinoceptors were classified into four subtypes: A_1, A_{2a}, A_{2b} and A_3 receptors. The type A_{2a} receptors are localised mainly in the brain, its highest expression is found in the striatum, nucleus accumbens and tuberculum olfactorium, whereas the A_{2b} receptors showed wide distribution, with high expression in the gastrointestinal tract. The recently identified A_3 receptors probably mediate the inhibition of adenylate cyclase.

Antagonist receptor ligands are especially beneficial in promoting a more complete understanding of the role of different sub-types of receptors in physiological responses. *In vivo* data indicate that 8-(3-chlorostyryl)-caffeine (CSC) is a high affinity antagonist specific to A_{2a} type of adenosine receptors (1). The CSC is a selective ligand having higher affinity for A_2 receptors (K_i=54 nM) than for A_1 receptors (K_i=28200 nM).

MATERIALS AND METHODS

Radiosynthesis of [^{11}C]CSC was carried out as shown in *Fig. 1* (*E*)-8-(3-Chlorostyryl)-1,3,-dimethylxanthine dissolved in DMF (1mg/0.4 ml) was methylated in the presence of potassium carbonate or caesium carbonate at 60 °C for 10 minutes. The specific activity was 50-150 mCi / μmol. Precursor content of the end-product was below the detection limit and the radiochemical purity was >99%.

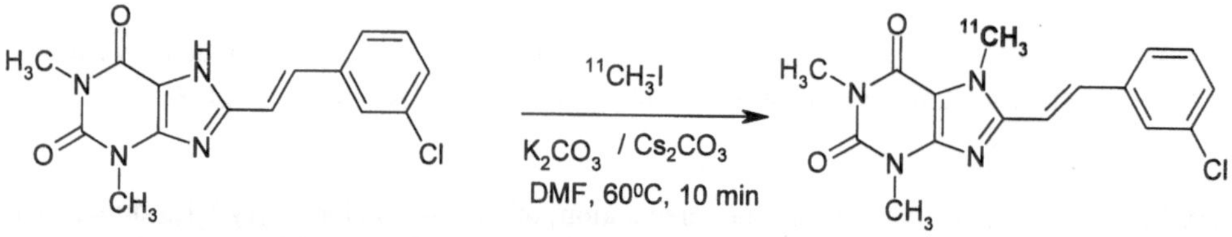

Figure 1 Reaction scheme of the synthesis of [^{11}C]CSC

Biodistribution of [^{11}C]CSC was studied on Swiss mice after i.v. injection of the ligand. [^{11}C]CSC [120 - 200 μCi / 1.2 - 8 nmol] was injected intravenously as a bolus. Uptake values were expressed as Differential Absorption Ratios (DAR = cpm recovered / g tissue / cpm injected / body weight).

In the autoradiography (ARG) studies storage phosphor screens (Molecular Dynamics) were used in combination with the PhosphorImager® scanner.

For anatomic correspondence a transparency scanner (TS [HP ScanJet 4c/T]) was used to obtain the color images of the sections. ARG and TS images were registered to fuse functional and anatomical information.

Dynamic PET scans were carried out on domestic rabbits using GE 4096 whole body PET camera. The animals were injected 1.5 - 2.5 mCi / 10-50 nmol [^{11}C]CSC in 2 ml physiologic salt solution intravenously as a 20-30 sec bolus. Transmission scans have been used to correct for tissue attenuation.

Regions of interests (ROI) were defined according to the different organs and time-activity curves (TAC) were constructed. The radioactivity of the blood samples was determined using a γ-counter cross-calibrated with the PET camera.

A 4-compartment kinetic model was used as the most general approach to fit experimental TAC data of different tissues (2). Measured time dependent tissue activities were also fitted using 2-, and 3-compartment models in some cases.

RESULTS AND DISCUSSION

Table 1 Tissue distribution of radioactivity (DAR) in mice after intravenous injection of $[^{11}C]$CSC. Data represent mean ± SD (n=3)

	10 min.	20 min.	40 min.	60 min.
Blood	0.18±0.06	0.19±0.06	0.36±0.20	0.26±0.06
Brain	0.83±0.42	0.70±0.44	0.41±0.18	0.18±0.06
Heart	0.76±0.05	0.76±0.15	0.89±0.18	0.46±0.15
Liver	2.88±1.46	1.22±0.16	3.2±0.72	1.1±0.35
Kidney	1.33±0.25	0.80±0.005	0.87±0.23	0.6±0.17
Muscle	0.30±0.05	0.12±0.01	0.32±0.05	0.12±0.07

The highest uptake at 10 min. after the injection was found in the liver followed by the kidney, heart and brain. The kinetics of the accumulation of radioactive CSC was different in the various tissues. The kinetics of the *brain* uptake was similar to the one of the *heart* uptake. The lowest radioactivity level was detected in the blood.

Foci of high CSC accumulation were clearly localized on the brain autoradiograms in several cases, with 15 min. post injection slicing, and were in accord with previous findings on specific spatial distribution of A_{2a} adenosine receptors in the CNS (3).

The binding of $[^{11}C]$CSC in mouse heart does not show differences in the ventricles and atriums, however, we found abrupt change in receptor density between the heart muscle and blood vessels originating from the former.

Gradually better fits of time-activity datas belonging to rabbit brain, heart and lung were obtained using 3-, or 4-compartment models instead of the simplest 2-compartment model. A fairly good fit was obtained for CSC accumulation in the kidney using the 3-compartment model.

We did not succeed in getting a good fit of time-activity data belonging to rabbit liver neither with 2-, and 3-compartment model nor with the 4-compartment model. The shape of the TAC and the calculated best fit-curves suggests kinetics described by more than four compartments. This phenomenon can be related to the special blood supply of the liver.

CONCLUSIONS

Biodistribution as well as autoradiographic and PET measurements showed pronounced differences between the measure and the kinetics of [^{11}C]CSC accumulation in the tissue of the different organs.

Time dependence of the tissue activity values is consistent with results of the data by biodistribution experiments.

Based on our results [^{11}C]CSC seems to be a very promising radiopharmacon for mapping adenosine receptors of type A_{2a} in various tissues, especially in the CNS. It is also suitable to perform investigations concerning time-dependent receptor expression changes (up- and down-regulation).

ACKNOWLEDGMENTS

This study was supported by OTKA Grants No. 16149, 16150 and ETT Grant No. 349/96.

REFERENCES

1. Jacobson, K. A.; Nikodijevic, O.; Padgett, W. L.; Gallo-Rodriguez. C.; Maillard, M.; Daly, J. W.: 8-(3-Chlorostyryl)caffeine (CSC) is a selective A_2-adenosine antagonist in vitro and in vivo. FEBS-Lett. 1993 May 24; 323(1-2): 141-4.

2. Feng, D.; Huang, S. C.; Wang, X.: Models for computer simulation studies of input functions for tracer kinetic modeling with positron emission tomography. Int. J. Biomed. Comput. 1993 Mar; 32(2): 95-110.

3. Johansson, B.; Georgiev, V.; Parkinson, F. E.; Fredholm, B. B.: The binding of the adenosine A_2 receptor selective agonist [^{3}H]CGS 21680 to rat cortex differs from its binding to rat striatum. Eur. J. Pharmacol. 1993 Oct 15; 247(2): 103-10.

Radioactive Isotopes in
Clinical Medicine and Research XXIII
ed. by H. Bergmann, H. Köhn and H. Sinzinger

IN-VITRO STUDIES ON THE USEFULNESS OF ^{99m}TC-TETROFOSMIN FOR SARCOMA DETECTION

G. Karanikas, P. Berghammer, Margarida Rodrigues, F. Chehne, H. Sinzinger
Departments of Nuclear Medicine and Oncology, University of Vienna, Austria

SUMMARY: ^{99m}Tc-tetrofosmin is a new lipophilic cationic tracer proposed as a myocardial perfusion agent. Recently, the usefulness of ^{99m}Tc-tetrofosmin in diagnosis of several tumors was reported. In order to evaluate the potential relevance of ^{99m}Tc-tetrofosmin for sarcoma detection, we investigated the sarcoma uptake (different cell lines) of ^{99m}Tc-tetrofosmin in-vitro. The influence of density of sarcoma cells, temperature and incubation time on the ^{99m}Tc-tetrofosmin-uptake (100µCi) were analysed. Different sarcoma cell-lines were examined. The sarcoma cell uptake of ^{99m}Tc-tetrofosmin was generally in the range of 1-3%. Our in-vitro data indicate that sarcoma cell uptake of ^{99m}Tc-tetrofosmin is reaching its maximum as early as after 10 minutes; the other optimal conditions have been characterized. The data are comparable to the findings with other tumours and therefore, in-vivo studies seem to be promising to investigate the potential value of ^{99m}Tc-tetrofosmin for scintigraphic detection of various sarcomas.

INTRODUCTION

Technetium-99m-1,2-bis [bis (2-ethoxyethyl) phosphino] ethane (tetrofosmin) has been introduced for myocardial perfusion imaging (1). It accumulates in viable myocardium and the uptake is proportional to regional blood flow. This radiopharmaceutical is now widely used in myocardial imaging and is commercially available (Myoview TM, Amersham International, Buckinghamshire, United Kingdom). It has several advantages compared with ^{201}Tl-chloride, which is also used as a tumour imaging agent (2). Recently, the usefulness of ^{99m}Tc-tetrofosmin in diagnosis of breast (3), lung (4) and thyroid cancer (5), among other tumours was reported. Systematic data for visualization of sarcomas with this tracer are lacking so far. In order to evaluate the potential usefulness of ^{99m}Tc-tetrofosmin for sarcoma detection, we investigated the sarcoma uptake (different cell lines) of ^{99m}Tc-tetrofosmin in-vitro.

MATERIAL AND METHODS

The sarcoma cell lines A-204 (rhabdomyosarcoma), SW684 (fibrosarcoma), SW872 (liposarcoma), SW982 (synovial sarcoma) and SW 1353 (chondrosarcoma) were cultured in Leibovitz's L-15 (PAA Laboratories GmbH., Linz, Austria) supplemented with 10% Mycoplex Fetal Calf Serum (FCS) (PAA Laboratories GmbH., Linz, Austria) at 37°C. For the uptake experiments cells were trypsinized, washed once in medium containing FCS in order to remove the trypsin and counted with a Coulter Counter. Cells were resuspended in Leibovitz's L-15 /10% FCS at different densities.

We analysed the influence of density of sarcoma cells (1.10^5 and 1.10^6 cells/ml.), temperature (4°C, 22°C, 37°C) and time (10, 20, 30, 40 and 60 min) of incubation, on the ^{99m}Tc-tetrofosmin-uptake (100µCi). Six probes of each combination of the above mentioned conditions were studied.

Results are presented as mean values ± standard deviation; calculation for significance was carried out by Student's t-test. A $p<0.01$ was considered as being significant.

RESULTS

The sarcoma cell uptake of ^{99m}Tc-tetrofosmin reaches the maximum after 10 minutes of incubation and at a density of 1.10^6 cells/ml. The uptake ranges from 1 to 3% (figures 1, 2, 3) comparable with the reported uptake of other tumours.

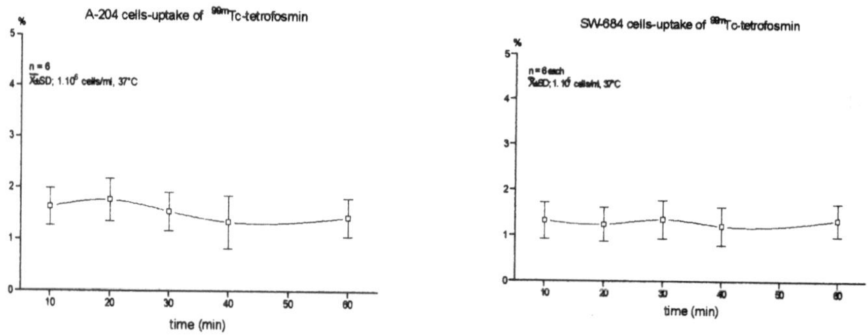

Figure 1. Cellular uptake is comparable, reaches a maximum at 10 minutes without significant change thereafter.

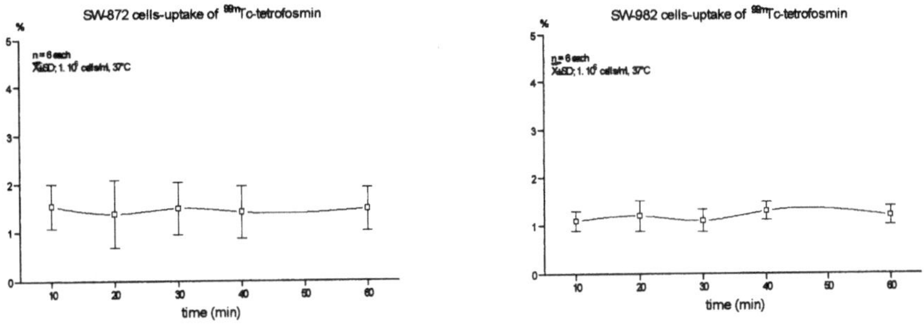

Figure 2. Already at 10 minutes incubation a constant uptake of ^{99m}Tc-tetrofosmin is achieved.

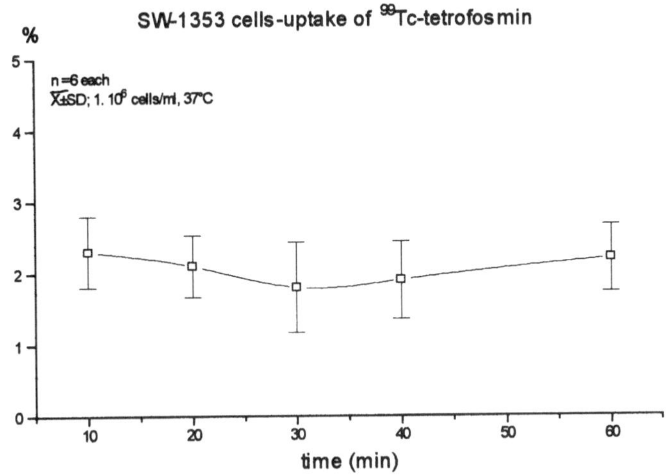

Figure 3. SW 1353 cells show the highest uptake among the tumour cells examined. The kinetics are identical.

DISCUSSION

^{99m}Tc-tetrofosmin is a lipophilic cation permeating cell membranes almost freely. In-vivo the tracer rapidly evades the circulation, with a blood clearance of more than 95%, 10 minutes after injection (6). Several groups of investigators have examined the tumour-seeking properties of tetrofosmin. Various tumour cell lines have been tested for tetrofosmin uptake kinetics, showing preferential uptake of tetrofosmin by cells rich in mitochondria, thus strengthening the hypothesis that malignant cells can be imaged with tetrofosmin due to the hight activity of mitochondria in these cells (7). Several studies described the imaging of lesions in patients with breast-, lung- and thyroid cancer, among others (3, 4, 5). In order to evaluate the potential usefulness of ^{99m}Tc-tetrofosmin for in-vivo detection of sarcomas, we investigated the uptake of different sarcoma cell lines of ^{99m}Tc-tetrofosmin in-vitro. Our in-vitro findings seem to be promising for clinical application of ^{99m}Tc-tetrofosmin for scintigraphic detection of sarcomas.

REFERENCES

1. Rigo P., Leclercq B., Itti R., Lahiri A., Braat S. Technetium-99m-tetrofosmin myocardial imaging: a comparison with thallium-201 and angiography. J Nucl Med 35: 587-593, 1994.
2. Cox P.H., Belter A.J., Power W.B. Thallium-201 chloride uptake in tumours, a possible complication in heart scintigraphy. Br J Radiol 49: 767, 1977.
3. Mansi L., Rambaldi P.F., Procaccini E., Gregorio F.D., Laprovitera A., Pecori B., Veccio W.D. Scintimammography with technetium-99m tetrofosmin in the diagnosis of breast cancer and lymph node metastases. Eur J Nucl Med 23: 932-939, 1996.
4. Ohtake E., Fukuda T. Small lung cancer demonstrated with Tc-99m tetrofosmin imaging. Clin Nucl Med 21: 576, 1996.
5. Klain M., Maurea S. Technetium-99m tetrofosmin imaging of differentiated mixed thyroid cancer. J Nucl Med 36: 2248-2251, 1995.
6. Berghammer P., Wiltschke C., Sinzinger H., Zielinski Ch. ^{99m}Tc-tetrofosmin soft tissue scanning and metastatic disease. Lancet 348: 1169-1170, 1996.
7. Arbab A.S., Koiyumi K., Toyama K., Araki T. Uptake of technetium-99m-tetrofosmin, technetium-99m-MIBI and thallium-201 in tumour cell lines. J Nucl Med 37: 1551-1556, 1996.

Acknowlegments

This study was supported by a grant from the “Kommission Onkologie der Medizinischen Fakultät der Universität Wien“.

Radioactive Isotopes in
Clinical Medicine and Research XXIII
ed. by H. Bergmann, H. Köhn and H. Sinzinger

THE EFFECT OF METABOLIC DEGRADATION ON RADIOTRACER DESIGN

I. Zolle, Ch. Halldin, C.-G. Swahn, Ch. Loc'h, L.A. Damani, B. Maziere

Dept. of Nuclear Medicine, Radiopharmacology, AKH Wien, 1090 Austria
European Cooperation COST Action B3

SUMMARY

Metyrapone, a potent inhibitor of 11β-hydroxylation in the adrenal cortex has been chemically modified to facilitate labelling with SPECT and PET radionuclides. The 2-substituted phenylmetyrapone derivatives 2-hydroxy- (2-OHPMP), 2-methoxy- (2-MPMP), and 2-bromo- (2-BrPMP) phenylmetyrapone were synthesized as precursors and as reference material. Two PET ligands, namely 2-[^{11}C]MPMP and 2-[^{76}Br]BrPMP and the SPECT radiotracer [^{123}I]iodophenyl-metyrapone were prepared and evaluated biochemically (in vitro) and in experimental animals.

INTRODUCTION

Biochemical evaluation of new ligands has been a valuable tool for choosing optimal precursors for labelling with SPECT and PET radionuclides. In case of metyrapone, 2-substituted phenyl-metyrapones have demonstrated high inhibitory potency of cytochrome P-450 11β-hydroxylation in vitro and a high binding capacity for adrenocortical binding sites. 2-Bromophenyl-metyrapone (2-BrPMP) and 2-hydroxyphenyl-metyrapone (2-OHPMP) have been labelled with radioiodine and carbon-11, respectively. For the synthesis of 2-[^{76}Br]bromophenyl-metyrapone (2-[^{76}Br]BrPMP), a stannylated precursor was used. When injected intravenously, adrenal uptake of the radiotracers differed considerably due to metabolic degradation.

MATERIALS AND METHODS

Determination of K_D- and IC_{50}-values

Homogenates of isolated mitochondria (100 µg protein) were incubated with 25 nM [^{3}H]metyrapol and different concentrations of metyrapone derivatives ranging from 3 nM to 1 µM. Metyrapone-mono-N-oxide was also subjected to this assay. A filtration technique was used for the separation of bound from free [^{3}H]metyrapol. The mitochondria retained on the filter were measured by liquid scintillation counting. Non-specific binding was determined in the presence of 0.1 mM metyrapol carrier, total [^{3}H]metyrapol binding (B_0) was achieved in the absence of inhibitor. Displacement curves were expressed by plotting B/B_0 versus the inhibitor concentration. Using the EBDA ligand program, K_D- and IC_{50}-values were calculated.

Biodistribution Studies

After the intravenous injection of 0.2 mL of the radiotracer (approx. 10 µCi/25 nmoles), rats were sacrifized at specified times and the excised organs measured in a well counter. The measured radioactivity was expressed as % dose/gram organ, in case of 2-[^{11}C]MPMP organ/blood ratios were plotted.

Pharmacokinetic Studies

Two groups of four conscious cannulated rats were dosed with either 2-MPMP or 2-BrPMP (25 mg/kg, i.v.), and urine collected 0-24 h, and 24-48 h. Serial arterial blood samples were taken for up to 7 h. Metabolites were identified in urine (1 mL) and blood samples (0.25 mL) after being extracted with dichloromethane (15 mL) by a gradient reversed-phase HPLC method, using reference material to generate a calibration curve. Detection limit about 1 µg/mL.

RESULTS AND DISCUSSION

Metyrapone derivatives have been evaluated by competitive displacement of [^{3}H]metyrapol binding to isolated adrenocortical mitochondria (1,2). A comparison of the binding affinities of metyrapone derivatives shown in Table 1 indicates that 2-substituted phenylmetyrapones exhibit the highest inhibitory potency.

Table 1. Relative Binding Affinity of Metyrapone Derivatives Determined by Competitive Displacement of [^{3}H]metyrapol Binding

Metyrapone Analogue	K_D - value (nM)	IC_{50} - value (nM)
2-Bromophenyl-metyrapone	30.10	59
2-Methoxyphenyl-metyrapone	33.16	65
2-Hydroxyphenyl-metyrapone	30.61	60
Phenylmetyrapone	60.71	119
Metyrapone	64.80	127
Metyrapol	60.71	119
Metyrapone-mono-N-oxide	361.7	709

Therefore, the 2-substituted phenylmetyrapone derivatives 2-OHPMP, and 2-BrPMP were labelled with ^{11}C, and ^{131}I or ^{76}Br, respectively, and their biodistribution and metabolism was studied in rats.

Labelling and Biodistribution of 2-[^{131}I]Iodophenyl-metyrapone

Labelling of 2-bromophenyl-metyrapone with iodine isotopes was performed by non-isotopic exchange in acetic acid using Cu^+-catalyst . Two methods were described by Yu et al. (3), and Schirbel and Coenen (4), respectively. The methods differ by the reaction conditions, resulting in effective radioiodination of the precursor with high specific activities (in case of 2-[^{123}I]iodophenyl-metyrapone 5300 ± 200 GBq/µmol, Ref. 4).

Radiochemical yields of approx. 95% have been obtained with both methods, however using Cu(I)-salt directly at 180 °C could reduce the reaction time to 5 minutes, whilest 1 h heating in a boiling water bath was necessary to produce a similar labelling yield with Cu(II)-catalyst.

After the i.v.-injection, 2-[^{131}I]IPMP showed accumulation in the adrenals, with high uptake in the liver. In vivo degradation of the radioactive label was indicated by thyroidal activity already 10 min after the i.v. injection (Figure 1). There is a gradual shift of radioactivity due to deiodination from the adrenals to the thyroid.

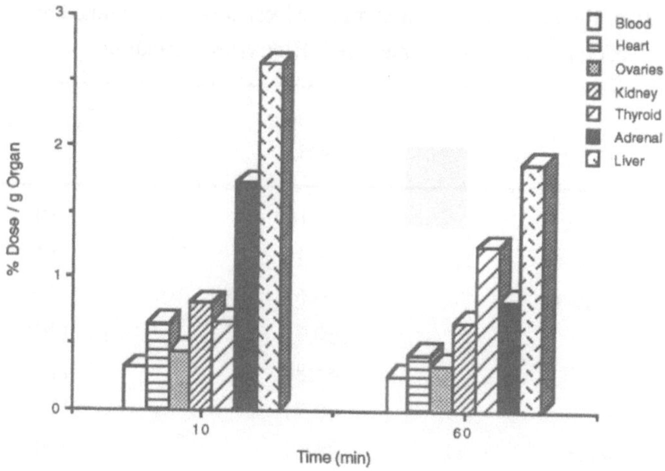

Figure 1. Biodistribution of 2-[^{131}I]iodophenyl-metyrapone in rats

Labelling and Biodistribution of 2-[^{11}C]Methoxyphenyl-metyrapone

2-Hydroxyphenyl-metyrapone was subjected to [$^{11}CH_3$]-methylation with a radiochemical yield of 50-60% (EOB), the radiochemical incorporation (based on [^{11}C]methyl-iodide) was >97% with a total synthesis time of 40-50 minutes (EOB). After HPLC-separation, the radiochemical purity was >99% with a specific activity of approx. 1 Ci/µmol of 2-[^{11}C]methoxyphenyl-metyrapone (5).

After the i.v.-injection, 2-[^{11}C]MPMP showed the highest accumulation in the lung, with increasing radioactivity in the kidney, indicating urinary excretion of 2-[^{11}C]MPMP (Figure 2).

Pharmacokinetic studies with 2-MPMP in rats have identified two demethylated metabolites in urine, namely 2-hydroxyphenyl-metyrapone (2-OHPMP) and 2-hydroxyphenyl-metyrapone-N-oxide (2-OHPMP-NO), representing approx. 75% of the injected dose. In blood, 2-OHPMP and 2-MPMP-NO were formed rapidly and excreted within 60 min. 2-MPMP was eliminated from blood with a $T_{1/2}$ of 23 min. Thus O-demethylation and N-oxidation are the major metabolic pathways, occuring rapidly (6-8).

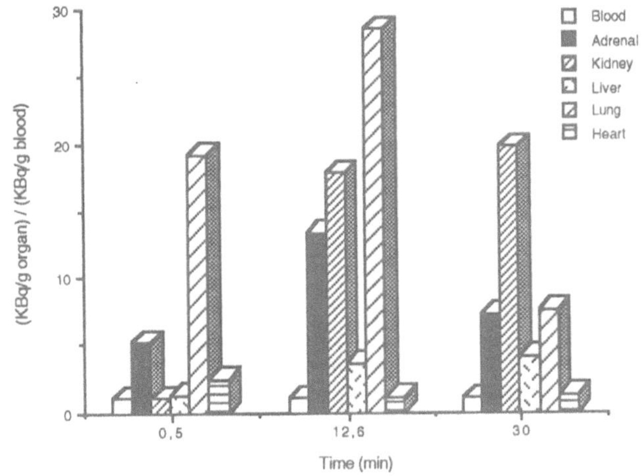

Figure 2. Biodistribution of 2-[^{11}C]methoxyphenyl-metyrapone in rats

In contrast, the elimination of 2-BrPMP from blood occured with a $T_{1/2}$ of 12 min, the only metabolite identified in blood, 2-bromophenyl-metyrapone-N-oxide (2-BrPMP-NO), showed a biological elimination half-time of 88.0 min. Less than 5% of the injected dose were recovered in the urine in 24 h.

Labelling and Biodistribution of 2-[^{76}Br]Bromophenyl-metyrapone

2-[^{76}Br]BrPMP was obtained by oxidative bromo-destannylation of the corresponding trimethylstannyl-precursor (2-StPMP). The highest labelling yield (80%) was obtained using 2-StPMP (0.2 mg), Chloramine-T (100 µL of 1 mg/mL), an aqueous solution of [^{76}Br]bromide (400 µL), and a reaction time of 10 min. The crude reaction mixture was placed onto an activated SEP-PAK C18 extraction cartridge (500 mg) and washed with 3 mL of water. 2-[^{76}Br]BrPMP was selectively bound to the matrix and eluted with 3 mL ethanol. Then the labelled product was evaporated and analyzed by reversed-phase HPLC (9).

After the i.v.-injection of 2-[^{76}Br]BrPMP, the kidney showed the highest accumulation of radioactivity, yet the mean total urinary excretion of the only metabolite, 2-BrPMP-NO in 24 hours was less than 5%. Adrenal uptake was very low. Considerable hepatic uptake was also observed (Figure 3).

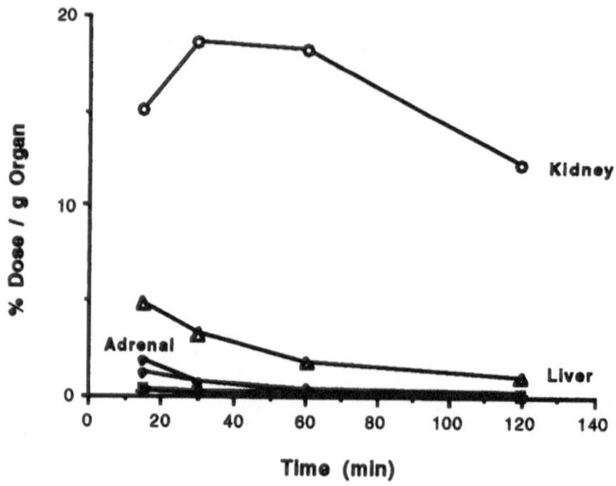

Figure 3. Biodistribution of 2-[^{76}Br]bromophenyl-metyrapone after i.v.- injection in rats

DISCUSSION

2-[^{123}I]iodo-PMP showed considerable deiodination indicated by a shift of radioactivity from the adrenals to the thyroid gland with time. The PET radiotracer 2-[^{11}C]MPMP showed high lung accumulation due to O-demethylation and formation of [^{11}C]CO_2 which is exhaled by the lung. The brominated derivative 2-[^{76}Br]BrPMP appeared to be metabolically stable, but most of the radioactivity was measured in the kidney. The low adrenal accumulation of 2-[^{76}Br]BrPMP may be explained by rapid formation of the N-oxide, which is biologically inactive (see Table 1).

CONCLUSIONS

Metabolic stability of the radioactive label is essential for medical application of a radiotracer. Our results have shown that enzyme binding studies provide sensitive parameters to demonstrate the effectiveness of functional derivatization. However, in vivo degradation had a considerable effect on the stability of the label, resulting in low adrenocortical binding and rapid elimination of radioactivity.

Acknowledgements - This work was supported by the Austrian Ministry of Science, Transport and the Arts, Vienna, and the European Commission, Unit XII-B-1: COST Secretariat, Scientific Missions, Brussels.

REFERENCES

1. Zolle I, Yu J, Robien W, Woloszczuk W, Höfer R. Biochemical Evaluation of Metyrapone Derivatives - Inhibition Kinetics and Affinity Studies. J. Labelled Compd. & Radiopharm. 1991; Vol. XXX: 420-422 (Abstract).

2. Zolle I, Woloszczuk W, Höfer R. Synthesis and in Vitro Evaluation of Metyrapone Derivatives as Potential Inhibitors of 11ß-Hydroxylase Activity, In: Radiopharmaceuticals & Labelled Compounds 1984, IAEA Vienna, 1985: 337-342.

3. Yu J, Zolle I, Mertens J, Rakias F. Synthesis of 2-[^{131}I]iodo-phenyl-metyrapone using Cu(I)-assisted nucleophilic exchange labelling: Study of the reaction conditions. Nucl Med Biol 1995; 22: 257-262.

4. Schirbel A, Coenen HH. Comparison of non-isotopic exchange methods for n.c.a. labelling of 2-iodophenyl-metyrapone. Nucl Med Biol 1995; 22: 1075-1079.

5. Zolle I, Halldin C, Yu J, Swahn CG. [^{11}C]-2-Methoxyphenyl-metyrapone for PET. J Labelled Compd & Radiopharm 1993; Vol. XXXII: 547-549.

6. Damani LA, Mitterhauser M, Zolle I, Lin,G, Oehler E, Ho YP. Metabolic and pharmacokinetic considerations in the design of 2-phenyl substituted metyrapone derivatives: 2-Methoxyphenylmetyrapone as a radioligand for functional diagnosis of adrenal pathology. Böttstein Colloquium, Villigen, Switzerland, October 6/7, 1994. Nucl Med & Biol 1995; 22: 1067-1074.

7. Damani LA, Mitterhauser M, Lin G, Ho YP, Zolle I. Urinary metabolic profile in rat of 1-(2-methoxyphenyl)-2-methyl-2-(3-pyridyl)-1-propanone: A potential radioligand for functional diagnosis of adrenal pathology. Xenobiotica 1996; 26: 211-219.

8. Ho YP, Lin G, Damani LA, Mitterhauser M, Zolle I. Spectral and chromatographic properties of 2-methoxyphenyl-metyrapone (2-MPMP) and its potential metabolites. J Pharm Biomed Anal 1997; 15: 479-486.

9. Mitterhauser M, Loc'h Ch, Halldin Ch, Swahn CG, Maziere B, Zolle I. Synthesis of 2-[^{76}Br]bromophenyl-metyrapone (1-(2-[^{76}Br] bromophenyl-2-methyl-2-(3-pyridyl)-1-propanone) by electrophilic substitution. COST B3 Conference on preclinical pharmacological studies with and for radiopharmaceuticals, Orsay, 1996 (Abstract).

Radioactive Isotopes in
Clinical Medicine and Research XXIII
ed. by H. Bergmann, H. Köhn and H. Sinzinger

INVESTIGATION OF RHENIUM COMPLEX FORMATION FOR DEVELOPMENT OF BONE-SEEKING KIT FOR 188-W/188-RE GENERATOR

O. Kolesnik, V. Basmanov

State Scientific Center of Russian Federation - Institute of Physics and Power Engineering, Bondarenko sq. 1, Obninsk, 249020, Russia

SUMMARY: Generator-produced carrier-free Re-188(E_{β}=2,12MeV,E_{γ}=155keV(15%), $T_{1/2}$=16,98h) is an attractive isotope for therapeutic use. Concentration stability constants (SCs) of rhenium complexes with phosphonic acids (PhAs): 1-hydroxyethane-1,1'-diphosphonic acid (HEDP) and 2,2'-diethylenediamine ether-N,N,N',N-tetrametylene phosphonic acid (oksabifor) were calculated based on pH-metric titration data: $lgK_{Re(Sn)L}$= 10,1 and 5,9 for HEDP and oksabiphor respectively. Radiolabelling studies were carried out using an eluate from $^{188}W/^{188}Re$ generator and lyophilized kits which contain HEDP, $SnCl_2 \bullet 2H_2O$ and in some cases HCl and ascorbic acid. Radiochemical purity (RCP) of ^{188}Re(Sn)HEDP was 95-99% about 1h after starting of the process of synthesis. Radiolabelled complexes were stable (RCP≥93-94%) in vitro (25°C) for at least one day. The influence of some conditions on RCP of complexes was investigated.

INTRODUCTION

There are many papers [1-9] concerning the preparation and in vivo investigations of the behaviour of rhenium (Re-186,188) complexes with PhAs. This interest stems from the wish to receive new bone therapeutic radiopharmaceuticals (RPhCs) for systemic radiotherapy of cancer diseases, which is possible thanks to similar chemistry of two elements: Tc and Re.

Rhenium isotopes Re-186(E_{β}=1,07 MeV, E_{γ}=137 keV(9,2%), $T_{1/2}$=90 h)and Re-188(E_{β}=2,12 MeV, E_{γ}=155 keV(15%), $T_{1/2}$=16,98h) are attractive ones for radiotherapeutic use because they have optimum energy of β^--particles which penetrate into tissue about 1,2 mm (Re-186). Besides, their ideal E_{γ} is similar to that of for diagnostic Tc-99m isotope (E_{γ}=140 keV) which enables one to trace easily the path of RPhC radiolabelled with Re-186,188 in organizm by means of gamma-camera. Generator-produced Re-188 is easily available and can be eluated from $^{188}W/^{188}Re$ generator by isotonic solution of NaCl.

If even Re(VII) forms complexes with ligands the kinetics of such reactions is very slow and unacceptable for rapid synthesis of RPhC by simple clinical procedure. The necessity of an introduction of reducing agent (mostly $SnCl_2 \bullet 2H_2O$) increases the rate of RPhC synthesis but complicates the process, so, the high yield of the radiolabelling complex will depend on many factors, namely: concentration and ratio of all components, kinetics of Re(VII) reduction and rate of the complex formation, temperature and pH of medium.

SCs are important physical-chemical characteristics of the complex strength. SCs determined at identical external conditions (t°, pressure, ionic medium, ionic strength) allow the propeties of two ligands or two metals to be compared.

MATERIALS AND METHODS

Stability constants. All chemicals were >95% assay. Potentiometric (pH-metric) titration was carried out in 0,1 M NaCl at 25°C using ionometer I-130. The calculation of concentration acid dissociation constants of PhAs for comparison with values reported by previous workers and SCs of normal and protonated rhenium complexes with HEDP and oksabiphor were determined using relationships obtained from equations of material balance and electroneutrality. The Bjerrum (*n*) functions of formation were calculated for each Re-HiL system and formation curves (*n* vs -lg[L]) were constructed. All calculations and plots were obtained using Excel 5.0. UV-visible spectra were recorded at 25°C in 1-sm quartz cell using SF-56 spectrophotometer.

Preparation of ^{188}Re(Sn)HEDP. The ^{188}Re isotope is obtained from ^{188}W/^{188}Re generator by elution with isotonic NaCl solution. The radiochemical purity was ReO_4^->99% and this value was obtained by gamma-counter measuring of a paper radiochromatogramma (1 x 10 sm) produced by thin layer chromatography in acetone. The ^{188}Re yield was >80% during 9 months of operation. Total amount of stable impurities in the ^{188}Re eluate (Al, Fe and etc) was <3-5 μg per ml. ^{188}W breakthrough was $\leq 10^{-4}$%. Lyophilized kits contained ligand (HEDP), reducing agent ($SnCl_2 \bullet 2H_2O$) and in some cases HCl (1M, 0,5M, 0,1M) and ascorbic acid. The preparation of ^{188}Re(Sn)HEDP was carried out by addition of up to 2 ml of the eluate with or without carrier ($KReO_4$, NH_4ReO_4) to the kit vial successively or simultaneously. The kit vials were placed in boiling water bath for 30 min and then were allowed to stand at room temperature for about 30 min for cooling. After this thin layer chromatography of the paper strip was carried out in acetone and RCP of the ^{188}Re(Sn)HEDP complex was determined. The RCP value was measured one day after ^{188}Re(Sn)HEDP preparation for estimating the complex stability in storage.

RESULTS AND DISCUSSION

The potentiometric titration curves indicate that rhenium forms stable watersoluble complexes with PhAs in Re(VII)-Sn(IV)-HiL-NaCl-NaOH-H_2O system in the whole pH range and, moreover, Re-HEDP complexes have better strength than Re-oksabiphor complexes do. The appearence of absorption peaks on UV-visible spectra at 380 and 430 nm for Re-HEDP and at 375 and 440 nm for Re-oksabiphor also demonstrates that the complexation take place. According to the formation curves for this component ratio about 45% and 20% of rhenium was bonded with ligand (with HEDP (Figure 1) and oksabiphor,respectively) at the beginning of acid-base titration. The reactions of a complex formation are accompanied by proton release. The formation curves indicate the presence of protonated rhenium complexes. They also show that hydrolysed complexes are likely to be present in the solution at pH >7 because a bend in the formation curves for Re-Sn-HEDP(Figure 1) and for Re-Sn-oksabiphor can be observed in this pH range. Since Sn(II) is present in the solution in equivalent ratio with Re is very likely to be formed the hydroxyheteronuclear complex $[Re(Sn)(OH)_nL]$ ($n \geq 2$).

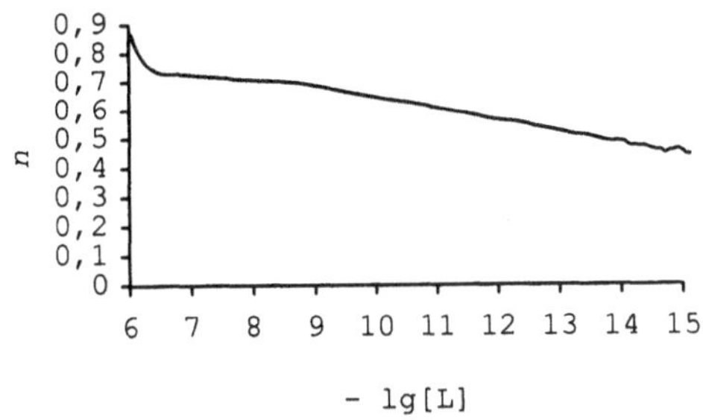

Figure 1. Formation curve for 1mM Re:1mM Sn:1mM HEDP

The concentration SCs were determined at stoichiometric ratio of components (1mM:1mM:1mM=Re:Sn:HiL) in conditions similar to those for radiolabelling reaction (the presence of $SnCl_2$, 0,1 M NaCl). The calculated concentration SCs of rhenium complexes with PhAs are listed in Table 1.

Table 1. Stability constants (lg K) of Re with HEDP and oksabiphor

Ligand	lg K_{ReL}	lg K_{ReHL}	lg K_{ReH2L}
HEDP	10,1	4,9	3,4
oksabiphor	5,9	-	2,2

The dependence of the radiolabelling yield on the Sn(II) content and excess of ligand (HEDP), the presence or the absence of carrier rhenium, the addition of 0,1 M NaOH for neutralization to achieve pH 5-6 have been investigated.

RCP of carrier-free $^{188}Re(Sn)HEDP$ complexes was 86-90% and it was lower than that of carrier-added ones which was 95-99%. The linear dependence of radiolabelling yield on Sn(II) content in the kit vial was observed. Moreover, the higher the ligand excess(>100-400 times) in the kit vial, the lower the RCP (55-65%). RCP did not depend on the variation of Sn(II) concentration if HEDP excess was ≤100 times. Because of the buffer solution formation under radiolabelling conditions the presence of HCl in the kit vial in concenration from 0 to 1M did not decrease the radiolabelling yield and pH of all solutions was almost equal before neutralization. The neutralization of the solutions did not influence RCP values. The radiolabelling yield of $^{188}Re(Sn)HEDP$ for the solutions containing ascorbic acid are given in Table 2. The radiolabelling complexes Re-188 with PhAs show a sufficient stability in vitro at least for one day. Its behavior in vivo will be analysed in our next studies.

Table 2. Radiolabelling yield of $^{188}Re(Sn)HEDP$ complexes

Time, h	Without carrier	With carrier($KReO_4$)
1	89,3	97,5
2,5	90,4	98,0
3 (with neutralization)	90,1	96,8
21 (with neutralization)	94,5	93,3

Without ascorbic acid the carrier-added $^{188}Re(Sn)HEDP$ complex was 70-85% in the solution after it had been stored for one day. The radiolabelling carrier-free $^{188}Re(Sn)HEDP$ complex was still less after a day(about 30%).

Cutler et al.[2] and Roodt et al.[?] carried out the comparative biodistributions in normal rats of several therapeutic bone-seeking agents $^{186}Re(Sn)HEDP$, $^{153}Sm(Sn)EDTMP$, ^{117m}Sn-DTPA, diagnostic $^{99m}Tc(Sn)HEDP$ complex and model $^{96}Tc(Sn)HEDP$ complex. All bone-seeking agents washed out from a bone differently. Re-186 agent washed out from normal bone most rapidly, technetium-99m,96 agents less rapidly. Sm-153 and Sn-117m agents did not wash out not at all or did, but only slightly. Tin(II,IV) forms a normal complex with DTPA having SC about 10^{18}-10^{20} [11]. Stability constant of samarium ($lgK_{Sm-EDTMP}$=22,39[12]) is still higher. As one can see, Sn and Sm form high stability complexes and they have the highest oxidation state (Sn^{4+}, Sm^{3+}) in complex compounds. The calculated Re(Sn)HEDP SC (about 10^{10}) corresponds to the formation of medium-stability complex. Besides in vivo redox conditions lead to oxidation of Re(V) to Re(VII), excretion of $^{186}Re(VII)$ as $^{186}ReO_4^-$ due to the complex destruction. Technetium behavior was similar to that of rhenium. Thus, rapid ^{186}Re washoff can be predicted from the knowledge of both SKs and of propeties of metals.

CONCLUSION

Rhenium can form stable watersoluble complexes with HEDP and oksabiphor in pH range 1-10. In the presence of $SnCl_2$ Re(VII) reduces to Re(V) and forms normal and protonated complexes with SKs of normal ones 10^{10} and 10^{6} respectively for HEDP and oksabiphor.

Our first results on radiolabelling HEDP with ^{188}Re for development of bone-seeking kit for $^{188}W/^{188}Re$ generator show that radiolabelling yield can be >90-95% both for carrier-free and the carrier-added $^{188}Re(Sn)$HEDP complexes within <1h after labelling starts. The presence of ascorbic acid increases the storage stability and after a day the RCP decrease was insignificant (only to 93-94%). The addition of a carrier increases the velocity of a complex formation reaction in comparison with carrier-free $^{188}Re(Sn)$HEDP and also it is the reason for higher stability of the carrier-added complexes Re-188 with HEDP in time for the solutions without ascorbic asid. The excess of the ligand led to a considerable decrease of radiolabelling yield to 55-65% and RCP was directly depent on $SnCl_2$ content in the kit vial.

The formation of bone-seeking radiopharmaceutical radiolabelled with Re-188 can be carried out by a simple routine procedure using the available $^{188}W/^{188}Re$ generator and lyophilized kit within less than 1h after the synthesis starts.

REFERENCES

1. Yeh SDJ, et al. Treatment of bone pain in patient with prostate carcinoma using Re-186-HEDP (hydroxyeththylidene diphosphonate) [abstract]. J Nucl Med 1992; 33:859.
2. Cutler C, et al. Comparative biodistribution of 186-Re, 96-Tc, 153-Sm and 117m-Sn bone seeking agents: mechanistic implications [abstract]. J Nucl Med 1992; 33:899.
3. Pipes D, et al. Radiolysis effects of the radiochemical and chemical stability of rhenium-186 etidronate injection [abstract]. J Nucl Med 1992; 33:1024-1025.
4. Maxon HR, et al. 186-Re(Sn)-HEDP for the treatment of painful osseous metastases: initial clinical experience. Technetium and rhenium in chemistry and nuclear medicine 3. New York: Corina Intenational-Raven Press; 1990: 733-739.
5. Yeh SJ, et al. The effect of reaction conditions on preparations of rhenium hydrohyethylidene diphosphonate complexes. Eur J Nucl Med 1996; 23:1245.

6. Kairemo KJA, et al. Quality control of bone seeking Re-188-labelled compounds using a gamma camera. Eur J Nucl Med 1996; 23:1266.
7. Palmedo H, et al. Re-188-HEDP for pain palliations of bone metastases: first clinical results. Eur J Nucl Med 1997; 24:962.
8. Han SH, et al. Efficacy of rhenium - 186 - etidronate in breast cancer patients with metastatic bone pain. Eur J Nucl Med 1997; 24:895.
9. Lin WY, et al. Rhenium-188 hydroxyeththylidene diphosphonate: a new generator-produced radiopharmaceutic drug of potential value for the treatment of bone metastases. Eur J Nucl Med 1997; 24:590-601.
10. Roodt A, et al. Studies on the mechanism of action of 186-Re(Sn)HEDP, a new agent for treament of painful skeletal metastases [abstract]. J Nucl Med 1989; 30:732.
11. Dyatlova NM, Tyomkina VY, Popov KI. Komplexony and komplexonaty metal-lov. Moscow: Chimia, 1988: 501, 362.
12. Dyatlova NM, Tyomkina VY, Kolpakova ND. Komplexony. Moscow: Chimia 1970: 179.

Radioactive Isotopes in
Clinical Medicine and Research XXIII
ed. by H. Bergmann, H. Köhn and H. Sinzinger

^{199}TL-DIETHYLDITHIOCARBAMATE - SPECT IN DIAGNOSIS OF BRACHIO-CEPHALIC ARTERIES ATHEROSCLEROSIS

Dygai I., Shvera I., Krivonogov N., Chernov V., Skuridin V., Lishmanov Yu.
Nuclear Medicine Department, Cardiology Institute, Tomsk, Russia, 634012

Summary. ^{199}Tl-diethyldithiocarbamate (^{199}Tl-DDC) - SPECT was performed in 36 stenosing brachiocephalic arteries (BCA) atherosclerosis and 16 control pts. ^{99m}Tc-HMPAO-SPECT was performed in 14 pts for comparison. The heating of the 9-10 mg DDC and ^{199}Tl-chloride solution (2,7-3,6 mCi/ml) mixture by t 85-90^{0}C during 20 min is necessary for ^{199}Tl-DDC preparation. The best tomoscintigramms and maximal brain tracer uptake were obtained in 25-30 min of ^{199}Tl-DDC injection. The brain imaging quality with ^{199}Tl-DDC was similar ^{99m}Tc-HMPAO. The sensitivity of ^{199}Tl-DDC SPECT in diagnosis of BCA atherosclerosis was 91,6%.

Introduction

Perfusion brain SPECT with lipophilic radiopharmaceuticals has the great importance in diagnostic of cerebrovascular insufficiency [1]. Nevertheless, the problem of optimal radiopharmaceutical selection remains to be defined. All known agents (^{99m}Tc-HMPAO, ^{123}I-iodoamphetamine, ^{201}Tl-diethyldithiocarbamate (^{201}Tl-DDC)) have some disadvantages [2,3,4,5,6,7,8] and are rather expensive. The main disadvantage of ^{201}Tl-DDC is high radiation dose to critical organs caused by long half-life of nuclide (73h) [7]. Ordinary and cheap method of ^{199}Tl production was developed by the Research Institute of Nuclear Physics by Tomsk Polytechnic University [9,10]. In our opinion, using of ^{199}Tl for DDC labeling will provide significant reduction of radiation dose to the patient with high quality of tomoscintigramms retention, since so that ^{199}Tl, as it is known, has half-life 10 times shorter than ^{201}Tl. The relatively low cost of ^{199}Tl production also can be considered as positive moment.

The aim of this study was to evaluate the possibility of ^{199}Tl-DDC - SPECT in diagnostic of brachiocephalic arteries (BCA) atherosclerosis.

Materials and methods

^{199}Tl-DDC-SPECT was performed in 36 stenosing BCA atherosclerosis and 16 control pts. ^{99m}Tc-HMPAO-SPECT was employed in 14 pts for comparison.

Regional cerebral perfusion was assessed using a rotating SPET single-head gamma camera ("Omega 500", Technicare Corp.) interfaced with dedicated computer system for scintigraphic data processing ("Scinty", "Gelmos" Corp., Russia).

^{199}Tl-DDC was prepared ex tempore in sterile conditions from 1,5-2,0 ml of a ^{199}Tl-chloridum solution (2,7-3,6 mCi/ml) and 9-10 mg of DDC. The dose injected to patients 3,5 MBq/ kg. Investigations were carried out with 20% window set at 72,5 keV by ^{199}Tl-DDC using and at 140 keV by ^{99m}Tc-HMPAO. Sixty four projections in a 64*64 matrix, of 30-60 s each, were acquired over 360^0. The spatial resolution (as full width at half maximum) was 14,6-14,8 mm in the center of the field of view. The count in each projection was more than 50 thousand.

Results and discussion

Hypoperfused zones of different localization and volume were observed in 33 stenosing BCA atherosclerosis pts (Figure 1.). The sensitivity of this method was 91,6%.

No reliably scintigraphy data confirming the presence of hypoperfusion areas were obtained in control group subjects.

The heating of the 9-10 mg DDC and ^{199}Tl-chloride solution (2,7-3,6 mCi/ml) mixture by t 85-90^{0}C during 20 min is necessary for ^{199}Tl-DDC preparation. These conditions allow to reach 95% DDC labeling, tested by means of ascending paper chromatography with methylethylketon as elution fluid.

The best imaging and maximal brain tracer uptake were obtained in 25-30 min of ^{199}Tl-DDC i.v. injection. This fact is in agreement with results of ^{199}Tl-DDC experimental investigation, which showed the stable level of indicator accumulation from the 30th to the 120th min after injection [11]. This time was defined for SPECT - procedure realization.

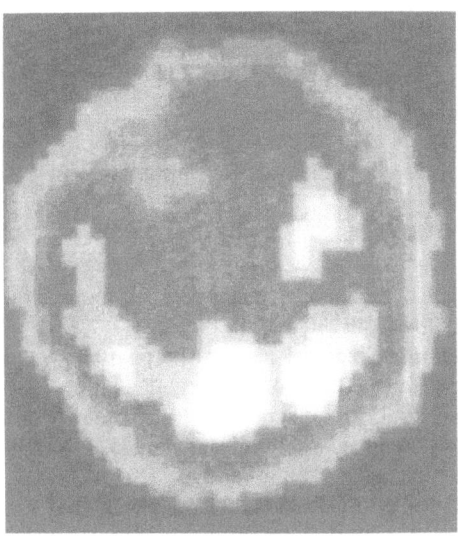

Fig. 1. SPECT of the brain using ^{199}Tl-DDC.

Zone of hypoperfusion is visualized in the left frontal area on tomographic slice performed at the level of lateral ventricles.

The quality of ^{199}Tl-DDC scintigramms was similar to ^{99m}Tc-HMPAO imaging both by visual and quantitative examination. The differences between «orbit/frontal lobe», «salivary glands/frontal lobe» coefficients and cerebral tracer uptake were not significant. Exclusion was only for «brain/background» coefficients, which were 6,27 ± 1,48 for ^{199}Tl-DDC and 10,58 ± 2,49 for ^{99m}Tc-HMPAO. Low «brain/background» coefficient by ^{199}Tl-DDC-SPECT was conditioned, probably, by Compton effect of high energy gamma - quantum, existence of which in 39,1% summarily was shown by ^{199}Tl spectrometric investigations. By using a high energy parallel collimator, short wave radiation was absorbed, thereby obviating the appearance of the Compton effect.

Perfusion defects were identified in 10 pts with cerebrovascular insufficiency investigated by using ^{99m}Tc-HMPAO as well as ^{199}Tl-DDC. Localization of hypoperfused zones in both radiopharmaceuticals imagings was identical. Hypoperfusion volumes ($V_{hypoperf}$) were differed not significantly by using of ^{199}Tl-DDC and ^{99m}Tc-HMPAO (51,55 ± 26,74 and 45,77 ± 24,98) with good correlation (r=0,93).

Thus, ^{199}Tl-DDC preparation conditions named above provide brain-tomoscintigramms of high quality receipt. Perfusion ^{199}Tl-DDC - SPECT can be used in cerebrovascular insufficiency diagnostic in stenosing BCA atherosclerosis patients.

REFERENCES

1. Holman B.L., Devous M.D. Functional brain SPECT: the emergence of a powerful clinical method. J Nucl Med 1992; 33: 1888-1904.
2. Neirinckx R.D. Evaluation of regional cerebral blood flow with 99mTc-d, 1 HM-PAO and SPECT. Neurosurg.Rev. 1987; 10: 181-184.
3. Neirinckx R.D., Canning L.R., Piper I.M. Technetium-99m d, l- HM-PAO: a new radiopharmaceutical for SPECT imaging of regional cerebral blood perfusion. J.Nucl.Med. 1987; 28: 191-202.
4. Creutzig H., Schober O., Gielow P. Cerebral dynamics of N-isopropyl-(123-I)-p-iodoamphetamine. J.Nucl.Med. 1986; 27: 178-183.
5. Takeshita C., Toyama H., Nakane K. Quantitative measurement of regional cerebral blood flow with I-123 IMP SPECT: a correction of the microsphere model by global extraction between artery and internal jugular vein. Ann.Nucl.Med.1991; 5: 145-148.
6. Van Royen E.A., de Bruine J.F., Hill T.C., Cerebral blood flow imaging with tallium-201 diethylditiocarbamate SPECT. J.Nucl.Med. 1987; 28: 178-183.
7. Vyth A., Fennema P., van der Shoot J. Tl-201-diethyl-dithicarbamate: a possible radiopharmaceutical for brain imaging. Pharm. Weekbl (Sci).1983; 5: 213-216.
8. Bruine J.F. de, Royen E.A. van, Vyth A. et al. Thallium-201 diethylditiocarbamate: an alternative to iodine - 123 N-isopropyl-p-iodoamphetamine. J. Nucl. Med. 1985; 26: 925-930.
9. Gluhov G., Komov A., Maslennikov Yu. et al. Thallium-199 production using accelerator U-120. In: Methods of thallium isotopes production and using in Nuclear Medicine 1989; 62-67 (in Russian).
10. Krivonogov N., Chernov V., Gluhov G., Lishmanov Yu. Spectrometrical and phantom investigations of thallium-199. In: Methods of thallium isotopes production and using in Nuclear Medicine 1989; 34-35 (in Russian).
11. Lishmanov Yu., Dygai I., Skuridin V., Krivonogov N., Shvera I., Chernov V., Vesnina Zh. The first experience with the use of ^{199}Tl-diethyldithiocarbamate for visualization of cerebral and myocardial perfusion. Angiology and vascular surgery (Moscow) 1997; 1: 8-20.

Radioactive Isotopes in
Clinical Medicine and Research XXIII
ed. by H. Bergmann, H. Köhn and H. Sinzinger

VINCRISTINE EFFECT ON THE DISTRIBUTION OF RADIOPHARMACEUTICALS IN MICE

D.M.M.Britto[1,2], M.L.Gomes[1,2], R.S.Freitas[1], P.Rodrigues[1], E.Paula[1] and M.Bernardo-Filho[1,2]

1 Instituto Nacional de Cancer, Brasil
2 Universidade do Estado do Rio de Janeiro, Instituto de Biologia, Departemento de Biofisica e Biometria, Rio de Janeiro, RJ,Brasil, 20551-030

SUMMARY: The distribution of radiopharmaceuticals is grossly and recognizably altered by drugs. We studied the effect of the chemotherapeutic drug vincristine on the distribution of ^{99m}Tc-DTPA of ^{99m}Tc-phytate in mice. After the last dose of vincristine, ^{99m}Tc-DTPA or ^{99m}TC-phytate were injected, the animals sacrificed and the percentage of radioactivity (%rad) in each organ calculated. ^{99m}Tc-DTPA, Vincristine increased the %rad in: thymus, ovary, uterus, spleen, kidney, heart, stomach, lung, liver and bone, ^{99m}Tc-phytate, the drug (a) decreased in ovary, uterus and kidney and (b) increased in pancreas, brain and bone. The results can be explained by its metabolization, therapeutic or immunosuppressive action.

INTRODUCTION

The discovery of technetium-99m (^{99m}TC) provided the first convenient radionuclide for labelling a large variety of radiopharmaceuticals [1,2]. Unexpected distribution patterns of radiopharmaceuticals provoke a flurry of questions regarding the quality of the administered agent.

However, the alterations in biodistributions may be related to the chemotherapeutic drug interaction [3,4,5,6].

Vincristine is a derivative of the periwinkle plant *Vinca rosea Linn* and has a broad spectrum of anti-tumor activity. This drug is used for the treatment of a variety of malignancies, among them leukemia, solid tumors, Hodgkin disease and other lymphomas [7,8].

As patients under chemotherapeutic treatment quite frequently undergo nuclear medicine procedures, we decided to study the effect vincristine on the biodistribution of the diethylenetriaminepentaacetic acid and sodium phytate labelled with the radionuclide technetium-99m (^{99m}Tc-DTPA and ^{99m}Tc-PHY) in mice.

MATERIAL AND METHODS

Vincristine (0.003mg, 0.3ml) was administered into female isogenic Balb/c mice (n=15), in three doses with an interval of 48 hours. One hour after the last dose, 0.3 ml of ^{99m}Tc-DTPA of ^{99m}Tc-PHY (7.4 MBq) were administered. After 0.5 hour, the animals were sacrificed, the various organs istolated and the radioactivity uptake determined in a well counter. The percentage of radioactivity administered. The results were compared with the control group, without vincristine, and statistical analysis was performed (Wilcoxon test, $p<0.05$).

RESULTS

Table 1 shows the uptake of ^{99m}Tc-DTPA in the group of the mice that was treated with vincristine and the control group. The analysis of the results reveals (a) no significant reduction of ^{99m}Tc-DTPA uptake in pancreas, thyroid and brain and (b) an increase in thymus, ovary, uterus, spleen, kidney, heart, stomach, lung, liver and bone.

Table 2 shows the uptake of ^{99m}Tc-PHY in the group of mice treated with vincristine and the control group. The analysis of the results reveals (a) no significant reduction of ^{99m}Tc-PHY uptake in thyroid, spleen, thymus, heart, liver, stomach and lung, (b) an increase in pancreas, brain and bone and (c) a decrease in ovary, uterus and kidney.

DISCUSSION

There is considerable evidence that the pharmacokinetics of radiopharmaceuticals may be altered by a variety of drugs, disease states and surgical procedures. If unknown, such factors may lead to poor organ visualization, a requirement to repeat the procedure resulting in unnecessary irradiation of organs or even misdiagnosis [1,2,3,5,6].

Vincristine has been used as a component of many chemotherapeutic regimens because of its

Table 1 - Effect of vincristine on the biodistribution of ^{99m}Tc-DTPA in mice

	% radioactivity	
Tissue	control	treated
Pancreas	0.0194±0.0018	0.0130±0.0021
Thyroid	0.0871±0.0123	0.0760±0.0151
Brain	0.0610±0.0132	0.0699±0.0211
Thymus	0.0103±0.0086	0.0353±0.0024
Ovary	0.0107±0.0016	0.0475±0.0112
Uterus	0.0204±0.0016	0.1350±0.0098
Spleen	0.0134±0.0068	0.0410±0.0112
Kidney	0.1587±0.0468	0.7891±0.0115
Heart	0.0165±0.0018	0.1632±0.0691
Stomach	0.0334±0.0192	0.2334±0.0142
Lung	0.0272±0.0095	0.4783±0.0181
Liver	0.0668±0.0122	0.3564±0.0102
Bone	0.0162±0.0036	0.1101±0.0311

Vincristine was administered into mice and after 96h ^{99m}Tc-DTPA. The animals were sacrificed, the organs isolated and the activities determined.

relative lack of hematologic toxicity. Its mechanism of action is by interfering with microtubule formation and exerts immunosuppressive activity [4,7,8]. The alterations in the u ptake of ^{99m}Tc-DTPA and ^{99m}Tc-PHY in kidneys can be due to the capability of vincristine to produce hyponatremia with abnormal water retention due (probably) to the nonasmotic release of ADH [7,11,12]. As vincristine is a immunosuppressive drug this effect can explain the increase of ^{99m}Tc-DTPA in thymus and spleen [4,8,9]. As vincristine is metabolized in the liver, this may contribute to the increase of uptake of ^{99m}Tc-DTPA in this organ [4]. As bone marrow suppression is the most frequent complication in the protocols using vincristine, this could influence the fixation of the ^{99m}Tc-DTPA and ^{99m}Tc-PHY in bone.

Table 2 - Effect of vincristine on the biodistribution of ^{99m}Tc-PHY in mice

Tissue	%radioactivity control	treated
Pancreas	0.0341±0.0018	0.0581±0.0011
Thyroid	0.0090±0.0012	0.0087±0.0015
Brain	0.0230±0.0163	0.0430±0.0021
Thymus	0.0110±0.0060	0.0130±0.0010
Ovary	0.0151±0.0021	0.0071±0.0015
Uterus	0.0590±0.0015	0.0301±0.0010
Spleen	1.7800±0.0270	1.8001±0.0503
Kidney	0.3980±0.0930	0.2060±0.0040
Heart	0.0630±0.0020	0.0500±0.0010
Stomach	0.1320±0.0010	0.1170±0.0470
Lung	0.0960±0.0070	0.1040±0.0200
Liver	3.0500±0.0122	3.0564±0.0102
Bone	0.0272±0.0090	0.0610±0.0020

Vincristine was administered into female mice Balb/c (n=15) and after 96h ^{99m}Tc-PHY was given. The animals were sacrificed, the organs isolated and the activities determined.

CONCLUSION

The results reported can be explained by the metabolization and/or therapeutic and immunosuppressive action of vincristine. The effect of thes chemotherapeutic drug on the biodistribution of other ^{99m}Tc-radiopharmaceuticals is now in progress and the renal excretion of patients under treatment with vincristine will be evaluated.

REFERENCES

1. Bernardo-Filho M, Nogueira JF, Sturm JA and Boasquevisque EM. Plasma proteins labelling with 99m-Technetium. Arquivos de Biologia e Tecnologia, 1190; 33: 811-817.
2. Saha GB. Fundamentals of Nuclear Pharmacy. Springer Verlag, New York, 1984: 100-120
3. Hladik III WB, Saha GB and Study KT (Editors). Essentials of Nuclear Medicine Science. Williams and Wilkins, Sidney, 1987: 50-85.
4. Rang HP and Dale MM (Editors). Farmacologia. Guanabara Koogan, Rio de Janeiro, 1991
5. Hung JC, Ponto JA and Hammes RJ. Radiopharmaceutical-related pitfalls and artifacts. Seminars in Nuclear Medicine 1996; 26: 208-255.
6. Sampson CB: Textbook of Radiopharmacy, Theory and Practice,1994
7. Mareel M and De Mets M. Effect of microtubule inhibitors on invasion and on related activities of tumor cells. Int Ver Cytol, 1984: 90-125.
8. Salloum E, Doria R, Schubert W et al. Second solid tumors in patients with Hodgkin's disease cured after radiation or chemotherapy plus adjuvant low-dose radiation. J Clin Oncol, 1996, 14: 2435-2443.

POSTER SESSION II

Radioactive Isotopes in
Clinical Medicine and Research XXIII
ed. by H. Bergmann, H. Köhn and H. Sinzinger

ASSESSMENT OF LEFT VENTRICULAR EJECTION FRACTION USING RADIONUCLIDE VENTRICULOGRAPHY IN PATIENTS WITH ACROMEGALY

R. Junik, K. Łącka , E. Manuszewska, R. Czepczyński, M. Gembicki

Dept. of Endocrinology, K. Marcinkowski University of Medical Sciences, Poznań, Poland

Summary: The aim of our study was to assess left ventricular parameters in acromegalic patients using radionuclide ventriculography. Ten patients and 20 controls underwent rest and exercise radionuclide angiography. During exercise, time to peak ejection rate (TPER) was longer in acromegalics without hypertension comparing to controls (150±22 msec vs 82±45 msec, respectively, $p<0.05$). Peak filling rate (PFR) was lower during exercise (6.0±1.3 vs 7.6±3.5) and time to peak filling rate (TPFR) was longer both at rest and during exercise(170 vs 126 and 144 vs 111 msec) in acromegalics than in controls.Conclusion: There are important alterations of systolic and diastolic function of left ventricle in patients with acromegaly.

Introduction

Cardiac complications are known to be major determinants of the shortened life expectancy of acromegalic patients (1, 2). In particular, left ventricular (LV) hypertrophy associated with impaired diastolic filling at rest is a common finding in patients with acromegaly, even in the absence of decreased systolic performance (2, 3). Hypertension of all forms is capable of producing left ventricular hypertrophy. The concomitant development of hypertension in patients with acromegaly may also play an important role in the etiology of heart disease. Data from experimental animal models suggest a possible direct affect of growth hormone (GH) on the heart, the indirect affects of GH and promotion of cardiac work in these model systems has not been rigorously excluded (4). In studies of patients with acromegaly who present with LV dysfunction, the presence of a disease-specific myopathy has been suggested (2, 4, 5).
Radionuclide ventriculography, being a noninvasive imaging method, offers the possibility of quantitative analysis of systolic and diastolic ventricular function (6). Moreover, this method is less operator-dependent than echocardiography (3, 5).

Therefore, the aim of our study was to assess left ventricular systolic and diastolic parameters at rest and during physical exercise in acromegalic patients using radionuclide ventriculography.

Patients and Methods

Ten patients with acromegaly (1 male and 9 female, mean age 50 yr) and 20 matched normal controls underwent rest and exercise radionuclide angiography. The diagnosis of acromegaly had been established by clinical examination and basal plasma human GH levels greater than10 μg/L. The mean GH concentration in blood serum of our patients was 20±5 μg/L. Administration of the oral glucose tolerance test had resulted in suppression of the elevated GH levels in all of the patients. The patients were subdivided according to the presence (5 pts) or the absence (5 pts) of arterial hypertension.

The test was performed using red blood cells labelled in vivo with 740 MBq 99mTc-pyrophosphate and a gamma camera (Diacam, Siemens) equipped with a low energy, high resolution collimator. Autologous red blood cells were labelled with 740 MBq 99mTc-pertechnate according to the in vivo labeling method. Left ventricular function was assesed in a left anterior oblique projection with caudal tilt.

Statistical analysis: One-way-analysis-of-variance and non-parametric tests (Mann-Whitney U test) were used to compare the acromegalic group with the control group, and the two subgroups of hypertensive and normotensive acromegalic patients with each other and with controls. Linear regression analyses were performed between duration of disease, GH levels and LV parameters.

Results and Discussion

During physical exercise, time to peak ejection rate (TPER) was considerably longer in acromegalic patients without hypertension comparing to controls (150±22 msec vs 82±45 msec, respectively, $p<0.05$). Acromegalic patients and controls did not differ with respect to ejection fraction (EF) and peak ejection rate (PER). Peak filling rate (PFR) was lower during exercise (6.0±1.3 vs 7.6±3.5, respectively) and time to peak filling rate (TPFR) was longer both at rest and during exercise(170 vs 126 and 144 vs 111 msec, respectively) in acromegalic patients than in controls.

Mean values of the scintigraphic parameters of the patients in comparison with the control group are given in table 1. Table 2 summarizes the hemodynamic data of acromegalic patients without and with coexisting arterial hypertension.

Table 1. Results of parameters obtained by radionuclide ventriculography at rest and during physical exercise in acromegalics and control subjects. Values are the mean +/- standard deviation (SD).

	rest		exercise	
mean±SD	patients	controls	patients	controls
EF (%)	65±7	62±9	70±10	72±9
PER	4.2±0.8	4.3±1.2	4.9± 0.7	7.1±3.0
TPER (msec)	122±32	95±44	108±52	82*±45
PFR	3.8±0.9	4.1±1.3	5.98±1.3	7.6±3.5
TPFR (msec)	170±33	126±68	144±21	111±54

Table 2. Comparison of parameters obtained by radionuclide ventriculography at rest and during physical exercise in acromegalics without and with coexisting arterial hypertension. Values are the mean ± standard deviation (SD).

* the difference statistically significant comparing to control group.

	rest		exercise	
mean±SD	acromegaly	acromegaly + hypertension	acromegaly	acromegaly + hypertension
EF (%)	61±6	64±12	71±13	68±10
PER	4.0±1.2	4.1±0.6	5.4±1.0	4.7±0.6
TPER (msec)	127 ±27	102±26	150* ±22	88±33
PFR	4.0±1.0	3.8±0.8	6.7±1.0	5.2±1.3
TPFR (msec)	161±34	196±21	134±24	154±18

Phase and amplitude analysis did not show any wall motion abnormality. No significant correlation was found between LV functional parameters and GH values or duration of the disease. No difference was observed between the subgrups of normotensive and hypertensive acromegalic patients. These findings are in agreement with previous observations by some of us (7) and those by Fazio (1) who did not observe significant difference in the indices of systolic and diastolic function between the subgroups of normotensive and hypertensive acromegalics, either at rest or during exercise.

TPER in our patients without arterial hypertension was significantly longer comparing to controls (150±22 vs 82±45 msec). The similar observation, namely increased speed of ejection fraction (PER) and the longer time taken to achieve it (TPER) in acromegalic patients comparing to controls was obtained by Sicolo (5) and Erbas (6). The increased maximum speed of EF , seems to indicate that the acromegalic hypertrophic myocardium is able to develope greater strenght in systole; however, probably at the beginning of the systolic phase there is a reduced speed in the ejection of ventricular blood (5).

Despite the others (1, 3, 5, 6), in our patients diastolic function were not found to be significantly different than those of the control group. However, mean value of PFR was lower and TPFR was longer in patients comparing to controls. Succesful disease treatment reverses changes in arterial smooth muscle (4, 8). Low incidence of impairment of myocardial function in patients with treated acromegaly suggests a possible effect of treatment on the prognosis of the disease (9). The mean GH concentration in blood serum of our acromegalics was 20±5 μg/L and was lower than in works of authors mentioned above; this may be an explanation of less pronounced changes in our patients. Conclusion: There are important alterations of systolic and diastolic function of left ventricle in patients with acromegaly.

References

1. Fazio S., Cittadini A, Cuocolo A, Merola B, Sabatini D, Colao A. Impaired cardiac performance is a distinct feature of uncomplicated acromegaly. J Clin Endocrinol Metab 1994; 79:441-446.
2. Sacca L, Cittadini A, Fazio S. Growth hormone and the heart. Endocr Rev 1994; 15:555-573.
3. Cuocolo A, Nicolai E, Fazio S, Pace L, Maurea S, Cittadini A, Sacca L, Salvatore M. Impaired left ventricular diastolic filling in patients with acromegaly: Assessment with radionuclide angiography. J Nucl Med 1995; 36:196-201.
4. Klein I, Ojamaa K. Cardiovascular manifestations of endocrine disease. J Clin Endocrinol Metab 1992; 75:339-342.
5. Sicolo N, Bui F, Sicolo M, Varotto L, Martini C, Macor C, Federspil G. Acromegalic cardiopathy: A left ventricular scintigraphic study. J Endocrinol Invest 1993; 16:123-127.
6. Erbas T, Erbas B, Usman A, Bekdik CF. Assessment of left ventricular dysfunction in acromegalic patients using radionuclide ventriculography parameters. Cardiology 1992; 80:172-179.
7. Łącka K, Piszczek I, Kosowicz J, Gembicki M. Echocardiographic abnormalities in acromegalic patients. Exp Clin Endocrinol 1988; 91:212-216.
8. Martins JB, Kerber RE, Sherman BM, Marcus ML, Ehrhardt JC. Cardiac size and function in acromegaly. Circulation 1977; 56:863-869.
9. O'Keefe JC, Grant SJ., Wisemant JC, Stiel JN, Wilmshurst EG, Cooper RA, Edwards AC. Acromegaly and the heart - echocardiographic and nuclear imaging studies. Aust N Z J Med 1982; 12:603-607.

Radioactive Isotopes in
Clinical Medicine and Research XXIII
ed. by H. Bergmann, H. Köhn and H. Sinzinger

TECHNETIUM-99m-PERTECHNETATE SCINTIGRAPHY IN SMALL THYROID NODULES

Ewald Kresnik, Peter Mikosch, Mario Molnar, Hans-Jürgen Gallowitsch,
Oliver Unterweger, Iris Gomez and Peter Lind.
Department of Nuclear Medicine and Endocrinology, Landeskrankenhaus Klagenfurt, Austria

Summary

The aim of our study was to compare the scinitgraphic pattern in different tumor stages of thyroid carcinoma. In addition, sonographic and cytologic results are evaluated.
In 140 patients ^{99m}Tc-pertechnetate scans were evaluated retrospectively by a visual inspection scoring method: Tumor size plays an important role in routinely used planar scintigraphy. Nodules greater 2cm in diameter tend to appear cold but microcarcinomas (≤1cm) are mostly warm on scan. Therefore not all cancers are cold. On ultrasonography, small nodules often have a similar echo structure. The echo structure tends to decrease when the nodules enlarge. Especially for the diagnosis of non palpable carcinomas, ultrasonographically guided FNAB is necessary.

Introduction

^{99m}Tc-pertechnetate has been widely and routinely used for imaging the gland. For further preoperative evaluation of cold thyroid nodules thallium 201 has been described with different sensitivity and specificity for malignancy. In the last years also the cationic complex molecules ^{99m}Tc-tetrofosmin and ^{99m}Tc-sestamibi were reported to be useful in thyroid scintigraphy as well as in thyroid cancer follow up (1-4). The study was performed to determine which thyroid nodules appear hypofunctional or cold on standardly used ^{99m} Tc- pertechnetate anterior images.

Material and methods

The data of 140 patients with thyroid carcinoma in different tumor stages were evaluated retrospectively (mean age 54.21±14.9 years, 112 female and 28 male). Ultrasonographic examination was performed in all patients and fine needle aspiration biopsy guided by ultrasonography in most of the patients. The ^{99m}Tc-pertechnetate scintigrams were obtained twenty minutes after intravenous injection of 74 MBq. Planar images in anterior-posterior projection were taken using a small field thyroid gamma camera (GAEDE® ,GKS I, Freiburg, Germany).

Visual interpretation was done using the following scoring method: A= no significant to D= uptake superior to that of normal thyroid tissue.

Results and discussion

The results are summarized in Table 1 and Table 2.

Table 1. Results in 140 patients with different tumor stages of thyroid carcinoma

Patients (n)	Histology	Diameter mean / SD in cm	Pertechnetate uptake A	B	C	D
5o	papillar carc. pT1	0.56±0.26	2	2	33	1[illegible]
2	follicular carc. pT1		1	1	-	-
30	papillar carc. pT2	1.66±0.49	4	10	12	4
6	follicular carc. pT2		1	1	1	3
4	papillar carc. pT3	3.58±1.07	3	-	1	-
7	follicular carc. pT3		4	1	1	1
38	papillar carc. pT4	2.16±1.45	12	5	14	7
2	follicular carc. pT4		1	1	-	-
1	nondiff. carc. pT4		1	-	-	-
Total	140 patients					
Mean age/ SD	54.21yr±14.9					
Male	28					
Female	112					

A= no significant uptake, B= higher uptake than background activity but less compared to normal thyroid, C= similar to thyroid, D= greater uptake than normal thyroid tissue; carc., carcinoma; nondiff., nondifferentiated; cm, centimeter; yr, year; SD, standard deviation.

Table 2. Cytological and sonographic findings in 140 patients with thyroid carcinoma in different tumor stages.

Histology	No. of patients	Sonography decr.	sim.	compl.	incr.	Cytology P	F	O	D	NA
pap. ca pT1	50	28	19	3	-	10	4	3	8	25
foll. ca pT1	2	1	1	-	-	-	1	-	-	1
pap. ca pT2	30	20	4	5	1	19	1	1	2	7
foll. ca pT2	6	2	4	-	-	-	3	1	-	2
pap. ca pT3	4	4	-	-	-	2	-	-	1	1
foll. ca pT3	7	3	-	4	-	-	2	1	-	4
pap. ca pT4	38	30	2	6	-	34	1	-	1	2
foll. ca pT4	2	2	-	-	-	-	1	-	-	1
nondiff. ca pT4	1	1	-	-	-	1	-	-	-	-

pap. ca, papillar carcinoma; foll. ca, follicular carcinoma; nondiff. ca, nondifferentiated carcinoma; decr., decreased echo; sim., similar echo; compl., complex echo; incr., increased echo; P, papillary carcinoma; F, follicular carcinoma; O, oxyphilic proliferation; D, degenerative changes; NA, not available

^{99m}Tc-pertechnetate anterior images are routinely used in evaluating thyroid nodules. Nodules with increased tracer uptake in relation to normal thyroid have a low probability of being malignant. Therefore, cancer should appear hypofunctioning or cold on scintiscan.

Microcarcinomas (≤1cm in diameter) are reported to be represent up to 30 per cent of all cancers. In our study the vast majority showed tracer uptake similar to surrounding thyroid tissue. It is reported that a small nonfunctional nodule can appear normofunctional entirely due to emissions from overlying tissue or gamma emissions passing through the nodule. Some authors report that oblique views can improve the evaluation of thyroid nodules, but because of problems in positioning the patients as well as difficulties in interpreting the images- oblique views were not routinely obtained.

Regarding to carcinomas in pT2 tumor stage, most of the nodules showed similar or less pertechnetate uptake compared to normal surrounding thyroid tissue. There were only five patients that were absolutely cold on scan. This is probably due to the small mean tumor size.

Tumor size plays an important role in planar scintigraphy. Nodules smaller than 2cm are often warm on scan and tend to be cold if they enlarge. Patients with pT4 carcinoma, 20 were classified as „A“ or „B“ on scan, but there were also fourteen patients that explained similar tracer uptake.

The incidence of hyperthyroidism and malignancy is rare, but several studies (5) report carcinoma in autonomously functioning thyroid. In our study there were nine patients with microcarcinomas, six patients in pT2 and six patients in pT4 tumor stage that were found in autonomously functioning nodules.

Ultrasound is an important diagnostic method to detect thyroid nodules. The diagnostic accuracy can probably be rated at 60 % (6). In our study, we also found that most of the thyroid nodules in pT2-pT4 tumor stage had a decreased echo structure, but in microcarcinomas, 20 had a similar echo structure.

FNAB guided by ultrasonography has a central role in the detection of thyroid cancer (7). In our study, cytology was available in 87 patients with papillary carcinoma. Cytology suspicious of malignancy was found in 66 patients. Cytology suspicious of malignancy could also be obtained in nine patients with a follicular carcinoma.

References

1. Lind P, Gallowitsch HJ, Langsteger W, Kresnik E, Mikosch P. Technetium-99m-tetrofosmin whole body scintigraphy in the follow up of differentiated thyroid cancer. J Nucl Med 1997; 38: 348-352.
2. Kresnik E, Gallowitsch HJ, Mikosch P, Molnar M, Pipam W, Gomez I, Lind P. Evaluation of thyroid nodules with technetium-99m tetrofosmin dual-phase scintigraphy. Eur J Nucl Med 1997; 24: 716-721.
3. Kresnik E, Gallowitsch HJ, Mikosch P, Lind P. Technetium-99m-MIBI scintigraphy of thyroid nodules in an endemic goiter area. J Nucl Med 1997; 38: 62-5.
4. Gallowitsch HJ, Mikosch P, Kresnik E, Molnar M, Gomez I, Lind P. Thyroglobulin, low dose I-131 and Tc-99m tetrofosmin WBS in the follow up of DTC: A direct comparison under endogenous TSH stimulation (Abstract). Eur J Nucl Med 1997; 24: 928.
5. Nicolusi A, Addis E, Calo PG, Tarquini A. Hyperthyroidism and cancer of the thyroid. Minerva Chir1994; 49: 491-495.
6. Riccabona G. Thyroid cancer. Ist epidemiology clinical features, and treatement. Springer company, Berlin, 1987; p 62.
7. Agrawal S. Diagnostic accuracy and role of fine needle aspiration cytology in management of thyroid nodules J Surg Oncol 1995; 58: 168-172.

Radioactive Isotopes in
Clinical Medicine and Research XXIII
ed. by H. Bergmann, H. Köhn and H. Sinzinger

THE IMAGING OF THYROID TUMORS: MRI VS. RADIONUCLIDE SCINTIGRAPHY AND ULTRASOUND

J. Mihailovic, M. Prvulovic, Lj. Stefanovic
Department of Nuclear Medicine and MRI Center, Institute of Oncology,
Institutski put 4, 21204 Sremska Kamenica, Yugoslavia

SUMMARY:

Thirty patients with unilateral thyroid tumors underwent this study. Radionuclide scintigraphy, ultrasound with fine-needle aspiration and MRI were performed. Scintigraphy detected cold nodes in all patients. Ultrasound could only detected cystic, solid, and mixed echo patterns. MRI was done at 1.5 T system using conventional SE pulse sequences and postcontrast T1w images. MRI could differentiate between cystic and solid benign thyroid nodes and characterized the cystic fluid. MR images showed enchancement with markedly increased signal intensity at postcontrast T1w images in thyroid cancer. MRI were able to detect tumor reccurences in medullary cancer in postoperatively follow up. Magnetic resonance, like radionuclide scintigraphy and ultrasound cannot reliably distinguish between benign and malignant thyroid tumors.

Key words: thyroid, thyroid tumors, magnetic resonance

INTRODUCTION:

Nodular goiters are one of the most frequent endocrine disorders. A prevalence of thyroid nodes in overall adult population is approximately 4-7% (1).Radionuclide scintigraphy and ultrasound are the most performed techniques in evaluation of thyroid tumors. The thyroid nodes are classified according to their ability to take up isotope at radionuclide scan to: cold, warm or hot. Malignancy was found in 20% in cold thyroid nodes (2).

More recently, magnetic resonance has been introduced in evaluation of thyroid tumors. Nowadays, it is generally recognized as imaging modality for the diagnosis of morphologic abnormalities of thyroid gland (3).

This study was aimed to compare the value of MR imaging of the thyroid tumors with radionuclide scintigraphy and ultrasound.

MATERIAL AND METHODS:

Thirty patients with solitary thyroid tumors were investigated. There were 4 (13.3%) male and 26 (86.7%) female, aged 23 - 76 years; mean 46.1 years. They underwent biochemical evaluations, radionuclide scintigraphy, ultrasound with fine needle aspiration (FNA) and magnetic resonance imaging (MRI). The final diagnoses were established either cytologically in 8 pts (cysts) and histologically in 20 operated pts (benign tumors included: 8 adenoma folliculare, 5 struma adenomatosa, 2 struma nodosa colloides and 1 Hashimoto thyroiditis and 4 malignant tumors included 4 medullary cancer). Two patients had anaplastic cancer which have been proven by characteristic clinical features and cytollogy.

Radionuclide scintigraphy was performed on rectilinear scanner (PHO/DOT II - Nuclear Chikago). Ultrasonography was performed using a 10 MHz linear array transducer (Siemens). The patients were examined in the supine position with the hyperextended neck and a cushion under the neck. Sonograms were obtained in standard transverse and longitudinal planes. Magnetic resonance was performed on a 1.5 T (Magnetom SP 63/4000, Siemens, Erlangen) imaging system using Helmholtz neck coil. The performed spin echo pulse sequences were: T1w (TR-450 ms, TE-15 ms) and PD/T2w (TR-2000 ms, TE-20-80 ms). Axial and coronal contiguous 4 mm slices were obtained utilizing a matrix grid of 256x256. There was a 230 mm field of view (FOV). Postcontrast T1w images were obtained after i.v. application of Gd-DTPA in 6 patients.

RESULTS:

All of investigated patients were euthyroid and had solitary, unilateral thyroid nodes, presented as „cold" at radionuclide scan. The control group was consisted of the opposite thyroid lobe without a node. MRI displayed normal thyroid tissue as homogeneous signal intensity on T1w and PD/T2w images. MR T1w images presented normal thyroid tissue as a slightly hyperintensity than the surrounding muscles. MR PD/T2w images showed a slightly higher signal intensity of the thyroid than on T1w images.

Benign thyroid nodes

Sonographic images showed 8 cystic, 12 solid and 4 mixed echo patterns. MRI showed 8 cysts (1 non-colloid and 7 colloid cysts), 6 parenchymal and 10 parenchymal-colloidal nodes. *Non-colloid cyst* was presented as hypointensity on T1w and hyperintensity on PD/T2w images. *Colloid cysts* were showed as hyperintense lesions at all pulse sequences. *Parenchymal nodes* were presented as heterogeneous isointensity on T1w and hyperintensity on PD/T2w images. *Parenchymal-colloidal nodes* were showed as distinctly bounded nodes with hypointense capsula. There was isointensity or slightly hyperintensity with heterogeneous signal distribution on T1w and slightly increased signal intensity on PD/T2w images.

Malignant thyroid tumors

Six patients with different types of thyroid cancer underwent this study: 3 before surgery (one medullary and two anaplastic cancer) and 3 after the surgery (three medullary cancer).

Medullary carcinoma

This study was performed in three patients in postoperatively follow-up. US detected thyroid tissue only in one patient. MRI didn't found reccurence in one case. MR detected unilateral enlargement lymph nodes in another case. A 35-year-old woman presented an isointense tumor on T1w images located in the right thyroid lobe and heterogeneous hyperintense lesion on T2w images, with retrotracheal spreading into the opposite thyroid lobe. The surroundings neck structures displayed higher signal intensity on T2w images. Postcontrast T1w images showed increased signal intensity in the tumor site, but central parts were necrotic and hypointense.

Preoperatively, this study was done in a 73-year-old woman. Ultrasound showed mixed echo patterns. MRI showed a great lobulated tumor in the left thyroid lobe with infiltration of capsule and compression of a trachea. Regional lymph nodes were enlarged. There was isointensity on T1w images mixed with some parts of hypo- and hyperintensity. There were slightly higher signal intensity on T2w images. The signal intensity was heterogeneous in all pulse sequences. Postcontrast T1w images showed enchancement with markedly increased signal intensity.

Figure 1: This is a 73-year-old woman with medullary cancer in the left thyroid lobe, preoperatively. A: MR axial T1w image shows isointensity mixed with some parts of hypo- and hyperintensity. B: MR axial T2w image displays slightly higher signal intensity. MRI showing heterogeneous signal intensity on T1w and T2w images. It also shows a capsule infiltration and lymphadenopathy. Trachea is compressed and dislocated by the tumor. C: Axial postcontrast T1w image displays enchancement with markedly increased signal intensity.

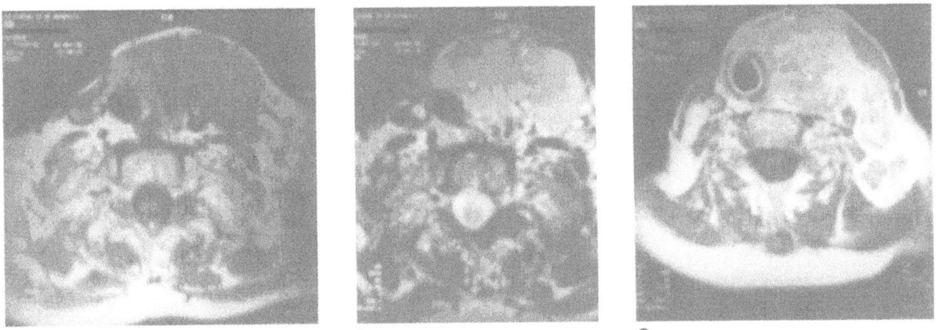

A B C

Anaplastic carcinoma

Two patients, a 76-year-old woman and a 58-year-old woman with anaplastic cancer were studied. They were not operated, but they received radiotherapy after the diagnostic investigation. Ultrasound found mixed echo patterns in both patients.

The 76-year-old woman presented on MRI with enormously large lobulated tumor of the thyroid. The tumor was irregularly shaped, distinctly bounded from the surrounding structures. The signal intensity was heterogeneous: there was isointensity with some parts of hypo- and hyperintensity on T1w images. The trachea was markedly dislocated and compressed as well as great blood vessels. There was lymphadenopathy on the right and left side of the neck. Postcontrast T1w images showed markedly increased signal intensity, heterogeneously distributed mixed with some necrotic hypointense and hemorrhagic hyperintense parts.

Figure 2: This is a 76-year-old woman with an anaplastic cancer of the thyroid. A: MR axial T1w image shows enormously large lobulated tumor irregularly shaped, distinctly bounded from the surrounding structures. There was heterogeneous signal intensity with some parts of hypo- and hyperintensity. The trachea was dislocated and compressed as well as great blood vessels. There were lymph node enlargements on the right and left side of the neck. B: Axial postcontrast T1w image displays markedly increased signal intensity, heterogeneously distributed mixed with some necrotic hypointense and hemorrhagic hyperintense parts.

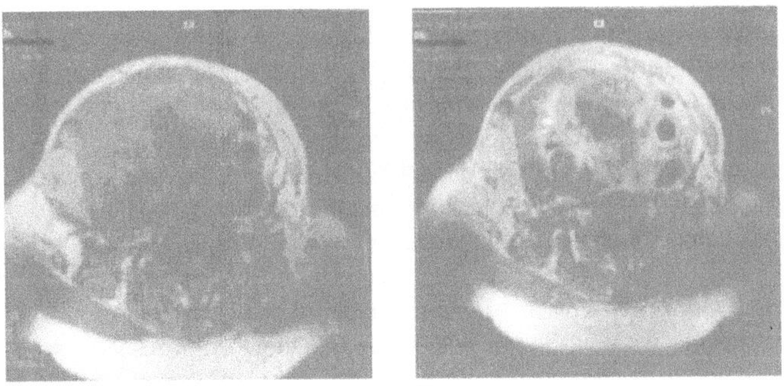

A B

The 58-year-old woman had a great thyroid tumor in the left lobe. MR T1w images displayed an isointense lesion irregularly shaped. T2w images showed slightly increased signal intensity without distinctly bounded margins. Postcontrast T1w images presented enchancement, with markedly increased signal intensity, mixed with multiple hypointense, necrotic parts. The surrounding muscles and fat were infiltrated by the pathologic process. Trachea was compressed and markedly dislocated to the right. Great blood vessels of the left side of the neck were compressed and dislocated, too. The lymph node on the left side of the neck and in the mediastinum were markedly enlarged.

Figure 3: This is a 58-year-old woman with an anaplastic cancer in the left thyroid lobe. A: Axial T1w image shows a great isointense tumor irregularly shaped. B: Axial T2w image displays slightly increased signal intensity. C: Axial postcontrast T1w image showing enchancement mixed with necrotic hypointense parts. There were compresseion and dislocation of the trachea and great blood vessels. MR images also shows lymphadenopathy on the left and in the mediastinum.

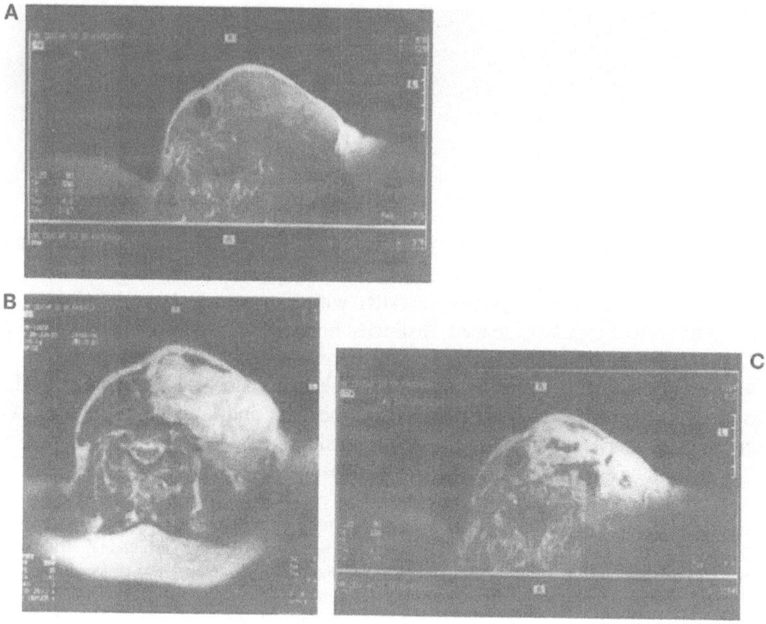

DISSCUSION

Patients with cold thyroid nodes present a risky group in regarding to malignancy and should be diagnosed properly (4,5,6). Radionuclide scanning is using as a „first line" diagnostic tool for assessment of functional status of the thyroid nodes (1). Ultrasound is non-invasive method that categorizes nodes as cystic and solid with more than 90% accuracy. This method is also able to determine the volume of the thyroid node (6). On the other hand, these both techniques has its limitations. Thus, radioisotope scan has poor spatial resolution and cannot present small nodes and nodes located in areas such as: istmus, anteriorly and posteriorly presented nodes. By this method it is not possible to detect lymphadenopathy and trachea or esophageal deviation. These imaging techniques cannot reliably distinguish between benign and malignant thyroid tumors (1).

MRI is a modern, non-invasive imaging modality producing high-resolution tomograms or three-dimensional images without the use of ionizing radiation. High resolution MR imaging permit excellent differentiation between muscles, lymph nodes, fat, blood vessels and thyroid gland (7).

In our study, MRI clearly distinguished between solid and cystic thyroid nodes and characterized between cystic fluid. Non-colloid cyst was displayed with low intensity on T1w images and high intensity on PD/T2w images. Colloid cysts or cysts with high proteinaceous content were showed with high signal intensity at all pulse sequences. This data have been already reported by several other authors (8,9).

In cases of carcinomas, MRI is able to evaluate the extent of invasive thyroid cancer and to detect muscle, tracheal or esophageal invasion as well as lymph node elnlargement. Our results shows that in all patients with thyroid cancer postcontrast T1w images showed enchancements. Some authors reported that postcontrast enchancements were seen in different malignant tumor(10).

MR images can detect small anatomical details, such as: presence or absence of distinct margins, regular contours and pseudocapsule or capsule infiltration and invasion of the surrounding neck structures. In postoperatively follow up, MR helps in detection of tumor reccurences. It is especially important in medullary cancer because the reccurences cannot be detected by the radioiodine scan. In such patients, with elevated serum thyrocalcitonin levels MRI should be done to locate the site and extent of tumor reccurence. These data are in accord with other reports (4,8,9).

CONCLUSION:

Absence of radiation and ability to obtain direct images in coronal and sagittal planes makes MRI as an excellent imaging diagnostic tool in evaluation of thyroid tumors. To date, MR imaging, like several others imaging techniques is nonspecific in distinguishing benign from malignant tumors. Beside radionuclide scintigraphy and ultrasound, magnetic resonance cannot reliably differentiate in histological characterization of the thyroid tumors.

REFERENCES:

1. Mafee MF, Capek V, Blend M, et al. Modern methodologies of differentiatin thyroid masses. Semin in Surg Onc 1991; 7: 67-75.
2. Harbert J. The thyroid. In: Harbert J, De Rocha AFG. Textbook of nuclear medicine. Volume II: Clinical applications. Philadelphia: Lea & Febiger, 1984: 3-52.
3. Higgins CB, Stevens SK. The thyroid and parathyroid glands. In: Higgins CB, Hricak H, Helms CA. Magnetic resonance of the body. Second edition. New York: Raven Press Ltd, 1992: 415-22.
4. Nelson LR, Wahner WH, Gorman AC. Rectilinear thyroid scanning as a predictor of malignancy. Ann Intern med 1987; 88: 41-4.
5. Ridgway EC. Clinical evaluation of solitary thyroid nodules. In: Braverman LE, Utiger RD. Werner and Ingbar's The thyroid. Seventh Edition. Philadelphia.New York: Lippincott-Raven, 1995: 966-72.
6. Mazzaferri EL. Management of a solitary thyroid nodule. N Engl J Med 1993; 25: 553-9.
7. Reading CC, Gorman CA. Thyroid imaging techniques. Clinics in Lab Med 1993; 13: 711-23.
8. Mountz JM, Glazer GM, Dmuchowski C, et al. MR imaging of the thyroid: Comparison with scintigraphy in the normal and diseased gland. J Comput Assist Tomogr 1987; 11: 612-9.
9. Eisenberg B, Velchick MG, Spritzer C, et al. Magnetic resonance imaging and scintigraphic correlation in thyroid disorders. Am J Physiol Imaging 1990; 5: 8-21.
10. Bydder GM. Clinical application of Gadolinium-DTPA. In: Stark DD, Bradley WG. Magnetic resonance imaging. St Louis: The CV Mosby Company, 1988: 182-200.

Radioactive Isotopes in
Clinical Medicine and Research XXIII
ed. by H. Bergmann, H. Köhn and H. Sinzinger

PULMONARY TUBERCULOSIS AND ITS THERAPY'S EFFECT ON THYROID FUNCTION. A SHORT-TERM PROSPECTIVE STUDY.

I Ilias[1] T Pappas[2], A Nikitas[2], D Nikolakakou[2], A Tselebis[2], A Boufas[2],
G Panoutsopoulos[1], N Filippou[2], J Christakopoulou[1]✉

[1] *Dept of Nuclear Medicine,* [2] *9th Dept of Pulmonary Medicine, «Sotiria» Hospital,*
152 Mesogion Avenue, Athinai GR-11527, HELLAS

Summary

Basal thyrotropin , TT_4, TT_3 and FT_3 were measured in 23 HIV(-) patients with focal pulmonary tuberculosis (TB) upon commencement and after 1 and 2 weeks of isoniazid, rifampicin and pyrazinamide therapy. Rapid elevations in FT_3 and TT_4 were noted respectively after 1 and 2 weeks of treatment. For most patients, however, hormone levels remained within normal limits throughout the study. Overall, the effects of TB and of its therapy on the thyroid function parameters examined, in otherwise healthy individuals, appear to be minimal.

Introduction

In recent years an increase in the incidence of tuberculosis (TB) has been observed worldwide, the main reason for this increase being the spread of HIV infection in Africa [1]. In most countries of the western world HIV played a small part in the disease's resurgence [1], though recently in the United States it was reported that 8% of TB patients were HIV(+)[2].

Few and conflicting reports exist on the effect of pulmonary tuberculosis and anti-TB therapy on thyroid function. Two recent research papers [3,4] have dealt with this problem. In the first all patients were over 50 years old and their HIV infection status was not ascertained [3], though overall mortality was very high, while in the second most of the patients with TB had either high HIV infection risk and/or were intravenous drug users and alcoholics [4]. HIV infection though is known to affect thyroid function [5]. The aim of the present study was to evaluate the effect of TB and of its concomitant therapy in a short-term prospective fashion in HIV(-) subjects.

Materials and methods

Sera from 23 HIV(-) patients (16 men, 7 women, mean age: 47 years old, SD: 12 years, mean BMI: 26.3) with focal pulmonary TB were collected upon commencement (0 week) and after 1 and 2 weeks of isoniazid (300 mg/day), rifampicin (600 mg/day) and pyrazinamide (30 mg/kg/day) po therapy. The patients' HIV infection status was assessed, with their consent, by ELISA (HIV-1/HIV-2 3rd Generation Plus EIA, Abbott GmbH, Deikenheim, Germany). The diagnosis of TB was sustained by sputum smears, biopsy specimens or bronchial washings. All the subjects were ambulatory, none was malnourished, no muscle wasting was evident and their serum albumin levels were > 3.9 g/dL. No patient was under known thyroid function altering medication, such as corticosteroids or amiodarone. Patients with a history of thyroid and/or autoimmune disease were excluded. Executed measurements (Table 1) included basal TSH (Gammacoat hTSH IRMA, INCSTAR, Stillwater, Minnesota, USA), TT_3 and TT4 (AMERLEX T3 and T4 RIA, Amersham Diagnostics, Amersham, UK) and FT_3 (Free T_3 Clinical Assay, INCSTAR, Stillwater, Minnesota, USA).

Table 1
Measurements (mean$\pm$SD) at 0, 1 and 2 weeks of anti-TB therapy

Parameter (normal range)	0 week	1 week	2 weeks
TSH in μIU/mL (0.40-3.10)	1.18$\pm$0.99	1.27$\pm$1.11	1.14$\pm$0.99
TT_3 in ng/mL (0.50-1.90)	0.99$\pm$0.43	1.15$\pm$0.45	1.33$\pm$0.53
FT_3 in pg/mL (1.50-3.20)	1.71$\pm$0.29	1.96$\pm$0.37	1.83$\pm$0.35
TT_4 in ng/mL (50-140)	105$\pm$26	102$\pm$31	104$\pm$26

Results

Measurements remained within normal limits for most subjects throughout the study (Table 2). A single patient presented initially (0 week) with the sick euthyroid syndrome (clinically euthyroid, with low FT_3 and TSH values within normal limits) which resolved following TB therapy. Two patients were found to be hyperthyroid (with low TSH, high TT_3 and high TT_4) at the end of the study. Overall statistically significant elevations were observed in FT_3 after the first week of treatment and in TT_3 after the second week of treatment (p_1=0.05 and p_2=0.01 respectively by the Friedman test).

Table 2
Characteristics of measurements' results

Parameter	0 week	1 week	2 weeks
TSH	2↑, 19 N, 2↓	1↑, 20 N, 2↓	1↑, 20 N, 2↓
TT_3	1↑, 21 N, 1↓	2↑, 21 N	2↑, 21 N
FT_3	4↓, 19 N	23 N	23 N
TT_4	1↑, 22 N	3↑, 20 N	2↑, 21 N

↑: higher than normal limits, N: within normal range, ↓: lower than normal limits

Discussion

To simplify the study's design measurements were kept to a minimum, hence no thyroid hormone binding protein or rT_3 levels were available; changes in these parameters have been described in patients with HIV infection [5]. On the other hand, based on earlier published work, where subnormal TT_3 and FT_3I values before TB therapy and a statistically significant increase and normalization in them after TB therapy were the principal findings [4], free triiodothyronine measurements were made. An undetectable FT_3 level when starting anti-TB therapy has been associated with very high subsequent mortality [3]. Triiodothyronine has a half life of one day so changes in its serum levels are more quickly discernible than these of T_4. If any significant changes in thyroid function were to occur though, the sensitive third generation TSH assay employed would most probably show them, since this is considered an adequate screening tool [6] of thyroid function. The observed changes in FT_3 could be attributed to the resolution of the low T_3 syndrome of nonthyroidal disease while the changes in TT_3 levels were probably the result of altered hepatic metabolism (including altered production of thyroid hormone binding proteins) due to the disease *per se* and/or the drug regimen [4].

Although rapid elevations were noted in FT_3 and TT_3 after initiation of anti-TB treatment, most hormone measurements remained within normal limits throughout the study. The effects of TB and of its concomitant therapy on the examined thyroid function parameters in otherwise normal individuals appear to be minimal.

Acknowledgments

We would like to thank Mr D Stravolaimos, Ms P Bakola and Ms A Anastassaki for their technical support.

References

1. Davies PDO Tuberculosis *Curr Opin Inf Dis* 1995; 8: 105-9

2. Cantwell MF, Snider DE, Cauthen GM, Onorato IM Epidemiology of tuberculosis in the United States, 1985 to 1992 *JAMA* 1994; 272: 535-9

3. Chow CC, Mak TW, Chan CH, Cockram CS Euthyroid sick syndrome in pulmonary tuberculosis before and after treatment *Ann Clin Biochem* 1995; 32: 385-91

4. Hill AR, Schmidt FJ, Schussler GC Rapid changes in thyroid function tests upon treatment of tuberculosis *Tub Lung Dis* 1995; 76: 223-9

5. Lambert M Thyroid dysfunction in HIV infection *Baillière's Clin Endocr Metab* 1994; 8: 825-35

6. Klee CG Biochemical thyroid function testing *Mayo Clin Proc* 1994; 69: 469-70

Radioactive Isotopes in
Clinical Medicine and Research XXIII
ed. by H. Bergmann, H. Köhn and H. Sinzinger

SERUM TOTAL T3-, T4- AND TSH-CONCENTRATIONS IN VIETNAMESE NEWBORN BABIES LIVING IN ENDEMIC NONGOITROUS (ENR) AND IN ENDEMIC GOITROUS (EGR) REGIONS DURING THE FIRST SEVEN DAYS OF LIFE

Mai Trong Khoa, Phan Sy An
Department of Nuclear Medicine, Bach Mai Hospital, Hanoi Medical School, Hanoi, Vietnam

SUMMARY: After 5 days of life, serum TSH concentrations were below 4mU/L in the newborn babies living in ENR and below 6mU/L in EGR. Therefore, measurement of TSH should be performed the 5th day of life for screening and diagnosis of congenital hypothyroidism.

INTRODUCTION

Iodine deficiency disorders especially congenital hypothyroidism still remains a serious public health problem in Vietnam. Simultaneous determination of serum TSH and thyroid hormones has not been carried out in neonates living in EGR. In Vietnam, early diagnosis of congenital hypothyroidism is difficult and overlooked.

The present study, therefore, was undertaken to investigate the changes in simultaneous serum TSH-, T4- and T3-concentrations of newborn babies living in ENR and in EGR during the first seven days of life. The aim of the study was to contribute to early diagnosis of congenital hypothyroidism in Vietnamese newborn babies.

MATERIALS AND METHODS

182 newborn babies offsprings of healthy mothers living in Hanoi-ENR (group 1) and 178 newborn babies offsprings of simple goiter mothers living in EGR (group 2) were examined. Cord blood samples and venous blood samples were obtained from newborn babies in group1 and 2. The postnatal age of all babies ranged from 2 to 168 hours. Serum total T3-, T4- and TSH-levels in babies of group 1 were compared to babies of group 2. Serum total T3- and T4-concentrations were measured by radioimmunoassay (RIA) and TSH by immunoradiometric assay (IRMA) in the RIA laboratory of the Nuclear Medicine Department - Bach Mai University Hospital, Hanoi-Vietnam supported by the WHO immunoassay D.P.Program. For statistical testing, analysis of Variance and Student's t-test were used.

RESULTS

1. Serum TSH (Table 1)

In both groups - 1 and 2 - maximum values of serum TSH of babies were seen within 24 hours after birth and subsequently a significant decrease with postnatal age was observed ($p<0.05$).

Table 1: Serum TSH-concentrations (mU/L) in newborn babies

		Postnatal period							
	Cord blood	0-12 hours	13-24 hours	48 hours	72 hours	96 hours	120 hours	144 hours	168 hours
Group 1									
Mean	5.38	8.14	9.67	7.03	4.85	4.44	3.20	0.03	2.98
SD	2.81	3.20	3.09	2.16	1.98	2.20	1.30	1.16	1.20
(n)	38	17	16	19	17	18	18	19	20
Group 2									
Mean	6.98	10.21	13.76	9.68	6.95	5.93	5.42	4.97	4.68
SD	3.01	3.92	4.26	3.78	3.20	2.89	2.34	1.46	1.48
(n)	32	18	17	18	18	19	17	20	19
Normal adult					2.06±0.98 (n=298)				

In the cord blood of both groups 1 and 2, serum TSH-values were higher than in normal adults ($p<0.001$). After the 5th day of life all TSH values below 4mU/L in group 1 and below 6mU/l in group 2.

2.Serum total T4

Table 2: Serum total T4-concentrations (nmol/l) in newborn babies

		Postnatal period							
	Cord blood	0-12 hours	13-24 hours	48 hours	72 hours	96 hours	120 hours	144 hours	168 hours
Group 1									
Mean	129.88	184.07	252.06	191.25	179.51	160.02	139.86	143.51	136.87
SD	22.60	28.19	25.41	26.87	25.78	22.48	26.71	20.35	27.08
(n)	38	17	16	19	17	18	18	19	20
Group 2									
Mean	84.58	128.35	165.31	120.31	114.51	100.38	108.25	95.47	94.81
SD	20.85	26.07	28.41	23.35	24.25	22.41	21.54	20.68	21.02
(n)	32	18	17	18	18	19	17	20	19
Normal adult					105.90±24.98 (n=297)				

In both groups, serum T4-levels reached a maximum about 24 hours after delivery. After the first day of life all T4 values were decreased significantly with postnatal age ($p<0.05$). The values of serum T4 in group 1 were significantly higher than in group 2 ($p<0.01$).

3.Serum total T3-concentrations

Table 3. Serum T3-concentrations (nmol/l) in newborn babies

		Postnatal period							
	Cord blood	0-12 hours	13-24 hours	48 hours	72 hours	96 hours	120 hours	144 hours	168 hours
Group 1									
Mean	0.78	0.3	3.78	2.89	2.15	2.04	2.06	2.21	2.24
SD	0.34	0.46	0.69	0.54	0.39	0.42	0.50	0.34	0.41
(n)	38	17	16	19	17	18	18	19	20
Group 2									
Mean	0.94	3.90	5.07	3.86	3.45	3.24	3.36	3.41	3.44
SD	0.36	0.50	0.58	0.51	0.46	0.49	0.35	0.41	0.51
(n)	32	18	17	18	18	19	17	20	19
Normal adult					2.03 ± 0.50 (n=298)				

The serum total T3-concentrations in group1 and 2 reached a maximum about 24 hours after birth; these values were about 5 times higher than in cord blood. Values of serum T3 in group 1 were significantly higher than in group 2 ($p<0.05$). After the 5th day of life the values of T3 in group 1 were within the normal adult range, but in group 2 they were lightly above the normal range.

DISCUSSION

In all the newborn babies of groups 1 and 2 there was a pronounced early increase of a maximum at about 24 hours after birth and a subsequent postnatal decrease in serum TSH values. TSH values in the cord blood were higher than in normal adults. In both groups the total serum concentrations of thyroid hormones were low in cord and increased during the first 24 hours after delivery. These results were in agreement with other authors and an own previous study (1,2,3).

In newborn babies of group 2 the serum levels of T3 and TSH were higher than the ones group1 the levels of T4, however, behaved contrary. Data on the human daily requirement of iodine in relation to age, growth, pregnancy, lactation and disease are still incomplete and conflicting (4). In this study, the mothers of newborn babies lived in EGR having simple goiters (grades I,II and III). The results of many studies proved that iodine deficiency disorders of mothers during pregnancy will influence directly their offsprings. In our study, the changes of

serum TSH-, T3- and T4-levels in the babies or group 2 were the same as their goitrous mothers i.e. higher TSH and T3 but lower T4 levels than in group 1.
In all babies of groups 1 and 2 the serum TSH and thyroid hormone levels decreased gradually during the postnatl period, however, after 5 days of life serum TSH levels of babies in group 2 were tendantially higher as compared to group1. This supports the role of TSH in the newborn screening and the diagnosis of congenital hypothyroidism in our country.

CONCLUSION

Newborn babies living in ENR and in EGR have serum T3-, T4- and TSH levels reaching the maximum about 24 hours after delivery; thereafter there is a gradual decrease in the postnatal period. Newborns living in EGR have lower T4 but higher TSH and T3 concentrations than newborn babies in ENR. After 5 days of life, serum TSH concentrations of babies were below 4mU/l in the group 1 and below 6mU/l in the group 2. So measurement of TSH should be performed from the 5th day of life for screening and diagnosis of congenital hypothyroidism.

ACKNOWLEDGMENTS

We are grateful for great assistance by the Hanoi Obstetric Hospital and some other hospitals in Hanoi-Vietnam.

REFERENCES

1. Eltom MA. Endemic goiter in the Sudan. UPPSALA, 1984: 7-9
2. Jacobsen BB, Andersen HJ, Peitersen B, Dige-Petersen and Hummer L. Serum levels of thyrotropin, thyroxine and triiodothyronine in full-term, small-for-gestational age and preterm newborn babies. Acta Pediatr Scand 1977, 66: 681-687
3. Khoa MT. Total concentration of T3, T4 and TSH in the blood of Vietnam healthy children. Pediatrics 1994, 1:1-5 (Published by Vietnam General Association of Medicine and Pharmacy)
4. Matovinovic J, Cild MA, Nichaman MZ et al. Iodine and endemic goiter. In Dunn JT Medeiros-Neto GA(eds): Endemic goiter and cretinism: Continuing Threat to World Health Vol 262: Washington,DC, Pan American Health Organization, 1974: 67

Radioactive Isotopes in
Clinical Medicine and Research XXIII
ed. by H. Bergmann, H. Köhn and H. Sinzinger

HIGH ACTIVITY RADIOIODINE THERAPY FOR ADVANCED DIFFERENTIATED THYROID CARCINOMA : EFFICACY AND MORBIDITY

D. Carnell, R. McCready, L. Vini and C. Harmer.
Thyroid and Isotope Therapy Unit, Royal Marsden Hospital,
Sutton, Surrey, SM2 5PT, U.K.

SUMMARY : High activities of radioiodine (9.0 GBq) were administered to 24 patients with a history of a poor response to radioiodine, locally advanced and/or metastatic differentiated thyroid cancer. The higher activities did not produce clinically significant side effects when related to the better than previous response to conventional activities. A complete response was seen in 9% with a partial response in 32% and stable disease in a further 32%. Thus 73% of all patients achieved stable disease or better.

INTRODUCTION

Traditionally therapeutic activities of radioiodine have not exceeded 5.5 GBq in order to limit side effects. However, some patients with advanced disease who respond poorly to 5.5 GBq may require higher activities to achieve an adequate dose to the tumour. A group of patients with a history of a poor response to conventional activities or with a poor prognosis was selected and given one or more administrations of 9.0 GBq and the efficacy and morbidity of the higher activity assessed. Poor prognostic features included older age, male gender and advanced stage of disease. Metastatic disease is found in 10 - 40 % of patients and is twice as likely with follicular thyroid carcinoma. The usual site is lung which carries a hazard ratio of 3.4:1 of death from the disease compared with the presence of bone metastases which has a hazard ratio of 10:1 and where the five year survival can be less than 10%. In the presence of distant metastases many patients eventually die of disease but prolonged disease free survival is possible, especially in younger patients with lung involvement alone (1).

The side effects from the traditional activities (3.5 GBq for ablation and 5.5 GBq for therapy) of radioiodine are well known. Nausea and vomiting occurs in approximately 33% of patients. Salivary gland swelling and discomfort, abnormal taste and xerostomia are found in 7% of patients (2). Severe radiation sialitis in the first 24 hours is rarely seen but in extreme cases salivary gland changes can become chronic leading to the development of a painful inflammatory mass which may require surgery. Dose-related changes in salivary gland function can be seen using Tc99m pertechnetate and gamma camera imaging several months after treatment (3). Transient bone marrow suppression is seen in 31 - 90 % of patients, described as a protracted suppressive effect which is seldom severe. A 50% reduction in bone marrow precursors over days 9 - 19 has been described (4). Rarely dysplasia or aplasia can occur particularly with high cumulative doses and especially in the presence of bone deposits. It has been recommended that blood counts are repeated monthly after cumulative doses of > 37 GBq (5). Lung fibrosis is extremely rare even with diffuse bilateral lung disease. Fertility in females does not appear to be affected (6), although a definite decline in male fertility is seen and is more pronounced as the cumulative dose rises. For activities >18.5 GBq sperm banking may be recommended (7). There is the potential for carcinogenesis. An excess of leukaemia has been seen in the first 3 years where total activities have exceeded 40 GBq, with an incidence of up to 2 % compared to that expected of 0.4% (8), although this has not been confirmed by others (9). There is also an excess of malignant tumours in those organs which concentrate radioiodine occurring with an incidence of 1.4% (9).

Early data suggested that when activities of > 10 GBq are used 28% of patients experienced complications in contrast to 6% if activities are kept below 10 GBq. At activities < 7.4 GBq this falls further to only 1.5% (2).

MATERIALS AND METHODS

A consecutive series of 24 patients were studied - 19 females and 5 males with a mean age of 45 (range 13-73 years). All had maximal surgical intervention which comprised total thyroidectomy, and lymph node excision when necessary, followed by ablation of thyroid remnants using up to 3 GBq radioiodine. 16 patients had papillary and 8 follicular thyroid cancer, all with locally advanced and/or metastatic disease. There was a predominance of stage T4 disease with extra thyroidal extension. The pattern of disease sites is shown in Figure 1. A high activity ^{131}I (9.2 GBq) was administered with a total of 31 treatments from 1/3/92 to 29/4/97. Cumulative activities ranged from 13 to 110 GBq (mean 33 GBq). Follow up after high activity was 3 to 36 months (mean 10 months). Follow up from initial diagnosis was 8 years (range 1-22 years).

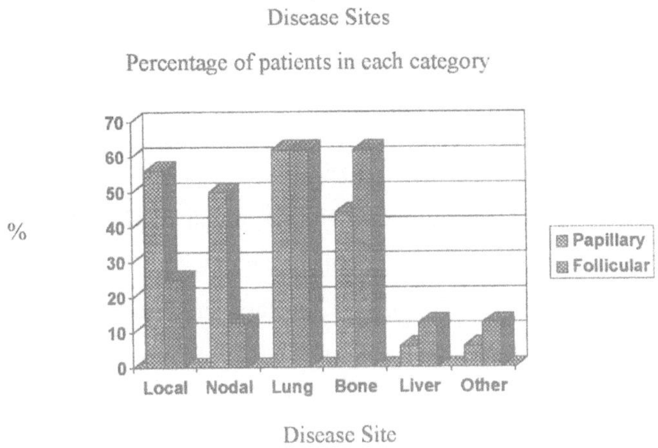

Figure 1

The side effects of the therapy were evaluated retrospectively using WHO toxicity criteria. The efficacy of treatment was assessed using clinical examination, plasma bound ^{131}I (PBI) 6 days post administration, thyroglobulin assay on suppressive doses of tri-iodothyronine or thyroxine, whole body ^{131}I scan and other radiological imaging when required. The 6 day PBI is used as a sensitive indicator of tumour mass. If found to be $> 0.006\%/L$ blood, tumour is likely to be present in the absence of any normal thyroid tissue. Therapy doses were repeated at intervals no less than 3 months provided that there was significant uptake into tumour tissue or until side effects precluded any further treatment. The majority of patients had received treatment with conventional activities of ^{131}I prior to receiving the higher activity.

Following the administration of the ^{131}I all patients received an antiemetic and a high fluid intake was encouraged. Lifelong follow up continues for all patients.

A diagnosis of complete response was made when there was no identifiable tumour and there was normalisation of thyroglobulin levels in the absence of significant neutralising antibody. A partial response was classified as a > 50% reduction in all tumour sites and thyroglobulin level. Stable disease was determined as no change in size, location of metastases or thyroglobulin level. Progressive disease was diagnosed when any site of disease had increased by 25% or the thyroglobulin had risen by 25% or a new disease site had been identified.

RESULTS

Acute bone marrow suppression up to grade 3 was seen in 18% of patients. Recovery was complete and was uncomplicated by sepsis. One patient did develop a dysplastic blood picture requiring blood and platelet support. This patient with metastatic follicular thyroid carcinoma initially received chemotherapy at the time of diagnosis and then a cumulative activity of 40.5 GBq ^{131}I. The patient eventually developed acute myeloid leukaemia as a terminal event having survived 22 years.

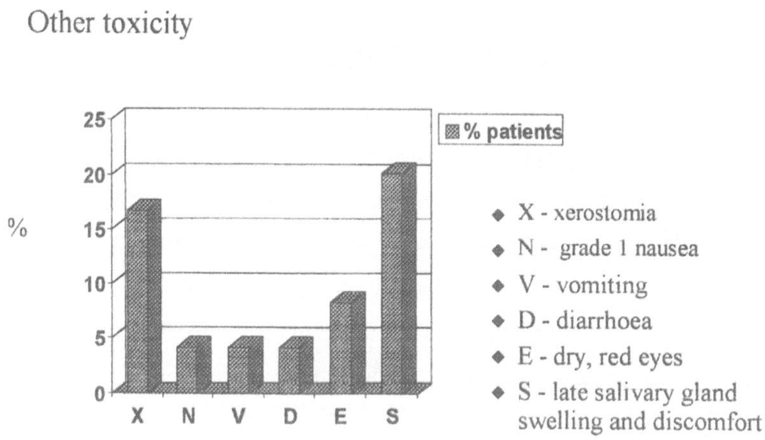

Figure 2

Other significant toxicity (Figure 2) was a 20% incidence of late salivary gland swelling and discomfort. In most cases this settled following a short course of anti-inflammatory medication. One patient who had received a single high activity dose of radioiodine and a cumulative dose of 19 GBq subsequently developed extreme xerostomia requiring reconstructive surgery using a free vascularised jejunal graft. There was a low incidence of all other side effects such as nausea and vomiting similar to that encountered with conventional activities of ^{131}I. No case of pneumonitis was seen.

Seventy three percent of all patients achieved stable disease or better : a complete response was documented in 9%, 32 % achieving a partial response and 32 % stable disease. Progressive disease occurred in 27% including 3 deaths and was more likely to occur with metastatic follicular carcinoma (Figure 3).

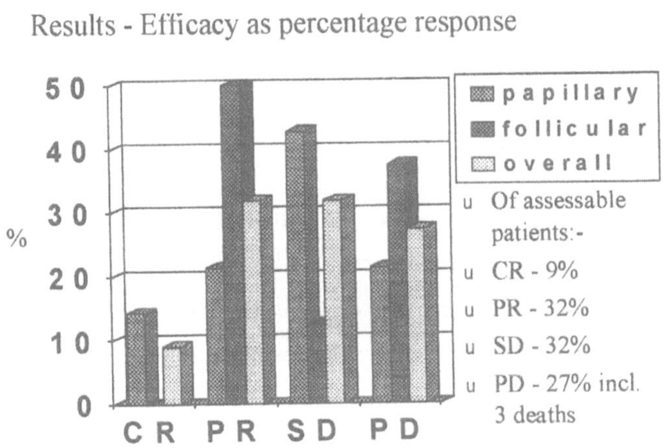

Figure 3

DISCUSSION

The majority of this series of patients were heavily pre-treated with conventional activities of radioiodine. A worthwhile response rate was seen in those patients who had failed to respond to the conventional activities. Greater side effects did occur but were manageable. It is thought that high activities of ^{131}I have the greatest potential when used early (10) and they have been advocated as an initial treatment possibly in pre-selected poor risk patients (11). Further detailed assessment of the toxicity of high activity radioiodine therapy is required particularly in regard to monitoring the haematological profile (especially around days 9 - 19 post administration and monthly thereafter), late salivary gland toxicity and the possible induction of a second malignancy. The possibility of reduced fertility in men requires further investigation with semen analysis and storage offered when appropriate. The use of laxatives and diuretics can reduce the radiation exposure of organs which excrete radioiodine (12). We expect that further dose escalation will increase the toxicity profile. The major limiting organ is the bone marrow. As in other types of high dose therapy, there may be a role for peripheral stem cell harvest and reinfusion for bone marrow rescue. Care will be required to reinfuse the cells at the most appropriate time when the residual radiation is lowest but before the nadir of the blood cell counts.

CONCLUSION

In a group of patients with a poor response to the traditional fixed activities of radioiodine we have shown that much higher activities can be given with relatively few side effects when the poor prognosis is taken into consideration. The determination of the optimum activity of ^{131}I will require more information on the dose delivered to the tumour by the administered activity. The problems of achieving reliable accurate dosimetry in this situation have yet to be solved (13).

REFERENCES

1. Vini L., Harmer C.L., McCready V.R.. Thyroid cancer: a review of treatment and follow up. Annals Nuc Med. 1996 10 : 1-7.
2. Benua R. S. et al. The relation of radioactive iodine dosimetry to results and complications in the treatment of metastatic thyroid cancer. Am J Roent Rad Ther Nucl Med 1962 ; 87 (1) : 171-182.

3. Malpani B. L., Samuel A. M., Ray S. Quantification of salivary gland function in thyroid cancer patients treated with radioiodine. Int J Radiat Oncol Biol Physics 1996 ; 35 (3) : 535-540.
4. Keldsen N. Haematological effects from radioiodine treatment of thyroid cancer. Acta Oncol 1990 ; 29 (8) : 1035-1039.
5. Grunwald F., Schomburg A., Menzel C., Steinecker S., Spath S., Bokisch A., Fimmers R., Hotze A.L., Biersack H.J. Blood count changes after radioiodine treatment in thyroid carcinoma. Med Klin 1994 ; 89 (10) : 522-528.
6. Sarkar S. D. et al. Subsequent fertility and birth history of children and adolescents treated with ^{131}I for thyroid cancer. J Nucl Med 1976 ; 17 : 460.
7. Pacini F et al. Testicular function in patients with differentiated thyroid cancer treated with radioiodine. J Nucl Med 1994 ; 35 : 1418-1422.
8. Edmonds C. J., Smith T. The long term hazards of the treatment of thyroid cancer with radioiodine. Br J Radiol 1986 ;59 :45-57.
9. Mazzaferri E.L., Young R.L. Papillary thyroid cancer : the impact of therapy in 576 patients. Medicine 1977 ; 56 : 171.
10. Maxon et al. Relation between effective radiation dose and outcome of radioiodine therapy for thyroid cancer. NEJM 1983; 309 (16) : 937-941.
11. De Groot L. J. Morbidity and mortality in follicular thyroid cancer. J Clin Endocrinol Metab 1995 ; 80 (10) : 2946-2953.
12. Seabold M. D. Diuretic enhanced radioiodine clearance after ablation therapy for differentiated thyroid cancer. Radiology 1986 ; 59 : 45-51.
13. Flower M.A., McCready V.R. Radionuclide therapy dose calculations: what accuracy can be achieved? Eur J Nucl Med 1997; 24: 1462

Radioactive Isotopes in
Clinical Medicine and Research XXIII
ed. by H. Bergmann, H. Köhn and H. Sinzinger

POSTTHERAPEUTIC CARE OF PATIENTS WITH MEDULLARY THYROID CARCINOMA – DIAGNOSTIC VALUE OF IN-VITRO-PARAMETERS AND IMAGING

J. Bredow, A. Kühne, L. Oehme, J. Kropp, and W.-G. Franke

Dept. of Nucl. Med., Univ. Hosp. Dresden, Germany

SUMMARY: In 8 of 20 patients all imaging methods failed to detect suspected recurrence or metastases in case of Medullary Thyroid Carcinoma (MTC). There is no „golden standard" of the imaging method and today no consensus exists about the radiotracer of choice and time to perform scintigraphy and/or CT/MRI.
Postoperative measurements of basal and stimulated levels of calcitonin and predisposed mutation of the RET-proto-oncogene are crucial for the diagnostic and therapeutic management and prognosis.

INTRODUCTION

The aim of this study was to determine the diagnostic value of in-vitro-parameters and different imaging methods in patients with surgically treated medullary thyroid carcinoma (MTC) in the posttherapeutic care. All the patients involved (20/30) had elevated calcitonin-levels.

MATERIALS AND METHODS

Basal calcitonin-, serum-calcium and CEA-levels were measured regularly. The RET-proto-oncogene of all patients was investigated in regard to a germ-line-mutation (hereditary MTC, MEN-II) or sporadic MTC. All patients underwent sonography (neck), ^{111}In-octreotide-scintigraphy, CT (head, neck, thorax), and MRI (neck).

In a number of patients scintigraphic studies (^{99m}Tc-MIBI, ^{99m}Tc-(V)-DMSA, ^{123}I-MIBG, ^{99m}Tc-anti-CEA-MoAB, ^{18}F-FDG-SPECT) were performed, in addition.

RESULTS

Only one hereditary form of MTC was found (proven mutation of the RET-proto-oncogene). In 8 patients all imaging methods failed to detect tumor recurrence or metastases. Sonography, especially in combination with fine needle aspiration cytology (FNAC) is supposed to be a very sensitive method to detect thyroid nodules. CT has a high sensitivity for suspect lesions in the lungs and the mediastinum; it has a lower sensitivity in the neck-shoulder area and abdomen (1). The majority of pathologic findings can be detected with MRI; a postsurgical differentiation of the tissue (scar?, recurrence?) is often not possible.

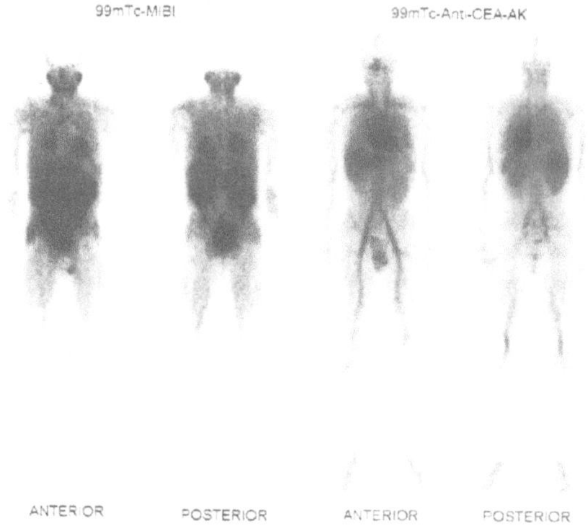

Figure 1: 46 years old man, suffering from metastatic MTC (neck, mediastinum, thorax). Whole body scintigraphy: left: the metastases show high uptake of ^{99m}Tc-MIBI right: low accumulation of ^{99m}Tc-anti-CEA-MoAB

The sensitivity of ^{111}In-octreotide-scintigraphy is found to be highly variable, depending especially on the tumor size or size of metastases. In case of „minor disease“ the sensitivity is about 33%; in case of progressive disease the sensitivity increases to 68% (2) (3). We found a pathologic accumulation of the radiotracer in 11 of 20 pts.

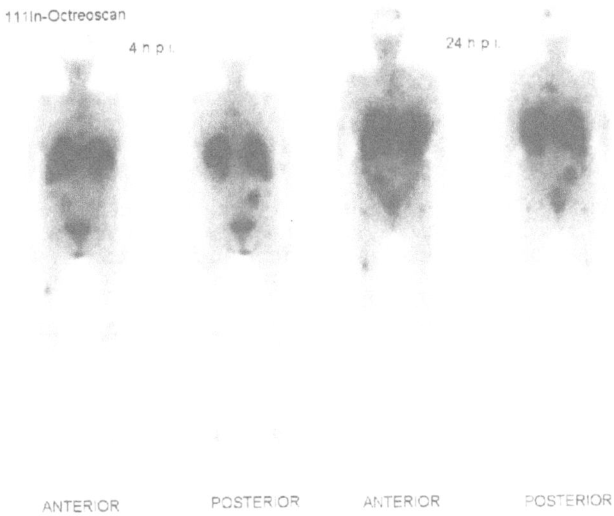

Figure 2: 58 years old woman with multiple metastases of MTC (mediastinum, lung, skeleton). Using ^{111}In--octreotide there is evidence of a high uptake in the metastases 4 h and 24 h p.i.

Using ^{99m}Tc-(V)-DMSA or ^{123}I-MIBG, a sensitivity of 95% can be obtained (depends on tumor mass). ^{99m}Tc-MIBI is widely used to detect tumors or metastases of different tissue; for MTC a sensitivity of about 47% was found by UGUR et al. (4).

If the CEA-level is also elevated and immunoscintigraphy with ^{131}I-MoAB is performed, a sensitivity of about 85% was described (5).

DISCUSSION

Our findings indicate that best results can be obtained with a combination of different radiopharmaceuticals, for example ^{111}In-Octreotide and ^{99m}Tc-(V)-DMSA. The highly variable individual time courses of the disease indicate biological differences of MTC. In some cases selective or systematic lymph node dissection could confirm malignant lymph nodes despite negative findings in all imaging methods used.

CONCLUSION

These findings indicate, that, especially in case of „minor disease", the imaging is of less sensitivity; better results can be obtained in case of progressive disease.

Until today, no consensus exists about the radiotracer of choice and time to perform scintigraphy and/or CT/MRI. Postoperative measurement of basal and stimulated levels of calcitonin and proof of a mutation in the RET-proto-oncogene are crucial for the diagnostic and therapeutic management and prognosis.

REFERENCES

1. Krausz Y., et al. Somatostatin-receptor imaging of medullary thyroid carcinoma. Clinical Nuclear Medicine 1990; 19 (5):416-21

2. Frank-Raue K, et al. Somatostatin receptor imaging in persistent medullary thyroid carcinoma. Clinical Endocrinology 1995; 42 (1):31-7

3. Esing EG, et al. Somatostatinrezeptor-szintigraphie bei medullaeren Schilddrüsenkarzinomen, GEP-Tumoren und Karzinoiden. Nuklearmedizin 1995; 34 (1):1-7

4. Ugur O, et al. Comparison of ^{99m}Tc(V)-DMSA, ^{201}Tl and ^{99m}Tc-MIBI imaging in the follow-up of patients with medullary carcinoma of the thyroid. European Journal of Nuclear Medicine 1996, 23 (10):1367-71

5. Behr T.M., et al. Improved Detection and Therapy of occult and metastatic Medullary Thyroid Cancer with radiolabeled anti-carcinoembryonic-antigen antibodies and peptides. oral presentation at ETA 1997, Munich

Radioactive Isotopes in
Clinical Medicine and Research XXIII
ed. by H. Bergmann, H. Köhn and H. Sinzinger

IMPROVED NEGATIVE PREDICTIVE VALUE OF MAMMOSCINTIGRAPHY IN PATIENTS WITH BREAST CANCER BY MEANS OF A „MALIGNANCY INDEX"

Mirzaei S.[1], Knoll P.[1], Bastati B.[1], Mirna A.[2], Salzer H.[2], Köhn H.[1]
[1]Institute of Nuclear Medicine, [2]Department of Gynecology and Obstetrics, Wilhelminenspital Vienna, Austria

Summary: Although mammoscintigraphy has a higher specificity than mammography, in praxis a negative mammoscintigraphy does not preclude (frequently unnecessary) biopsy. To further improve the negative predictive value of mammoscintigraphy, we calculated a "mamma malignancy index" (MMI) taking into account the results of mammoscintigraphy (MS), mammography (M) and mammo-sonography (S), respectively. The respective results of these modalities were scored from 0 to 2 (0=negative; 1=indeterminate; 2=positive). A MMI was calculated by simply adding the respective scores of each investigation. The study comprised 64 prospectively studied patients with suspect lesions in the breast. M, S and MS were performed in each patient within 4 weeks of excisional biopsy. Our preliminary results suggest that a malignancy index seems to have a high negative predictive value (100%) for patients with MMI of < 2.

Introduction:

Technetium-99m methoxyisobutylisonitrile (MIBI), 99mTc-Tetrofosmin were introduced for myocardial imaging, but found additional applications as they taken up by different tumours, enabling imaging of these lesions in patients [1,2]. Recent publications, have reported favourable sensitivity and specificity results, 84%-96% and 72%-94%, respectively, for Tc-99m-sestamibi scintigraphy in the diagnosis of breast cancer [1,4-7]. The major goal of this study was to find a key indicator for the open biopsy of suspect lesions in the breast in order to reduce the number of unnecessary biopsies.

Materials and methods:

64 consecutive patients (mean age 51 y, range 21-82 y) with suspicious palpation and/or mamographic findings were investigated. 10 min. after i.v. injection of 555 MBq Tc-99m MIBI planar prone imaging (256x256 matrix; LEUHR collimator) in anterior-posterior and lateral projections using a high resolution double head gamma camera (Elscint Helix HR, Haifa) was performed . Afterwards SPECT was performed in supine position (64x64 matrix, 6°/step, 20 sec/step, 180° / head, LEUHR collimator). Scintimammography was evaluated by two experienced nuclear medicine physicians blinded to the history of the patient.

Results:

In all of the patients a final histological diagnosis by open biopsy was established. Tc-99m scintimammography was negative in 40 (38 true negative, 2 false negative) and positive in 24 (18 true positive, 6 false positive) cases. The tumour size ranged from 6 to 35 mm in diameter, while the smallest lesion detected by scintimammography was 9 mm in diameter. Three out of the six false positive cases were inflammatory infiltrated. The two wrong negative cases were multicentric intraductal cancer , and a high differentiated neuroendocrin tumour of a carcinoid type. The other histopathologic findings in patients with malignancy were as follows: 9 ductal, 6 lobular, 1 mucinous and 2 ductal carcinoma in situ.

Discussion:

Routine breast self examination, physical examination and mammography are despite their diagnostic limitations still the most common methods of early cancer detection. Due to its high sensitivity and availability, mammography is the method of choice in screening of asymptomatic woman [10-13]. However, mammography has major problems in additional assessment of patients with dense breast tissue, unclear microcalcifications and in differentiating between scar and recurrency [10,11]. In women with dense breasts, mammography has a false negative rate of 25%-45% accordingly to several studies [14,15]. Ultrasonography has very good ability to differentiate between cystic and solid masses, but its sensitivity for the detection of small carcinomas is not high. Its ideal use is in young women with full glandular breasts, owing to their intrinsic radiopacity, while it can also be used for guidance in obtaining aspiration material for cytology [16].

A few paper in the literature discuss the superior role of SMM in the preoperative diagnostic of breast cancer in reducing unnecessary biopsies, because of the high sensitivity and specificity of this test [4-6,18-21]. Up to now, however, there is no report of a criterion or investigation, which could recognise a lesion as benign and make the biopsy unnecessary.

We defined the following formula retrospectively and therefore categorised the patients in seven different groups: [Mamma-Malignancy-Index (MMI)] = [MM-Factor] + [MMS-Factor] + [SMM-Factor]. Each factor can obtain a value of 0, 1 or 2 as followed:

MM-F / MMS-F was: a) "0" if the investigation yielded a normal or a benign lesion; b) "1", if MM / MMS yielded a probably benign lesion, but biopsy was recommended (indeterminate); c) "2", if MM / MMS yielded a malign lesion or suspect microcalcifications.

The [SMM-F] was: a) "0", in case of negative SMM; b) "1" , in case of an indeterminate finding in SPECT or in planar images, in other words in case of a probably positive finding c) "2", if a pathological uptake was diagnosed in SPECT and/or planar images.

In this study there were 16 cases with MMI of 0 (table 1), 18 cases with MMI of 1, while in these cases no malignancy was diagnosed after biopsy (n= 34). In other mean the biopsy in these patients, 53% of the whole collective, was not necessary. Breast cancer was confirmed by histopathology in 20 patients with a MMI of 2 or more (n=30). The tumour size ranged from 6 to 35 mm in diameter, while the smallest verified tumour by SMM was 9 mm in diameter. The overall sensitivity and specificity of SMM for diagnosing breast cancer were 90% and 86%, respectively.

Table 1

MMI	0	1	2	3	4	5	6
cases	16	18	16	7	2	2	3
malignancy rate	0	0	7	6	2	2	3

MMI = Mamma Malignancy Index

We believe, that the mamma-malignancy-index (MMI), as defined above, is a criterion with a high negative predictive value for the patients with a score of 0 or 1 (in this study of 100%) and these patients should not be routinely reffered for biopsy but rather could be observed and undergo a follow-up. The prevalence of the malignancy raises in this study nearly linear with the MMI and reaches a plateau by MMI of 4 (diagram 1).

Diagramm 1

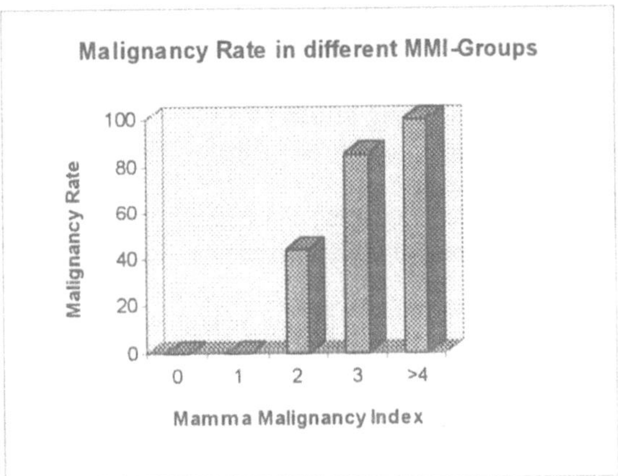

MMI = Mammamalignancy Index

References:

1) Burak Z, Argon M, Memis A, Erdem S, Balkan Z, Duman Y, Ustun EE, Erhan Y, Ozzkilic H. Evaluation of palpable breast masses with 99m Tc-MIBI: a comparative study with mammography and ultrasonography. Ncl Med Commun 1994; 15: 604-612.
2) Mansi L, Rambaldi PF, La Provitera A, Di Gregorio F, Procaccini E. Tc-99m tetrofosmin uptake in breast tumours. J Nucl Med 1995; 36: 83P.
3) Müller S, Guth-Tougelides B, Creutzig H. Imaging of malignant tumours with Tc-99-m-MIBI [abstract]. J Nucl Med 1987; 28; 562.
4) Khalkhali I, Mena I, Jouanne E et al. Prone scintimammography in patients with suspicion of breast cancer. J Am Coll Surg 1994; 178: 491-497.
5) Palmedo H, Grünwald F, Bender H, et al. Scintimammography with technetium-99m methoxyisobutrylisonitril: comparison with mammography and magnetic resonance imaging. Eur J Nucl Med 1996; 23:940-946.
6) Lind P., Umschaden H., Forsthuber, et al. Scintimammography using Tc-99m Tetrofosmin. Acta Med. Austriaca; 1997; 2:50-54.
7) Tiling R, Sommer H, Pechmann M, et al. Comparison of Technetium-99m-Sestamibi Scintimammography with Contrast-Enhanced MRI for Diagnosis of Breast Lesions. J Nucl Med 1997; 38: 58-62.
8) Wingo PA, Tong T, Bolden S: Cancer statistics 1995. CA Cancer J Clin 1995; 45: 8-30.
9) Miller BA, Feuer FJ, Hankey BF: The increasing incidence of breast cancer since 1982; relevance of early detection. Cancer Causes Control 1991; 2: 67-74.
10) Bird RE, Wallace TW, Yankanskas BC. Analysis of cancer missed at the screening mammography. Radiology 1992; 184:613-617.
11) Jackson VP, Hendrick RE, Kerg SA, et al. Imaging of the radiographically dense breast. Radiology 1993; 198: 297-301.
12) Kopans DB. Positive predictive value of mamography. Am J Roentgenol 1992; 158: 521-526.
13) Humphry LL, Ballard DJ. Early detection of breast cancer in women. Prev Pract 1989; 16: 115-132.
14) Niloff PH, Sheiner NM; False negative mammograms in patients with breast cancer. Can J Surg 1981; 24: 50-52
15) Pollei SR, Mettler FA, Barstow SA, Moradian G, Moskowita M: Occult breast cancer: Prevalence and radiographic detectability. Radiology 1987; 163: 459-462.
16) Teubner J. Echomammography: technique and results. In: Friedrich M, Sickels EA, eds. Radiological diagnosis of breast diseases. Berlin Heidelberg New York: Springer; 1997: 181-220.
17) Jacob D, Brombart J, Muller C, et al. Analysis of the results of 137 subclinical breast lesions. Value of ultrasonography in the early diagnosis of breast cancer. J Gynecol Obstet Biol Reprod 1997; 26: 27-31
18) Khalkhali I, Cutrone J, Mena I, et al. Scintimammography: the complementary role of 99mTc-sestamibi prone breast imaging for the diagnosis of breast carcinoma. Radiology 1995; 196: 421-426.
19) Khalkhali I, Cutrone J, Mena I, et al. Technetium-99m-sestamibi scintimammography of breast lesions: clinical and pathological follow-up. J Nucl Med 1995; 36: 1784-1789.
20) Goldenberg DM, Larson SM: Radioimmundetection in cancer identification. J Nucl Med 1992; 33: 803-814.
21) Clifford E, Lugo-Zamudio C. Scinitimammography in the diagnosis of breast cancer. Am J Surg 1996; 172: 483-486.

Radioactive Isotopes in
Clinical Medicine and Research XXIII
ed. by H. Bergmann, H. Köhn and H. Sinzinger

QUANTITATIVE Tc-99m TETROFOSMIN SCINTIGRAPHY IN THE DIFFERENTIATION OF MALIGNANT FROM BENIGN BREAST MASSES

Erhan Varoglu, Yasemin Akin, Müfide N.Akcay, Ali Sahin, Fatih Akcay, Önder Özcan.
Ataturk University, Medical School, Depts. of Nuclear Medicine, General Surgery, and Biochemistry
Erzurum-Turkey

SUMMARY

The aim of this study was to evaluate the diagnostic value of Tc-99m tetrofosmin scintigraphy in the differentiation of malignant from benign breast lesions. Total twenty-five patients (20 malignant and 5 benign) were studied. The sens. and the spesif. of tetrofosmin scintigraphy were 85 % and 80 %, respectively. Quantitative evaluation showed that the tetrofosmin uptake of malign lesion was greater than benigns, and benign lesions have rapid tetrofosmin washout than malignant ones. Our results indicated that tetrofosmin scintigraphy might have an important role in the differentiation of malignant from benign breast masses.

INTRODUCTION

Several radiotracers including Ga-67 citrate, Tl-201 chloride, Tc-99m MDP and Tc-99m sestamibi have been widely used in an attempt to help discriminate benign from malignant breast lesions (1,2). Tc-99m tetrofosmin, a myocardial imaging agent, has also been used to detect various malignant tumors and to distinguish malign from benign breast lesions as well (3-5). This study was designed to differentiate malignant from benign breast lesions and to show their lymph node metastasis with Tc-99m tetrofosmin scintigraphy.

MATERIALS AND METHODS

Twenty-five patients (20 malignant and 5 benign lesions) were included in this study. Mean ages of patients with malignant and benign breast masses were 51.9 ± 10.8 and 35.5 ± 9.4 years, respectively. All patients with breast masses were evaluated with mammography and ultrasonography. In histopathologic examination, 14 invasive ductal, 2 intraductal, 2 lobular, 1 medullary and 1 mixed carcinoma cases were identified. Mean diameters of malignant lesions were 4.6 ± 1.2 cm. Histopathologic results of benign lesions were fibrocystic disease (3), adenoma (1), and mastitis (1). After radiologic examination, Tc-99m tetrofosmin sintigraphy was performed. Twenty-five mCi of Tc-99m tetrofosmin was injected intravenously to the patients' opposite site of the palpable breast mass. After 15. and 180. minutes of injection, planar breast images for 10 minutes were acquired. Anterior, right and left lateral and oblique images were obtained at the sitting position. A large field of view gama camera peaked to 140 keV with a 15 % energy window with a low-energy, parallel-hole collimator was used for image acqusition. All images were interpreted by two nuclear medicine physician without knowledge of the pathologic results. Visual interpretation was performed with the grading of Tc-99m tetrofosmin uptake, the activity was scored from 0 to 4. Two different methods were used for quantitative evaluation. The first was quantitative Tc-99m tetrofosmin uptake and the second was washout method. A free region of interest (ROI) was drawn on the breast lesions and the contralateral background area, and the mean counts of these ROI's were used for calculating lesion to background ratio (quantitative tetrofosmin uptake) and washout rate. Lesion to background ratios of early (15. min) and delay (3.hour) images, and the washout rates of tetrofosmin with time were used for identifying malign from benign lesions. The Tc-99m tetrofosmin uptake and washout ratios of histopathologic tumor types were also compared.

The results of visual scintigraphic interpretation were used to calculate sensitivity and spesificity of tetrofosmin scintigraphy with comparing scintigraphic results to histopathologic results. The quantitative Tc-99m tetrofosmin uptakes and washout ratios of malign and benign breast lesions were compared using Mann-Whitney U teset. The Kruskall Wallis analysis was used to compare the tetrofosmin uptake and wash-out ratios of different tumor types.

RESULTS

Seventeen of 20 patients with malign breast lesions had pathologic Tc-99m tetrofosmin accumulation on the lesion area and 3 had no pathologic accumulation. The histopathologic results of these 3 patients without tetrofosmin accumulation were intraductal carcinoma (2 pts) and lobular carcinoma (1 pt). Mammographic findings of those patients were compatible with malignant lesion similar to the remaining 17 patients. Palpable axillary lymph node metastasis were found in 7 of 20 patients with malign breast masses. Only 4 of 7 lymph node metastasis were detected with tetrofosmin scintigraphy. The scintigraphic images of patients with pathologically proven medullary carcinoma were shown in Figure 1.

Figure 1: Anterior (A) and right oblique (B) images of a patient with medullary carcinoma of breast showed increased Tc-99m tetrofosmin accumulation in the right breast and the right axillary region.

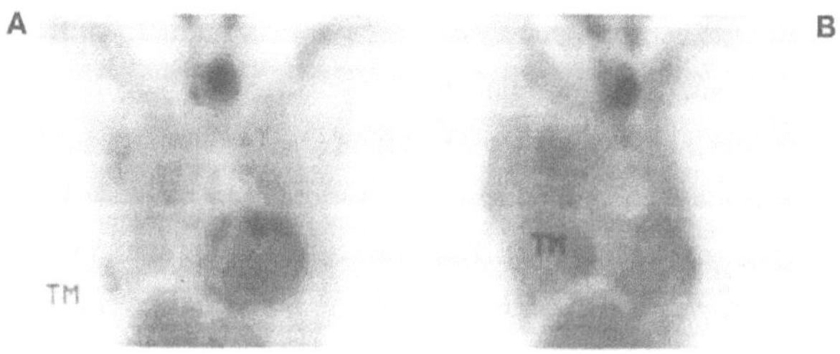

Only one of 5 patients with benign breast lesions showed Tc-99m tetrofosmin accumulation and the histopatologic result was mastitis. The sensitivity and the specificity of the Tc-99m tetrofosmin scintigraphy were calculated as 85% and 80%, respectively. There was higher tetrofosmin accumulation in the malignant breast masses than benign lesions in terms of visual scorring system.

In the quantitative evaluation; the tetrofosmin uptake and washout ratios of malign and bening lesions were calculated in early and late phases. The quantitative uptake ratios of malignant lesions were significantly greater than benign lesions at the 15.min ($p<0.001$) and 3.h ($p<0.001$), (2.10±0.85*, 3.63±1.25**) and (0.99±0.04*, 0.99±0.182**), The benign lesions had higher Tc-99m tetrofosmin washout ratios (41.2 ± 6.0) than those of malignant lesions (20.3 ±14.8), ($p<0.001$) There were no significant difference between the different tumor types with respect to the quantitative tetrofosmin uptake and washout ratios.

DISCUSSION

Several radionuclide imaging approaches have been proposed for detecting breast cancer and differantiating malignant and benign breast masses. Presently, two of these techniques have been more extensively applied in humans: Tl-201 and Tc-99m sestamibi images. F-18 FDG PET has also been used for imaging breast tumors and their metastatic spread (6). Nowadays, Tc-99m tetrofosmin has also been started to use for evaluating breast masses and differentiating malignant and benign breast tumours as well as other techniques (7).

Various studies performed with Tc-99m sestamibi were shown that scintimammography had a great importance for detection malignant breast lesion. Burak et al. reported that the sensitivity and the specificty of scintimammography were 93 and 86 % (2). These results are greater than our results, 85 and 80 %. The investigators used a visual scorring system to evaluate malignant and benign lesions and they found higher visual uptake score in the malignant lesion. We also showed that the malignant lesions had more prominent tetrofosmin uptake in the visual interpretation scorring. In addition to visual interpretation, we used quantitative tetrofosmin uptake and washout rates to eliminate inter-observer variability. The quantitative tetrofosmin uptake ratios of malignant breast lesions was significantly higher than benigns and the benign lesions had more rapid tetrofosmin washout than malignant lesions.

Although the mammography, a sceening test for diagnosis of breast cancer, has very high sensitivity (100 %), it has relatively poor sfecificity (30-75 %) and positive predictive value to identify malignancy in the breast lesions because only the 20 to 23 % of patiens having suspected malignancy with mammography have breast carcinoma in histopathologic examination. Furthermore, 25 % of women, especially in the younger, have increased breast density which influences accuracy of the results of mammography (8). Therefore, a sensitive and noninvasive method should be introduced to help clinician for identifying malignant from benign lesion and to guide for selecting patient who needs biopsy and histopathologic examination. Our data sugessted that tetrofosmin scintigraphy seems to be a suitable diagnostic technique for this purpose and additional studies are needed to be done to assess diagnostic accuracy of tetrofosmin scintigrapy, and to determine the possibility of tetrofosmin scintigraphy for using as a diagnostic test in the pre treatment evaluation of patients with palpable breast masses.

In conclusion, we showed that Tc-99m tetrofosmin was non-invasive and easy to perform scintigraphic method with high sensitivity and specificity in the differentiation of malignant from benign breast lesions. Furthermore, it should be used to complement the use of anatomical imaging techniques of the breast and may be of value in patients where mammography is difficult or non diagnostic.

REFERENCES

1-Waxman AD, Ramanna, Mensic L et al. Thallium scintigraphy in the evaluation of mass abnormalities of the breast. J Nucl Med 1993; 34:18-23.

2-Burak Z, Argon M, Memiß A et al. Evaluation of palpable breast masses with Tc-99m MIBI: a comparative study with mammography and ultrasonography. Nucl Med Comm 1994; 604-612.

3-BaßoÛlu T, Þahin M, Coßkun C et al. Tc-99m tetrofosmin scintigraphy in malignant lung tumours. Eur J Nucl Med 1995; 687-689.

4-Ak□ay G, Uslu H, VaroÛlu E et al. Assessment of thyroid nodules by technetium 99m tetrofosmin scintigraphy. Br J Clin Pract 1997; 51: 5-7.

5-Rambaldi PF, Mansi L, Procaccini E et al. Breast cancer detection with Tc-99m tetrofosmin. Clin Nucl Med 1995; 20: 703-705.

6-Adler LP, Crowe JP, Al-Kaisi NK et al. Evaluation of breast masses and axillary lymph nodes with (F-18)2-deoxy-2-fluoro-d-glucose PET. Radiol 1993; 187: 743-750.

7-Batista JF, Solano ME, Oliva JP et al. Usefulness of Tc-99m tetrofosmin scintimammography in palpable breast tumours. Nucl Med Comm 1997; 18: 338-340

8- Khalkali I, Cutrone J, Mena I et al. Technetium-99m sestamibi scintimammography of breast lesions: clinical and pathological follow up. J Nucl Med 1995; 36: 1784-1789.

Radioactive Isotopes in
Clinical Medicine and Research XXIII
ed. by H. Bergmann, H. Köhn and H. Sinzinger

THE RELATIONSHIP BETWEEN PROLIFERATION AND DEOXYGLUCOSE UPTAKE BY BREAST TUMOUR CELLS

T.A.D. Smith, J.C. Titley and V.R. McCready

Departments of Nuclear Medicine and Cell and Experimental Pathology, The Royal Marsden NHS Trust and Institute of Cancer Research, Sutton, Surrey SM2 5PT UK

SUMMARY: Proliferative index (S-phase fraction) and the uptake of 2-Deoxy-D-[1-^{3}H]glucose (^{3}H-DG) by logarithmic MCF7 and T47D breast tumour cells was measured when cells were grown in the presence of serum and 24 hours after serum-deprivation. Removal of serum from early log phase cells was associated with a decrease in both S-phase and the uptake of ^{3}H-DG compared with cells maintained in the presence of serum. As cells progressed through log phase growth the effect of serum-deprivation on S-phase fraction was less pronounced. No significant change in the uptake of ^{3}H-DG between serum deprived and serum maintained cells in late log phase.

INTRODUCTION

The use of 2-deoxy-D-glucose labelled with ^{18}F (FDG) in combination with PET, exploiting enhanced glycolysis by tumours (1), has been shown to be useful in the detection of many different tumour types (reviewed in 2). Serial quantitative FDG-PET scanning studies (3,4) suggest that therapeutic responsiveness may be detected using this technique. The clinical role of PET-FDG in differencial diagnosis and therapeutic response will depend on which feature of malignancy is most related to its uptake. Some in-vivo studies (5,6), though not all (7,8), have observed strong correlations between DG uptake and proliferative indices. In the present study the effect of removing serum for 24 hours from log phase MCF7 and T47D breast tumour cells at various time points after seeding in tissue culture has been examined. S-phase fraction (Spf) was determined as a measure of proliferation. We present evidence suggesting that DG uptake, in some situations, reflects proliferative status.

MATERIALS AND METHODS

Cells and treatment: MCF7 and T47D cell lines were grown in Dulbecco's MEM containing 4.5 mM glucose (Gibco, UK), 10% foetal bovine serum (Sigma Chemical Co, UK) and penicillin /streptomycin. Trypsinized cells from confluent populations were (about 3 x $10^{5)}$ were seeded in 25 cm^3 tissue culture flasks (Nunc, UK) in 3ml of complete medium and maintained at 37°C in 5%Co_2:95% air. Between 2 and 8 days later, medium was removed from each of 3 flasks, replaced with unsupplemented medium and incubated for a further 24 hours. Incorporation of ^{3}H-DG was determined in cells grown in serum-supplemented and after 24 hours in unsupplemented medium.

Determination of ^{3}H-DG incorporation: Medium replaced in each flask prior to determination of ^{3}H-DG incorporation. After 1 hour 128 KBq of 2-Deoxy-D-[1-^{3}H]glucose (^{3}H-DG) (326 Gbq/mmol, 37 Mbq/ml) was added to each flask and incubated at 37°C for 30 min. Medium then poured off and flasks washed 5 times with PBS. Cells then trypsinized and after neutralizing the trypsin with 1 ml of complete medium, were dissagreggated by aspirating the suspension up and down a 1 ml pipette tip. ^{3}H-DG uptake (disintegrations/minute (D/M) determined in aliquots in a beta-counter. A further 0.5 ml sample of cell suspension was centrifuged at 400g for 10 min and after removing supernatant the cells were resuspended in 200 µl of PBS. After addition of 0.7 ml of ice cold ethanol the fixed cells were stored at 4°C for determination of Spf using cell cycle analysis. Viable cell numbers were determined on 100 µl aliquots of the cell suspension.

RESULTS

S-phase fraction: In 24 hour serum deprived samples (S-) was 49% and 39% lower on days 3 ($p<0.005$) and 4 ($p<0.005$) when compared with serum-maintained cultures (S+) (see table). On day 5 the difference in Spf between serum-maintained and 24 hour serum deprived T47D was not significant. On day 9 serum-deprived cells were found to have a significantly higher Spf than serum-maintained cells although this difference was marginally statistically significant ($p<0.05$). Removal of serum for 24 hours from MCF7 cells resulted in 38% and 50% lower Spf on days 4 ($p< 0.05$)and 6 ($p< 0.005$). On day 8 the difference in Spf between serum maintained and 24 hour deprived cultures was not significant.

Table: Mean ±SD Spf and ^{3}H-DG uptake (D/M) in presence (S+) and absence (S-) of serum

Cell type	T47D				MCF7		
Day	3	4	5	9	4	6	8
Spf (S+)	29±2.2	29±2	28±2.9	27±2.4	32±3.5	32±1.6	18±0.8
Spf (S-)	18±1.1	20±2.4	24±4.2	33±2.8	21±2.0	19±2	15±2.0
D/M (S+)	13.6±1	12.9±1.3	13.1±3.3	11.2±0.5	8.2±6.5	6.5±0.2	6.9±0.1
D/M (S-)	9.7±1.6	9.4±1.0	10.4±1.6	10.9±0.4	4.5±5.0	4.1±0.5	6.0±0.4

Uptake of ^{3}H-DG: The uptake of ^{3}H-DG per 10^3 viable cells is shown in the table. ^{3}H-DG uptake by T47D cells was significantly lower in serum-deprived cells compared with serum-maintained cultures on days 3 ($p<0.005$) and 4 ($p<0.005$) i.e. when there was a large difference in S-phase fraction between serum-starved and serum-maintained cultures. The difference in ^{3}H-DG uptake between serum-maintained and 24 hour serum-deprived T47D cultures was not significant on days 5 and 9. The uptake of ^{3}H-DG per viable cell is significantly lower in 24 hour serum deprived MCF7 cells compared with serum-maintained cells on days 4 and 6 but not on day 8 again paralleling changes in proliferative index.

DISCUSSION

Depriving early log phase MCF7 and T47D cells of serum resulted in a decrease in proliferative fraction and in the uptake of ^{3}H-DG. Removal of serum from late log phase cells, however was found not to produce a significant change in either Spf or deoxyglucose uptake. These findings suggest that changes in the uptake of DG correlates with changes in cell cycle distribution after certain anti-proliferative treatments. Serum contains a variety of growth factors, some of which interact with receptors associated with protein kinase C (PKC) activation. Treatment of cells with oncogenes associated with phosphatidylinositol turnover and hence activation of PKC, such as src and ras oncogenes, cause large increases in the uptake of DG (9). Similarly, treatment of rat 3T3 fibroblasts with TPA which also activates PKC increases the uptake of DG (9). Thus changes in DG uptake and proliferation induced by serum deprivation may be mediated via the effect of down regulation of PKC. Proliferative changes induced by anticancer therapies that act by interfering with growth factor stimulation, which represents the basis of a number of biological therapies (10) may therefore be detectable by monitoring DG uptake.

REFERENCES

1. Wienhouse S. The Warburg hypothesis fifty years later (guest editorial). Z Krebsforsch. 1976; 87:115-126

2. Strauss LG and Conti PS. The applications of PET in clinical oncology. J Nucl Med 1991; 32:623-648

3. Hoekstra OS, Ossenkoppele GJ, Golding R. Early treatment response in malignant lymphoma, as determined by planar fluorine-18-fluorodeoxyglucose scintigraphy. J Nucl. Med 1993; 34:1706-1710

4. Wahl RL, Zasadny KR, Hutchins GD, Weber M, Cody R. Metabolic monitoring of breast cancer chemohormonotherapy using positron emission tomography (PET): initial evaluation. J Clin Oncol 1993; 11:2101-2111

5. Watanabe A, Tanaka R, Takeda N, Washiyama K. DNA synthesis, blood flow, and glucose utilization in experimental rat tumors. J Neurosurg. 1989; 70:86-91

6. Minn H, Joensuu H, Ahonen A, Klemi P. Fluorodeoxyglucose imaging:a method to assess the proliferative activity of human cancer in vivo. Cancer 1988; 61:1776-1781

7. Haberkorn U, Ziegler SI, Oberdorfer F, et al. FDG uptake, tumor proliferation and expression of gltcolysis associated genes in animal tumor models. Nucl Med Biol 1994; 21:827-834

8. Brown RS, Leung JY, Fisher SJ, Frey KA, Ethier SP and Wahl RL. Intratumoral distribution of tritiated fluorodeoxyglucose in breast carcinoma: I, are inflammatory cells important? J Nucl Med 1995; 36:1854-1861

9.Flier JS, Mueckler MM, Usher P, et al. Elevated levels of glucose transport and transporter messenger RNA are induced by ras and src oncogenes. Science 1987; 235:1492-1495

10. Langton SP and Smyth JF. Inhibition of cell signalling pathways. Cancer Treatment Rev 1995; 21:65-89

Radioactive Isotopes in
Clinical Medicine and Research XXIII
ed. by H. Bergmann, H. Köhn and H. Sinzinger

POTENTIAL ROLE OF WHOLE-BODY ^{18}FDG-PET IN THE ROUTINE STAGING OF MALIGNANT MELANOMA

Bender H[1], Frohmann, JP[2], Grapow M[1], Schomburg A[1], Biersack H.-J[1].

Departments of [1]Nuclear Medicine and [2]Dermatology;
University of Bonn, Germany.

SUMMARY: In order to evaluate the clinical importance of positron-emission tomography, intermediate and high-risk melanoma patients (n=96) were enrolled for routine staging. Lesions with intense FDG-uptake proved to be predominantly malignant tissue, with a sensitivity and specificity of 97% and 96%. In contrast, lesions with moderate uptake, were mostly non-malignant processes (positive predictive value 37%). FDG-PET proved to be more sensitive mainly in lymph node assessment as compared to CT/MRI.

INTRODUCTION

Several studies have demonstrated that melanoma show a high rate of fluoro-18-deoxyglucose (FDG) uptake (1,2). Clinical studies have shown promising results suggesting a benefit of FDG-PET in the staging of melanoma patients under study conditions (3-5). The aims of our prospective, ongoing study are (a) to assess the feasibility of FDG-PET as part of available staging modalities in intermediate- and high-risk melanoma patients, and (b) to evaluate its diagnostic accuracy as compared to routinely used staging methods

PATIENTS, MATERIALS and METHODS

Patients were prospectively enrolled a few days after surgical tumor resection and histological confirmation. High-risk patients were defined as cutaneous melanoma having a penetration level according to Clark level >II and/or a tumor-thickness according to Breslow >0.75 mm). Tumor staging included physical examination, ultrasound of lymph node groups and abdomen, CT head, thorax and abdomen, MRI (selected areas), bone scintigraphy and immunoscintigraphy.

Patients fasted overnight (12-18 hrs), but were allowed to drink sugar-free liquids ad libitum. Blood-sugar was monitored prior to FDG-injection and was usually ^{2}130 mg%, with few exceptions.

PET-studies were performed on an ECAT Exact 921/47 scanner (Siemens/CTI) and consisted of a body-trunk (5-7 bed positions) transmission scan (7-10 min. per bed position), followed by an emission scan (10 min./bed position), 45-60 min. after injection of 185-300 MBq FDG. FDG was commercially obtained from the Nuclear Research Centers Karlsruhe (Germany) or Jülich (Germany). Tomograms were reconstructed by filtered-backprojection and attenuation-corrected based on the measured transmission matrix. FDG-uptake was qualitatively evaluated by a 4-point scoring system: FDG-uptake (1) intense (>>liver) = malignancy-typical; (2) moderate (>liver) = malignancy-suspect; (3) minimal (^{2}liver) = unspecific; (4) none (=background) = no-evidence of disease. All lesions with moderate or high FDG-uptake were verified by CT/MRI, histology and/or clinical follow-up (3-monthly intervals, including complete physical examination, ultrasound and/or CT/MRI). Primary image assessment (PET, CT/MRI etc.) was done without knowledge of the respective findings of the other modalities. The final institutional diagnosis was used as gold-standard.

RESULTS

A total of 96 patients have been evaluated, 39 females and 57 males with a mean age of 58 years (range 18-90 years.). Histology showed nodular (n=19), superficial-spreading (n=42), amelanotic (n=5) and various other melanoma types (n=30). No melanoma manifestation was found in 50 patients and confirmed by clinical follow-up of at least 6 months. In 46 patients, a total of 214 focal areas with enhanced FDG-trapping were identified. Multiple areas at the same site e.g. axilla were counted as 1 lesion and 8 lymph node regions per patient were assessed (neck 2x, axilla 2x, thorax/mediastine 1x, abdomen 1x, and inguinal 2x). In 72 lesions intense, in 57 moderate and in 85 minimal glucose-utilization was observed, respectively. Overall, sensitivity, specificity and accuracy ranged from 89-100%, 60-97%, and 90-99%, respectively.

Primary assessment of our data indicated a high sensitivity but an unacceptable rate of false-positive findings, with a positive predictive value (PPV) of approximately 68%. A further analyses, comparing the diagnostic safety of lesions with intense versus moderate FDG-utake significantly improved the results (Table 1).

Our data clearly demonstrate, that lesions with high FDG-utilization are indicative of a malignant process, demonstrating a positive predictive value of 92% and a negative predictive value (NPV) of 99%. In contrast, lesions with moderate uptake seem to be mostly non-malignant processes

(PPV 12%, NPV 98%). Further analyses are currently performed, in order to improve the differentiation of malignant versus non-malignant processes in moderately accumulating lesions, were 7/57 (12%) were confirmed melanoma sites.

Table 2: Diagnostic safety as a function of FDG-uptake: Intense (n = 72/214) versus moderate (n=57/146) glucose-utilization in 46 patients.

FDG-uptake	TP	FP	TN	FN	Sens.	Spec.	Acc.
Intense	66	6	138	2	97	96	96
Moderate	7	50	87	2	78	64	64

TP:true positive; **FP**:false positive; **TN**:true negative; **FN**:false negative; **Sens.**:sensitivity; **Spec.**:specificity; **Acc.**:accuracy

When the PET-results were directly compared with CT/MRI, overall, FDG-PET was distinctly more sensitive (82% vs. 74%) and accurate (90% vs. 89%) and most beneficial in the evaluation of lymph node involvement (PET vs. CT: sensitivity 81% vs. 62% and accuracy 96% vs. 93%).

DISCUSSION

We have studied melanoma patients for primary tumor staging employing FDG-PET under clinical routine conditions. Qualitative image assessment (hot-spot imaging) allowed the grading of glucose-utilization (intense, moderate, minimal, none) in reference to normal organs (mediastine and liver). Our data clearly demonstrate, that malignant involvement is associated with intense FDG-accumulation, in contrast to lesions with moderate uptake. Various groups have previously reported, that FDG-PET is a sensitive and accurate method in the staging of melanoma patients under study conditions (3-7). Our results substantiate these findings and suggest the feasibility also in the clinical routine.

Direct comparison of FDG-PET with conventional imaging (CT/MRI) underscores the utility of FDG-PET and its advantage in the assessment of lymph-node involvement, including normal-sized nodes. These findings are in accordance with previous reports (5,7,9), indicating a detection limit of malignant processes of around 3-5 mm (7, 9). This underscores the potential of FDG-PET in the evaluation of normal-sized lymph-nodes (5).

CONCLUSIONS

Melanoma show regularly intense FDG-utilization, thus allowing the identification also of small lesions. The introduction of a rigid scoring system for image evaluation, improves the predictive values and accuracy of interpretation and allows application in the clinical routine. FDG-PET is suitable for the primary staging of intermediate- and high-risk melanoma patients (Breslow >0.75 mm and Clark >II) and suspicious findings should be complemented by ultrasound and/or CT/MRI.

REFERENCES

1. Kern KA. [14C]deoxyglucose uptake and imaging in malignant melanoma. J. Surg. Res. 1991, 50: 643-7

2. Wahl RL, Hutchins GD, Buchsbaum DJ, Liebert M, Grossman HB, Fisher S 18F-2-deoxy-2-fluoro-D-glucose uptake into human tumor xenografts. Feasibility studies for cancer imaging with positron-emission tomography. Cancer. 1991, 67: 1544-50

3. Damian DL, Fulham MJ, Thompson E, Thompson JF Positron emission tomography in the detection and management of metastatic melanoma. Melanoma Res. 1996, 6: 325-9

4. Valk PE, Pounds TR, Tesar RD, Hopkins DM, Haseman MK Cost-effectiveness of PET imaging in clinical oncology. Nucl. Med. Biol. 1996, 23: 737-43

5. Wagner JD, Schauwecker D, Hutchins G, Coleman JJ,3rd. Initial assessment of positron emission tomography for detection of nonpalpable regional lymphatic metastases in melanoma. J. Surg. Oncol. 1997, 64: 181-9

6. Modorati G, Lucignani G, Landoni C, Freschi M, Trabucchi G, Fazio F, Brancato R Glucose metabolism and pathological findings in uveal melanoma: preliminary results. Nucl. Med. Commun. 1996, 17: 1052-6

7. Steinert HC, Huch Boni RA, Buck A, Boni R, Berthold T, Marincek B, Burg G, von Schulthess GK Malignant melanoma: staging with whole-body positron emission tomography and 2-[F-18]-fluoro-2-deoxy-D-glucose. Radiology. 1995, 195: 705-9

8. Gritters LS, Francis IR, Zasadny KR, Wahl RL Initial assessment of positron emission tomography using 2-fluorine-18-fluoro-2-deoxy-D-glucose in the imaging of malignant melanoma. J. Nucl. Med. 1993, 34: 1420-7

9. Boni R, Boni RA, Steinert H, Burg G, Buck A, Marincek B, Berthold T, Dummer R, Voellmy D, Ballmer B, et al Staging of metastatic melanoma by whole-body positron emission tomography using 2-fluorine-18-fluoro-2-deoxy-D-glucose. Br. J. Dermatol. 1995, 132: 556-62

Radioactive Isotopes in
Clinical Medicine and Research XXIII
ed. by H. Bergmann, H. Köhn and H. Sinzinger

THE POSSIBLE PLACE OF FDG-PET INVESTIGATIONS IN THE DIFFERENTIAL DIAGNOSIS OF FOCAL PANCREATIC LESIONS

M. Papós, T. Takács, L. Trón, G. Farkas, E. Ambrus, J. Lonovics, L. Csernay, L. Pávics

Department of Nuclear Medicine, 1st Department of Medicine, Department of Surgery, Albert Szent-Györgyi Medical University, Szeged, DOTE PET Centre, Debrecen, Hungary

SUMMARY: The values of different diagnostic modalities (measurement of the CA 19-9 level, abdominal ultrasonography (US) and computed tomography (CT), endoscopic retrograde cholangiopancreatography (ERCP) investigations and fluorodeoxyglucose positron emission tomography (FDG-PET)) were analysed retrospectively in the differential diagnosis of focal pancreatic lesions. FDG-PET was found to be the most effective tool for differentiation between malignant and benign focal pancreatic lesions. It is suggested that in cases where focal pancreatic lesions detected by CT or US, and there is a simultaneously elevated CA 19-9 level, FDG-PET should be the next step in the diagnostic strategy.

INTRODUCTION

The differential diagnosis of focal pancreatic lesions is often difficult. It is not easy to distinguish the focal abnormalities due to chronic pancreatitis from malignancy on the basis of the morphological signs observed by means of US, CT or ERCP (1,2). FDG-PET, based on visualization of the increased glucose metabolism of tumours, is a method that affords high accuracy in the evaluation of malignancy. It is also effective in the assessment of pancreatic malignancy (3). The aim of the present study was to compare the values of different diagnostic modalities and to establish the exact potential of FDG-PET in the differential diagnosis of focal pancreatic lesions.

PATIENTS AND METHODS

Sixteen patients (11 males, 5 females, aged 29-59 years, mean: 42 years) with focal pancreatic lesions were investigated. Atypical abdominal pain and weight loss were the main symptoms in all cases; 2 of them had chronic pancreatitis in the history. Acute pancreatitis was excluded on the basis of a non-elevated serum amylase level. In all patients, the CA 19-9 level was measured, and US, CT and ERCP investigations were performed. Following these diagnostic procedures, FDG-PET investigations were carried out. After an overnight fasting, 232-418 MBq of 18-FDG was administered to the patients, and 60 min later a PET investigation concentrating on the pancreatic regions was performed with a PET device (GE 4096 plus, General Electric, UK). The results of the different diagnostic modalities were compared with the final diagnosis (verified by surgery in 7 patients and on the basis of a 6-month clinical follow-up in 9 cases).

RESULTS

Malignant lesions were found in 5 cases whereas 11 focal cases of pancreatic disease proved to be benign. Elevated CA 19-9 levels were measured in all patients with malignancies, but also in 4 patients with benign lesions. The diagnostic values of CT and US were found to be the same. CT and US were informative for malignant disease in only one patient (liver metastases were detected). In 2 cases, the characteristic pattern of calcification as a sign of benign disease was detected. In the other cases, CT and US localized the focal lesion, but these methods were ineffective in the differential diagnosis. ERCP was unsuccessful in 4 patients in 2 cases, a calcification was detected. ERCP was definitely negative in only one of the 11 patients with benign lesions. In the remaining 7 cases, it could not clearly differentiate between malignant and benign disease.

FDG-PET revealed an increased metabolism in all patients with malignancies. Nine negative FDG-PET results were in agreement with the surgery findings or with the clinical follow-up. In two cases, however, the PET finding proved to be false-positive.

TABLE 1.

	Final diagnosis	
	malignant	benign
CA 19-9		
elevated	5	4
normal	-	6
CT		
focal lesion	4	9
calcification	-	2
metastasis	1	-
US		
focal lesion	4	9
calcification	-	2
metastasis	1	-
ERCP		
unsuccessful	2	2
stop/stenosis	3	4
calcification	-	2
negative	-	2
FDG-PET		
positive	5	2
negative	-	9

DISCUSSION

In current clinical practice, ERCP is the most important tool for the diagnosis of pancreatic malignancy because of the predominance of ductal adenocarcinoma (4). US and CT are often the first diagnostic modalities which raise the suspicion of focal lesions in the

pancreas, but these methods are not sufficiently specific. The tumour antigen CA 19-9 is likewise not sensitive and specific enough for the diagnosis of pancreatic malignancies (5). FDG-PET is a method that affords high accuracy in the evaluation of malignancy (3).
In the present study, FDG-PET proved to be the most sensitive and specific method in the differential diagnosis of pancreatic malignancy. Determination of CA 19-9 was found to be a method with good sensitivity but, the large number of false-positive investigations lead to the diagnostic value of the procedure being low. CT and US were found to be useful only for the localization of focal lesions. In contrast with the previously published results, in this study the value of ERCP was similarly found to be ambiguous due to the large number of unsuccessful examinations.

CONCLUSIONS

FDG-PET is an effective tool for differentiation between malignant and benign focal pancreatic lesions. Our results suggest that in cases with focal pancreatic lesions detected by CT or US, and with a simultaneously elevated CA 19-9 level, FDG-PET should be the next step in the diagnostic strategy. The application of ERCP is suggested following FDG-PET.

REFERENCES

1. Hawkins R. Pancreatic tumors: imaging with PET. Radiology 1995; 195: 320-322.
2. Megibow AJ, Zhou XH,Rotterdam H et al. Pancreatic adenocarcinoma: CT versus MR imaging in the evaluation of resectability - Report of the radiology diagnostic oncology group. Radiology 1995; 195: 327-332.
3. Klever P, Bares R, Fass J et al. PET with fluorine 18 deoxyglucose for pancreatic disease. Lancet 1992; 340: 1158-1159.
4. Ralls PW, Halls J, Renner I, Juttner H. Endoscopic retrograde cholangiopancreatography (ERCP) in pancreatic disease. Radiology 1980; 119: 347-352.
5. Malesci A, Tommasisni MA, Bonato C et al. Determination of CA 19-9 antigen in serum and pancreatic juice for differential diagnosis of pancreatic adenocarcinoma from pancreatitis. Gastroenterology 1987; 92: 60-67.

Radioactive Isotopes in
Clinical Medicine and Research XXIII
ed. by H. Bergmann, H. Köhn and H. Sinzinger

FDG PET IN THE FOLLOW-UP OF PATIENTS WITH DIFFERENTIATED THYROID CANCER

Szakáll S. jr., Ésik O., Emri M., Füzy M., Tóth E., Forrai G., Trón L.

PET Center, University Medical School of Debrecen, Bem tér 18/c., H-4026 Hungary
Departments of Radiotherapy, Nuclear Medicine, Molecular Pathology and Radiology of National Institute of Oncology, Ráth Gy. u. 7-9., Budapest, H-1122 Hungary

SUMMARY: The results of fluorine-18 fluorodeoxyglucose (FDG) positron emission tomography (PET) were compared with images of other modalities to survey the diagnostic value of FDG PET. Radiologic and isotope examinations were performed in 29 patients with a history of differentiated thyroid cancer and monitorized by serum tumour marker levels. The FDG PET scans were instrumental in localizing lymph node metastases particularly in cases with elevated serum tumour marker level.

INTRODUCTION

Serum tumour marker, such as thyroglobulin, calcitonin and carcinoembryonic antigen (CEA), measurements combined with structural (computed tomography - CT, magnetic resonance imaging – MRI, ultrasonography - US) and functional (whole-body scintigraphy – WBS - with ^{131}iodine or meta-^{131}iodobenzylguanidine - MIBG) imaging modalities are widely used for detection of local recurrence and lymph node or distant metastases during the follow-up of differentiated thyroid carcinomas (1-3). However, recurrent differentiated thyroid tumour tissue especially in lymph nodes can often not be localized by conventional radiological and nuclear medicine methods. In these cases, functional maps provided by fluorine-18 fluororodeoxyglucose (FDG) positron emission tomography (PET) may result in diagnosis (4-5). The retain of FDG in malignant tissue is well known, and the uptake is influenced by the proliferative capacity/grade of malignancy (6).

In this study, results of FDG PET scans were compared with serum tumour marker levels and findings of other imaging methods to survey the diagnostic value of FDG PET examinations in differentiated thyroid cancers.

PATIENTS AND METHODS

This study included 29 patients (8 male and 21 female) mean age 43 (range: 17-68) with a history of medullary (17 cases), papillary (10 cases) and follicular (2 cases) carcinoma. The serum tumour marker levels (thyroglobulin, calcitonin and CEA) were determined systematically during the follow-up. Each patient had regular posttherapeutic (surgery and radiotherapy) CT and/or MRI and/or US scans and whole-body planar $Na^{131}I$ or radioiodinated MIBG scintigraphy. The inclusion criteria for FDG PET examinations were the negative scintigraphy or a small extent of the tumour as compared to the elevated level of the tumour markers; or the discrepancy between the clinical observation or the findings of conventional imaging methods and the measured normal marker level.

FDG PET studies were performed after 5 weeks or more following surgery, external irradiation or radionuclide therapy and within 2 months from tests by other imaging procedures. The FDG accumulation maps were provided by a GE 4096 PLUS whole-body PET scanner. The patients received 191-480 (mean: 352) MBq FDG intravenously 40 min prior to the static PET scans. Using 10 min aqusition time for each frame, whole-body (5-8 frames) scan was made in 21 patients, and the rest of the studies were performed in regions most probably involved (neck, mediastinum with 1-4 frames). Table 1. gives an overwiew of clinical data and the results of the diagnostic assessments.

RESULTS

Elevated serum tumour marker level was measured during the follow-up in 20 patients (15 medullary, 3 papillary and 2 follicular cases). Out of the 20 patients, FDG PET localized tumour tissues in 19 cases. CT/MRI/US results were conclusive only in 8 cases. Scintigraphy yielded positive results in 4 cases, including also the one (patient 12) with the negative FDG PET and CT/MRI/US scans (it was a solitary vertebral metastasis proved by histology).

Table 1. The results of the diagnostic assessments

Patient No.	Histol-ogy	Marker level	CT/MRI/US	WBS Na-^{131}iodine	WBS ^{131}I-MIBG	FDG PET
1	M	Elevated	Normal	-	Normal	C(m) SC(m) ME(m)
2	M	Elevated	Normal	-	Normal	C(m) SC(m) ME(m) B(m)
3	M	Elevated	Normal	-	Normal	C(m) ME(m)
4	M	Elevated	Normal	-	Normal	C(m) ME(s)
5	M	Elevated	Normal	-	Normal	C(m)
6	M	Elevated	Normal	-	Normal	C(s)
7	M	Elevated	Normal	-	Normal	SC(s) ME(m)
8	M	Elevated	Normal	-	Normal	C(m) ME(m)
9	F	Elevated	Normal	Normal	-	C(m) ME(s)
10	F	Elevated	Normal	Normal	-	C(s)
11	M	Elevated	Normal	-	C(s)	C(m) SC(m) ME(m)
12	***P***	***Elevated***	***Normal***	***B(s)***	-	***Normal***
13	M	Elevated	C(s)	-	Normal	C(m) SC(m) ME(m)
14	M	Elevated	C(s)	-	Normal	C(m) SC(m) ME(m)
15	M	Elevated	C(m)	-	Normal	C(m) ME(m)
16	M	Elevated	ME(m)	-	Normal	C(m) ME(m)
17	M	Elevated	SC(m)	-	Normal	C(m) SC(m) ME(m)
18	P	Elevated	C(m) ME(m)	Normal	-	C(s) ME(m) L
19	M	Elevated	C(s) ME(m)	-	C(m)	C(m) SC(m) ME(m)
20	P	Elevated	L	C(m) L	-	C(m) ME(m) L
21	M	Normal	C(s)	-	C(s)	C(m) SC(s) ME(m)
22	P	Normal	ME(s)	Normal	-	C(m) ME(m)
23	P	Normal	C(m)	Normal	-	C(m)
24	P	Normal	ME(m)	C(m) ME(m)	-	C(s) SC(m) ME(m)
25	P	Normal	L	Normal	-	C(m) ME(m)
26	P	Normal	C(m) SC(s) ME(s)	Normal	-	C(m) SC(m) ME(m)
27	P	Normal	Normal	C(s)	-	C(m)
28	M	Normal	Normal	-	Normal	Normal
29	P	Normal	Normal	Normal	-	Normal

M – medullary, P – papillary, F – follicular, C – cervical lymph node metastasis, SC – supraclavicular lymph node metastasis, ME – mediastinal lymph node metastasis, B – bone metastasis, L – lung metastasis, s – single focus, m – multiple foci

Normal tumour marker level was found in 9 patients (2 medullary and 7 papillary cases). Out of them 6 cases were positive with CT/MRI/US (including also the 2 cases of positive scintigraphy in this group) and 7 with FDG PET. In spite of the clinical suspicion, no lesion was detected with any of the imaging methods in 2 cases and the clinical follow-up confirmed the results of the imaging modalities.

In the case of 26 FDG PET positive patients, the findings of FDG PET were confirmed later during the follow-up by histology/cytology in 9 cases, and by other imaging modalities and clinical data in 7 patients. In 10 cases the pathological FDG PET results have remained unproven. In the case of 25 patients PET resulted in more information localizing additional lesions undetected by other imaging modalities. At the same time FDG PET failed to detect tumour tissue in one case with positive scintigraphy.

CONCLUSION

FDG PET scans may be instrumental in diagnosing recurrent differentiated thyroid cancer tissue in cases with elevated serum tumour marker levels accompanied by negative results of traditional imaging methods or with normal serum tumour marker level accompanied with clinical symptoms indicating viable tumour.

ACKNOWLEDGEMENTS

This study was supported by OTKA 16149, OTKA F16504, ETT 12/96 and ETT 362/96 grants.

REFERENCES

1. Grünwald F, Schomburg A, Bender H, Klemm E, Menzel C, Bultmann T, Palmo H, Ruhlmann J, Kozak B, Biersack HJ. Fluorine-18 fluorodeoxyglucose positron emission tomography in the follow-up of differentiated thyroid cancer. Eur J Nucl Med 1996; 23:312-319

2. Troncone L, Rufini V, Montemaggi P, Danza FM, Lasorella A, Mastrangelo R. The diagnostic and therapeutic utility of radioiodinated metaiodobenzylguanidine (MIBG). 5 years of experience. Eur J Nucl Med 1990; 16:325-335

3. Freitas JE, Freitas AE. Thyroid and parathyroid imaging. Semin Nucl Med 1994; 24:234-245

4. Feine U, Lietzenmayer R, Hanke JP, Held J, Wöhrle H, Müller-Schauenburg W. Fluorine-18-FDG and iodine-131-iodide uptake in thyroid cancer. J Nucl Med 1996; 37:1468-72

5. Simon GH, Nitzsche EU, Laubenberger JJ, Einert A, Moser E. PET imaging of recurrent medullary thyroid cancer. Nuklearmed 1996; 35:102-104

6. Strauss LG, Conti PS. The applications of PET in clinical oncology. J Nucl Med 1991; 32:623-648

Radioactive Isotopes in
Clinical Medicine and Research XXIII
ed. by H. Bergmann, H. Köhn and H. Sinzinger

APROTININ 99mTc MYOCARDIAL SCAN : RISK STRATIFICATION OF CARDIAC EVENTS IN PATIENTS WITH AL/ATTR AMYLOIDOSIS

Aprile C, Merlini G,Saponaro R, Cannizzaro G, Calsamiglia G, Anesi E, Garini P

Fond. «S.Maugeri»,IRCCS- Nuclear Med. Serv.
S.Matteo University Hosp.,IRCCS- Biotechnology Res. Lab.
Pavia – Italy

SUMMARY

Myocardial scan with 99m Tc Aprotinin was performed in 89 pts with primary amyloidosis. Negative results allowed to rule out myocardial involvement in pts with a pre-test probability of involvement, while deaths attributable to cardiac causes or deterioration of cardiac function were observed only in pts with positive scan. Therefore, Aprotinin scan seems to be able to stratify pts with amyloidosis as far as organ failure and/or cardiac deaths are concerned.

INTRODUCTION

Amyloid involvement of the heart represents the most powerful prognostic factor in pts. with light chain (AL) and familial (ATTR) amyloidosis, since organ involvement leads either to sudden death due to fatal arrhythmias or to congestive heart failure (CHF), with a median survival time of 6-12 months (1). We previously reported the possibility to image myocardial involvement with the bovine lung antiprotease aprotinin (Trasylol) labelled with 99mTc (2,3) before than the classical echo and ECG signs are evident. The aim of this paper was to test the possibility to stratify the risk of myocardial events on the basis of the scintigrafic results.

MATERIALS & METHODS

One hundred eleven studies were performed in 89 pts. with biopsy proven amyloidosis, 76 with the AL and 13 with the ATTR form, 90 minutes after iv. administration of about 600-800 MBq of 99m Tc- Aprotinin (TcA), in the anterior and LAO projection. The intensity of uptake was visually graded with a 4 points scale: 0-no uptake, 1-faint, 2-moderate, 3-

prominent uptake. The pre-test likelihood of cardiac involvement was assessed according to the clinical and instrumental findings of the Italian Society of Amyloidosis : A-no evidence of involvement, B- suspected, C-high probability/clear without CHF, D- as C with CHF. Median follow-up time was 12 months. In 11 pts endomyocardial biopsy was available.

RESULTS

The results of pre-test classification and scintigraphic results as well as the outcome at the end of follow-up are reported in table 1. Final data comprise 76 fully evaluable pts, excluding therefore those who had a follow-up <6 mo. without any change of the cardiac status and those lost for follow-up.

pre-test	Score	ALIVE			DEAD		Lost or n.e.
		no involv	=	+	CARDIAC CAUSES (SCD / HF)	Other causes	
A	*0*	22				4	5
n 33	*1*				1		
	2				1		
	3						
B	*0*	6				2	1
n 18	*1*		1	1	1		
	2		1	1	1		
	3		1	1			1
C	*0*	4				1	1
n 19	*1*						
	2		3	1	5		
	3		1	1		1	1
D	*0*						
n 19	*1*						
	2		1		1	1	1
	3			4	7	1	3

Tab.1 Clinical evolution of pts with amyloidosis according to the pre-test classification and results of the aprotinin 99mTc scan. (= no change , + deterioration of cardiac conditions, SCD sudden cardiac death, HF heart failure, n.e. not evaluable).

No deaths attributable to cardiac causes were observed in pts with negative scan while, in general, pts with positive scan deteriorated their cardiac function or died for cardiac causes. It is interesting to note that 3 pts treated with iodo-doxorubicin (1 class B score 1, 1 class B score 2 and 1 class D score 2) did not showed sign of further deterioration (4). As expected, survival, as far as cardiac causes were concerned, and slower evolution of the cardiac disease was observed in pts with the ATTR form.

DISCUSSION

Current conventional assessment of cardiac involvement in pts with amyloidosis is complicated by the fact that the diagnosis is based on the classical echo and ECG findings which are more indicative of organ failure rather than being an early index of tissue deposits(1,2,5). Therefore , when these signs are present, there are few therapeutical possibilities (6,7). We previously reported the high accuracy of TcA to depict organ deposits. Prominent uptake (score 2 or 3) , indicating a conspicuous amyloid burden, is frequently associated with the presence or with a rapid development of CHF, leading to death for heart failure, while lower uptake (score 1) indicates the risk of sudden cardiac death due to fatal arrhythmias.

In our group of pts no change of the cardiac function associated with TcA uptake was observed only in pts submitted to more aggressive therapies (4,6) and in pts with the ATTR form, where a different myocardial distribution of the deposits was responsible for a less unfauvorable prognosis (8).

On the other side, the absence of significant myocardial uptake allowed us to rule out myocardial involvement and, in this subgroup of pts, the deaths observed were due to non-cardiac causes.

REFERENCES

1. Falk RH,Comenzo RL,Skinner M. The systemic amyloidosis. N Engl J Med 1997;337:898-909.
2. Aprile C, Marinone G, Saponaro R.Cardiac and pleuropulmonary AL amyloid imaging with technetium -99m labelled aprotinin. Eur J Nucl Med 1995;22:1393-1401.
3. Aprile C, Marinone MG, Saponaro R et al. Detection of myocardial amyloid involvement with Tc-99m Aprotinin. J Nucl Med 1996;37(suppl):185P
4. Gianni L, Bellotti V, Gianni AM, Merlini G. New drug therapy of amyloidoses: resorption of AL-type deposits with 4′-iodo-4′-deoxydoxorubicin. *Blood* 1995; 86: 855-861.
5. Dubrey S,Falk RH. Heart transplantation in AL amyloidosis.. Amyloid:Int J Exp Clin

Invest 1995;2:284-287
6. Merlini G. Treatment of primary amyloidosis. *Semin Hematol* 1995; 32: 60-79.
7. Dubrey S,Mendes L,Skinner M,Falk RH. Resolution of heart failure in patients with AL amyloidosis. Ann Intern Med 1996;125:481-484.
8. Van de Walle JP,Fourcade L,Panagides D et al. apport de la biopsie myocardique et de l'etude immunoistochimique a l'evaluation pronostique des amyloses cardiaques. Arch Mal Coeur 1994;87:235-239

Radioactive Isotopes in
Clinical Medicine and Research XXIII
ed. by H. Bergmann, H. Köhn and H. Sinzinger

DISTURBED MYOCARDIAL ENERGY METABOLISM IN PATIENTS WITH NONTRANSMURAL CHRONIC MYOCARDIAL INFARCTION.

D. Moka, U. Sechtem, P. Theissen, E. Voth and H. Schicha
Departments of Nuclear Medicine and Cardiology, University of Cologne, Germany

SUMMARY

To characterise energy metabolism after nontransmural myocardial infarction (NtMI), 19 patients (A) with a LAD stenosis and anterior wall hypokinesia were examined using ^{31}P MRS. To separate the influence of coronary stenosis from that of the ischemic insult, also 4 patients (B) with LAD-stenosis but without LV dysfunction were examined. Mean PCr/ATP-ratio was significantly lower in A (1.24 ± 0.18) than in healthy volunteers (1.74 ± 0.23; $p < 0.01$). B showed nearly normal PCr/ATP-ratios (1.64 ± 0.22). Hypokinetic myocardium after NtMI is characterised by a decrease of the cellular energy buffer PCr. This may be caused by degenerative changes of myocytes in vital areas of the infarct, disturbed microperfusion and remodelling of the vital myocardium in these regions.

INTRODUCTION

Recent advances in cardiovascular applications of phosphorus 31 - spectroscopy are reported (1, 2). Cardiac contraction and cellular function requires the availability of energy represented mainly in the human organism by phosphocreatine (PCr) and adenosintriphosphate (ATP). ^{31}P-NMR-spectra trace high energy phosphate metabolism, which may be altered in abnormal / ischemic heart disease (3).

When coronary flow is limited by arterial stenosis, myocardial perfusion becomes transmurally non-uniform. If there are additional alterations of the myocardial wall like fibrotic changes after a nontransmural infarction, the subendocardial layer may not be sufficient by supplied with oxygen or blood. This may affect the PCr / ATP - ratio as a marker of an ischemic heart disease even at rest (4, 5).

The purpose of this study was to characterize myocardial energy metabolism after nontransmural infarction using ^{31}P-MRS, to determine whether the alterations correlated mainly to the coronary stenosis or to the hypokinesia of the myocardial wall after NtMI and to establish whether ischemic changes represented by the PCr / ATP - ratio can be improved by anti-ischemic medication.

This maybe of prognostic and therapeutic significance.

PATIENTS AND METHODS

Magnetic resonance spectroscopy

^{31}P-NMR spectroscopy is a non-invasive tool for investigation of high-energy metabolism in the heart. 3D localised ^{31}P-spectra can be obtained from the myocardium using a single 14-cm-diameter surface coil, serving as both transmitter and receiver coil, placed on the chest over the cardiac apex. Measurements were performed in a 1.5-T (resonance frequency for ^{31}P: 25,84 MHz) whole-body Philips Gyroscan MR system (1).

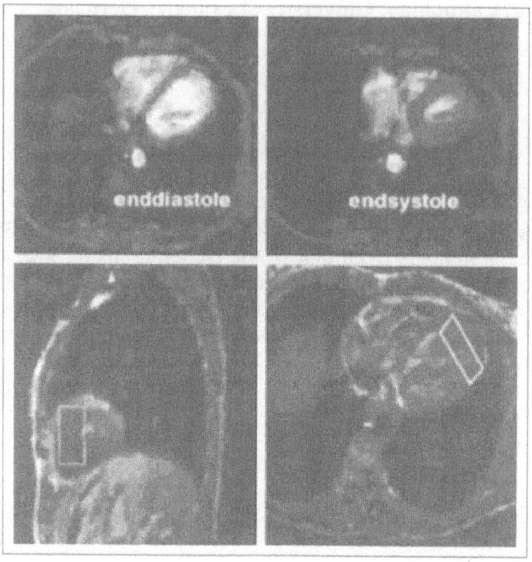

Localisation of the cube-shaped volume of interest (VOI - 50 x 50 x 30 mm) in the anterior myocardial wall using ISIS software and ^{1}H-gradient-echo-images (above) and spin-echo-images (below) of the heart.

Coronary stenosis and anterior wall hypokinesia versus healthy volunteers **(patient group A)**

Examinations were performed in 19 patients with LAD-stenosis and anterior wall hypokinesia, shown by laevocardiography, and in 10 healthy volunteers. All patients had a minimum wall thickness of 6 mm as assessed by gradient-echo MRI. Patient spectra were recorded under optimal anti-ischemic medication. To minimize the influence of blood-ATP, all spectra were recorded at end-systole and were corrected for blood-contamination and T_1-effects.

LAD-stenosis versus hypokinesia **(patient group B)**

To eliminate the possibility that the detected alterations of the PCr / ATP -ratio were mainly caused by the LAD-stenosis, 4 additional patients with critical LAD-stenosis (> 90 % diameter stenosis) but normal ventricular function were examined following the same protocol.

Influence of glycerol trinitrate on the ischemic heart metabolism **(patient group C)**

The effect of glycerol trinitrate (GTN) on ^{31}P-spectra was evaluated in 4 further patients who had the same clinical features as patient group A. Spectroscopy was performed without anti-ischemic medication (washout period > one day) and during i.v. application of GTN.

RESULTS

In patient group A (LAD-stenosis und anterior wall hypokinesia after NtMI) mean PCr/ATP ratio (1.24 ± 0.18) was significantly lower than in normal controls (1.74 ± 0.23; p = 0.01).

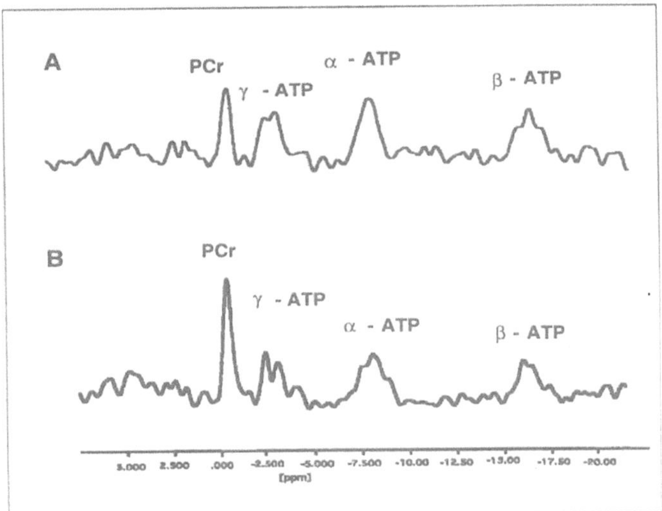

Cardiac ^{31}P magnetic resonance spectra from a healthy volunteer (**B**) compared with a patient with LAD-stenosis and hypokinesia of the anterior myocardial wall after NtMI (**A**).

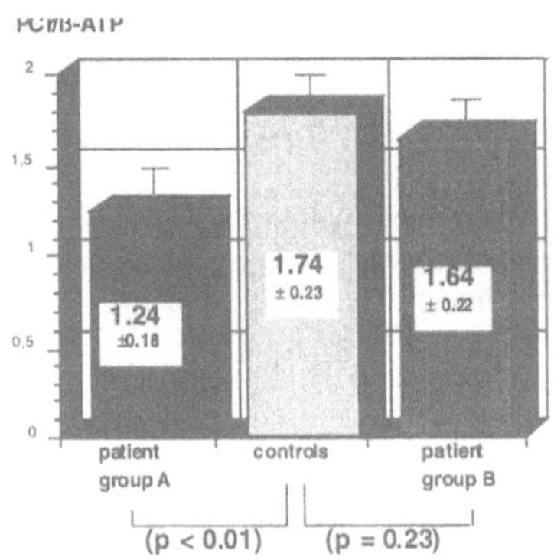

Comparison of the mean PCr / ß-ATP-ratio (± SD) of patients with LAD-stenosis and NtMI (A), and patients with LAD-stenosis without MI and normal left ventricular function (B) with healthy controls.

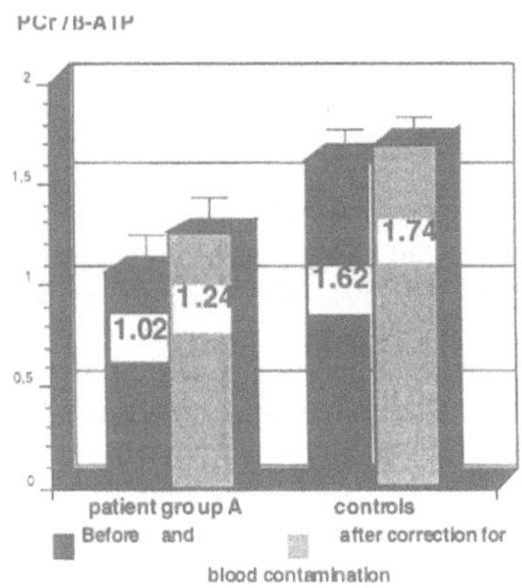

Comparison of the mean PCr / ß-ATP-ratio of patients with LAD-stenosis and NtMI with healthy controls before and after correction for blood contamination.

Patient group B (critical LAD-stenosis and normal ventricular function) had PCr / ATP - ratios similiar to those of normal controls: 1.64 ± 0.22 (p = 0.23 unpaired t-test).

PCr / ATP - ratio of patient group C rose from 1.12 ± 0.08 (without anti-ischemic medication) to 1.32 ± 0.13 (p = 0.04 paired t-test) after 10 min. i.v. infusion of GTN.

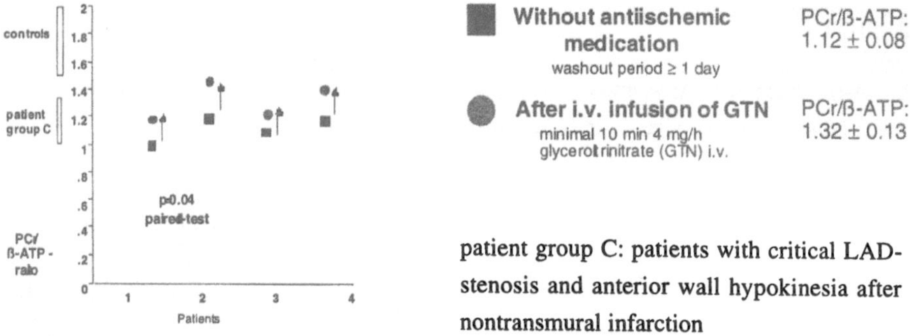

patient group C: patients with critical LAD-stenosis and anterior wall hypokinesia after nontransmural infarction

Conclusion

The reduction of the PCr / ATP - ratio in patients after NtMI correlated with the hypokinesia in this area (6). Patients with critical LAD-stenosis without any history of MI had a normal PCr / ATP - ratio. These results may have arisen from a disturbance of microperfusion due to degenerative and fibrotic changes of the myocardial wall after NtMI. The observation that improving myocardial perfusion with GTN leads to better myocardial energy metabolism support this explanation. Another possible reason for the reduction of PCr / ATP - ratio could be remodelling processes and alterations of myocardial enzyme concentrations in vital residual myocardium (7). Our study shows that in vivo ^{31}P MRS of the heart is playing an increasing important role in the evaluation of ischemic myocardial disease (1, 8).

REFERENCES

1. Moka D, Sechtem U, Theissen P, Voth E, Schicha H. Nontransmural infarction: Alerations of myocardial energy metabolism in vital residual myocardium. Z. Kariol. 1997; 86: 113-120.
2. Bottomley PA. MR spectroscopy of the human heart: The status and the challenges. Radiology 1994; 191: 593-612.
3. Neubauer S, Krahe T, Schindler R, Horn M, Hillenbrand H, Entzeroth C, et al. 31P magnetic resonance spectroscopy in dilated cardiomyopathy and coronary artery disease. Altered cardiac high-energy phosphate metabolism in heart failure. Circ. 1992; 86: 1810-8.
4. Fedele FA, Gewirtz H, Capone RJ, Sharaf B, Most AS. Metabolic response to prolonged reduction of myocardial blood flow distal to a severe coronary artery stenosis. Circulation 1988; 78: 729-35.
5. Flameng W, Suy R, Schwarz F, Borgers M, Piessens J, Thone F, et al. Ultrastructural correlates of left ventricular contraction abnormalities in patients with chronic ischemic heart disease: Determinants of reversible segmental asynergy postrevascularization surgery. Am Heart J 1981; 102: 846-57.
6. Schaefer S, Schwartz GG, Gober JR, Wong AK, Camacho SA, Massie B, et al. Relationship between myocardial metabolites and contractile abnormalities during regional ischemia. J. Clin. Invest. 1990; 85: 706-713.
7. Sharkey SW, Murakami MM, Smith SA, Apple FS. Canine myocardial creatine kinase isoenzymes after chronic coronary artery occlusion. Circulation 1991; 84: 333-340.
8. Pohost GM. Is 31P-NMR spectroscopic imaging a viable approach to assess myocardial viability? Circulation 1995; 92: 9-10.

Radioactive Isotopes in
Clinical Medicine and Research XXIII
ed. by H. Bergmann, H. Köhn and H. Sinzinger

QUANTITATIVE, MULTIVARIATE ANALYSIS - BASED ASSESSMENT OF MIBI PLANAR HEART PERFUSION STUDIES.

J. Kuśmierek[1], A. Płachcińska[1], M. Bieńkiewicz[1], M. Kośmider[2]
[1]Department of Nuclear Medicine
[2]Division of Angiocardiography and Haemodynamics
Medical University, Łódź, Poland.

SUMMARY

A quantitative assessment of myocardial perfusion scintigrams was performed on the basis of analysis of circumferential profile curves, after adoption of perfusion defect severity measures resulting from comparison of curves with normal trends (separately for both sexes) and application of a multivariate analysis and a discriminant analysis to the process of patient classification. The method secures a reliable criterion for detection of coronary artery disease and is especially valuable for evaluation of scintigrams of females.

INTRODUCTION

MIBI, a technetium-99m labeled methoxyisobutylisonitryle, is the most widely used radiotracer of a myocardial perfusion. Cardiac perfusion studies are performed making use of two techniques: tomographic and planar, the latter being theoretically less accurate, but also less expensive and not so complex as the tomographic one and in many countries much more available.

The purpose of the study was to elaborate a quantitative method for evaluation of planar MIBI cardiac perfusion scintigrams and to work out an objective, statistics - based criterion for classification of patients to groups with normal and impaired perfusion in order to select patients with coronary artery disease.

MATERIALS

Group I - a reference group - 53 individuals (29 males and 24 females) with low (<10%) probability of coronary artery disease (acc. to Diamond).

Groups II and III - 90 and 83 patients suspected of having coronary artery disease, without history of myocardial infarction. Patients were included into group II or III acc. to the date of the scintigraphic study. Group II was used for elaboration of the method, group III - for verification of its results on an independent group of patients. All patients from these groups were subjected to coronary angiography.

METHODS

Two day (stress and rest) scintigraphic study protocol was applied, in three standard projections: anterior, LAO 45, LAO 70. Administered activity amounted to 550-740MBq.

Scintigrams of all patients from groups II and III were inspected visually and assessed quantitatively making use of our method, which is described below.

After subtraction of extracardiac background from scintigrams, by means of Goris-Watson method [2] as modified by Sinusas [3] and transformation of myocardial uptake of the tracer into circumferential profile curves, our method [1] generated normal trends for all projections (patients from group I).

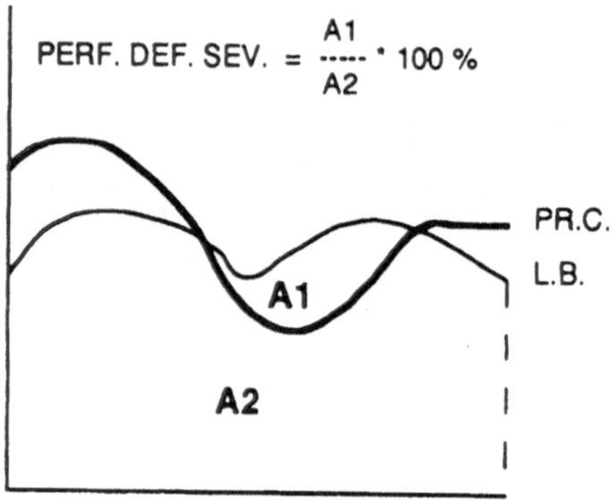

Fig. 1. Quantified evaluation of perfusion defect from a scintigram. PR.C.- profile curve, L.B.-lower boundary of the trend.

After fitting of curves of patients from group II into normal trends the quantitative measure of perfusion defect severity was adopted (fig.1) and its ability to differentiate patients with and without stenosed main coronary arteries (groups IIa and IIb) was tested by means of a multivariate analysis [4]. At the next step a discriminant analysis was applied by introduction of a discriminant function, a basis for patient classification, being a result of transformation of the tracer uptake in 6 scintigrams into one numeric value:

$v = d_1 * PDS_1 + d_2 * PDS_2 + \ldots + d_6 * PDS_6$,

where $PDS_1, \ldots, PDS_6$ denote perfusion defect measures in six (three stress and three rest) scintigrams and $d_1, \ldots, d_6$ - resp. weights calulated by means of discriminant analysis.

After selection of an optimum discriminant threshold this classification was verified on an independent group of patients (group III).

RESULTS

Mean values (trends) of normal profile curves (patients from the reference group) with confidence intervals for three projections, turned out different for males and females, especially in LAO 45 and LAO 70 projections.

Vectors of mean values of perfusion defect measures differed between subgroups IIa and IIb (with stenosed and normal arteries) at a significance level of $p<10^{-5}$.

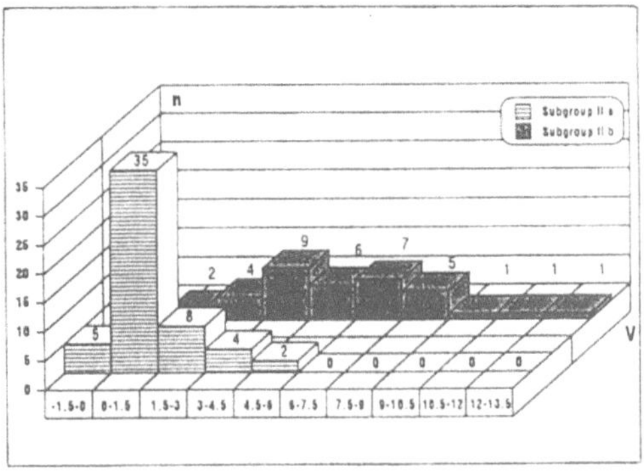

Fig. 2. Histograms depicting distribution of values of discriminant function v in subgroubs IIa and IIb.

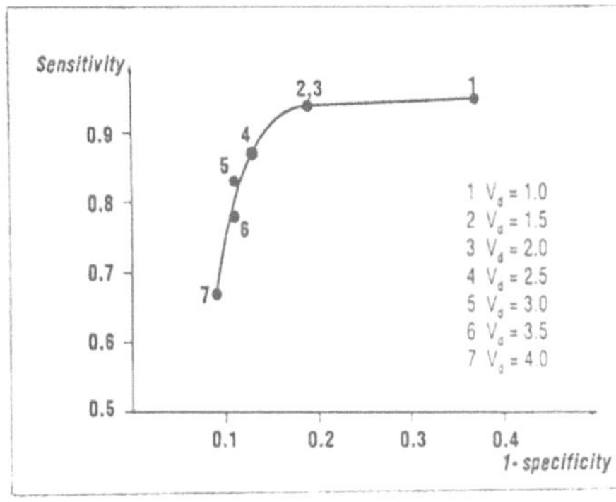

Fig. 3. An ROC curve resulting from stepwise shift of the discriminating threshold between distributions of v values in subgr. IIa and IIb (Fig.2).

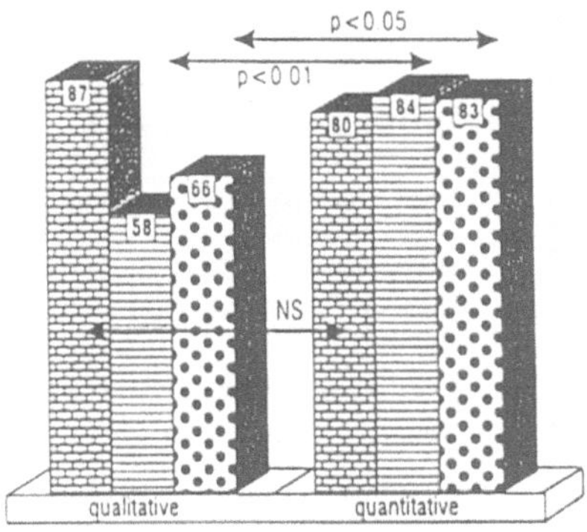

Fig.4. Comparison of diagnostic efficacy of the qualitative and quantitative evaluating procedures in detection of CAD in females (n=58)

After application of a quantitative diagnostic criterion - an optimum discriminant threshold (v_d=2.5), selected as a result of ROC curve inspection (figs.2 and 3), the sensitivity, specificity and accuracy of detection of perfusion impairment reached 86%, 87% and 87%, respectively.

Verification of this diagnostic criterion on the independent group of patients (gr. III) confirmed its high efficacy - sensitivity, specificity and accuracy amounted to 84%, 83% and 83%, respectively.

After subdivision of pooled patients from groups II and III into subgroups of males (n=115) and females (n=58), the basic indices of diagnostic efficacy amounted to 88%, 83% , 85% and 87%, 58%, 66% for qualitative method and 87%, 86%, 86% and 80%, 84%, 83% for the quantitative one, resp. The higher specificity and accuracy of the quantitative method (fig. 4)was mainly due to the reduction of the number of false positive results of the qualitative method in women.

DISCUSSION

Our method of quantitative assessment of planar MIBI perfusion scintigrams is apparently different from the methods published earlier [5,6,7,8], mainly in taking advantage of differences in profile trends associated with patients' sex and application of a multivariate analysis and a discriminant analysis to the process of quantification of scintigrams and classification of patients.The present method secures high indices of the diagnostic efficacy in detection of coronary artery disease, confirmed in a study of the independent group of patients. This method is especially valuable for the assesment of scintigrams of female patients being subject to mistakes in preliminary diagnostics of coronary artery disease, resulting in improper selection to coronary angiography.

REFERENCES

1. Plachcinska A, Kusmierek J Kosmider M et al. Quantitative assessment of technetium-99m methoxyisobutylisonitryle planar perfusion heart studies: application of multivariate analysis to patient classification. Eur J Nucl Med 1995;22:193-200.
2. Watson DD, Campbell NP, Read EK, et al. Spatial and temporal quantitation of plane thallium myocardial scintigraphy. J Nucl Med 1981;22:577-584.
3. Sinusas AJ, Beller GA, Smith WH, et al. Quantitative planar imaging with technetium-99m methoxyisobutyl isonitrile: comparison with uptake patterns with thallium-201. J Nucl Med 1989;30:1456-1463.
4. Ahrens H, Lauter J. Mehrdimensionale Varianzanalyse. Berlin:Akademie: 1974:95.
5. Watson DD, Smith WH, Beller GA et al. Blinded evaluation of planar technetium-99m-sestamibi myocardial perfusion studies. J Nucl Med 1992;33:668-675.
6. Dilsizian V, Rocco TP, Strauss HW et al. Technetium-99m-isonitrile myocardial uptake at rest.I Relation to severity of coronary artery stenosis. J Am Cardiol 1989;14:1673-1677.
7. Koster K, Weckers FJ, Mattera JA et al. Quantitative analysis of planar technetium-99m-sestamibi perfusion images using modified background subtraction. J Nucl Med 1990:31:1400-1408
8. Verzijlbergen JF, Oudheusden D, Cramer MH et al. Quantitative analysis of planar technetium-99m-sestamibi myocardial perfusion images;clinical application of a modified method for the subtraction of tissue crosstalk. Eur Heart J 1994;15:1217-1226.

POSTER SESSION III

Radioactive Isotopes in
Clinical Medicine and Research XXIII
ed. by H. Bergmann, H. Köhn and H. Sinzinger

DETECTION OF FISTULAE IN CROHN'S PATIENTS WITH IMMUNOSCINTIGRAPHY (IS)

A Kroiss, Ch Auinger, D Tschabitscher, W Weiss, Ch Kölbl-Schrutka, A Neumayr.

Institute of Nuclear Medicine, 4th Medical Department,
Ludwig Boltzmann Institut für Geriatrie,
KA Rudolfstiftung, Vienna, 1030 Austria

SUMMARY: The antibody we used was the BW 250/183 produced by the Behringwerke, Germany and labelled with Tc-99m. We did planar scanning and SPECT studies 4 hours and 24 hrs with a rotating digital camera (Elscint). A total of 16 patients (6 male, 10 female; age ranging from 19-67 years) were investigated. In 1 patient the investigation was performed 3 times and in 2 patients twice. Diagnosis of fistulae was established by surgical, endosopic and X-ray procedures. We found no false-positive result, a false-negative result in 2 patients, a true positive result in 16 and a true negative result in 2 patients. This would mean a sensitivity of 88%. SPECT studies are necessary to achieve these good results.

INTRODUCTION

Crohn´ s disease is characterized by transmural inflammation which may lead to the formation of fistulae in up to 40% of patients (1). Radiologic imaging modalities, particularly barium examinations are commonly obtained in Crohn´s patients and be the first to identify fistulization. Recent studies reported enhanced CT scans and MRI to be useful for the demonstration of fistulae (2). The role of 111-In-white blood cell (WBC) scintigraphy and antigranulocyte-antibodies in the assessment of disease activity and extent in Crohn`s patients has been cited in a large number of publications (3,4,5). In a retrospective study we wanted to determine the role of an antigranulocyte - antibody in this clinical setting.

PATIENTS AND METHOD

16 patients with Crohn's disease (10 female, 6 male; with an average age 39,7 years (range 19-67) entered the study after having given informed written consent. In one patient the investigation was performed 3 times and in two patients twice. Diagnosis of fistula was established by surgical procedures.

The antibody we used was the BW 250/183 produced by Behringwerke/Germany (distributed in Austria by Biocis). This is an immunoglobulin IgG1 isotype and binds to an epitope of NCA 95. 0.5 - 1 mg of this monoclonal antibody was labeled with 20 mCi (540 MBq) Tc - 99m in a simple labeling procedure which lasts about 20 min and is performed by a technician.

After slow intravenous injection of the labeled Ab without premedication - except blockade of the thyroid with perchlorate - imaging was performed with a rotating digital camera (Elscint; Apex 401 A).

We did planar scanning (256x256 matrix) and SPECT studies (64x64 matrix) 4 - 6 hr and 24 hr post injection.

RESULTS

Table 1

Patients with fistulae

Diagnosis	n
Ileosigmoid fistulae	6
Ileocecal fistulae	2
Enterovesicle	2
Anal fistulae in pt with colostomy	3
Enterovaginal	2
Enteroscrotal	1
	16 pt

In one patient the investigation was performed 3 times (Fig. 1) and in two patients twice. Doing 4-6 and 24 hours planar and SPECT investigations we achieved these good results: We found no false positive result, a false negative result in 2 patients, a true positive result in 16 and a true negative result in 2 patients. This would mean a sensitivity of 88%.

The results were concordant with endoscopic, X - ray and surgical results.

FIGURES

FIG. 1:

A 40 year old male patient with Crohn' s disease and status post ileostoma and status post Miles operation suffered from extraintestinal manifestations: fever, uveitis, arthritis.

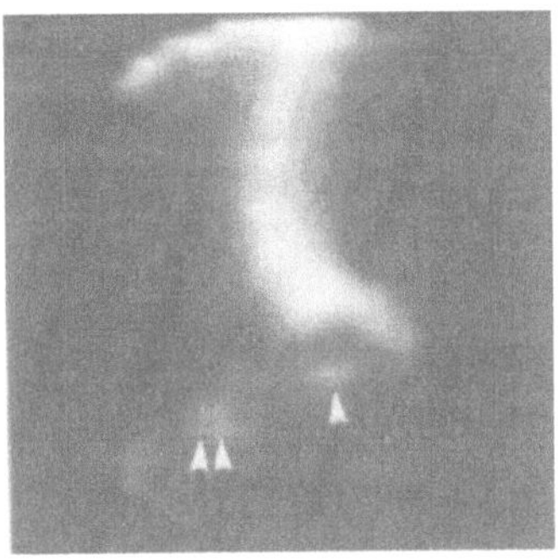

1A: Sagittal SPECT image shows the close connection of this fistula (↑) and the urinary bladder (↑↑).

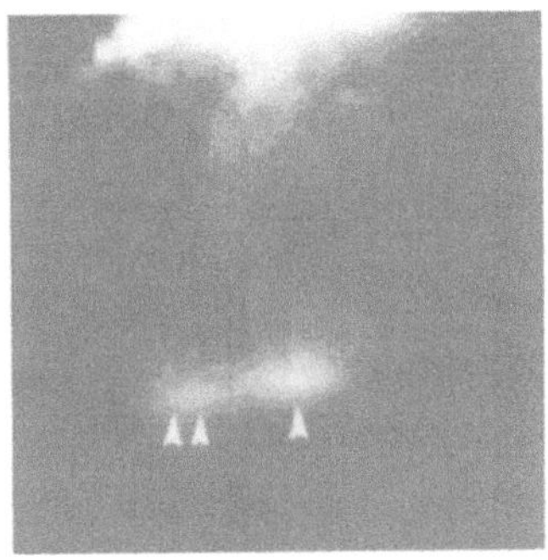

2B: The same patient after several fistula operations. This was the third investigation and the fistula is still detected but the contrast is not as good as in the pictures before. In the meantime the HAMA (human anti - mouse antibody)- levels were elevated.

DISCUSSION

The application of the antibodies permits imaging of an active bowel disease, therefore, differentiation between an active inflammatory disease and scarred strictures is possible. Imaging of fistula can be done, but 24 hours imaging and SPECT imaging are necessary.
A major drawback is, that in patients with repeated investigations the HAMA - levels (human anti - mouse antibody) could be elevated, so that the contrast of the pictures is not as good as in patients without HAMA`s

CONCLUSION

In patients with Crohn`s disease who are clinically or radiographically suspected of having fistulae, antigranulocyte - antibody scintigraphy may add information which is essential for appropriate clinical management and therefore should be included especially in preoperative investigations.

REFERENCES

1. McNamara MJ, Fazio FW, Lavery IC et al. Surgical treatment of entero-vesical fistulas in Crohn`s disease. Dis Colon Rectum 1990; 33:271-276.
2. Koelbel G, Schmiedl U, Majer MC et al. Diagnosis of fistulae and sinus tracts in patients with Crohn`s disease: value of MR imaging. AJR 1989; 152:999-1003
3. Becker W, Fischbach W, Reiners C, Börner W. Three-phase white blood cell scan: diagnostic validity in abdominal inflammatory diseases. J Nucl Med 1986; 27:1109-1115.
4. Kroiss A, Weiss W, Auinger Ch, Kölbl Ch, Weidlich G, Feichtenschlager T,Neumayr A. Immunoscintigraphy (IS) with Tc-99m labeled granulocytes antibody (Ab) in patients with inflammatory bowel diseasis. Schmidt HAE, van der Schoot JB, editors.Nuclear Medicine 1990: 259-261.
5. Lind P, Langsteger W, Költringer P, Dimai HP, Passl R, Eber O. Immunoscintigraphy of inflammatory process with a technetium-99m-labeled monoclonal antigranulocyte antibody (Mab BW250/183). J Nucl Med 1990; 31:417-423.
6. Even-Sapir E, Barnes DC, Martin RH, LeBrun PG. Indium-111-white blood cell scintigraphy in Crohn`s patients with fistulae and sinus tracts. J Nucl Med 1994; 35:245-250.

Radioactive Isotopes in
Clinical Medicine and Research XXIII
ed. by H. Bergmann, H. Köhn and H. Sinzinger

IMMUNORADIOMETRIC ASSAY OF TOTAL PSA, FREE PSA AND PSA RATIO CALCULATION IN PROSTATIC CANCER (PCa) DIAGNOSIS

Luca Giovanella, Paola Erba, Luca Ceriani, (*)Patrizia Vio, Silvana Garancini

Departments of Nuclear Medicine and (*) Urology - Azienda Ospedaliera"Ospedale di Circolo e Fondazione Macchi"-Varese - University of Pavia - II Faculty of Medicine,Varese - Italy

SUMMARY: Total PSA assay is a well established procedure for biochemical evaluation and management of PCa which usefulness in its diagnosis is limited by its weak specificity with regard to BPH. Recently the assay of Free- PSA and the calculation of Free/Total-PSA Ratio has been suggested to improve the specificity of PSA in the range of concentrations between 2.5 and 20 ng/mL. We evaluated the diagnostic performance of PSA-Ratio among untreated patients with PSA levels ranging from 2.5 to 20 ng/mL and histological diagnosis of PCa or BPH. As the ROC curves analysis showed PSA-Ratio is the better parameter to discriminate between PCa and BPH: PSA-Ratio could be employed to enhance the diagnostic performance of PSA alone in PCa diagnosis.

INTRODUCTION

The immunometric assay of Prostatic Specific Antigen (PSA), represents an important diagnostic instrument for prostatic adenocarcinoma (PCa) evaluation and follow up. Major limitations are present for its use at the diagnosis time especially for PSA values minor than 10-20 ng/mL, where benignant and malignant pathology superimposed and the marker specificity is critical. PSA biochemical structure is characterised by a single glycoproteic chain (33-kDa) synthesised from the prostatic ephitelium. This molecule belong to the seric extracellular proteinase family and it has chymotrypsin-like activity. Therefore PSA enzymatic activity can be delete from the major circulating proteinase inhibitor: we know PSA forms stable complexes with alpha1-antichymotrypsin (ACT) and alpha2-macroglobulin (a2M). PSA-ACT reaction produce eqimolar complexes (90kDa) letting some epitopes exposition and, then, the immunological recognition of the molecule. Viceversa PSA-a2M complexes are characterised from the total inclusion of PSA which become unapproachable to the immunological reaction. A little PSA share is present in the blood in free form, circulating without any carrier. So, the immunological PSA assay methods evaluate both Free-PSA and PSA-ACT. Recently the PSA assays were standardised against international equimolar reference preparations. The development of PSA-ACT quantification methods using direct techniques or Free-PSA determination, underlined that the molar excess of complexed PSA is about 1000 times higher in PCa than BPH while in PCa circulating Free-PSA is a subliminal part of circulating PSA /1/. Although the reasons are not definitely explained, Free-PSA and Free-PSA/Total PSA (PSA Ratio) determinations seem to be able to improve the diagnostic performance of PSA alone and the discrimination between PCa and BPH /2,3,4/. Aim of our work was the evaluation of diagnostic significance of PSA-Ratio in a group of patients with Total-PSA concentration between 2.5 and 20 ng/mL and histological diagnosis, obtained trough prostatic eco-guided biopsy, of PCa and BPH respectively.

MATERIALS AND METHODS

We selected 245 patients (age 45-84, medium age 58 years) with Total-PSA between 2.5 and 20 ng/mL. We left out all the patients pharmacological treated for BPH or affected with infective-inflammatory urinary diseases. A blood sample was obtained from all the patients in order to determinate Total and Free PSA and eco-guided transrectal prostatic biopsy was performed. The histological diagnosis was of PCa in 104 patients and BPH in 141. Total and Free PSA were detected by immunoradiometric methods (IRMA, Tandem-R PSA e Tandem R-FreePSA, Hybritech Italia Sesto Fiorentino, Italia) and Free-PSA/Total-PSA Ratio was calculated from analytical data. The markers were not distributed normally: data were expressed as median and interquartile range while non parametrical analysis was employed. Mann-Whitney U test was used to compare two independent groups: a p value minor than 0.05 was considered significant.
Total-PSA and PSA-Ratio ROC curves were plotted and compared.

RESULTS

Table I show the markers distribution in the two groups: Total-PSA and Free-PSA distributions are not significantly different between the two groups while PSA-Ratio is significantly lower in PCa group of patients respect BPH group ($p<0.0001$). ROC curve analysis demostred that the area under PSA-Ratio curve is higher than Total-PSA one showing that PSA-Ratio is able to discriminate Pca and BPH better than Total-PSA (Figure 1). Ensuing the more diagnostic accuracy point on the ROC curve, we obtained a clinical cut-off value of 0.18 (sensitivity 0.65, specificity 0.94).

Table I. Distribution of Total-PSA, Free-PSA and Free-PSA/Total-PSA concentrations in patients suffering from PCa and BPH and comparison through U Mann-Whitney Test

Parameter		BPH	PCa	p
Total-PSA	(ng/mL)	7.60 (2.46-16.90)	6.95 (2.90-19.75)	ns
Free-PSA	(ng/mL)	1.20 (0.15- 2.94)	0.95 (0.07- 1.85)	ns
PSA-Ratio		0.23 (0.12- 0.34)	0.11 (0.03- 0.22)	<0.0001

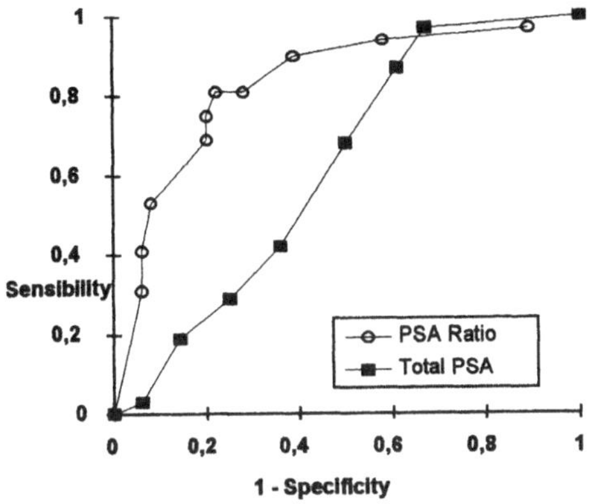

Figure 1: ROC CURVE of PSA-RATIO AND TOTAL-PSA

DISCUSSION

PSA clinical role in PCa evaluation and follow up is well established and it represents one of the more useful biomarkers in clinical practice. The diagnostic role of this marker is still discussed, 'cause of the overlap phenomena between PCa and BPH: anyway it's worthwhile to underline that the association of PSA, rectal exploration and/or trans-rectal ultrasound allows an high diagnostic sensitivity. The demonstration of different PSA isoforms, and the determination of complexed PSA forms and Free-PSA permit the deepening of PSA biochemical and fisiopatological knowledges and to obtain important diagnostic informations. Lilija and Stenman experiences demostred that PSA-ACT complexes are more represented in serum of patients suffering from PCa respect patients with BPH /5,6/. The following development of Free-PSA quantification techniques turned the interest on PSA-Ratio determination: different Authors demostred this parameter is able to increase significantly the diagnostic specificity and to improve the discrimination between PCa and BPH /7/. In our experience we evaluated patients selected on the basis of PSA concentration in the range of 2.5 and 20ng/mL which had been selected according to literature and clinical experience of our team and all those patients underwent echo-guided biopsy in order to obtain the histological characterisation. The analysis of PSA-Ratio distribution between the two groups and the ROC curves comparison show that also in our population PSA-Ratio allows a significant improvement of discriminative capability between PCa and BPH, better than the only Total-PSA. *Using a cut-off level of 0.18 we were able to identify 7 PCa over 10 and 9 BPH over 10:* so, PSA-Ratio represents an interesting evolution of laboratory medicine, even if it cannot be considered an absolute parameter of discrimination. In fact, further epidemiological and economical studies are needed in order to evaluate the cost/effectiveness balance before validating the rutinary use of this test. Nevertheless, on a laboratory and clinical point of view, we can settle that PSA-Ratio is a useful parameter in the differential diagnosis between PCa and BPH in patients with seric PSA values included in the so called "Gray Area".

REFERENCES:

/1/ Christensson A, Bjork T, Nilsson O et al. Serum prostate-specific antigen complexed to alpha1-antichymotrypsin as an indicator of prostate cancer. J Urol 1996, 156: 1042-1049.

/2/ Elgamal AA, Cornillie FJ, Van poppel HP et al. Free to total prostate specific antigen as a single test for detection of significant stage T1c prostate cancer. J Urol 1996, 156: 1042-1049.

/3/ Bangma CH, Kranse R, Blijenberg BG et al.. The free to total serum prostate specific antigen ratio for staging prostate carcinoma. J Urol 1997, 157: 544-547.

/4/ Prestigiacomo AF, Stamey TA. Can free and total serum prostate specific antigen and prostatic volume distinguish between men with negative and positive systematic ultrasound guided prostate biopsies? J Urol 1997, 157: 189-194.

/5/ Lilja H, Christensson A, Dahlen U et al. Prostate-specific antigen in human serum occurs predominantly in complex with alpha1-antichymotrypsin. Clin Chem 1991, 37: 1618-1623.

/6/ Stenman UH, Leinonen J, Alfthan H et al. A complex between prostate-specific antigen and alpha1-antichymotrypsin is the major form of prostate-specific antigen in serum of patients with prostatic cancer: assay of the complex improves clinical sensitivity for cancer. Cancer Res 1991, 51: 222-226.

/7/ Catalona WJ, Smith DS, Wolfert RL et al. Evaluation of percentage of free serum prostate-specific antigen to improve specificity of prostate cancer screening. JAMA 1995, 274: 1214-1220

Radioactive Isotopes in
Clinical Medicine and Research XXIII
ed. by H. Bergmann, H. Köhn and H. Sinzinger

3-D- IMAGING AND VOLUME MATHEMATICS VERSUS COMMON STATIC IMAGING IN COMBINED INHALATION / PERFUSION LUNG SCINTIGRAPHY

M. Wenger, R. Moncayo, J. Zaknun, Claudia Bacher Stier, Eveline Donnemiller, A. Theurl*, C. Decristoforo, M. Oberladstätter and G. Riccabona

Dept. of Nuclear Medicine, University Hospital of Innsbruck, Austria
* Dept. of Nuclear Medicine, County Hospital of Lienz, Eastern Tyrol, Austria

SUMMARY: The purpose of the present study was to assess the diagnostic value and the practical usefulness of inhalation-/ perfusion SPET of the lung applying Multimodality three-dimensional (3-D-) data analysis. Lung perfusion scintigraphy (LP) is a common method for detecting sites of decreased perfusion. Lung inhalation scintigraphy (LI) is routinely performed when perfusion defects are visualized by LP. Visual analysis of studies showing abnormalities both in LP as well as in LI, can sometimes be difficult to carry out. The comparison of the images can be difficult in cases with inhalation and perfusion defects. Combined LI/LP in planar and SPET 3-D- technique was investigated in 33 patients having known or suspected lung disorders. Our data demonstrate an equal sensitivity of the 3-D-SPET in patients with pure pulmonary embolism (PE) and a better sensitivity in patients with chronic obstructive pulmonary disease (COPD) and PE compared with planar scans. Both methods require similar acquisition time, the time needed for 3-D- processing generally depends on the performance of the computer equipment.

INTRODUCTION

Combined inhalation-/perfusion lung scintigraphy is an established method for the differential diagnosis of lung perfusion defects [1]. When applying the same isotope for both radiotracers, a central problem is the sequence of the investigations [2]. Using Technegas™ for the inhalation scan, the achievable count rates usually remain lower than these of the corresponding perfusion study. Therefore inhalation scans are done mostly prior to perfusion scans. Interpretation problems may arise when both investigations show similar, but not identical distribution of the radioactivity. Furthermore, varying projection angles in planar studies may change the appearance of the resulting image. We intended to develop a simple method for an objective assessment of inhalation- /perfusion mismatches taking advantage of 3-D- reconstruction techniques.

PATIENTS

Thirty three patients were studied. Pulmonary embolism was suspected in 8 patients having no previous lung diseases; 13 patients suffering from chronic obstructive pulmonary disease developed symptoms of pulmonary embolism; 5 patients with progressive emphysema were expecting volume reduction surgery of the lung; 3 were scheduled for lung transplantation, and 4 patients were routinely examined after lung transplantation.

METHODS

Inhalation studies were done using ^{99m}Tc-Technegas (370 MBq). After tracer inhalation, planar images with 200 kcts each were collected in six projections (SIEMENS ZLC™), followed by the SPET study on a dual head camera equipped with LEAP collimators (ELSCINT HELIX™, 60 projections, 20 sec each, matrix size 64 x 64). This was immediately followed by i.v. injection of 111 MBq ^{99m}Tc-MAA, while the patient rested in the same supine position on the camera table. A second SPET was then started, however, the acquisition time was reduced to 7 sec. After completion of the SPET studies, planar images, 400 kcts each, were acquired. Twenty six patients (78.8%) had a planar LP scan up to 24 h prior to SPET. The raw data were transferred to a SUN™ Spark Station equipped with special multimodality software (HERMES™ from Nuclear Diagnostics Ltd., UK).

A pixel-based comparison between the pure SPET perfusion data and the inhalation-SPET data was accomplished by subtracting the decay-corrected and acquisition time compensated inhalation SPET from the combined LI/LP data. The 3-D- calculation of the transverse slice data was done choosing a 256 x 256 matrix, volume rendering, gray gradient shading, 25% lower threshold for both inhalation and perfusion raw data. After normalization to the same maximum pixel counts before subtraction, subtracted 3-D- images LI - LP were drawn in 16 projections each. The 3-D- images and the planar images were compared by three independent observers. Match or mismatch presence was considered when the interobserver agreement was 100%.

RESULTS

All mismatches found in the static images were also identified in the 3-D-images. In 2 patients which were considered to have matched defects in the static images, mismatched areas were observed by the 3-D- studies, therefore classifying them correctly as having PE. The results are summarized in the Table. Considering the technical aspects of the investigations, the total acquisition time of the combined SPET is only 30 minutes, while that of static image sampling varies between 30 to 60 minutes.

Table: Comparison of planar and 3-D imaging techniques

Scan results	n = 33	normal	mismatch	match	match and mismatch
	Static	3	8	13	9
	3 - D	3	9	11	10

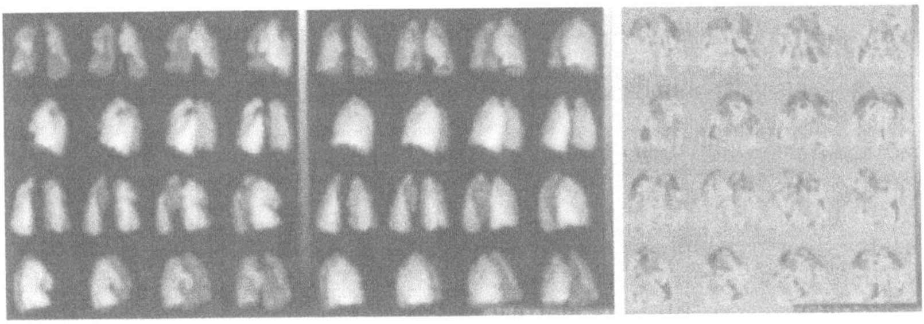

Fig. 1: 3-D- display of COPD and PE (LP left, LI middle, subtracted right)

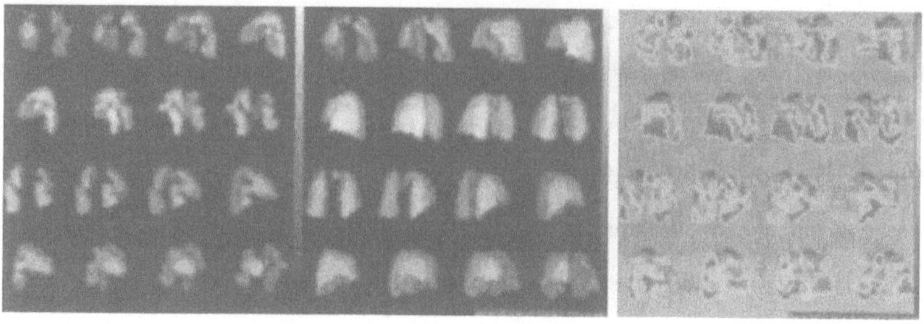
Fig. 2: 3-D- display of pure PE (LP left, LI middle, subtracted right)

DISCUSSION

Three dimensional multimodality imaging of inhalation- /perfusion lung SPET provides a reliable additional tool for the detection of mismatched areas in LI/LP scans. The feature of pixel based subtraction of the inhalation data from the perfusion data offers the facility of gaining a pure perfusion SPET. The „Subtracted Image Display" is able to visualize even small mismatched sites of lung parenchyma. In contrast to the dual isotope technique with ^{81}Kr Gas, the present method is carried out with one single isotope for both scintigraphies which positively influences costs and procedure requirements.

In conclusion, our results suggest that 3-D- Multimodality subtraction imaging is superior to convenient planar imaging in patients with pathologic perfusion and inhalation scans. The method does not exceed accuracy of conventional planar imaging in patients with perfusion defects and normal inhalation scans. Currently, a method which could provide quantification of the mismatched parenchymal volume is being developed. This might be of interest in the control of therapy success in patients with pulmonary embolism and in patients after lung surgery.

REFERENCES

1. James-JM; Testa-HJ: The use of 99Tcm-Technegas in the investigation of patients with pulmonary thromboembolism. Nucl-Med-Commun. 1995 Oct; 16(10): 802-10

2. Isawa-T; Teshima-T; Anazawa-Y; Miki-M; Soni-PS: Technegas versus krypton-81m gas as an inhalation agent. Comparison of pulmonary distribution at total lung capacity. Clin-Nucl-Med. 1994 Dec; 19(12): 1085-90

Radioactive Isotopes in
Clinical Medicine and Research XXIII
ed. by H. Bergmann, H. Köhn and H. Sinzinger

INVESTIGATION OF PLAZMINOGEN ACTIVATOR EFFECTS ON PROGRESSIVE ISCHEMIA INTO THE TISSUE ADJACENT THE BURN INJURY BY TC-99m MIBI SCINTIGRAPHY AND AUTORADIOGRAPHY IN AN EXPERIMENTAL LOCAL BURN MODEL

Bengül Günalp[1], Seyfettin Ilgan[1], Selçuk Işık[2], Ünal Þahin[2]
[1]Department of Nuclear Medicine and [2]Department of Plastic and Reconstructive Surgery
Gülhane Military Medical Academy and Faculty 06018 Turkey

This study was designed to determine the effect of recombinant tissue-type plasminogen activator (r-tPA) on vessels thrombosis in zones of stasis postburn. Standardized full-thickness burns of the experimental group were treated with r-tPA. To evaluate perfusion of panniculus carnosus muscle, which is beneath the burned area of skin, 99m-Tc MIBI scintigraphy and autoradiography were performed.. The percentage of survived interspace areas in the experimental group was 87.8%, while it was 31.8% in the control group ($p<0.05$). The results confirm that treatment with this selective fibrinolytic agent (r-tPA) after burn injury would have some benefits on saving the zone of stasis in burns.

Introduction

Vessel-thrombosis under or near burned areas is an well-observed postburn complication. Two to three hours following a scald injury, hypercoagulability of the lymph and plasma occur (1,2). During the burn wound healing process, these initially formed blood clots have to be removed by enzymatic digestion usually with plasmin. Tissue-type plasminogen activator (tPA) is known as one of the second-generation thrombolytic agents, which have the theoretical possibility of achieving selective thrombolysis (3,4). It is suggested that these drugs can be used for selective lysis of pathological fibrin because of their specificity for it. Recombinant tPA (r-tPA) which is biotechnologically synthesized from eukaryotic cells has the same biochemical and enzymatic properties as does natural t-PA.

Saving the 'zone of stasis' which surrounds the thermally injured dermis region has been the goal of burn research. Diminished circulation in this region results in progressive ischemia in this zone. Maintaining adequate blood flow and vessel patency can save the viable tissues and dermis of this zone of stasis (1). An experimental study has been devised to show the r-tPA treatment maintained patent vessels in the zone of stasis and prevented further necrosis of this region.

Material and methods

Animals and the burn model: Adult Sprague-Dawley rats (350-400g) were used. Anesthesia was achieved by pentobarbital [35 mg/kg intraperitoneally (i.p.)]. The entire backs of the rats were shaved with clippers. The 'comb burn' model as described by Regas and Erhlich was carried out on the back of the rats with a special brass probe containing four rows (1x2cm) and three interspaces (0.5x1cm) (1). This special device was immersed in boiling water until thermal equilibrium was achieved. The heated brass band was placed on the back of the rats 0.5cm lateral and parallel to the midline and held for 20s without any pressure. The same burn model was made the other side of the backs again, 0.5 cm lateral and parallel to the midline, 15 min. later (Figure 1).

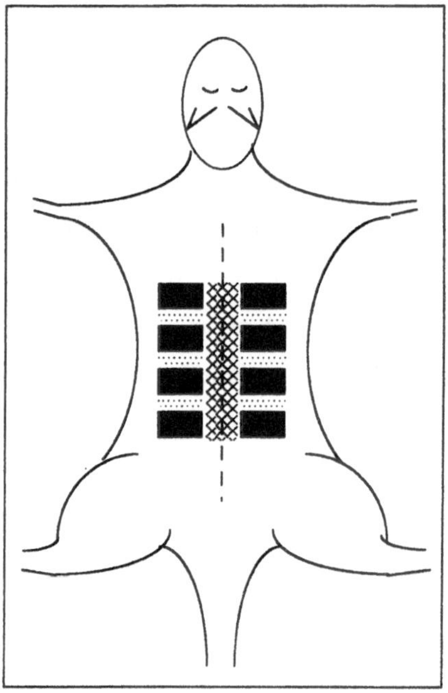

Figure 1: The comb burn model. The vertical space area (1x5.5cm) (hatched area) between two sets of burn rows were evaluated as well as the interspace areas (0.5x1cm each) (dotted areas).

Twenty rats were randomly assigned to experimental or control groups (n = 10 rats per group). Each group was then subdivided into subgroups according to assessment time, either 24h or 7 days (n = 5 in each subgroup).

Treatment: After the creation of full-thickness skin burns, rats were held for 2h under anesthesia. In the experimental group, freshly prepared r-tPA (1 mg/kg) (Actilyse, Boehringer Ingelheim, Germany) was administered by intravenous route via the exposed femoral vein with an insulin needle. The contol group rats were given same amount of saline by the same route.

Assessment of muscle perfusion: Twenty-four hours after the burn injury, the experimental and control subgroups (n=5 in each) under pentobarbital anesthesia were injected with 3 mCi of technetium-99m methoxyisobutylisonitrile (Tc-99m MIBI) via the femoral veins. After 30 min the rats were killed by decapitation. The entire back skin including the panniculus carnosus muscle layer was incised and dissected away from the body. The specimen was laid on a translucent film layer (0.2mm in thickness) which was used as a carrier in order to prevent distortion of the specimen and spreading of the radioactive agent by extravasated fluids. The skin was placed so the outer skin surface contacted the carrier. On the day 7, the method was repeated for five more experimental and five more control subgroups. The specimens were immediately put under the gamma camera (Starcam 400 ACT, General Electrics, USA) and images were obtained with a pinhole collimator for 15 min with a 256x256 matrix. Tc-99m MIBI uptake was expressed as percentage of activity taken up in the interspaces compared to that taken up in the burned areas. After imaging, specimens were used for direct autoradiography. Specimens were placed in intimate contact with the film (Hyperfilm-MP, Amersham) and, then, placed in authoradiography cassette (Hypercasette, Amersham). After 24h exposure at -70^0C, the films were developed using an automatic processor (Cronex T-G Processor, Dupont). The total necrotic and viable areas of interspaces and vertical space area between the two groups of burn rows were counted after transferring the images to sheet with $1mm^2$ grids.

Statistical analysis: Average blood flow measurements, Tc-99m MIBI uptake percentages and average survived interspace percentages were statistically compared using one-way analysis of variance (ANOVA) and unpaired two-tailed Student's t-test.

Results

Tc-99m MIBI Scintigraphy and Autoradiography: Uptake of Tc-99m MIBI by interspace areas was higher than by burn areas in both the experimental and the control groups. At 7 days, Tc-99m MIBI images revealed 60-90 % more uptake in interspaces than in the burned areas while uptake ranged between 20 and 50 % in the control control group. The necrotic area patterns were in accordance with autoradiography patterns but it was difficult to map out the borders. Autoradiographs gave excellent results that showed the necrotic area borders exactly (Figure 2) The mean percentage of survived interspace and vertical space areas was higher in the experimental group than in the control group at either 24h or day 7. On day 7, the average surviving interspace and vertical space areas was 87.8 % of the total evaluated area of 8.5 cm^2 (2 x 1.5 cm^2 of interspaces + 5.5 cm^2 of the vertical space area). The average surviving percentage was 31.8 % in the control group at this time. These results were significantly different ($P<0.05$).

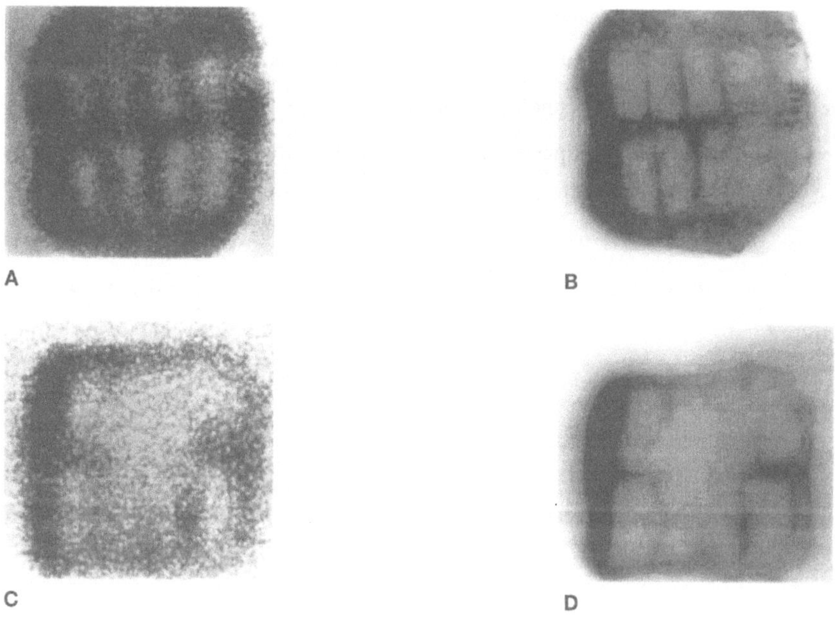

Figure 2: A) Tc-99m MIBI images of entire back skin of treated group had higher uptakes in the vertical space and interspace areas compared with burned areas. **B)** Autoradiography of the specimen seen in A. Note the significant borders between necrotic and viable areas. **C)** Tc-99m MIBI image of the back skin of control group revealed extended necrotic areas. **D)** Autoradiography of specimen seen in C

Discussion

The 'comb burn' model first described by Regas and Ehrlich was found to be ideal for research about the 'zone of stasis' (1,5). Among the evaluation methods, Laser Doppler blood flowmetry and Tc-99m MIBI images gave knowledge about the skin and muscle perfusion of each area, respectively. Autoradiography gave the exact borders between necrotic and survived areas. This simple technique is the method of choice when spatial resolution is more important than absolute sensitivity. Autoradiography produces quantitative images in which the absorbency of the film image is directly proportional to the amount of radioactivity. If given access to a digital autoradiography system, the results would have been quantitated.

Alterations in blood flow and vessel patency in the interspaces are predictive of whether or not the interspace dermis will retain viable or become incorporated into the acutely killed region (1). The fibrinolytic effect of r-tPA resulted in patent vessels in zone of stasis in the present study. That restoration of both vascular patency and blood flow of this area was achieved by r-tPA treatment was significantly confirmed by skin blood flow measurements, Tc-99m MIBI scintigrams and autoradiography. Thus, experimental group had significant survival rates of interspaces and vertical space areas than did the untreated group. The circulating zone of stasis achieved by this agent ensured the survival rate by an average of 87%. It is believed that the major pathology in the zone of stasis is thrombus formation that restricts the blood circulation and, that the effective agent in this situation should be the fibrinolytic one which has a clinical usage. As a result, this study confirms that treatment with this selective fibrinolytic agent (r-tPA) 2 h after burn injury would have some benefits on saving the zone of stasis in burns.

References

1. Regas F.C., Ehrlich H.P. Elucidating the vascular response to burns with a new rat model. J Trauma 1992; 32: 557-563.

2 Arturson G. Pathophysiology of the burn wound and pharmacological treatment. The Rudi Hermans Lecture, 1995. Burns 1996; 22: 255-274.

3. Agnelli G. In: Agnelli G., ed. Thrrombolysis Yearbook 1995. Amsterdam: Excepta Medica, 1195; pp. 41-48.

4. Collen D. On The regulation and control of fibrinolysis. Thromb Haemost 1980; 43: 77-89

5. Çetinkale O., Demir M., Sayman H. B., et al. Effects of allopurinol, ibuprofen and cyclosporin A on local microcirculatory distrurbances due to burn injuries. Burns 1997; 23: 43-49.

Radioactive Isotopes in
Clinical Medicine and Research XXIII
ed. by H. Bergmann, H. Köhn and H. Sinzinger

IMPROVEMENT IN SPECT IMAGING AND REDUCTION OF THE ABSORBED DOSE USING AN ADDITIONAL COMPTON ENERGY WINDOW FOR ^{18}FDG

[1]C. Haas, [3,4]M. Ljungberg, [2]H. Fritzsche, [4]J. Dahlström, [3]S.-E. Strand and [1]E. Hillbrand.
[1]Dept. of Medical Physics and [2]Dept. of Nuclear Medicine, Landeskrankenhaus, Feldkirch, Austria, [3]Dept. of Radiation Physics, Lund University, Sweden, [4]Dept. of Clinical Physiology, Helsingborg Hospital, Sweden.

SUMMARY
A method that adds data acquired in a secondary Compton window to the data obtained from the photopeak window has shown to produce images of similar quality for a reduction in the administered ^{18}FDG activity from 450 MBq to 300 MBq. The underlying justification for this method is that primary events that are correctly positioned appear in the Compton region due to partly absorption in the crystal. The method does not only reduce the cost but also reduce the absorbed dose to the patient by 23%. The protocol has been used clinically for 12 month. Both phantom experiments with comparative Monte Carlo simulations and clinical examples are shown.

INTRODUCTION
When simultaneously imaging ^{99}Tc^{m}MIBI/^{18}FDG for myocardial perfusion/viability studies, the use of ultra-high energy collimators is necessary. The sensitivity is low due to the thin crystal resulting in high noise levels in the projection data. Earlier Monte Carlo (MC) studies have shown that a significant fraction of the primary photons (not scattered in the patient) is not registered in the photo-peak window (PW) due to Compton interaction in the crystal [1]. Thus, 'correctly positioned' events are lost. Using a second Compton window (CW), such 'lost' events can be added to the PW data. The present study compares phantom studies with MC simulations and gives examples of patient studies with and without addition of the CW.

MATERIAL AND METHODS
Phantom studies: A Data Spectrum cardiac phantom with a cold defect at a 90° location was inserted in a 11-cm radius cylindrical water phantom. SPECT data was collected in 64x64 matrix mode, 64 views, 360°, and 50s/view on a Siemens MultiSPECT system and reconstructed by filtered backprojection (Butterworth pre-filter 4th order, cut-off=0.3 cm^{-1}). Studies were made

with 16.5 MBq ^{18}FDG in the cardiac insertion only and with 17.9 MBq in the cardiac and 77.3 MBq in the whole cylindrical tank, respectively. Separate acquisitions were made for PW (472-550 keV) and CW (250-390 keV. MC studies were made [2] to compare simulations with measurement.

Patient studies: Adding a CW has been applied in routine ^{99}Tc^{m}-MIBI/ ^{18}FDG studies at the Feldkirch hospital during a period of 12 month. Before, a single 15% PW was used for imaging ^{18}FDG. The administered activity was then 450 MBq 18FDG and 625 MBq ^{99}Tc^{m}-MIBI. In the current protocol, 300 MBq ^{18}FDG and 550 MBq ^{99}Tc^{m}-MIBI is administered 1h prior to acquisition. The camera system allows four energy windows, which can be stored in three separate studies. For the perfusion study with ^{99}Tc^{m}, a 20% window is centred around 140 keV. Additionally, a 20% window is set around 170 keV to correct for the ^{18}FDG contribution to the ^{99}Tc^{m}-photopeak window. The events from the ^{18}FDG PW (511 keV, 15%) and the CW (320 keV, 44%) are added together during acquisition. Therefore, we cannot present studies comparing slices with PW alone and PW+CW of the same patient.

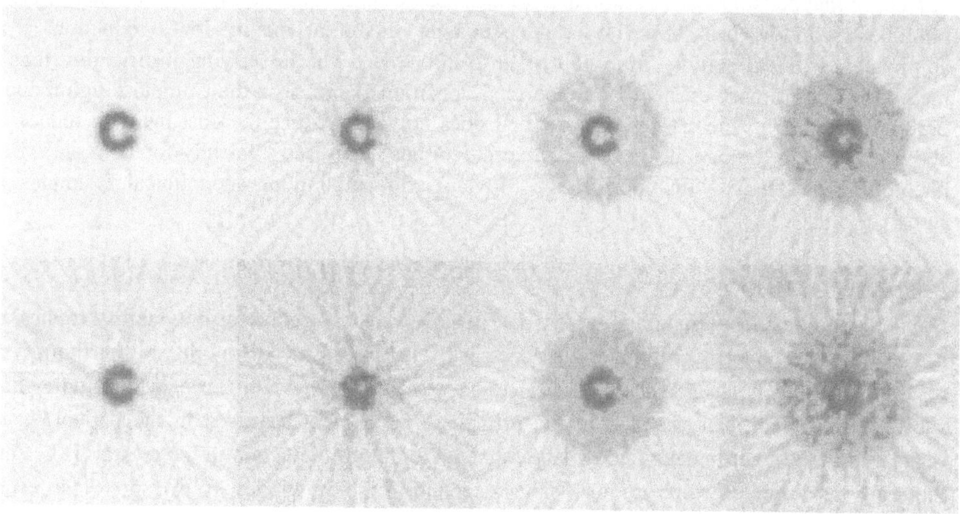

Fig 1: Reconstructed images for the MC simulation (upper row) and the phantom studies (lower row). The columns show from the left, reconstructed images for PW and CW with no background and PW and CW with background, respectively

RESULTS AND DISCUSSION

Fig. 1 shows reconstructed images for the phantom measurements and corresponding MC simulations. There is a good agreement between simulated and measured images. In Fig. 2, circumferencial profiles calculated from the images in Fig 1. are shown. Fig. 3 shows examples of ^{18}FDG heart studies for PW imaging only (A-B) where 420 MBq ^{18}FDG have been administered and PW+CW imaging (C-D) where 300 MBq ^{18}FDG have been given. The images with PW+CW contain about twice as much events for the same acquisition time as those with PW only despite the lower administered activity

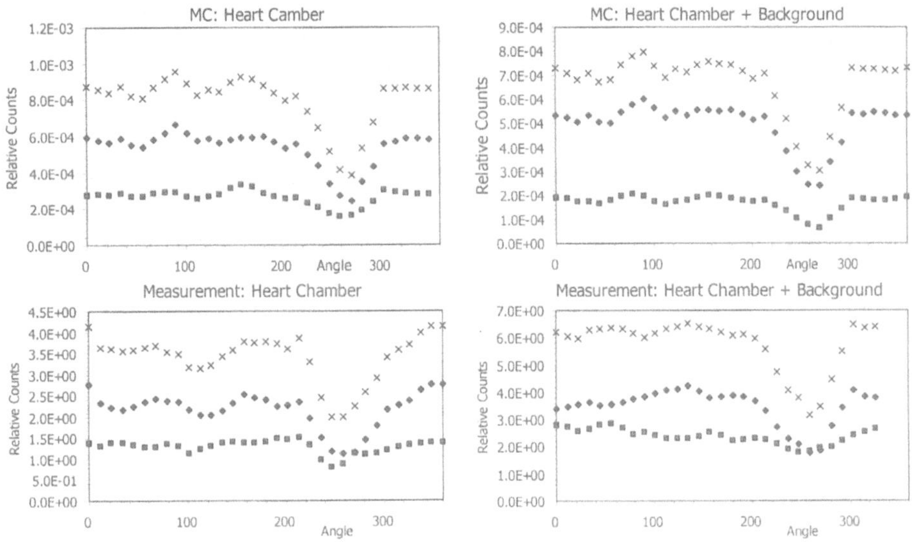

Fig 2: Circumferencial profiles, calculated from the images in Fig.1 The different curves represent PW (diamonds), CW (squares) and PW+CW (crosses).

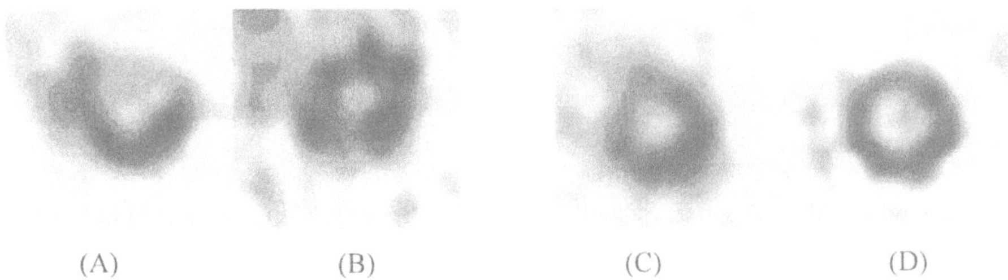

Fig 3: (A) 74 years male, inferior wall infarction. Matching of defects in MIBI and FDG images, thus area of scar in inferior wall (B) 58 years male, scar in inferior wall, defect in MIBI uptake (perfusion) in the scar area but FDG uptake inferior, thus sign of viable myocardium. (C) 72 years male, inferior wall infarction. Matching of defects in MIBI and FDG images, thus area of scar in inferior wall. (D) 62 years male, stenosis of RCA / CX, scar apical, inferior, lateral. Defect in MIBI uptake, but FDG uptake in the inferior and posterolateral area, thus sign of viable myocardium.

The direct addition of the events in the CW adds scatter to the image, which may degrade image contrast and quantification. Our hypothesis is that the degradation from CW scatter depends on the source distribution. In cardiac imaging, the area-of-interest is the heart region only. High-energy scattered photons have a relative long mean-free path length and thus result in events in the image outside the evaluation region. Therefore, these scatter events might not significantly influence the evaluation of the heart uptake. More work, based on MC simulations, is necessary here. Furthermore, in the dual isotope method the diagnosis is regularly found by comparing scar areas in the perfusion and metabolism images by looking at match/mismatch patterns in the areas of interest. To our experience, so far this possibility is not affected by the additional scatter component in the PW+CW images.

For both radiopharmaceuticals, the effective dose was calculated from reported organ doses using the tissue weighting factors for the different organs and tissues which are documented by ICRP [3]. The effective dose for the $^{99}Tc^{m}$-MIBI studies (evaluated from the information paper to the Cardiolite® MIBI preparation set from DuPont Pharma) is 15.1 μSv/MBq giving an effective dose equivalent of 9.4 mSv per investigation for the old protocol and 8.3 mSv for the new protocol. For ^{18}FDG, the whole body dose equivalent [4] is 20.4 μSv/MBq, which results in an effective dose of 9.2 mSv for the old protocol and 6.1 mSv for the new protocol. Summarising the effective dose is 18.6 mSv per investigation for the old protocol and is now 14.4 mSv per investigation for the new protocol, which represents a total effective dose reduction of 23 %. In summary, adding events in the PW from the CW enhances the image quality and reduces the effective dose. We recommend that this method should be used when applicable.

ACKNOWLEDGEMENT

This work has been funded by Stig and Ragna Gorthons Foundation #100/97, the Swedish Radiation Protection Institute #963.96, the Gunnar Nilsson Foundation and the Kamprad Foundation.

REFERENCES

1. Ljungberg M, Ohlsson T, Sandell A, Strand S. Scintillation Camera Imaging of Positron-emitting Radionuclides In The Compton Region. *Conference Records of the IEEE Medical Imaging Conference* 1996;**2**:977-81.
2. Ljungberg M, Strand S. A Monte Carlo Program Simulating Scintillation Camera Imaging. *Comput Meth Programs Biomed* 1989;**29**:257-72.
3. International Comission on Radiological Protection (ICRP). ICRP Publication 60: 1990 Recommendations of the International Commission on Radiological Protection Oxford: Pergamon Press, 1991.
4. Jones SC, Alavi A, Christman D, Montanez I, Wolf AP, Reivich M. The radiation dosimetry of 2-[F-18]Fluoro-2-Deoxy-Glucose in man. *J Nucl Med* 1982;**23**:613-7.

Radioactive Isotopes in
Clinical Medicine and Research XXIII
ed. by H. Bergmann, H. Köhn and H. Sinzinger

USABLE COUNTRATES FOR A COMMERCIALLY AVAILABLE DUAL-HEAD-PET SYSTEM

M. Oberladstätter, U. Noelpp*, J. Zaknun, G. Riccabona

Univ.Clinic for Nuclear Medicine, Anichstraße 35, A-6020 Innsbruck, Austria
* University of Berne, Insel Hospital, Dept.of Nuclear Medicine, CH-3010 Bern, Switzerland

SUMMARY: Two gammacameras of the same type with coincidence detection options were tested with regard to the usable or allowable countrates. The countrate features are particularly important as very high singles countrates are necessary to gain high enough true coincidence countrates to keep the patient study duration acceptably short.

INTRODUCTION

Dual-head gammacameras with an add-on option for coincidence detection provide an interesting further possibility to perform PET-studies with fluorodeoxyglucose (FDG).
When compared with PET ring systems, the physical limitations of the dual-head systems are concentrated mainly in the following features: countrates, efficiency and attenuation correction (see fig.1).
During installation tests the system in Berne was exposed to extremely high countrates and was found to produce artefacts in the reconstructed slices. We therefore subjected the systems in Berne and Innsbruck to controlled tests to find the range of countrates which can be used safely in a clinical environment without the risk of artefacts due to too high countrates.

MATERIAL AND METHODS

To switch the operation mode for the given dual-head-system (ADAC VERTEX MCD) from single-photon mode to coincidence mode one has to exchange the collimator set used for single-photon-mode studies for a socalled scatter shield set as well as to load a different set of correction tables. These actions altogether need about 5 minutes, whereby the collimator exchange after its initialization is done without any user interaction.
A 3D-phantom (JASZCZAK-phantom) with the cold rods insert in place (in Innsbruck) was filled with 120 MBq of F-18 FDG and tap water and mounted on the pallet with its axis of symmetry parallel to the patient axis but offset from the center of rotation axis by about 7 cm. For the series of measurements in Berne the phantom was used without any insert.
The acquisition parameters were 30 s/azimuth and 32 azimuths, 2 windows centered at the annihilation peak and at an energy of 300 keV (which is within the Compton range) for each detector and window widths of 30 % each.
A series of acquisitions was performed starting every half hour for a duration of about 5 hours altogether.

	SPECT- Systems		PET-Systems	
	2-head-SPECT	2-head-PET option	Partial Ring-PET	Ring-PET
Number of usable SPECT-tracers	++	++ [1]	- -	- -
Number of usable PET-tracers	- [2]	+	+ [3]	++ [4]
System spacial resolution	-	++	++	++
Sensitivity	-	+ [5]	+	++
Countrates	-	- [6]	+	++
Dynamic studies	- -	- -	+	++
Attenuation correction	-	- (+) [7]	++	++
Quantification of activity/volume	-	- (+) [7]	++	++
System costs	++	+	-	- -

- -	very disadvantageous resp. not applicable	1	all SPECT tracers including Tl-201
-	disadvantageous	2	using 511 keV-Collimators
+	advantageous	3	operated without cyclotron
++	very advantageous	4	operated with cyclotron
		5	3D acquisition modus
		6	although singles countrates two orders of magnitude higher can be processed
		7	with attenuation correction option

Fig.1: Dual-head-PET system versus Ring-PET systems, comparison of selected features

RESULTS

The asymetrical position of the phantom resulted in different singles countrates for the two detector heads in Innsbruck. The activity content of the phantom was chosen in a way that the countrate slightly exceedes the maximal singles countrate per detector specifications of the system, stated as ≥ 2,4 Mc/s, namely 2,5 Mc/s for the nearer head.

Every single acquisition was reconstructed in a standard manner, using the built-in iterative reconstruction algorithm, Butterworth-filter with cutoff 0,5 and order 5 as well as averaging 3 slices.

We found that the coincidence countrates saturated at values of < 30 kc/s for the system in Berne, whereas the system in Innsbruck allowed coincidence countrates of ≥ 35 kc/s.

Connected with the saturation of the coincidence countrate we saw pronounced artefacts along the COR line and less pronounced ones parallel to that line most visible in the sagittal and coronal slices, which were named 'pearlstring'-artefacts or 'fishnet'-artefacts (see fig. 2). Fig. 3 shows the course of singles countrate and coincidence countrate versus activity content within the phantom, as well as the presence or absence of the artefacts.

DISCUSSION

Associated with the onset of artefacts during phantom-studies in coincidence mode are singles countrates in the range of about 1,5 Mc/s per detector head, which is well below the specified maximum countrate.

To establish certain safety margins for patient-studies we therefore limited the *usable* singles countrates per detector for the faster system in Innsbruck to ≤ 1,3 Mc/s, the coincidence countrates to ≤ 20 kc/s when using photopeak-photopeak as well as photopeak-Compton coincidences (PP + PC, 30 % window). The usable coincidence countrates for photopeak-photopeak only coincidences (PP only, 30% window) were limited to ≤ 10 kc/s.

Especially within lateral or coronal slices through the spine under bad conditions the artefacts could mimic hot lesions. But using the established limits, no artefacts within the patient studies did show up. Until now we performed more than 150 patient studies in coincidence mode.

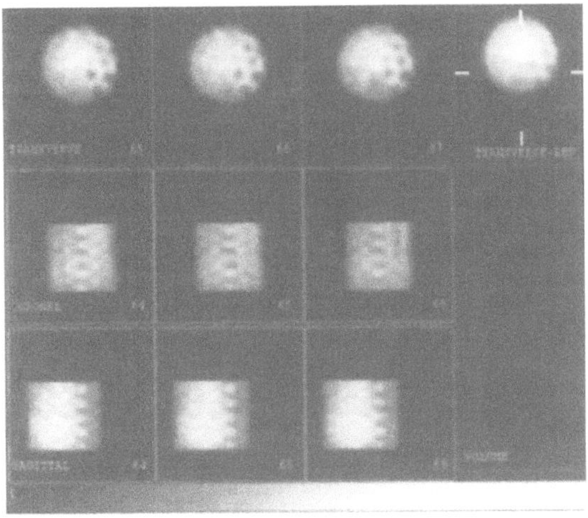

Fig.2: Coincidence mode study of JASZCZAK-phantom with cold-rods-insert in upper half, artefacts in reconstructed slices at very high countrates.
Singles countrates CR(detector 1) = 2,2 Mc/s; CR(detector 2) = 1,5 Mc/s; coincidence countrates CR = 35 kc/s.

CONCLUSION

With a recently developed, commercially available dual-head system the extent of functional diagnostic imaging using gammacameras was enhanced by incorporating new concepts of counting and positioning the events within NaJ(Tl)-scintillation detectors. On the basis of spending one analog-to-digital converter per photomultiplier, of fast pulse clipping methods and non-Anger methods of position calculation is was possible to speed up the camera electronics in a way that, besides the standard planar or SPECT scintigraphy, coincidence-detection techniques are now available.

These systems however must be sensitive as well as fast enough. They ought to produce a high enough (coincidence) countrate, to be able to finish patient studies in time with a good enough statistical quality.

The very high countrates, the detector heads operate with in coincidence mode, are quite unusual for NaJ(Tl)-scintillation techniques. To avoid artefacts due to high countrates, studies have to be acquired within a range of countrates, which must be well within certain limits, although the systems are able to detect far higher (singles) countrates.

The usable countrates of the given dual-head system permit FDG-patient studies to be performed within a schedule similar to some SPECT studies.

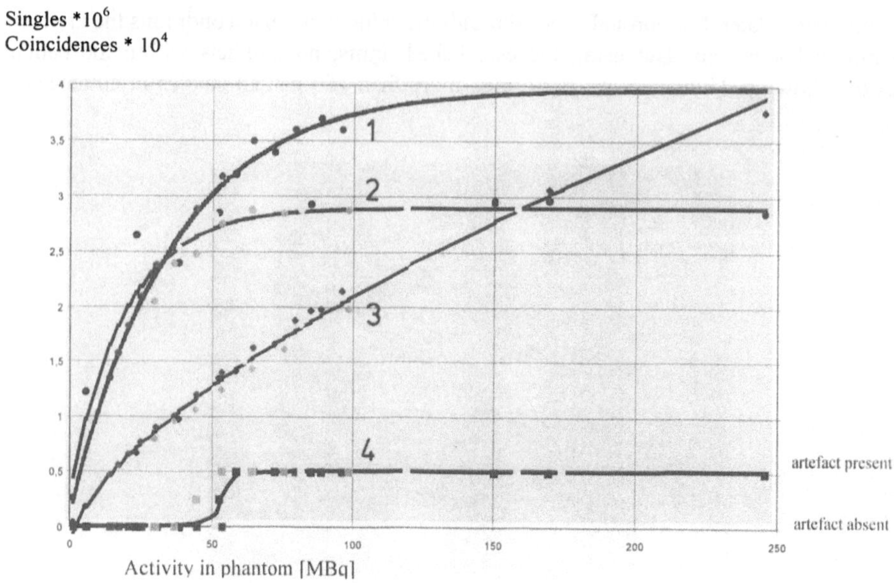

Fig.3: Coincidence mode study of JASZCZAK-phantom countrates and onset of artefacts versus activity

1 ... coincidence countrate for faster system (Innsbruck)

2 ... coincidence countrate for slower system (Berne)

3 ... singles countrate

4 ... presence or absence of 'pearlstring'-artefacts

ACKNOWLEDGEMENTS

We gratefully acknowledge the cooperation and help provided by the colleagues in Milano, Munich and Utrecht.

REFERENCES

1. Jarrit PH., Acton PD.: PET imaging using gamma camera systems: a review. Nucl-Med-Comm. 1996 Sep; 17(9): 758-66
2. Karp JS., Muehllehner G., Qu H., Yan XH.: Singles transmission in volume-imaging PET with a 137-Cs source. Phys-Med-Biol. 1995 May, 40(5): 929-44.
3. Dell MA.: Radiation safety review for 511-keV emitters in nuclear medicine. J-Nucl-Med-Technol. 1997 Mar, 25(1): 12-7

Radioactive Isotopes in
Clinical Medicine and Research XXIII
ed. by H. Bergmann, H. Köhn and H. Sinzinger

INTERNAL EXPOSURE TO RELATIVES OF RADIOIODINE THERAPY PATIENTS FROM I-131 INHALATION AT HOME

W. Eschner, U. Wellner, H.-W. Hillger and H. Schicha

Clinic for Nuclear Medicine, University of Cologne, D-50924 Köln, Germany

SUMMARY: We studied the exposure to relatives of radioiodine therapy (RIT) patients from inhalation of ^{131}I exhaled by the patients at home after their discharge from the hospital. Whole-body ^{131}I activity was measured in 17 volunteers, all relatives of patients who had undergone RIT for benign thyroid disease, a few days after the patients' discharge. In 9 out of these, thyroidal ^{131}I activity was measured, too. The measured activity was compared with the result of calculations based on a three-compartment model of iodine kinetics. A good correlation ($r = 0{,}88$) was established between measured and predicted thyroidal activities under the assumption that 2 μg from a daily iodine intake of 60 μg are being exhaled. Effective dose from inhaled ^{131}I did never exceed 100 μSv. Using the same model parameters effective doses of more than 8 mSv are predicted for out-patient RIT under worst-case assumptions.

INTRODUCTION

Patients undergoing radioiodine therapy exhale some portion of the administered ^{131}I, while most of the activity is excreted via the urinary pathway. Measurements of the amount of exhaled iodine, however, are sparse and inconclusive (1-4).

European and national recommendations have recently been published concerning the release of patients after radioiodine therapy (5, 6). They take into account exposure to persons in the vicinity of the patients from external radiation but not from inhalation of ^{131}I exhaled by the patient.

The aim of this study was to measure the amount of ^{131}I inhaled by family members after the RIT patients had returned home, compute resulting doses, and compare the measured values with predictions from a kinetic model for iodine.

MATERIALS AND METHODS

In n = 17 volunteers (all adult partners of patients who had undergone RIT for benign thyroid disease, administered activities ranging from 300 to 1400 MBq) we measured whole-body iodine activity in a whole-body counter between 1 and 3 days after discharge of the patient. In n = 9 out of these, activity in the thyroid was measured separately.

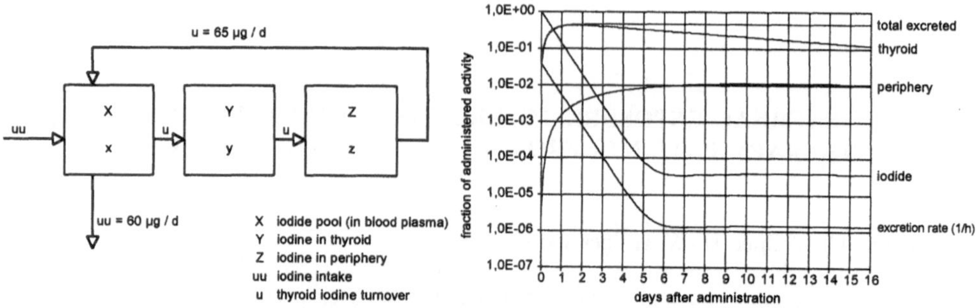

Fig. 1: Three-compartment model of iodine kinetics (left) and distribution of iodine to the model compartments (right).

The measured values were compared with calculations based on a three-compartment model of iodine kinetics. The model (Fig. 1) assumes iodine to be exhaled only in inorganic form (from the iodide pool) and with a rate proportional to total iodide excretion (2 µg/d). The model approach (7) was extended to take into account the time that patient and partner spent together, as well as room volumes and air throughput in the patients' homes. Those data were recorded from the volunteers via a questionnaire. Effective half-life of iodine excretion was determined for each patient during the period of stay in the hospital (minimum 72 hours in this group).

RESULTS AND DISCUSSION

Computed and measured activities correlate well (r = 0,88 for thyroidal activities, Fig. 2).

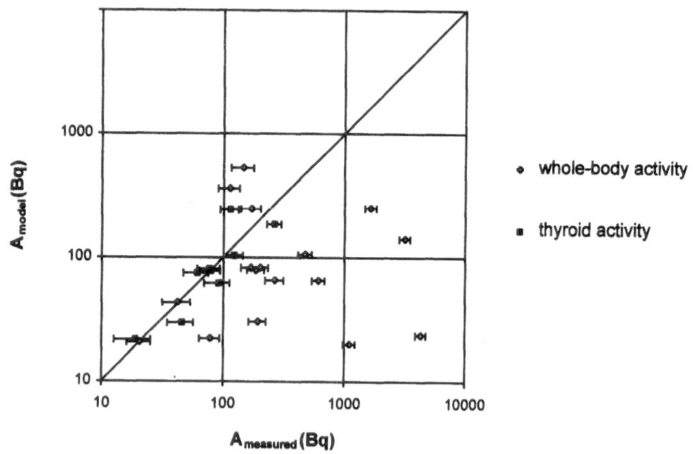

Fig. 2: Predicted vs. measured I-131 activity

The amount of inhaled iodine was computed from measured activities using the above model and the recorded patient data. From that iodine intake, effective doses were calculated using tabulated dose coefficients (8). Effective doses did not exceed 100 μSv in any case (Table 1).

patient	administered activity (MBq)	effective dose (μSv) from whole-body measurement	effective dose (μSv) from thyroid measurement	predicted dose (μSv) assuming release after 48h	predicted dose (μSv) assuming out-patient therapy
GQ	296	24,6	5,3	28	1433
UK	370	3,4	1,6	37	1864
GB	444	0,8	-	37	1878
IM	444	3,4	1,2	36	1818
ZU	481	4,9	1,7	54	2722
IH	518	0,3	-	45	2277
ES	555	2,2	-	66	3320
GK	555	2,3	-	68	3427
HS	666	10,5	2,8	80	4018
WC	720	3,9	1,0	38	1927
EW	740	64,1	-	53	2662
MK	777	1,6	0,4	78	3932
KE	925	64,0	-	78	3850
MT	1036	11,1	-	165	8301
KF	1184	3,5	2,3	148	7454
DS	1332	3,7	1,5	112	5635
CJ	1406	22,3	-	152	7631

Table 1: Measured and predicted effective doses

The model was then used to compute internal doses to relatives which would have resulted in case the patients had left the ward after 48 hours (which is the minimum time of hospitalization in Germany). Assuming „worst-case“ conditions otherwise, namely 12 hours being spent together in the living room plus an extra 8 hours in a common bedroom, the model predicts a maximum of 165 μSv effective dose from ^{131}I inhalation (Table 1). As can be seen from Fig. 1, radioiodine excretion (and thus exhalation) decreases exponentially during the first few days, such that under otherwise similar assumptions effective doses exceeding 8 mSv are predicted from the model for the case of out-patient therapy.

Our model gives good agreement with the measured values when exhalation is assumed to account for approx. 3% of total excreted iodine, resulting in an integral exhalation of more than 1% of the total administered activity. That value is between one and two orders of magnitude higher than reported by other authors (1-3). Certainly, more experimental evidence is needed to substantiate these findings, particularly for the first couple of days after administration.

Furthermore, the whole-body counter cannot discriminate between incorporation and contamination. Measurements of thyroidal ^{131}I activity are less likely to be influenced by contamination than whole-body measurements, which leads us to conclude that a significant amount of the detected whole-body activity is probably contamination, especially in those cases where the measured activity outweighs the predicted one by an order of magnitude or more (Fig. 2). But even in the case of incorporation the cause does not have to be inhalation but can also be ingestion, e.g. from contaminated cutlery and crockery.

CONCLUSION

Internal exposure is well below 1 mSv when the radioiodine therapy patient stays in the hospital for at least 48 hours as recommended by the Strahlenschutzkommission (6). In out-patient RIT, however, significant exposures from inhaled I-131 alone are possible unless recommendations for the patients' behaviour (5) are strictly followed.

REFERENCES

1. Nishizawa K, Ohara K, Ohshima M, Maekoshi H, Orito T, Watanabe T. Monitoring of I excretions and used materials of patients treated with ^{131}I. Health Physics 1980; 38: 467-481.
2. Laßmann M, Hänscheid H, Alt P, Börner W. Messung der ^{131}I-Aktivität in der Fortluft einer Radiojod-Therapiestation. In: W. Koelzer RM, ed. Strahlenschutz: Physik und Meßtechnik. Köln: Fachverband für Strahlenschutz, 1994:719-722.
3. Krzesniak J, Chomicki O, Czerminska M, Gorowski T. Airborne radioiodine contamination caused by ^{131}I treatment. Nuklearmedizin 1979; 18: 246-251.
4. Ibis E, Wilson C, Collier B, Akansel G, Isitman A, Yoss R. Iodine-131 contamination from thyroid cancer patients. J Nucl Med 1992; 33: 2110-2115.
5. Expert Group ex art 31 EURATOM. Guidance for radiation protection following iodine-131 therapy concerning doses due to out-patients or discharged in-patients (Final Draft). 1997.
6. Strahlenschutzkommission (SSK). Strahlenschutzgrundsätze für die Radioiodtherapie. Bundesanzeiger Nr. 68: 1997: 4769.
7. Wellner U, Alef K, Schicha H. Der Einfluß physiologischer und pharmakologischer Iodmengen auf den ^{131}I -Uptake der Schilddrüse - eine Modellrechnung. Nuklearmedizin 1996; 35: 251-263.
8. International Commission on Radiological Protection (ICRP). Age-dependent Doses to Members of the Public from Intake of Radionuclides: Part 4. Inhalation Dose Coefficients. ICRP Publication 71. Oxford: Elsevier Science Ltd., 1995.

Radioactive Isotopes in
Clinical Medicine and Research XXIII
ed. by H. Bergmann, H. Köhn and H. Sinzinger

THE USAGE OF GATED SPECT IN LUNG SCINTIGRAPHY PHANTOM STUDIES AND CLINICAL RESULTS

M. Andreeff *, J. Kropp *, B. Beuthin-Baumann *, L. Oehme *,
S. Schellong **, Y. Prescher**, J. Pinkert *, W.-G. Franke *,
W.-G. Daniel**

Department of *Nuclear Medicine and **Internal Medicine, University of Technology Dresden,
Fetscherstr. 74, Dresden, D-01307, Germany

SUMMARY: „Normal" SPECT (nSPECT) aquisition might be helpful to improve this limitation but the images of this acquisition method are still hampered by movement artifacts because movement of lungs reduce both resolution and contrast. Phantom studies with a moving individually filled sphere (diameter 25mm; shift 25mm; „cold" Lesion) is resolved with a gated SPECT study only. The phantom studies demostrated that gated SPECT is more efficient for detection of small defects in lung scintigraphy. The clinical gated SPECT studies showed a clear increase of resolution and contrast (>20%) compared with non-gated SPECT. By gated pulmonary SPECT there is an improvement of spatial resolution and contrast which leads to a more reliable diagnosis of pulmonary embolism in V/Q scintigraphy.

INTRODUCTION

Planar pulmonary scintigraphy is limited to diagnose subsegmental pulmonary embolism (PE). „Normal" SPECT (nSPECT) acquisition might be helpful to improve this limitation but the images of this acquisition method are still hampered by movement artifacts because movement of lungs reduce both resolution and contrast. We thereful were interested in the question if it is possible to improve nSPECT slices by gating of the SPECT acquisition by the breath cycle.

METHODS

As a first step a prepared body phantom was used for simulation of the setup and the feasability of the method was tested (Figure 1). The cyclic movement of a shere in an appropriate activity containing medium (negative contrast) was acquired in coincidence with a trigger pulse (TTL-pulse) for camera control.

For clinical purposes gated SPECT (gSPECT) was realized by a thermosensor of an electrical flowmeter registering the temperature difference of the in- and exheald air from which gating was derived (1). A TTL-pulse enabled breath cycle corresponding imaging (Figure 2).

A dual head LFOV gamma camera was used. The gSPECT acquisition parameters - 64x64

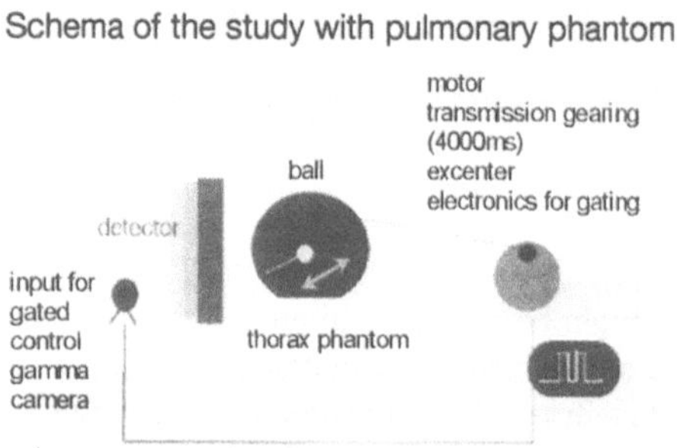

Figure 1. Principles of gated phantom studies

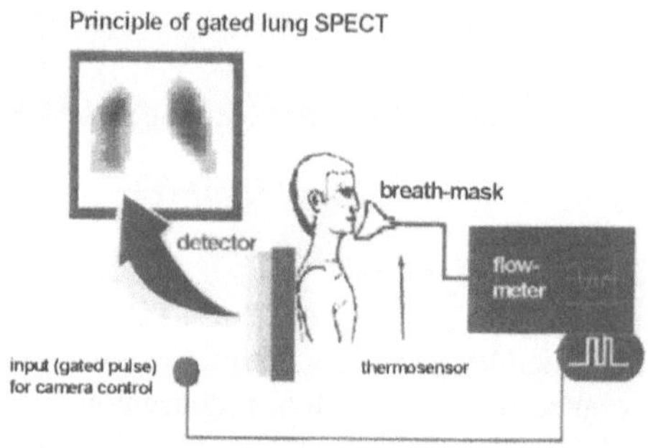

Figure 2. Principles of clinical gated V/Q studies

matrix , 64 views with 8 timebins and 15 accepted breath cycles per views- result from compromising count statistics and total acquisition time tolerated by the patient. For data analysis the time bin representing the beginning of inhalation was reconstructed by filtered back projection. These slices were compared to the nSPECT slices (sum of all time bins).

RESULTS

The gated phantom studies showed a significant increase of resolution and contrast compared with non-gated SPECT (nSPECT) readed by visual analysis (Figure 3). If realistic acquisition parameters and activity concentrations were used the detection of the defects were quite similar compared to those of the non-gated studies if the sphere was fixed.

In 36 pts suffering from deep vein thrombosis (proven by duplex sonography) V/Q scintigraphy was performed using Tc-99m-labeled Technegas and MAA using n- and gSPECT immediately before and 10 days after initialization of two different therapy regimes (standard or low-molecular-weight heparin; early versus late mobilization) (2). All scans were

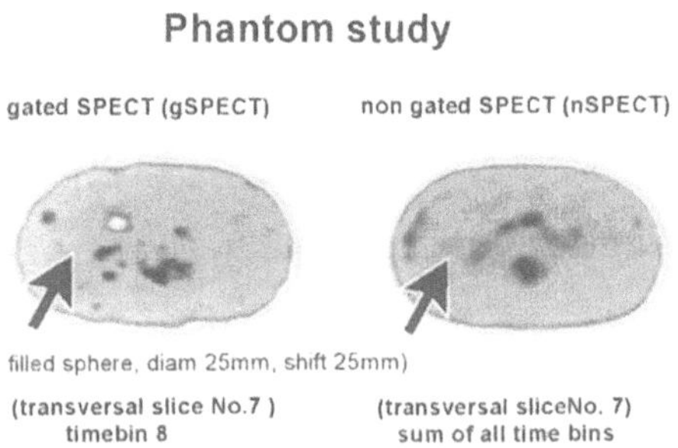

Figure 3. Transversal slices of gated SPECT to non-gated SPECT Phantom study with a moving individually filled sphere is resolved with a gated SPECT study only.

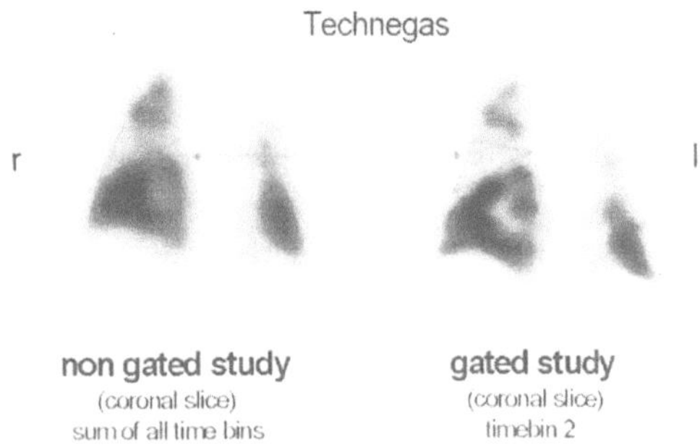

Figure 4. Example of a coronal slice of a gated und ungated SPECT ventilation scan. Improvement of resolution of the gated study is obvious (arrow).

blindly readed by two experienced physicians. Interobserver agreement was 82% an 94% for

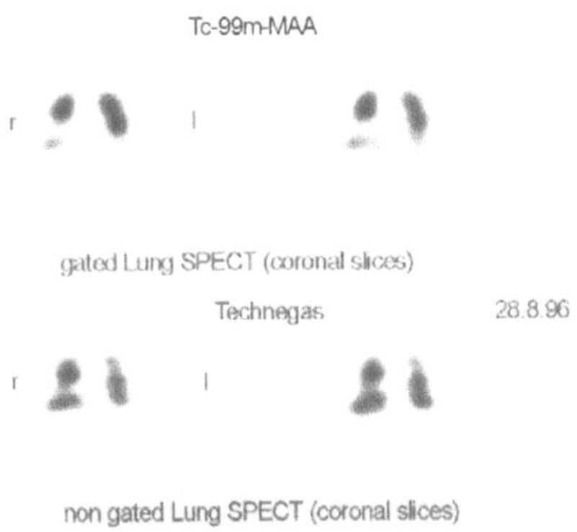

Figure 5. Coronal slices of the gated V/Q SPECT of a patient with matched V/Q defects and mismatch V/Q defects indicating disturbed ventilation/perfusion and PE

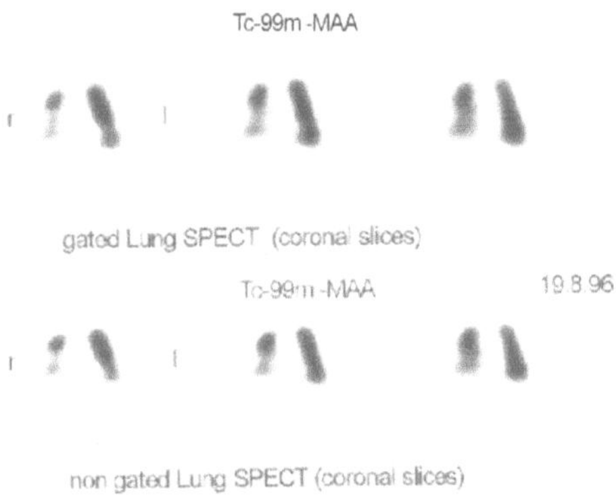

Figure 6. Example of coronal slices of a gated and ungated SPECT perfusion scan. Improvement of resolution of the gated study is obvious (arrows).

nSPECT and gSPECT, respectively. Initially 58% of pts had PE. 55% of pts showed no clinical change. In the two groups with different therapies improvement of PE was diagnosed in both groups in 6 (17%) of the pts whereas in 2 pts (5.5%) a worsening was found. Some clinical examples are displayed in Figure 4-6.

CONCLUSION

Phantom studies with a moving individually filled sphere (diameter 25mm; shift 25mm; „cold“ Lesion) is resolved with a gated SPECT study only. The phantom studies demostrated that gated SPECT is more efficient for detection of small defects in lung scintigraphy.

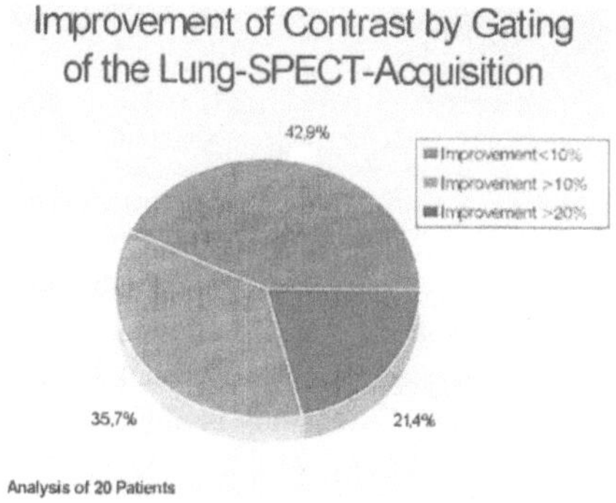

Figure 7. Improvement of Contrast by gating of the V/Q SPECT scan in 20 patients.

The clinical gated SPECT studies showed a clear increase of resolution and contrast (Figure 7) compared with non-gated SPECT. Therefore by gated pulmonary SPECT there is an improvement of spatial resolution and contrast which leads to a more reliable diagnosis of pulmonary embolism in V/Q scintigraphy.

REFERENCES

1. Water W, Neeb W. Eine Methode zur Atemtriggerung und ihre Anwendung bei der atemgetriggerten Sequenzszintigraphie. NucCompact 1983;14;130-132.

2. Eichlinsberger R, Frauchinger B, Jäger K. Neue Trends in der Behandlung der tiefen Venenthrombose. Schweiz.Rundschau Med. 1994;83;183-188

Radioactive Isotopes in
Clinical Medicine and Research XXIII
ed. by H. Bergmann, H. Köhn and H. Sinzinger

THE DEPARTMENT OF NUCLEAR MEDICINE, SZEGED, ON THE INTERNET

A. Kuba Jr., L. Pávics

Department of Nuclear Medicine, Albert Szent-Györgyi Medical University, Szeged, Hungary

SUMMARY: In response to the demand of an easy-to-use information system at the Department of Nuclear Medicine, Szeged, a complete web-site has been developed. The web pages are in HTML 3.0 language, which is well known by all Internet browsers. The system covers almost all aspects of the departmental activities. However, students and nuclear medicine scientists can profit most from it.

INTRODUCTION

The demand arose at our department for an information system that would facilitate the information exchange within the department and operate as a bulletin board for the outside world. We wanted to present references of the department (e.g. the main activities, research fields, personal data, and history of the department), and help the university students in collecting educational information. It also seemed useful to create an information base where news and orders would be available for both divisions of the department. The ready availability of details on recent conferences and professional meetings under organization by the department was a further demand.

The most important material facilities had already been installeded : the computers and the local (departmental) network with connections to the university network. The Internet connection and the software required to browse trough the web were also given.

The aims were to develop an easy-to-use information system for the staff, students, colleagues and persons interested in the department, consideration being given to the extremely different hardware and software conditions.

The intended functions of the system were: a personal section, a research section, an educational section, general information on the department, and a history section.

MATERIALS AND METHODS

The following hardware items were available: a SUN workstation, PCs (i386 and i486) mainly with color SVGA monitors, medical imaging systems, and the Ethernet network.

The following software was used : SUN OS, OpenWindows; MS-DOS; Novell Netware 3.X and 4.X; MS Windows 3.1, and 3.11; Trumpet Winsock 1.0, 2.0, 3.0; Netscape for all platforms (except VAX); Word for Windows 2.0, 6.0 and other text editors, data processors and data management tools.

The system is based on HTML 3.0 language and Netscape Navigator. GNN Press was used as a main tool during the development period. Some features, such as the JavaScript-powered pages, required manual programming. The pages were tested in two stages: first by a SUN system, and secondly on PCs. Netscape Navigator was the test-browser on both platforms.

RESULTS

The developed web-site meets our goals. The prepared pages are now available at **http://ss10.numed.szote.u-szeged.hu**. The main system is ready, although many supplementary features are planned. The system is integrated into the web-system of Albert Szent-Györgyi Medical University in Szeged.

The pages are arranged into a multi-level tree. It has 8 parts. The section "Education" provides information on lectures and examinations. The section "Employees" contains personal data on the employees of the department, e.g. CVs and e-mail addresses. In the "Scientific activities" section, publication lists, grants and scholarships are to be found. The "Patient care" section contains statistics on the investigations performed through the years. The instrumentation and the infrastructure of the department are also presented, together with information on the books and journals accessible in the library section of the department. "The first 20 years" is the network publication of the departmental history.

DISCUSSION

The advantages of the system have become clear. The largest group of visitors on the web-site is the staff. Through the system they can leave messages or inform each other about important facts. They also have the possibility to create their own home-pages.
The second largest user group is the researchers from other institutes and other people interested in the department or only in the web-site. The services they can use vary from checking the CVs, through searching in the publication list to glancing through the educational structure of the department. Currently the most frequented pages are those relating to the scientific meeting to be held in Budapest in September 1998. Besides the general information about this meeting, a registration form is available, whereby anyone can register. It is our intention to display hot information on current conferences and meetings in central and eastern Europe in the future too.
The third group comprises the students. They can find on the pages timetables and other details on the courses, including links to the lecturers. The students can now contact the teaching staff via the network without any e-mail or web address they must keep in mind.
Since 01.06.1997, more than 8300 http requests have been recorded on the pages. 55% of those were local or other Hungarian ones, the other requests came from abroad.

The first problem with the system is the lack of suitable computers both in the students' homes and at the department. Fortunately, this will change as time goes by. The second problem is that there are no constant ways to update the information presented on the web. Because of this, some details are absent, such as CVs in certain cases. The rate of reliability is relatively high: only in one case were we alarmed that the site is not available.

CONCLUSION

It is clear that the system is useful. It promotes contacts with similar institutes and increases the quality and flexibility of the information exchange within the department. It helps with the solutions of organizational problems (e.g. registration at meetings), and the institution management can also use it with benefit. Our virtual guests can collect information on the department much more easily than previously.

REFERENCES

1. Index dot HTML: The Advanced HTML Reference.
   http://www.blooberry.com/html/
2. Netscape: JavaScript Guide
   http://home.netscape.com/eng/mozilla/3.0/handbook/jevescript/
3. EFF's (Extended) Guide to the Internet
   http://www.eff.org/papers/eegtti/

Radioactive Isotopes in
Clinical Medicine and Research XXIII
ed. by H. Bergmann, H. Köhn and H. Sinzinger

NUCLEAR MEDICINE IMAGE DATA EASY TRANSFER VIA E-MAIL

Lyra M., Skouroliakou K., *Stratis I.
Athens University, Department of Radiology
*** Athens University, Department of Mathematics**
Athens, Greece.

SUMMARY

The opportunity of exchange of images and knowledge between scientists has been facilitated by net technology development. Internet offers alternative services that provide the Nuclear Medicine world with means for communication. The authors present their experience in utilising the e-mail service for the transfer of patient data between medical specialists.

INTRODUCTION

Exchange of ideas and knowledge between scientists has always been of vital importance in all scientific fields. Especially in medicine a particular difficulty encountered was the secure and quick transportation of diagnostic images. The advent and development of net software and hardware has enabled the immediate exchange of images as well as all required patient data between scientists and medical centres. Additionally the opportunity offered by the WWW of immediate access to scientific sites has contributed to the notion of a global community in medicine [1-3].

However, when the quick and simple transfer of particular patients' data is required the authors have found the e-mail service to be very satisfying and reliable.

MATERIALS - METHODS

Internet offers the service of electronic mail that can be used for personal exchange of individual patient images and data safely and instantly. The use of e-mail as the mean of image exchange ensures security of transportation. The process is easy and quick and does not require any particular software or hardware knowledge from the user. It also does not require any sophisticated computer systems.

The problem encountered is the transfer of images from the γ-camera dedicated computer to a PC and then the image can be manipulated as any image file [4,5]. The γ-camera used is a GE STARCAM camera working under a RMX Operating System. The data are transferred to the local PC via a Local Area Network and are modified to *.TIF type image files through STARLAB software (Figure 1).

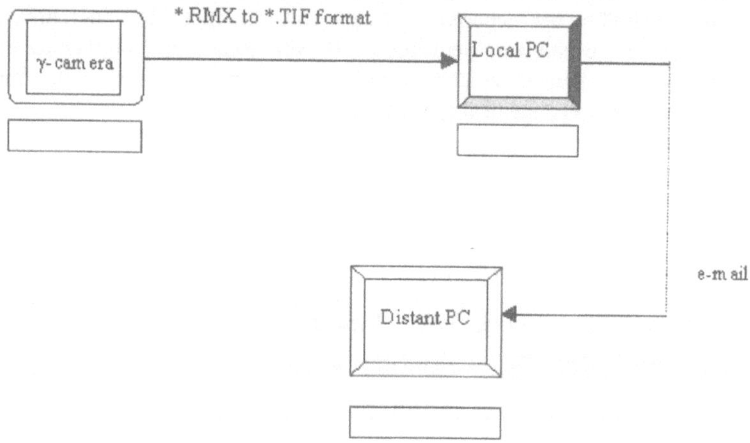

Figure 1: File modification and transfer process

After the image has been transferred to the PC as a *.TIF file it can be manipulated by means of an image processing programme in order to change the colour scale or emphasise at certain details. Medical record data are combined with the image in a hypertext file that can be sent as an attachment via an e-mailer functioning under Windows environment. The other mailing part should be equipped with a similar e-mailer and can view or print the image through a suitable browser. The mailed images are characterised by diagnostic quality analogous to the one of the original image. The quality is of diagnostic value not only for planar but also for tomographic and 3-dimensionally reconstructed images.

Subject: **Αποστολή ζητούμενου αρχείου**
Date: Sun, 11 Jan 1998 21:34:09 +0200
From: askourol@atlas.uoa.gr
To: istratis@eudoxos.uoa.gr
CC: askourol@atlas.uoa.gr

Part 1	**Name:** unif.html **Type:** Hypertext Markup Language (text/html) **Rncoding:** 8bit

---

Figure 2: E-mail transfer of the hypertext file unif.html resulting in the receipt of figure 4.

The e-mail service is been used by the authors for the transfer of particular patient data (Figure 3), as well as for the transfer of teaching files (figure 4). The hyperlinks in this case are opening the e-mailer for the request of the particular teaching file.

Patient #1

Στοιχεία ασθενούς και σύντομο ιστορικό : 12 ετών, κορίτσι, εμπύρετο 39°C προ εβδομάδος
Κυστεογραφία και υπερηχογράφημα εντός Φ.Ο.

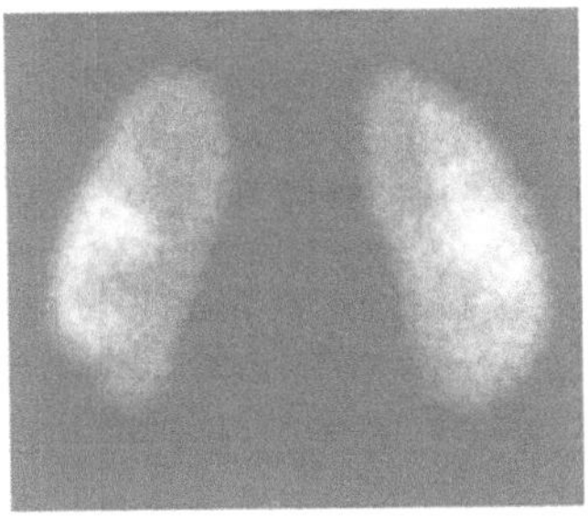

Οπίσθια λήψη. Αριστερός νεφρός:μειωμένη καθήλωση άνω έσω χείλος. Σχετική πρόσληψη: Αρ.Νεφρός 47%, Δε. Νεφρός 53%

Figure 3: Posterior planar view of a Tc99m-DMSA scan as received in hypertext format by e-mail

UNIFORMITY

Uniformity is a measure of the slightly different response of different areas of the detector to irradiation by a uniform source. The parameter is measured with or without the collimator. The calculations are carried for the Geometrical and the Central Fields of View (GFOV and CFOV respectively). Uniformity is checked daily with the acquisition of an image containing at least 3.000.000 counts. Additionally a uniformity check image of 30.000.000 is acquired per week. From these images the integral and differential non-uniformity as well as the coefficient of variation of the pixel counts are calculated

Uniformity check procedure

Home Page | Quality control parameters

Figure 4: Uniformity teaching file.

CONCLUSION

Transfer via e-mail has been used in our centre for the exchange of images to and from our colleagues when particular patients are concerned. The transferred images are characterised by diagnostic quality, and are not distorted by the transfer process. Electronic mail is also used for the transfer of teaching files in hypertext format. E-mail transfer enables the archiving of particular files from the authors' Institute database ensuring the security desired and it has been proven to be a quick and safe mean of exchange of images between scientists and scientific centres. The process is easy, immediate and valuable for the transfer of large number of images. At the same time it does not result in any significant distortion of the transferred images.

REFERENCES

[1] Glodi LM, Challenges and opportunities of the Internet for medical oncology. J Clin Oncol, 1996.

[2] Pouliquen B, Using World Wide Web multimedia in medicine. Medinfo, 1995.

[3] Lowe HJ The World Wide Web: a review of an emerging internet-based echnology for the distribution of biomedical information. J Am Med Inform Assoc, 1996.

[4] Burgard M.J., Dos-Unix Networking and Internetworking (Wiley professional Computing),1994.

[5] Fortier P.J., Handbook of Lan Technology (McGraw-Hill Series on Computer Communications) , 1992.

Radioactive Isotopes in
Clinical Medicine and Research XXIII
ed. by H. Bergmann, H. Köhn and H. Sinzinger

TALK TO YOUR PATIENTS VI@ INTERNET! PATIENT INFORMATION IN A COMMUNITY NETWORK

W. Schröttle, E. Püls, F. Paul and D. Picker

Departments of Nuclear Medicine and Internal Medicine, Klinikum Ingolstadt, Germany

SUMMARY: Patient information and health education is getting more important in the twenty-first Century. Publishing in the Internet is a fast and cheap opportunity. There are still problems because the target group of this public-relation does not have access to the electronic network yet. The Bavarian community networks provide a cheap Internet access and support for Internet newbies. After one year experience with a medical webside we recognised the need of special public-relation for patient groups and healthcare workers.

OBJECTIVES

The world population is increasing exponentially. For economic reasons the prevention of disease will get the greatest challenge of medicine in the twenty-first Century. Better health education is an important cobble-stone on this way.

Patient information is very important, not only because of the patients have to give informed consent to medical procedures now. Especially with the care for young patients suffering from AIDS or cancer the role of the physician is changing. The former leader developed to a partner of the well-informed patients.

With the loose of the absolute authority the gowns of some doctors became polluted by press reports. Physicians are forced to be concerned with the public relation of the high-tech medicine.

BACKGROUND

With over 20% Internet users in the North American population (1) Internet is getting a mass-medium. Not more than 10% of the population use Internet (2) in Germany. As a part of the program "Bayern Online" the Bavarian government wanted a cheap Internet-access for every citizen. Over 60 community networks were formed based on private initiatives and with the financial support of interested local governments and firms.

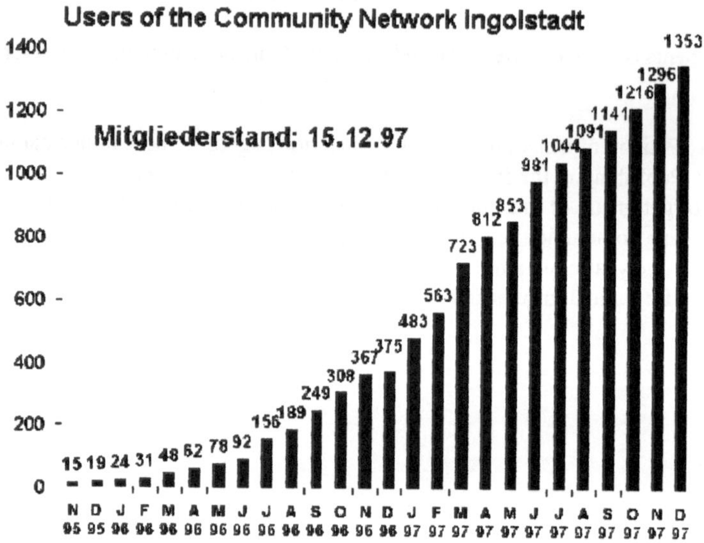

There is too much information on the Internet. Publishing in the Internet is cheap and easy for everyone. There is no quality control. How can the patients find reliable information? Who should separate the wheat from the chaff?

There is also a lack of good medical information on the net for people who do not understand English. Information resources like the PDQ cancer net of the NIH (3) still do not have a counterpart in German language.

CONCEPTION

There are many hindrances on the way to the information highway. So as a first step the authors were engaged in the construction of a community network. In a course called the Internet driving-licence people learn how to connect to the Internet and how to find information. For advanced users our webside (4) provides further information about the different Internet services and the configuration of the client programs.

Links to reliable medical information-sides in German language dealing with prevention, disease and disability are collected in our health-forum. This is complemented by the information of local patient groups. Contributes of physicians and other health-care workers shall complete this webside (5). If there are further questions the patients can ask in our interactive WWW health forum.

One of our first contributors were the coming up radiology technicians of the "Ingolstädter MTRA Kurs 94-97". They compiled information about radiation exposure in nuclear medicine, radiology and radiotherapy. We transformed it into HTML web pages and stored it on our webside (6).

EXPERIENCE

We did not have to spend any money for publishing of patient information in our community network until now. Because of the public attention we hope to get financial support from the Bavarian government for the expansion of our webside.

In December 1997 there were 4417 hits on our health-forum. This is not too much compared with the 1205862 hits (7) on the whole bingo webside in the same period. The typical Internet user is male and aged between 30 and 35 (8). These healthy users are more interested in culture than in medicine. Therefore the counter on our local cinema homepage (9) is running more than fivefold faster.

There were only few contributes to our interactive WWW health-forum. We think many people are still afraid of writing in a mass medium.

Most patient groups in our town appreciated our initiative. Because they do not have a Internet-access they do not care for updates or expansions of their homepages.

CONCLUSION

Publishing in the Internet is a fast and cheap opportunity for patient information. When they get older a greater part of the Internet users will be interested in medicine.

With special themes and Java games we have to make our webside more funny for young people. We plan to use a part of the financial support for the programming of more tricky applications.

With the change of our culture more people will be interested to communicate via Internet. We recognised the need of special public-relation for patient groups and healthcare workers.

ACKNOWLEDGEMENTS

Many thanks to and best wishes for Dr. med. Bettina Müller and Prof. Dr. med. Günter Hennersdorf. Prof. Hennersdorf established one of the first German medical mailbox systems (Medmail, Völklingen) . In 1991 he and Mr. Mohr supported my first steps in electronic communication with a 2400-Baud-Modem. Dr. B. Müller formed MedNet, the first medical network in Germany. Very early she tried to establish things like an electronic Balint group or gateways on her system (Neurobox, Würzburg). This gave me an idea about the enormous opportunities of electronic communication in medicine.

REFERENCES

1. http://www.commerce.net/work/pilot/nielsen_96/
2. http://www.door.ch/Internet-Survey.ZH96/presse/auswahlv.html#A09
3. http://imsdd.meb.uni-bonn.de/cancernet/cancernet.html
4. http://www.bingo.baynet.de/
5. http://www.bingo.baynet.de/gesund/
6. http://www.bingo.baynet.de/~ep777/strahlng/vorwort.htm
7. http://www.bingo.baynet.de/statistik/
8. http://www.door.ch/Internet-Survey.ZH96/presse/sozdem.html#Uage_k
9. http://www.bingo.baynet.de/~hs279/kino/

FREE PAPERS

Radioactive Isotopes in
Clinical Medicine and Research XXIII
ed. by H. Bergmann, H. Köhn and H. Sinzinger

FACTORS INFLUENCING MYOCARDIAL UPTAKE OF MIBG IN-VITRO

S. Mayer, G. Karanikas, Margarida Rodrigues, Susanne Granegger and H. Sinzinger

Department of Nuclear Medicine, University of Vienna, Austria

SUMMARY

Metaiodobenzylguanidine (MIBG) is an aralkylguanidine with certain structural similarities to the neurotransmitter norepinephrine. Due to its ability to concentrate in various neuroendocrine tumors, scintigraphy with ^{123}I- and ^{131}I-MIBG is frequently performed for diagnostic reasons. Recently, ^{123}I-MIBG has been applied to characterize the sympathetic innervation of the heart. In order to assess the myocardial uptake of MIBG, we conducted an in-vitro study with incubation series using rabbit myocardial tissue with MIBG at varying conditions, such as temperature, incubation period, amount of radioactivity and the amount of tissue. Our findings show that the myocardial tissue-uptake of ^{123}I-MIBG is quite high, ranging between 15% and 25%, and increases with the time of incubation and the amount of tissue, but is independent of temperature and the amount of radioactivity. These uptake characteristics as well as an eventual influence of cardiovascular drugs on myocardial ^{123}I-MIBG uptake should be carefully considered when interpreting imaging results in patients.

INTRODUCTION

MIBG

Metaiodobenzylguanidine (MIBG) is an aralkylguanidine with certain structural similarities to the neurotransmitter norepinephrine (1). Due to its ability to concentrate in various neuroendocrine tumors, scintigraphy with ^{131}I-MIBG is routinely performed for diagnostic reason in pheochromocytoma (2), neuroblastoma (3) and several other tumors of similar origin. MIBG has a strong affinity for and a long retention in the adrenal medulla, which plays an important role in the synthesis and storage of catecholamines, as well as early high myocardial concentrations (4). This radiopharmaceutical is also applied in high doses as a therapeutic agent (5). The exact uptake mechanism of MIBG still remains unclear. It is believed to share the uptake- and storage-mechanism with NE. In a comparative study of MIBG-and NE-uptake into cultured human cell lines, two mechanisms of uptake in the human cytoplasm were identified: an active, sodium- and energy-dependent type I-uptake mechanism with a high-affinity, but a low capacity being easily saturable, and a sodium-independent, apparently unsaturable process of passive diffusion (6). A subsequent active uptake mechanism, different from the one at the cell membrane, is responsible for the translocation of intracellular MIBG into the storage granules (7).

In the last years, 123I-MIBG imaging has been applied to examine the sympathetic cardiac innervation in several pathophysiologic conditions of the heart, such as ischemic heart disease (8), diabetes mellitus (9) and cardiomyopathies of different origin (10, 11).

MATERIALS AND METHODS

Rabbit hearts were obtained from the Department of Pharmacology (University of Vienna). They were cleaned from blood by injecting NaCl-solution (0,9%) into the aortic trunk. The hearts were then prepared using a sterile scalpel removing as much fat and connective tissue elements as possible. The tissue was cut into pieces of about 1mm in diameter and stored immediately at -70°C until examination.

^{123}I-MIBG was purchased from the Department of Chemistry, Seibersdorf, Austria and diluted in NaCl-solution(0,9%) to a concentration of 0.04mg/ml. The amount of radioactivity in the stock-solution was 0.2mCi/ml.

From six hearts one thawed piece each was incubated with 0,1 ml of ^{123}I-MIBG in plastic test tubes. Incubation was stopped by removing the tissue from the tube with an i.v. injection-needle(20G x 2´´). The tissue was then washed in NaCl-solution and transferred into a new tube. The uptake of ^{123}I-MIBG into the tissue was determined by comparative measurement of the radioactivity in the tissue and the remaining ^{123}I-MIBG-solution in a gamma counter.

The influence of the following conditions on the ^{123}I-MIBG-uptake into the myocardial tissue was examined:

a) time of incubation (10, 20, 30, 40, 50 and 60 minutes as well as 2, 3, 4, and 5 hours)
b) temperature (4°C, 22°C and 37°C)
c) amount of radioactivity (0.2, 2 and 20 μCi)
d) amount of tissue (1 and 3 pieces)

Statistical analysis: From the six results in each experiment the mean values and standard-deviations were calculated. A value of $p<0.01$ was considered as being significant.

RESULTS

The rabbit myocardial tissue uptake of ^{123}I-MIBG:

* is independent of the amount of radioactivity,
* is temperature-independent (figure 1),
* increases with the incubation time, reaching ist maximum at 1hour, and
* increases with the amount of the tissue (figure 2)

Myocardial ^{123}I-MIBG-uptake: influence of incubation time

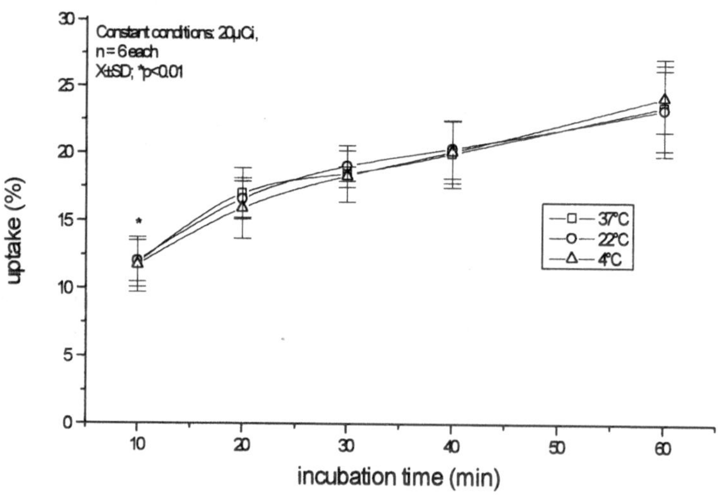

Fig. 1 Rabbit myocardial tissue uptake of ^{123}I-MIBG is dependent on the incubation-time and independent of the temperature.

Amount of tissue influences ^{123}I-MIBG-uptake

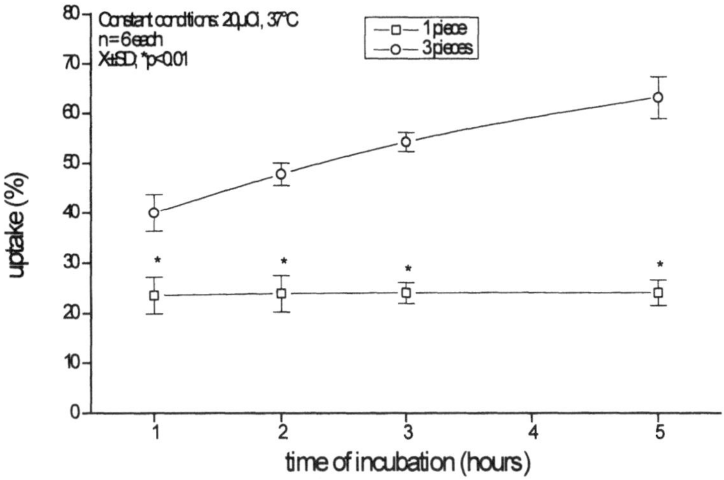

Fig. 2 The triple amount of rabbit myocardial tissue shows a significantly higher uptake of ^{123}I-MIBG.

DISCUSSION

Although the use of ^{123}I-MIBG for diagnosis of myocardial adrenergic function gained increasing interest (8, 9, 10, 11), data on isolated myocardial tissue in-vitro are not yet available. The knowledge of the uptake behavior under normal and pathological conditions, however, and in particular the influence of the most widely used drugs in these patients, i.e. β-blockers, calcium antagonists and angiotensin-converting enzyme inhibitors is of utmost importance for quantitative functional imaging. Interestingly enough, going through the methodology in the papers available, the patients intake of drugs is not described in detail, if at all. This clearly shows that their relevance was completely neglected so far.

The presented findings indicate a surprisingly high in-vitro myocardial ^{123}I-MIBG-uptake. However, they show that the concomitant administration of various drugs usually given to these patients itself might affect the uptake. Thus, an altered uptake might either reflect a therapeutic effect or a direct influence of the respective substance only. The relative contribution of these two potential effects on myocardial ^{123}I-MIBG-uptake is under investigation at present in an experimental animal perfusion model. Furthermore, class effects and substance-specific effects still need to be defined in detail for each drug before this test can enter the clinical routine program.

If there is any kind of change in therapy with a drug known to interfere with myocardial uptake, this should be considered. By the way, also an influence on platelet uptake as reported earlier (12) may significantly influence the available circulating concentration of the compound and thus secondarily result in an altered myocardial uptake as well.

Our data are presented in %-uptake, which actually more reliably reflects „net content" at the time of investigation balancing tissue uptake and parallel ongoing elution (washout) of the tracer.

Uptake studies in-vivo using para-fluorine-18-fluorobenzylguanidine (13) during application of various drugs might help to clarify this issue in-vivo in the future.

REFERENCES

1. Beierwaltes W.H.: Update on basic research and clinical experience with metaiodobenzylguanidine.Med Ped Oncol 15:163-169, 1987.
2. Lynn M.D. , Shapiro B. , Sisson J.C. , Swanson D.P. , Mangner T.J. , Wieland D.M. , Meyers L.J. , Glowniak J.V. , Beierwaltes W.H.:Portrayal of pheochromocytoma and normal human adrenal medulla by m-123I Iodobenzylguanidine: concise communication. J Nucl Med 25:436-440,1984.
3. Mueller-Gaertner H.W. , Montz R.: ^{123}I-Meta-iodobenzylguanidine MIBG scintigraphy in diagnosis of neuroblastoma. Nuclear Medicine 25:A 56, 1986.
4. Wieland D.M. , Wu J.L. , Brown L.E. , Mangner T.J. , Swanson D.P. , Beierwaltes W.M.: Radiolabeled adrenergic neuron blocking agents: Adrenomedullary imaging with ^{131}I-iodobenzylguanidine. J Nucl Med 21:349-353, 1980.
5. Hoefnagel C.A. , Voute P.A. , de Kraker J. , Marcuse H.R.: Radionuclide diagnosis and therapy of neural crest tumors using iodine-131 metaiodobenzylguanidine. J Nucl Med 28:308-314, 1987.
6. Jaques Jr.S. , Tobes M.C. , Sisson J.C. , Baker J.A.: Mechanisms of uptake of norepinephrine(NE) and meta-iodobenzylguanidine (MIBG) into cultured human pheochromocytoma cells. J Nucl Med 25:P122, 1984.
7. Sisson J.C. , Wieland D.M. , Sherman P. , Mangner T.J. , Tobes M.C. , Jacques Jr.S.: Metaiodobenzylguanidine as an index of the adrenergic nervous system integrity and funcion. J Nucl Med 28: 1620-1624, 1987.
8. Dae M. , Herr J. , Botvinick E. , Huberty J. , O´Connell W. , Davis J. , Chin M.: Scintigraphic detection of denervated myocardium after infarction (Abstract). J Nucl Med 27: 27, 1986.
9. Nagaoka H. , Ilzuka T. , Kubota S. , Kato N. , Suzuki N. , Inoue T. , Endo K. , Nagai R.: Depressed contractile response to exercise in diabetic patients in the absence of cardiovascular disease: Relationship to adrenergic dysinnervation. Nucl Med Comm 18: 761-770,1997
10. Yamazaki J. , Muto H. , Ishiguro S. , Okamoto K. , Hosoi H. , Nakano H. , Morishita T. Quantitative szintigraphic analysis of ^{123}J-MIBG by polar map in patients with dilated cardiomyopathy. Nucl Med Comm 18: 219-229, 1997.
11. Nakajima K. , Bunko H. , Taki J. , Shimizu M. , Muramori A. , Hisada K.: Quantitative analysis of 123J-metaiodobenzylguanidine (MIBG) uptake in hypertrophic cardiomyopathy. Am Heart J 119: 1329-1337, 1990.
12. Karanikas G. : Platelet uptake of MIBG diagnostic and therapeutic relevance? Thesis. Facultas Vol 6, 1994.
13. Berry C.R. , Garg P.K. , Zalutsky M.R. , Coleman R.E. , DeGrado T.R. : Uptake and retention kinetics of para-Fluorine-18-Fluorobenzylguanidine in isolated rat heart. J Nucl Med 37:2011-2016, 1996.

Radioactive Isotopes in
Clinical Medicine and Research XXIII
ed. by H. Bergmann, H. Köhn and H. Sinzinger

BINDING STUDIES WITH OXIDIZED AND GLYCATED ^{125}I-LDL TO DETECT MACROPHAGE SCAVENGER- AND AGE-RECEPTORS IN ATHEROSCLEROTIC LESIONS.

Grazyna Sobal, J. E. Menzel, and H. Sinzinger.

Department of Nuclear Medicine, and *Institute of Immunology, University of Vienna, Austria

SUMMARY: In this study we describe binding studies performed with the ligand ^{125}Iodine-oxidized and glycated-LDL to demonstrate the presence of scavenger and AGE-receptors (RAGE) on monocytes/macrophages from peripheral blood. Oxidation of LDL at a concentration of 0,25 mg /ml Apolipoprotein B in PBS buffer pH 7,4 was performed at 37°C in the presence of 5 μM Cu^{2+} for 24h. Glycation of LDL was performed by incubation of LDL with 500mM glucose in 0.2M phosphate buffer pH 7,4 at 37°C for 31 days. LDL was labelled according to the method of McConahey and Dixon. The influence of cell activation by lipopolysaccharide (LPS) was investigated. Scatchard analysis of binding data was performed. We found on quiescent monocytes $6{,}02 \times 10^{5}$ receptors/cell and a Kd=$0{,}55 \times 10^{-8}$M for oxidized LDL as compared to activated monocytes with $1{,}32 \times 10^{6}$ receptors/cell and Kd=$1{,}65 \times 10^{-8}$M. In case of glycated LDL as ligand we found $1{,}5 \times 10^{6}$ receptors/cell and a Kd=$3{,}1 \times 10^{-7}$ M as compared to $3{,}0 \times 10^{6}$ receptors/cell and Kd=$1{,}8 \times 10^{-8}$M for activated monocytes. Thus, activation of monocytes resulted in a clearcut increase of receptors.

INTRODUCTION

Oxidation and glycation of low-density lipoprotein (LDL) has been proposed to play a central role in the pathogenesis of atherosclerosis. The non-enzymatic reaction of glucose with proteins and lipoproteins, i.e. glycation, results in attachment of glucose to amino-groups forming first reversible Amadori products which are than slowly transformed into irreversible advanced glycosylation end products (AGEs). The modified (glycoxidized) LDL are centrally involved in the pathogenesis of late complications in diabetes mellitus (2). The atherosclerotic risk for the development of vasculopathy in diabetic patients with elevated glucose levels is increased several times (3).These diabetic or renally impaired patients show elevated levels of circulating protein- and lipid-bound AGEs. In the vascular wall, formation of AGEs can influence the vasodilation by both reduced elasticity of AGE-modified structural proteins (4) or by „quenching" of nitric oxide. Macrophages possess specific AGE-receptors and uptake of AGEs via these receptors could contribute to foam cells formation. Also endothelial cells, smooth muscle cells exhibit such receptors for AGEs.In this study we investigate binding of oxidized and glycated LDL on quiescent monocytes and endothelial cells as compared to lipopolysaccharide-activated cells.

METHODS:

LDL was isolated from normolipidemic overnight fasting volunteers (n=12, age range 22-60 yr, 8 females, 4 men, non-smokers, non-diabetics, not taking any drug since at least 2 weeks)

by sequential centrifugation according to the method of Havel et al.(5). The in-vitro oxidation of LDL was performed using a modification of the method by Esterbauer et al.(6). TBARS after oxidation of LDL were assayed according to a microtiter plate-modified method by Buege and Aust (7).The glycation of LDL was performed by incubation of LDL with 500mM glucose in 0.2 M phosphate buffer (pH 7.4) at 37°C for varying periods of time ranging from 10 up to 31 days. As a protection against microorganisms 0.01% natrium azide was used and sterile filtration was performed. The fluorescence of the advanced glycosylation end product AGE-LDL was determined (370 nm excitation and 440 nm emission).

1. Monocytes: Monocytes were activated by lipopolysaccharide (LPS) or tumor necrosis factor (TNF).
2. Endothelial cells: Cells were activated over night by incubation with 1 µg/ml lipopolysaccharide (Sigma). Cytokines were quantitated using commercial ELISA IL-6 and IL-8 assays (Medgenix).

The labelling of AGE-LDL was performed with iodine-125 (Amersham) and Chloramine-T (Merck) according to the method of Mc Conahey and Dixon (8). Reaction time was one minute. The final specific radioactivity of AGE-LDL was 6,4 mCi/µmol protein. Labelling yield was 86 %, purification was performed using immune adsorption on an anti-AGE column, containing antibody bound to cyanobromide-activated Sepharose (Sephadex). Radiochemical purity was determined by thin layer chromatography (TLC) with silica gel plates, developed in a solvent of methanol/10% ammonium formiate/0,5 M citric acid (20:20:10) (vol/vol/vol). The electrophoretic mobility of native and glycated LDL was determined by agarose gel electrophoresis, using Rapidophor equipment (Immuno AG, Vienna, Austria), at 60 V for 1 h in phosphate buffer pH 8.6. After drying the gel was stained by Amido-Black. Glycated LDL showed an increased relative electrophoretic mobility (REM) of 1.9.

Binding studies were performed using long-term glycated LDL (AGE-LDL) in 125-I-labeled form. Monocytes (10^6 cells) and endothelial cells (0.5×10^6) were incubated at 4°C for two hours with increasing amounts of iodinated AGE-LDL. After three rapid washings with medium, cell-bound radioactivity was determined in a Packard Gamma-Counter. Evaluation of the binding data was performed using Scatchard analysis.

RESULTS

We show the presence of AGE-receptors (RAGE) on endothelial cells from human umbilical vein cells (HUVEC) and monocytes/macrophages from peripheral blood.
The time course of copper-catalysed oxidation of LDL indicates that maximal oxidation as measured via TBARS is obtained after 4 hours (data not shown).

As presented in figure 1 the glycation can be performed by glucose or by glucose 6-phosphate, which is an activated form of glucose and accelerates this process. In this case the modification of amino groups on both ApoB and phospholipids as well was so extensive that the amount of remaining polyunsaturated fatty acids (PUFA) in modified LDL was very low. As a consequence, the concentration of MDA, a product of PUFA decomposition measured by TBARS assay, was very low; therefore, we prefered glycation with glucose.

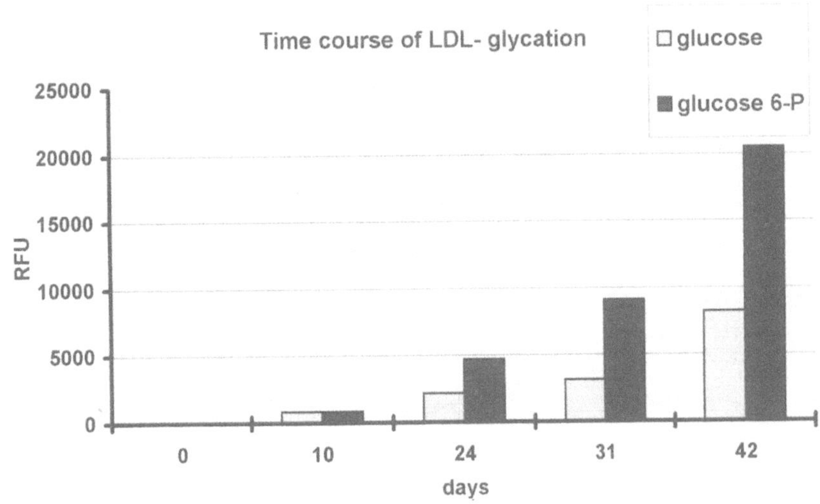

Figure 1. Time course of glycation of LDL. The fluorescence of the advanced glycosylation end product AGE-LDL was determined (370 nm excitation and 440 nm emission) and expressed as relative fluorescence units (RFU).

On HUVEC we found $3.0x10^6$ RAGE /cell and $Kd=2.5x10^{-7}M$ as compared to LPS-activated HUVEC with $6.7x10^6$ RAGE / cell and $Kd=2.7x10^{-7}M$ (figure 2).

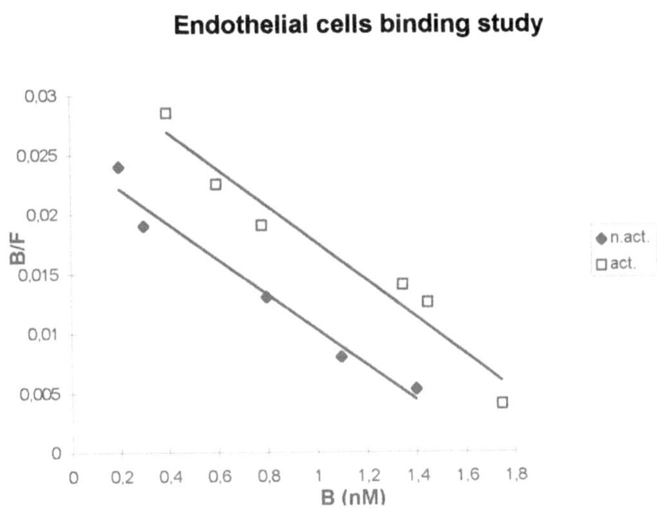

Figure 2. Scatchard data comparing binding of AGE-LDL to quiescent and LPS-activated endothelial cells.

On monocytes we found $6{,}02x10^5$ receptors/cell and a $Kd=0.55x10^{-8}M$ on quiescent monocytes for oxidized LDL as compared to activated monocytes with $1.32x10^6$ receptors/cell and $Kd=1.65x10^{-8}M$. Using oxidized LDL as ligand we found $1.5x10^6$ receptors/cell and a $Kd=3.1x10^{-7}$ M as compared to $3.0x10^6$ receptors/cell and $Kd=1.8x10^{-8}M$ for glycated LDL using activated monocytes (figure 3).

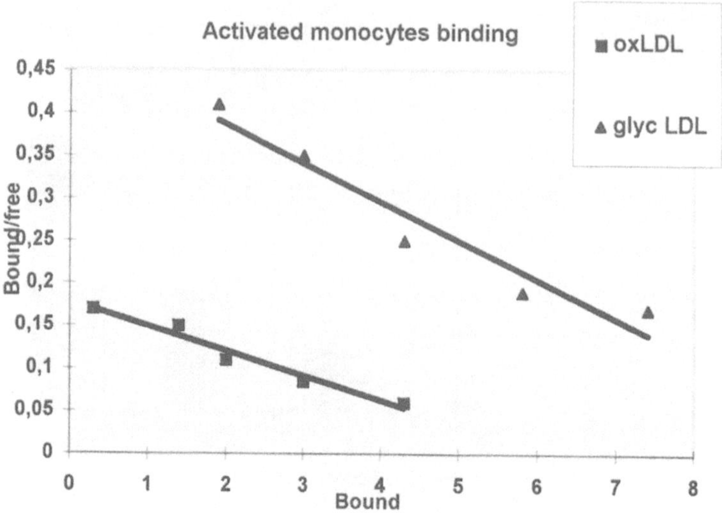

Figure 3. Scatchard data of binding experiments using LDL and glycated LDL as ligands for monocytes.

Activation of monocytes resulted in a clearcut increase of receptors. Total and non-specific binding was investigated using labeled AGE-LDL in presence or absence of a hundredfold excess of unlabeled AGE-LDL. The specific binding curve was constructed by substracting unspecific binding from total binding The state of activation of HUVEC was studied by determining the production of cytokines such as IL-6 and IL-8 (data not shown).

DISCUSSION

Our data show that ^{125}-I-AGE-LDL binds in a specific and saturable manner to endothelial cells and monocytes. This finding seems to be in agreement with the studies by A.M. Schmidt et al. who found two proteins, termed AGE-binding proteins , displayed on the endothelial cell surface: a 35-kDa polypeptide, and a lactoferrin-like 80-kDa polypeptide. Also evidence for AGE- receptors on monocytes has been reported . Both types of receptors are different from normal albumin-binding and scavenger receptors.Our data also prove, that activation of HUVEC and monocytes by lipopolysaccharide (LPS) resulted in a clearcut increase of AGE-receptor numbers. For monocytes only an increase in K_d value was shown for oxidized LDL, which indicates that the binding affinity of the AGE-receptor is lower on activated cells in contrast to glycated LDL.

It is well known that AGE-receptors are strongly expressed in atherosclerotic lesions, causing accumulation of AGEs. Further studies should be performed using ^{111}In- modified LDL injected i.v. into hypercholesterolemic rabbits for RAGEs-scintigraphy in the arterial tissue. Therefore, our results may be used to create an imaging method for RAGEs in arterial tissue to evaluate and quantitate AGE-receptors in diabetes patients developing atherosclerosis.

REFERENCES

1. Steinberg D, Parthasarathy S, Carew TE, Khoo JD, Witzum JL. Beyond cholesterol:modification that increases ist atherogenicity. New Engl J Med. 1989;320:915-924.

2. Lyons TJ. Glycation, oxidation, and glycoxidation reactions in the development of diabetic complication. Maeda K, Shinzato T(eds): Dialysis-Related Amyloidosis. Contr Nephrol Basel Karger. 1995;112:1-10.
3. Kortland W, van Rijn HJM, Erkelens DW. Glycation and lipoproteins. Diab Nutr Metab. 1993;6:231-239.
4. Cerami A, Vlassara H, Brownlee M.Role of advanced glycosylation products in complication in diabetes. Diabetics care. 1988;11:73-79.
5. Havel, R.J.,Eder, H.A.,and Bragdon, J.H. The distribution and chemical composition of ultracentrifugally separated lipoproteins in human serum. J Clin Invest. 1985;34:1345-1353.
6. Esterbauer, H., Striegl, G.,Puhl, H., and Rotheneder, M. Continuous monitoring of in vitro oxidation of human low-density lipoproteins. Free Rad Res Comm. 19816:67-75.
7. Buege, J.A., and Aust, S.D. Lactoperoxidase-catalyzed lipid peroxidation of microsomal and artificial membranes. Biochim Biophys Acta . 1976;444:192-201.
8. P.J.Mc Conahey and F.J.Dixon. A method of trace iodination of proteins for immunologic studies. Int Arch Allergy. 1966;29:185-187.

Radioactive Isotopes in
Clinical Medicine and Research XXIII
ed. by H. Bergmann, H. Köhn and H. Sinzinger

AUGER AND CONVERSION ELECTRON THERAPY WITH In-111 PENTETREOTIDE IN HEPATOCELLURAL CARCINOMA

GS Limouris[1], M Lyra[1], D Skarlos[2], A Hatzioannou[1], A Gouliamos[1], A Moulopoulou[1], L Vlahos[1]
[1]Radiology Department, Athens University
[2] Anticancer Hospital, Kifissia
Athens, Greece

Introduction: In a 42 year male, with hepatocellural carcinoma, confirmed by biopsy and a positive for somatostatin receptor liver scan, without any symptoms of neuroendocrine activity, it was decided to be treated with high therapeutic doses of [In-111-DTPA-D-Phe^1] Octreotide [Mallinckrodt Br, Petten] and to abandon the conventional and, in the majority of the cases, hopeless cytostatic therapy.

Method/Results: So far, 4 months after the first [110 mCi] and 2 months after the second [110 mCi] infusion of the tracer via an intrahepatic artery catheterization, the patient is in excellent clinical condition without any side-effect from renal, pituitary, bone marrow and thyroid function.
On MRI sequential imaging liver size remains stable. A progressive increase of the cystic/necrotic element is markedly observed in dispense of the surrounding thick pericystic/perinecrotic tissue.
Dosimetric calculations are presented in page 2.

Conclusion: Auger and conversion electron treatment seems to open new horizons in the effective management of the oncology. In the present case major problem will soon appear if this cystic/necrotic augmentation continues to grow progressively, since an expected cystic rupture has to be effectively confrontated.

Reference:
1. E Krenning et al: Peptide receptor radionuclide therapy with [Indium-111-DTPA-D-Phe] - Octreotide, J Nucl Med 38(5): 47P, 1997 [abstract]
2. Radiation Internal Dose Information Center, Oak Ridge Institute of Science and Education: MIRDOSE software version 3.0, J Nucl Med 37: 538-546, 1996

Dosimetry of In 111 & In 111 Octreotide Treatment

Radioactivity administered: 110 mCi In-111 (Octreoscan)
Two administrations for therapy purposes
8 Sep 97 and **10 Nov 97** of 110 mCi In-111 each

Fractional distribution of radioactivity to liver is considered practically =1
Dose Estimations by MIRDOSE3 of RIDIC Oak Ridge

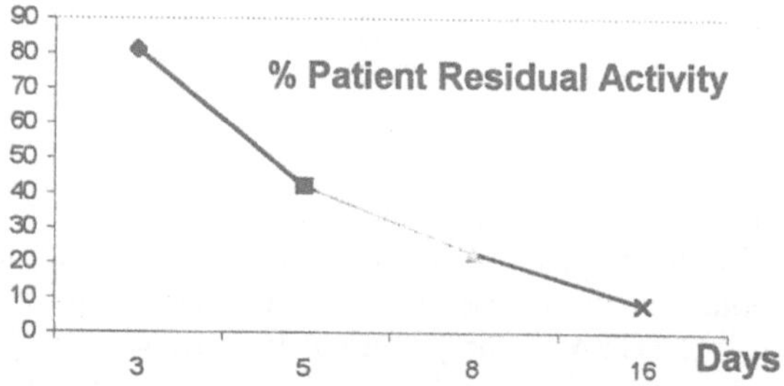

Whole body data from γ- camera in a follow up of 16 days normalized for scanning parameters gave the % residual activity curve and the effective time T_{eff} of the tracer catheterized intra hepatically.

Absorbed Dose Estimations in tumour and surrounding organs

Organ	**Absorbed dose (rads)**
Tumor	**4346.2**
Liver	**1241.5**
Kidneys	**440.6**
GI-tract	**361.08**
Spleen	**141.3**
Red marrow	**272.34**

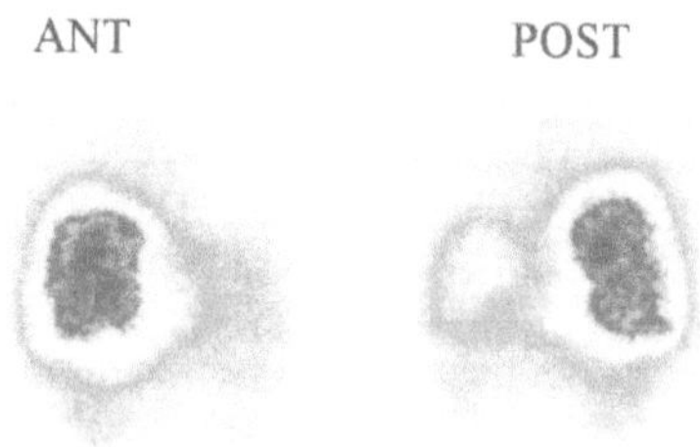

Tumour volume and mass were determined by the γ-camera anterior and posterior scintigrams [edge effect software was used]

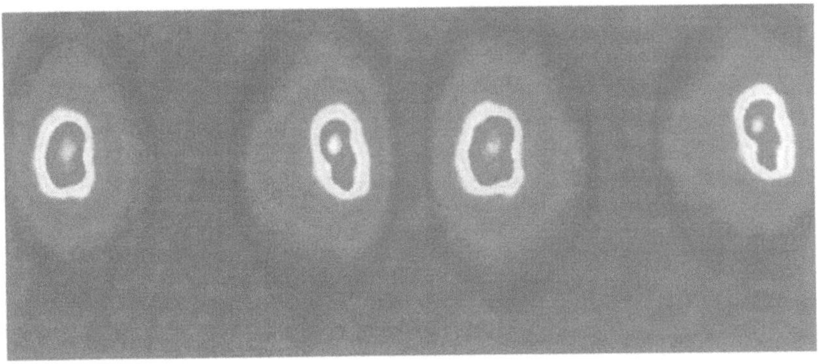

In 111 Octreotide Whole Body Scintigraphy. From left to right: Ant & Post images 3 days post, Ant & Post images 8 days post catheterization.

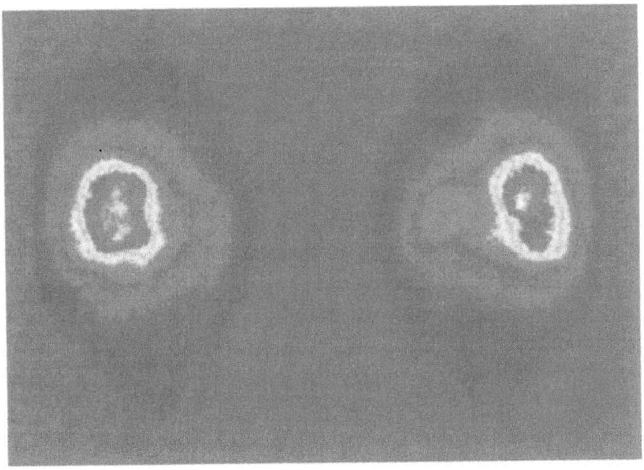

16 days post Ant & Post images

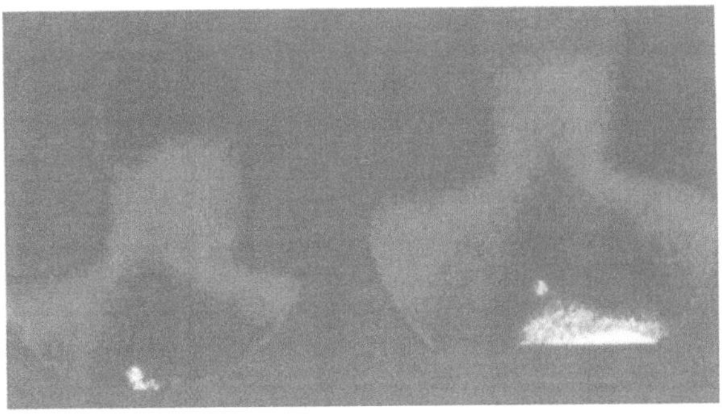

In 111 Octreotide meta detection. Thorax Ant & Post Profiles [edge enhancement technique] from left to right

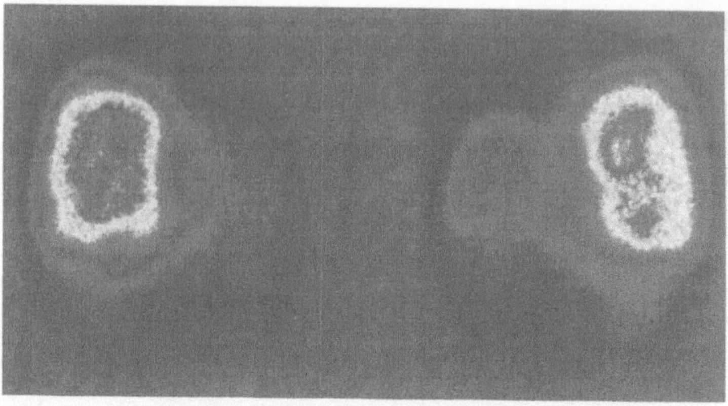

ANTERIOR POSTERIOR

STATIC SCINTIGRAMS
LIVER PROJECTIONS 5 DAYS POST ADMINISTRATION
In 111 TREATMENT DOSE

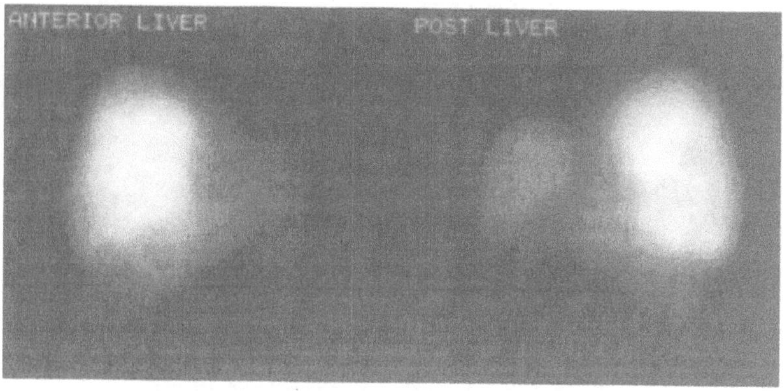

Author index

Subject index